D1269111

TEXTBOOK IN PSYCHIATRIC EPIDEMIOLOGY

SECOND EDITION

TEXTBOOK IN PSYCHIATRIC EPIDEMIOLOGY

SECOND EDITION

Edited by

Ming T. Tsuang
Department of Epidemiology
Harvard School of Public Health
and
Pediatric Psychopharmacology Unit
Psychiatry Service
Massachusetts General Hospital

Mauricio Tohen
Lilly Research Laboratories
and
Department of Psychiatry
McLean Hospital
Harvard Medical College

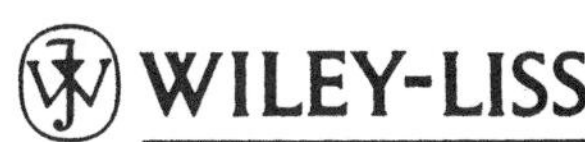

A John Wiley & Sons, Inc., Publication

This book is printed on acid-free paper. ♾

Published simultaneously in Canada.

For ordering and customer service, call 1-800-CALL-WILEY

Library of Congress Cataloging-in-Publication Data:

Textbook in psychiatric epidemiology / edited by Ming T. Tsuang,
Mauricio Tohen. - - 2nd ed.
p. cm.
Includes bibliographical references and index.
ISBN 0-471-40974-X (cloth : alk. paper)
1. Psychiatric epidemiology. I. Tsuang, Ming. T., 1931-
II. Tohen, Mauricio.
[DNLM: 1. Mental Disorders - - epidemiology. 2. Epidemiologic
Methods. 3. Mental Disorders - - diagnosis. WM 100 T3545
2002]
RC455.2.E64T49 2002
614.5′989--dc21

2002072646

Printed in the United States of America

10 9 8 7 6 5 4 3 2 1

CONTENTS

CONTRIBUTORS

Jules Angst, Research Department, Psychiatric University Hospital, P. O. Box 68, 8029 Zurich, Switzerland

James C. Anthony, Johns Hopkins University, 624 North Broadway, Room 893, Baltimore, MD 21205

Shelli Avenevoli, Mood and Anxiety Disorder Program, National Institute of Mental Health, 15K North Drive, MSC #2670, Bethesda, MD 20892

Jerry Avorn, Division of Pharmacoepidemiology and Pharmacoeconomics, Brigham and Women's Hospital Medical School, Boston, MA 02115

Dan G. Blazer, Department of Psychiatry and Behavioral Sciences, Duke University Medical Center, Durham, NC 27710

Michaeline Bresnaham, Department of Edpidemiology, Mailman School of Public Health, Columbia University, New York, NY, and New York Psychiatric Institute, New York, NY 10032

Evelyn J. Bromet, State University of New York at Stony Brook, Stony Brook, NY 11794

Stephen L. Buka, Departments of Maternal and Child Health and Epidemiology, Harvard School of Public Health, Boston, MA 02115

Jack D. Burke, Jr., Department of Psychiatry, Harvard Medical School, The Cambridge Hospital, Cambridge, MA 02139

Mary Cannon, Division of Psychological Medicine, Institute of Psychiatry, London, UK SE5 8AF

Rose S. Cohen, College of Physicians and Surgeons of Columbia University, New York, NY 10032

Nancy L. Day, Western Psychiatric Institute and Clinic, University of Pittsburgh School of Medicine, Pittsburgh, PA 15213-2593

Mary Amanda Dew, Johns Hopkins University, Baltimore, MD 21205

Felton Earls, Harvard School of Public Health, Boston, MA 02115

William W. Eaton, Department of Mental Hygiene, Bloomberg School of Public Health, Johns Hopkins University, Baltimore, MD 21205

Stephen V. Faraone, Department of Psychiatry, Massachusetts Mental Health Center, 750 Washington Street, Suite 255, South Eaton, MA 02375

Michael B. First, New York State Psychiatric Institute, New York, NY 10032

Jerome A. Fleming, Harvard Medical School, Department of Psychiatry at Massachusetts Mental Health Center, Harvard Institute of Psychiatric Epidemiology and Genetics, and Brockton/West Roxbury Veterans Administration Medical Center, Psychiatry Service, Brockton, MA 02301

Jill M. Goldstein, Harvard Medical School at Massachusetts Mental Health Center, Harvard Institute of Psychiatric Epidemiology and Genetics, Massachusetts General Hospital, Massachusetts Mental Health Center, Boston, MA 02115

John E. Helzer, Health Behavior Research Center, 54 West Twin Oaks Terrace, Suite 14, South Burlington, VT 05403

Stephen L. Hillis, Department of Statistics and Actuarial Science, University of Iowa College of Liberal Arts, Iowa City, IA 52242

Gregory G. Homish, Program in Alcohol Epidemiology, Western Psychiatric Institute and Clinic, University of Pittsburgh School of Medicine, Pittsburgh, PA 15213-2593

Ewald Horwath, College of Physicians and Surgeons of Columbia University, New York State Psychiatric Institute, New York, NY 10032

Chang-Cheng Hsieh, Division of Biostatistics and Epidemiology, University of Massachusetts Cancer Center, Worcester, MA 01605

Matti Huttunen, Department of Mental Health and Alcohol Research, National Public Health Institute, Helsinki, Finland

Celia F. Hybels, Department of Psychiatry and Behavioral Sciences, Duke University Medical Center, Durham, NC 27710

Beth A. Jerskey, Department of Psychology, Boston University, Boston, MA 02115

Peter B. Jones, Department of Psychiatry, University of Cambridge, Adenbrooke's Hospital, Cambridge, UK

Ronald C. Kessler, Department of Health Care Policy, Harvard Medical School, Boston, MA 02115

Bruce Link, Department of Epidemiology, Mailman School of Public Health, Columbia University, New York, NY, and New York State Psychiatric Institute, New York, NY 10032

Tuhina Lloyd, University of Nottingham, Duncan Macmillan House, Nottingham, UK

Michael J. Lyons, Cemter for Clinical Biopsychology, Department of Psychology, Boston University, and Harvard Institute of Psychiatric Epidemiology and Genetics, Boston, MA 02215

Kathleen Ries Merikangas, Mood and Anxiety Disorder Program, National Institute of Mental Health, 15K North Drive, MSC #2670, Bethesda, MD 20892

Michael Monuteaux, Harvard School of Public Health, Boston, MA 02115

Jane M. Murphy, Department of Psychiatry, Harvard Medical School, Department of Epidemiology, Harvard School of Public Health, and Psychiatric Epidemiology Unit, Department of Psychiatry, Massachusetts General Hospital, Charlestown, MA 02109

Robin Murray, Division of Psychological Medicine, Institute of Psychiatry, London, UK SE5 8AF

Lee N. Robins, Department of Psychiatry, Washington University School of Medicine, St. Louis, MO 63110

Patrick E. Shrout, Department of Psychology, New York University, New York NY 10003

John C, Simpson, Harvard Medical School Department of Psychiatry, Harvard Institute of Psychiatric Epidemiology and Genetics, Massachusetts Mental Health Center, Boston, MA, and VA Boston Healthcare System, Mental Health Careline, Boston, MA 02115

Ezra Susser, Department of Epidemiology, Joseph L. Mailman School of Public Health, Columbia University, College of Physcians and Surgeons, and New York State Psychiatric Institute, New York, NY 10032

Mauricio Tohen, Lilly Research Laboratories, Indianapolis, IN, Department of Psychiatry, McLean Hospital, Harvard Medical School, Boston, MA 02184

Debby Tsuang, VAPSHCS (116) MIRECC, 1660 South Columbian Way, Seattle, WA 98108

Ming T. Tsuang, Department of Epidemiology, Harvard School of Public Health and Pediatric Psychopharmacology Unit, Psychiatry Service, Massachusetts General Hospital, Boston, MA 02115

Alexander M. Walker, Department of Epidemiology, Harvard School of Public Health, Boston, MA 02115

Ellen Walters, Harvard Medical School, Boston, MA 02115

Philip S. Wang, Division of Pharmacoepidemiology and Pharmacoeconomics, Brigham and Women's Hospital, Boston, MA 02115

Myrna M. Weissman, Department of Epidemiology in Psychiatry, College of Physicians and Surgeons of Columbia University, New York, NY 10032

Robert F. Woolson, Department of Biostatistics, The University of Iowa, College of Public Health, Iowa City, IA 52242

PREFACE

It has been seven years since the publication of our first edition of the *Textbook of Psychiatric Epidemiology*. The field has continued to expand and important new findings have been published.

The intent of the first edition was to produce a textbook for our students at the Harvard Program in Psychiatric Epidemiology and Biostatistics as well as for students from other training programs across the United States. We have received extremely positive feedback about the first edition from students and faculty from training sites across the United States. Our expectations were actually surpassed, as general psychiatrists, epidemiologists, and other mental health professionals have been very favorable of the textbook. The interest in our textbook, especially from Western Europe, has expanded our geographical boundaries.

The second edition includes an update of the chapters by the same distinguished faculty. We have extended our list of contributors to include our European experts who are contributing as co-authors or, in some cases, with chapters that were not included in the first edition. We have also added two chapters on the epidemiology of child mental disorders.

The textbook is prepared in four separate sections. The first focuses on study design and methods, the second on assessment, and the third on epidemiology of major psychiatric disorders. The fourth section focuses on the epidemiology of special populations, such as the elderly and children.

As in our first edition, our objective is to provide a comprehensive, easy to understand overview of research methods for the nonmethodologist. Our targeted audience is students of psychiatric epidemiology, psychiatric residents, general psychiatrists, and other mental health professionals.

We would like to acknowledge three individuals; Alexander Leighton, Gerald Klerman, and Brian MacMahon who were the foundation of the Harvard Program in Psychiatric Epidemiology.

MING T. TSUANG
MAURICE TOHEN

PART I

Study Design and Methods

CHAPTER 1

Introduction to Epidemiologic Research Methods

JEROME A. FLEMING and CHUNG-CHENG HSIEH

Harvard Medical School, Department of Psychiatry at Massachusetts Mental Health Center, Harvard Institute of Psychiatric Epidemiology and Genetics, and Brockton/West Roxbury Veterans Administration Medical Center, Psychiatry Service, Brockton, MA 02301 (J.A.F.). Correspondence to JAF: (116A) 940 Belmont Street (508) 583-4500/fax 586-6791; Division of Biostatistics and Epidemiology, University of Massachusetts Cancer Research Center, Worcester, MA 01605 (C.C.H.).

INTRODUCTION

Epidemiology is the study of the distribution and determinants of disease frequency in humans (MacMahon and Pugh, 1970). Classic epidemiologic research designs developed to study chronic diseases are being used increasingly in investigations of psychiatric disorders. In turn, efforts to study psychiatric conditions have introduced new methodologic challenges for epidemiologists. Despite many advances in psychiatric classification in the last three decades, case definition, the sine qua non of many facets of epidemiologic research, remains an area of controversy in psychiatry. The complex manifestations and courses of psychiatric syndromes are often difficult to capture in basic epidemiologic study designs involving data collection at one or two points in time. In addition, risk factors for psychiatric conditions can be as difficult to conceptualize and assess as psychiatric outcomes.

Notwithstanding these methodologic challenges, epidemiology offers some of the best available research strategies for addressing critical questions in psychiatry concerning the nature, etiology, and prognosis of mental disorders. Psychiatric cases seen in treatment represent a small, highly self-selected segment of the full spectrum of psychopathology found in the general population. Epidemiologic study designs enable inferences to be made about the total population at risk, even when study subjects are drawn from treatment settings. Also, many putative determinants of mental disorders, such as gender, marital status, social class, and stress, cannot be randomly assigned to study groups for ethical or practical reasons.

Textbook in Psychiatric Epidemiology, Second Edition, Edited by Ming T. Tsuang and Mauricio Tohen.
ISBN 0-471-40974-X

Experimental methods used in medicine and psychology that rely on randomization therefore cannot be used to study these types of risk factors. In comparison, observational epidemiologic designs are fully appropriate.

In this chapter, we review some of the common approaches to quantifying the occurrence of psychiatric outcomes in a population and will present basic epidemiologic research designs used to identify the determinants of psychiatric conditions. Biases associated with observational epidemiologic study designs, and factors to consider in interpreting findings from these studies, are discussed. Attention is also given to the special problems faced in the application of these methods to the study of psychiatric conditions.

EPIDEMIOLOGIC MEASURES OF OUTCOME OCCURRENCE IN POPULATION GROUPS

The frequency of outcome occurrence in a population group can be measured several ways. The two principal approaches involve measures of proportions and measures of densities (rates). The distinction and relation between these two types of measurements have been discussed in detail in the context of psychiatric research (Kramer, 1957). They are described briefly here.

Incidence Density (Force of Morbidity or Mortality)

Incidence refers to new events (outcomes) occurring over time among members of the population who are candidates for such events. There are two commonly employed incidence measures: incidence density and cumulative incidence.

An incidence density quantifies the number of events occurring per unit of population per unit of time. It is not dimensionless because time is retained in the unit of measurement. In estimating incidence density, the population under study should exclude all individuals with the health outcome at the start of the period of observation. This candidate population is often referred to as the population at risk. In practice, when the number of cases in the population under study is very small, such as in studies of rare diseases in general population samples, the total population can be used for the population at risk. In small study cohorts, however, it is important to remove all current cases from the baseline sample before calculating incidence.

Incidence density can be assessed for an instantaneous time point by the slope of a curve measuring change in disease-free population size over time. This instantaneous rate of change is often referred to as the hazard rate or the force of morbidity. Incidence density is also often expressed as an average rate of change over a time interval. For example, if a group of 300 manic-depressive patients is followed for an average of 10 years with 12 deaths (the outcome event) occurring during the follow-up, the numerator of the average incidence density of death (the mortality rate) would be 12 deaths, and the denominator would be 300 patients times 10 years, or 3,000 person-years. After division, the mortality rate would be reported as 4 per 1,000 persons per year (or 4 per 1,000 person-years).

A density-type measure is usually referred to as a rate. However, in common usage, rates can also refer to proportions, such as unemployment rate, tax rate, and prevalence rate. To avoid confusion, it is important to know the context in which rate is being used and to specify the method by which it has been calculated (Elandt-Johnson, 1975).

Cumulative Incidence, Risk, and Survival

Cumulative incidence, risk, and survival rates are estimates of the probability of the occurrence of an outcome event over a specified period of time. Cumulative incidence is usually used to describe the probability of outcome occurrence among a group or population. Risk is usually used to predict an individuals chance of such an event. Risk is also commonly expressed by its mathematical complement, the probability of surviving or the survival rate. Cumulative incidence, risk, and the survival rate are dimensionless measures.

Cumulative incidence can be either an observed probability or a theoretical quantity estimated from the incidence density function. The observed cumulative incidence is a simple proportion and is calculated as the number of health outcomes occurring over a time interval divided by the size of the population at risk. If the outcomes of all members of a candidate population are observed without any loss to follow-up from causes other than the event under study, cumulative incidence can be used as an estimate of individual risk for the time interval under study (e.g., five-year risk of dying) or, in a complementary fashion, as the survival rate.

In practice, however, loss to follow-up or censoring through subject dropouts or death by other causes is common. The interpretability of the observed cumulative incidence measure when such loss occurs is seriously compromised. For example, an observed five-year survival rate for a group of manic-depressive study subjects can be distorted by censoring, even if those who were lost had the same probability of surviving as the remaining study participants. This distortion will take place because outcomes occurring among subjects lost to follow-up are excluded from the numerator of the observed cumulative incidence calculation. Cases lost to follow-up are still retained in the denominator, however, which equals the total size of the candidate population at the start of the study with no adjustment for reduction in the size of the study cohort over the observation period. Consequently, observed cumulative incidence, and risk and survival estimates based on it, is only appropriate for studies in which there is negligible loss to follow-up over the course of the study. The types of studies for which these observed measures are best suited involve closed or fixed cohorts (that is, cohorts in which the disease course of each subject in the study is individually monitored over the period of observation) in which there is no loss to follow-up and the follow-up interval is short.

When loss-to-follow-up occurs, or when incidence is estimated for a dynamic community population (i.e., where the disease experience of each individual is not monitored), a more appropriate measure of the probability of disease occurrence is derived from the observed incidence density function (Chiang, 1968). The estimate of the observed incidence density is not affected by the competing causes of subject removal (e.g., loss to follow-up) from a candidate population since those who are lost will no longer be among the candidates for the occurrence of the next outcome event. For the prognosis of an individual patient in this study, the complement of a five-year survival rate derived from the incidence density can be appropriately interpreted as the risk of dying in five years.

Prevalence

Simply put, a prevalence or prevalence rate is that proportion of persons in a population who have a particular health condition at a point or period in time. For example, the point prevalence of major depression in a community is the number of persons fulfilling diagnostic criteria for depression at a stated point in time divided by the number of persons in the community. As a proportion, prevalence is a dimensionless quantity; that is, it is not expressed in units of another characteristic, such as time.

Both newly onset cases and cases that begin prior to the study period contribute to prevalence. In a community population in which the numbers of entries and exits (from births, deaths, migrations, and so forth) are balanced and the disease rates are stable (a steady state), prevalence is proportional to the frequency of development of new cases of the condition (the incidence density) multiplied by the average duration of the condition. Exact relationships between prevalence, incidence, and duration have been presented by Freeman and Hutchison (1980, 1986).

Prevalence rates are frequently reported for population subgroups, such as age- or sex-specific rates. In these stratum-specific estimates, the numerator of the prevalence is formed by the number of cases within the population subgroup, and the denominator is the total size of the subgroup.

In psychiatric studies, "period" prevalence rates are also often reported. A period prevalence rate uses the same denominator as a point prevalence rate, but expands the numerator to include all cases present during a selected time period, such as one month, six months, one year, or a lifetime. Period prevalence has gained popularity in psychiatric epidemiology because of the complex, episodic course of many psychiatric conditions. Use of a period prevalence allows individuals with chronic psychiatric conditions who are temporarily in remission to be included in prevalence counts. Also, the diagnostic criteria for many psychiatric disorders requires the occurrence of clusters of symptoms over extended time intervals, such as one month (e.g., generalized anxiety) or one year (e.g., dysthymic disorder). A time period is therefore implicit in any prevalence measure involving these conditions, even a point prevalence.

Although period prevalence has several practical advantages, there are a number of limitations associated with this hybrid measure. In extended time periods, patients who remit early in the time interval without recurrence are likely to be missed in the period prevalence counts, especially when the information by disease status is gathered by recall (Aneshensel et al., 1987). In addition, empirical estimates of lifetime prevalence frequently exhibit a counter-intuitive age distribution. Over the age distribution of a population, lifetime prevalence should increase during age intervals associated with disease onset and remain constant at other ages. However, lifetime prevalences of many psychiatric disorders have been observed in several population surveys (Weissman and Myers, 1978; Robins et al., 1984) to decrease sharply in the older age groups. Several explanations have been offered for this artifact. In addition to recall bias, high case fatality rates (i.e., patients do not survive until older ages), increasing rates of psychopathology in recent cohorts, and changing diagnostic practices have been suggested as explanatory factors (Robins, 1985; Klerman, 1988).

Measures of Association and Impact: Relative Risk, Odds Ratio, and Attributable Risk

Epidemiologic studies yield statistical associations between a disease and exposure. We must interpret the meaning of these relationships, since an association may be artifactual, noncasual, or casual. An artifactual or spurious association may arise because of bias in the study. When an outcome is affected by multiple variables, in order to examine the influence of a single one, it is necessary to adjust for the effects of the others. A simple technique for isolating a specific effect due to one variable is to examine the outcome rates, at several levels of this variable, while holding the other variables constant. A more sophisticated approach involves the use of multiple regression analysis to measure the independent effect of the contribution of each of a series of variables on an outcome. Casuality is assumed when one factor is shown to contribute to the development of disease and its removal is shown to reduce the frequency of disease (Morton et al, 2001).

If there is an association between a study factor and a psychiatric disorder, the frequency with which the disorder occurs will differ in groups that vary on the study factor, such as groups who are exposed and not exposed to an environmental agent or a trait. Therefore, a measure of the association can be obtained by comparing the rates of disease occurrence in exposed and unexposed groups. Group comparisons can be expressed as a difference or as a ratio of rates. The magnitude of the difference or ratio is an indicator of the strength of association between the study factor and psychiatric outcome. In psychiatric epidemiology, ratios of disease rates are typically used to express the strength of the association. The ratio between two rates (or "rate ratio") is often referred to as the relative risk. Since relative risk can also be a risk ratio and rates and risks are different measures of disease occurrence (see "Cumulative Incidence, Risk, and Survival," mentioned earflier), it is important to know the context in which relative risk is used.

To illustrate, suppose an investigator is interested in comparing the mortality rates of adults with and without a psychotic disorder in a community of 120,000. In this population, 1,200 persons (1%) meet diagnostic criteria for a psychotic disorder, and 118,800 do not. Over a 1-year period, 312 deaths occur, including 15 individuals with a diagnosis of psychosis and 297 without. The rate (density) of dying for the group with psychosis (15 of 1,200 psychotics) and without this disorder (297 of 118,800) expressed as a mortality rate ratio (relative risk of dying) would be 5 (15/1,200 divided by 297/118,800).

Certain types of epidemiologic studies do not directly assess the disease experience in a population and compare estimated disease rates for individuals with and without exposure. Instead, the exposure histories of samples of individuals with (cases) and without (controls) the disease from the population are compared. This type of subject selection is commonly referred to as retrospective or case–control sampling. It is possible, nevertheless, to estimate the rate ratio of disease occurrence among cases and controls in these studies if certain conditions are met.

TABLE 1. Results of a Case–Control Study of Relative Risk of Mortality Among Psychotics and Nonpsychotic Adults

Exposure Status	Cases	Controls
With psychotic disorder	15	6
Without psychotic disorder	297	594
Total	312	600

Suppose in the example above that available resources do not allow the investigator to determine the mental health status for each of the 120,000 residents in the community. With a retrospective (case–control) sampling approach, cases would be the complete or partial sample of the 312 subjects with the outcome event (death), and controls would be a sample of the 120,000 residents who were candidates of the outcome event. If the available resources allowed for sampling approximately two times the number of controls as cases, an investigator might decide to select 600 subjects as the controls. With a random sample of the population, the distribution of the exposure (the psychotic disorder) among these 600 controls would be proportional to the distribution in the original population. Therefore, 6 controls (1%) would be expected to have a psychotic disorder and 594 would not after an examination of their mental health status. Table 1 displays the cross-tabulation of the outcome and exposure status from this sampling design.

To estimate the relative risk of dying among those with and without a psychotic disorder in this case–control study, the odds of exposure among the cases (15/297) is contrasted to the odds of exposure among the controls (6/594). The result of the division of these two odds, known as an "odds ratio," is 5. Note that the odds ratio computed from the case–control study in this example yields the same result as the mortality rate ratio among psychotics and nonpsychotics in the total population. An odds ratio is frequently computed as an estimate of relative risk or incidence rate ratios in case–control studies. The accuracy of this approximation depends on a number of factors, including the nature of the source population (i.e., whether it is a dynamic population with a "steady state" of in- and out-migration), the rarity of the outcome, the use of incident versus prevalent cases, and the length of the risk period between exposure and disease occurrence. The reader is referred to Chapter 3 (this volume) and to Kleinbaum et al. (1982) for a detailed description of the conditions under which an odds ratio equals or approximates a rate ratio or relative risk in the retrospective sampling schemes used in case–control studies. For the most common types of case-control studies involving incident cases, the odds ratio estimates the rate ratio exactly.

Another commonly employed epidemiologic measure is attributable risk (AR), which is also known as the etiologic fraction or population attributable risk percent (Kleinbaum et al., 1982). The AR describes the proportion (or percent) of new cases arising in a population that are attributable to the exposure under study. The AR depends on the prevalence of the exposure in the population and on the strength of the association between the exposure and outcome. The AR can be estimated by the following formula: $AR = p_e(RR - 1)/(p_e(RR - 1) + 1)$ where p_e is the proportion of the source population that is exposed and RR is the relative risk estimate. The AR ranges in value from 0 (none of the outcome occurrence is attributable to the exposure) to 1 (all occurrences take place in the presence of the exposure, i.e., the exposure is a "necessary" cause). The accuracy of this measure depends on the extent to which component measures used to calculate AR reflect current population characteristics. This index is useful for planning and policy purposes because it describes the potential impact of removing an exposure upon the frequency of disease occurrence.

Attributable risk can also be calculated specifically for individuals who have a positive history of exposure. This estimate, known as the attributable risk among the exposed (AR_e) or attributable risk percent, is computed as $AR_e = (RR - 1)/RR$.

The AR_e can be interpreted as the probability that an exposed case developed the condition as a result of the exposure. As a hypothetical example, in a study where exposure is family history and the outcome is schizophrenia, an AR_e of 0.75 would indicate that 75% of the schizophrenic cases with a positive family history for this disorder developed their condition because of their familial loading.

OVERVIEW OF STUDY DESIGNS

Epidemiologic research in its most elementary form involves studying the relationship between a risk factor and a health outcome. The risk factor is often referred to as the exposure or treatment. To learn about its relationship to a health outcome, a comparative study is undertaken in which the experience of disease occurrence in a group of individuals with one characteristic (e.g., exposed) of the risk factor is contrasted with that of another group differing on the characteristic (not exposed).

Although the epidemiologic approach focuses on comparisons of the relative magnitudes of rates of disease occurrence between two groups, in practice a variety of research designs can be invoked. These designs can be distinguished by a number of characteristics. The most important distinctions involve the timing of data collection in relation to risk factors and disease occurrence, the separation between risk factor and disease occurrence in time, and the methods used in sampling study subjects (Miettinen, 1985a). In addition, studies vary in cost, feasibility, and quality of information gathered. The study designs listed below are in common use in psychiatric epidemiology, although there is some variation in the terminology employed at different research centers. We briefly describe each type of the study in turn and provide examples of studies examining psychiatric outcomes:

- Experimental
- Nonexperimental (observational)
  - Cross–sectional
  - Cohort
    - Prospective
    - Retrospective
  - Case–control
    - Case–crossover
    - Case–cohort

Hybrid studies
  Repeated cross-sectional
  Multistage
  Panel

In addition to these basic epidemiologic study designs, the reader is referred to Chapters 4 through 8 (this volume) for reviews and illustrations of other research designs currently employed in psychiatric epidemiology.

Experimental Studies

In an experimental study, the investigator controls the allocation of subjects to different comparison groups and also regulates the experimental conditions of each group. Study subjects are randomly assigned to comparison groups and followed up over time to record the outcome event of interest, such as the recurrence of a psychiatric illness or the occurrence of death. Clinical trials and intervention studies are the most common forms of experimental studies in human populations. To ensure the comparability between groups and obtain valid results, an experimental study employs three basic research strategies: randomization, placebo, and blinding.

Randomization. When an investigator randomly assigns subjects to different experimental conditions, differences between groups are determined by chance. If the randomization is carried out properly and the sample sizes are sufficiently large, the groups are likely to be similar in all regards other than the conditions under study. Consequently, if the experimental conditions have no effect the rates of disease occurrence are expected to be the same in the comparison groups.

Even with random allocation it is possible that the groups will be imbalanced with respect to extraneous factors that may influence the rates of disease occurrence, particularly if the sample sizes are small. Before analyzing the results of randomized experiments, it is generally recommended that investigators test whether the groups are balanced on all known or suspected determinants of the outcome under study. If an imbalance is detected, the investigator can use statistical methods to adjust for the effects of these factors on the distribution of disease occurrence across groups. For unknown determinants, it is usually assumed that randomization will achieve a balanced distribution on these factors in the long run over hypothetical repetitions of the same study. The confidence in this assumption increases if the number of study subjects is adequate.

Placebo. One complication of experimental studies is that extraneous aspects of the treatment procedure may influence the outcome under study. For example, psychiatric patients who are given a new medication may show improvements because they receive special attention from study staff monitoring the treatment trial. Participating in an experiment in and of itself can also influence outcomes, an artifact that is commonly known as the Hawthorne effect. To control for these unwanted effects, one comparison group is usually administered a placebo that, under optimal conditions, mimics the extraneous features of the experimental condition or treatment under study but does not otherwise influence the rates of disease occurrence. Differences in disease rates between the placebo and experimental groups can be attributed to the effect of treatment per se rather than to the effect of other aspects of the procedure, activity, or environment associated with the treatment. Differences between placebo groups and groups that are not assigned to any experimental condition are also measured in some randomized trials, and these differences are referred to as placebo effects.

Blinding. For many of the reasons previously discussed, with placebo treatments it is important that participants in a randomized trial be unaware of the group to which they are assigned. It is equally important to withhold this information from the investigator and other professionals who manage the trial. Knowledge that an individual has been assigned to the experimental treatment may influence the handling, treatment, and measurements of participants in the randomized trial. Standardization of the study procedures are also easier to enforce when both the investigator and the patient are unaware of the group assignments. The process of "double blinding," in which neither investigators nor study participants are given information about the group assignment, helps to ensure that group conditions are similar and that identical study procedures are followed with every study subject. Although double blinding is desirable in every randomized experiment, it is not always feasible, especially when the treatment produces other effects that are observable or require monitoring to protect participants, such as changes in blood pressure.

Even though experimental studies are considered a paradigm in many research fields, the randomized trial has several shortcomings for use in studying human populations. Ethical considerations dictate that experimental studies involving human subjects can only be used to study exposures (treatments or medications) that are likely to be beneficial. It is unethical to randomize human subjects to harmful exposures. Furthermore, constitutional characteristics such as inherited or congenital traits cannot be randomized. It is also not feasible to randomize groups into many other sociodemographic conditions that may influence mental health outcomes, such as marital status or religious denomination. Therefore, the effect of many putative risk factors for major psychiatric disorders cannot be evaluated by an experimental study. Also, if the follow-up period for the ascertainment of outcomes of an experimental procedure is long, the treatment assessed may be obsolete by the time the results are available (Elwood, 1988).

A Randomized Clinical Trial in Psychiatry. Random assignment of study participants to intervention and control groups is the procedure that will give the greatest confidence that the groups are comparable. If you have two groups of patients, and you apply a different treatment to each group (clinical trial), you can only attribute a difference in outcome to the differing treatment if that is the only factor that differs between the groups (Morton et al., 2001). This goal can only be achieved if group membership is determined randomly. There is usually a logical sequence to clinical trial analysis. It begins with a comparison of the intervention and control groups to demonstrate comparability, showing that randomization works. Finally, the main analysis is to test whether the hypothesized health effect resulted.

Gibbons et al. (1993) present results from a longitudinal analysis of a randomized clinical trial of two forms of psychotherapy using the NIMH Treatment of

Depression Collaborative Research Program Dataset. The objectives of this clinical trial were to evaluate and compare the effectiveness of cognitive behavior therapy (CBT) and interpersonal psychotherapy (IPT) in comparison to a standard reference treatment, imipramine plus clinical management group (IMI-CM). A placebo plus clinical management group was also enrolled to control for effects of standard treatment (PLA-CM). Subjects (n = 250) were randomized into each of these four experimental conditions; 239 subjects entered treatment and 219 received measures after baseline. Depressive symptoms were assessed over 16 weeks with a modified Hamilton (1960) rating scale completed by clinical evaluators who were blind to treatment conditions. Contrasts between the experimental groups were made to test three main null hypotheses: (1) no difference between the two psychotherapies (IPT compared with CBT); (2) no difference between psychotherapy (IPT and CBT combined) and the standard treatment (IMI-CM); and (3) no difference between the standard treatment (IMI-CM) and the placebo (PLA-CM). No significant differences were found between the two psychotherapies (Hypothesis 1) or between psychotherapy and standard treatment (Hypothesis 2), but rate of improvement for the standard treatment (IMI-CM) was significantly greater than for the placebo. This detailed report also describes methods taken to control for potential bias introduced by attrition after randomization, missing data, differences between collaborating research sites, and assumptions in statistical modeling.

Nonexperimental (Observational) Studies

In a nonexperimental study, the investigator has no control over the group designation of each study subject. The investigator generally selects subjects for the different exposure conditions from previously existing groups and then observes the resulting health outcomes. Hence, epidemiologic nonexperimental studies are sometimes called observational studies. The three most common epidemiologic observational studies designs are cross-sectional, cohort, and case–control studies. Our discussion of observational designs begins with these classic methodologies.

Cross-Sectional Studies. In a cross-sectional study, the data on exposure and outcome are obtained at the same point in time, and both usually relate to the current period. The information is typically gathered through sample surveys of geographically defined populations. The current disease status of groups with and without the exposure, expressed as prevalence rates, are compared in analysis. By providing a "snapshot" of the current levels of illness in the total population and in different exposure groups, this design has been found to be useful for describing the health care needs of different populations.

Cross-sectional studies have enjoyed considerable popularity in psychiatric epidemiology for a number of reasons. A population survey allows investigators to gather information on all cases of disorder occurring in a defined area, including syndromes in an asymptomatic phase and conditions for which treatment is not routinely sought. Because current diagnostic procedures in psychiatry rely heavily upon the verbal report of symptoms, the interview methods used in most surveys can be used to obtain some of the basic information commonly used in formulating diagnoses. Also, prevalence rates obtained by cross-sectional surveys are widely used in psychiatry because onset (incidence) is difficult to demarcate. The chronicity of many psychiatric disorders also facilitates prevalence estimation, which, as will be recalled, is proportional to the product of incidence times duration. Therefore, even though the incidence rates for most psychiatric disorders are believed to be very low, the number of prevalent cases detected in a cross-sectional survey of moderate size is often sufficient to obtain precise estimates of rates and measures of association.

For an illustration of a major cross-sectional study in psychiatric epidemiology, the reader is referred to Chapter 5 (this volume) on the Epidemiologic Catchment Area study.

Cross-Sectional Survey Sampling. A study sample that is representative of the target population is an essential feature of cross-sectional surveys. To achieve representativeness, subjects are selected as probability samples of the population using sample survey methods (Kish, 1965; Cochran, 1977). A variety of different sampling methods are in current use that vary in complexity. Before designing a cross-sectional survey, it is important to consult a statistician about the appropriate method to employ. The sampling method will influence the number of subjects required for the survey, and certain sampling designs will also require special data analytic procedures such as weighted data and variance adjustments. Although a comprehensive overview of sampling methods is beyond the scope of this text, we will mention some of the major approaches and highlight some of the major factors that influence selection of one method over another.

Before describing the sampling methods, some terminology must be defined. The target population is the group to which results are to be generalized. This may be inclusive of all individuals in a geographic area or may exclude certain groups, such as individuals above or below a certain age or institutionalized individuals. Elementary units are the elements or members of the target population to be studied. Individuals are usually the elementary units in epidemiologic studies, but examples of other elementary units include households, neighborhoods, or hospitals. A list of all of the units in the target population used to draw the sample is known as the sampling frame, and the entries (e.g., names or addresses) on the sampling frame are called enumeration or listing units. Examples of sampling frames include telephone directories, voter registration or tax lists, town censuses, and utility listings.

Before selecting a sampling scheme, the investigator should examine the available sampling frames. Ideally, there should be a one-to-one correspondence between the enumeration units on the sampling frame and the elementary units in the target population. In practice, this is rarely the case. Some frames only contain clusters or groupings of elementary units. For example, an investigator may wish to survey all individuals in a town, but only has access to a frame (e.g., utility listings) that enumerates households. Examples of other problems with sampling frames include missing elements (failing to provide coverage of all individuals in the target population), duplicate entries, and blanks or foreign elements (e.g., out-of-date lists that include individuals who have died or emigrated, or overly inclusive lists, containing individuals outside the target population or individuals whose primary residence is outside the geographic area under study). Before the sample is drawn, the investigator should review and correct errors in the list. The list may need to be updated by contacting current residents in the survey area, a process referred to as enumeration.

There are several types of sampling plans used in cross-sectional surveys. Choice of a sampling plan depends on a number of issues, including the information contained in the sampling frame, the rarity of the characteristic under study, the desired precision of the prevalence estimates or prevalence ratios, the size of the area to be studied, and the cost of the study.

One of the most commonly cited sampling methods but infrequently employed in actual practice is simple random sampling. This method requires the availability of a complete listing of the population to use as a sampling frame. The usual method of drawing a simple random sample is to number each element on the sampling frame from 1 to N, where N is the size of the target population, assuming that the frame is completely accurate. A set of n unique random numbers, where n is the desired number of elements to be contacted for the survey, is then obtained either from a random number generator on a computer or from a published table of random numbers. The frame is then searched for elements whose numbers correspond to each of the n random numbers. These elements are chosen to be the study sample. If random numbers are not available, a lottery method can also be used by preparing N cards or tokens representing enumeration elements on the frame and drawing the desired n number of tokens at random.

In simple random sampling, the probability that any individual element is chosen is the ratio of the sample size to the size of the population: n divided by N. Although this sampling method is intuitively easy to understand, a complete listing of the population is not always available. In addition, it is possible that rare characteristics will not be represented in a simple random sample. This method is also very expensive for large study areas because interviewers will be required to travel throughout the survey region.

A modification of simple random sampling is known as stratified random sampling. In this method, the sampling frame is divided into different strata (such as age, sex, and ethnic-race groups), and simple random samples are drawn within each stratum. This approach ensures adequate representation of different groups under study. Under most conditions, it will also improve the precision of prevalence estimates. To carry out stratified random sampling, as with simple random sampling, a listing of the population is required. In addition, the characteristics to be used in stratification must also be available on the frame.

When a list of the population is not available, two commonly employed sampling methods are systematic sampling and cluster sampling. Systematic sampling is one of the most widely used methods in practice and has the advantage of being easily taught to individuals who have little knowledge of survey methods. It can also be used for samples that accrue over time, such as patient enrollments. In this method, sample members are drawn at fixed intervals, as, for example, every fifth household or every seventh name on a class enrollment list. The sampling interval, k, can be calculated by dividing the projected total population size (N) by the desired sample size (n). For example, if it is estimated that there will be 100 houses in a community and a sample of 25 is desired, the sampling interval is 100/25 or 4, and interviewers can be instructed to go to every fourth household.

Despite its simplicity, an investigator should consult with a statistician before using this method, because it may yield biased, imprecise prevalence estimates. If the population (N) and sample size (n) are reasonably large and the elements randomly ordered, the estimates can be assumed to be unbiased with variances approximating simple random sampling.

Cluster sampling is the most complex survey sampling procedure of the four methods described here. As previously described, a cluster is a listing element that may contain more than one elementary unit. Examples of clusters of individuals include hospitals, classrooms, and households. Geographic areas, such as states, counties, cities, or blocks, also represent clusters in many sampling schemes. In cluster sampling, a probability sample of clusters is drawn. In a single-stage cluster sample design, information is then gathered on all elements in each sampled cluster. Alternatively, multistage sampling may take place, in which probability samples of elements are drawn at each stage until a sample of the desired elementary units is obtained. To illustrate the multistage cluster sampling process, consider the following example of a five-stage design for a probability sample of adults in the United States: In stage 1, a random sample of counties is drawn; stage 2 consists of a random sample of towns within each selected county; in stage 3, a random sample of blocks is drawn from each selected town; stage 4 consists of a random sample of households in each sampled town; and the process concludes with a random selection of one adult from each household (stage 5).

There are several advantages to this approach. First, the investigator does not need a list of all of the elementary units (e.g., all adults in the United States) in order to sample. Second, data collection is concentrated in small areas, decreasing the fieldwork costs. These potential benefits have to be weighed against two principal disadvantages. First, there is frequently a loss in precision of the population estimates obtained by cluster sampling, which is reflected by larger standard errors, broader confidence intervals, or a decreased statistical power to detect differences between groups in the sample compared with simple random sampling. This loss in precision is commonly measured by a design effect, which is the ratio of variances obtained under cluster sampling versus simple random sampling. Another related disadvantage of cluster sampling is that special statistical software for complex survey samples may be needed in order to obtain correct variance estimates.

Measures of Disease and Exposure Status in a Cross-Sectional Survey. Study participants in a cross-sectional survey are not enrolled on the basis of their exposure or disease status. All information regarding these factors is obtained during the investigation and is usually limited to survey interview information. There are three common methods of conducting surveys: mail surveys, telephone surveys, and face-to-face interviews. [These methods vary in expense and quality. Dr. Robins reviews the relative merits of these approaches in Chapter 11 (this volume).]

We limit our discussion of measurement in cross-sectional studies to one problem concerning the time frame for information obtained in survey interviews. Cross-sectional surveys are conventionally viewed as assessing both disease and exposure data at the current point in time. Cause and effect cannot be distinguished for true cross-sectional data of this type. However, many cross-sectional surveys also attempt to obtain some information about events predating the current point in time. This historical information is usually based on the respondent's recollection and may be subject to considerable error (Neugebauer, 1981). Severe or salient events that are not embarrassing to report, such as death of a parent, birth of a child, or marriage, may be recalled with reasonable accuracy (Funch and Marshall, 1984; Kessler and Wethington, 1991). However, past emotions or behaviors are difficult to recall accurately, and historical reports of psychiatric symptoms may be biased by the current mental health of the respondent (Aneshensel et al., 1987; Schrader et al., 1990). A researcher should exercise considerable caution in attempting to assess life history information through respondent recall. Time lines, visual cues such as medication charts, or organization of questions around concrete events or by social contexts (e.g., home, work, school) may be used as memory aides (Kessler and Wethington, 1991).

Cohort Studies. Cohort studies in epidemiology have two essential features. First, study subjects are defined by characteristics present before disease occurrence, and these individuals form the study cohort. This is in contrast to case–control studies, where subjects are selected according to their disease status, and to cross-sectional studies, where subjects are selected by neither disease nor exposure status, but, instead, are selected to be representative of a target population.

The second characteristic of a cohort study is that real time is allowed to elapse before disease status is ascertained. Cohort members are followed through time to determine the frequency of new outcomes or events in each group. Measures of exposures and outcomes thus are both gathered at the time of their occurrence. This type of study design thereby offers the greatest potential of the epidemiologic observational studies to separate cause and effect. However, if the time elapsing between exposure and disease onset is long, and if the exposure levels vary over time, this type of study can be extremely costly and difficult to undertake.

There are two types of cohort studies that differ primarily in regard to the timing of study in relation to the occurrence of exposure and disease outcomes. The experience of a cohort can be studied prospectively or retrospectively, as is described in the following section.

Prospective Cohort Studies. In prospective cohort studies, groups of initially disease-free people are classified in terms of their exposure and are then followed forward in time. It should be noted that "disease free" is a relative term. For disorders with a poorly defined onset, such as psychiatric disorders, it may be difficult to guarantee that all members of the cohort are truly disease free at the outset of the investigation. [This issue is explored in greater detail in Chapter 9 (this volume) on studying the natural history of psychopathology.] Also, in practice, some retrospective information on exposure history may also be collected at baseline in addition to assessing current exposure levels.

Prospective cohort studies can be further subdivided into two study types based on whether the cohort is selected with or without regard to exposure status. Selection without regard to exposure status is frequently undertaken by following a study cohort sampled in a cross-sectional population survey over time. Three major cross-sectional study samples that have formed longitudinal cohorts in psychiatric epidemiology include the U.S. Epidemiologic Catchment Area study (Eaton et al., 1989), the Stirling County study in Canada (Murphy et al., 1988), and the Lundby study in Sweden (Hagnell et al., 1982). [Eaton details the methodologic problems encountered in assessing the course of psychiatric disorders in these studies in Chapter 9 (this volume).]

The other major form of prospective cohort study involves stratification on exposure, that is, selection of an exposed cohort and appropriate comparison series. There have been several different types of exposure groups that have been studied in relation to psychiatric and psychosocial outcomes, including occupational groups such as workers in plants that are closing (Cobb and Kasl, 1977) or nuclear plant workers (Kasl et al., 1981); veterans exposed to combat stress (Helzer, 1981; Decoufle et al., 1992); and population-wide environmental exposures, such as the nuclear accident at Three Mile Island (Cleary and Houts, 1984). In a prospective cohort study stratified on exposure, an appropriate comparison group of unexposed individuals must be identified for follow-up, such as other occupational groups that are not under stress, or workers who are not at risk of losing their jobs, or community samples drawn from an area with low rates of exposures. Published incidence rates for the general population that are available for comparisons with exposed cohorts for many chronic diseases are not routinely available for psychiatric disorders.

Prospective cohort studies, although appealing because exposure and disease onset are monitored in real time, are not without methodologic problems. Comparability of exposed and unexposed groups may present a problem, particularly if subject selection involves stratification by exposure. It is also difficult to obtain pre-exposure (baseline) measures on confounding factors.

Procedures for follow-up and ascertainment of disease status over time may also be complicated in prospective studies. It is essential that the time frame for follow-up closely mirrors the disease induction period. For diseases with long latency periods, a follow-up interval spanning several decades may be required. Extended follow-up periods are costly from both a financial and a professional perspective. Additionally, as a study cohort ages over time it may not be representative of younger cohorts in the population. Changing knowledge of disease over time may identify new risk factors that were not measured at baseline. Definitions of "disease" and "disease free," influenced largely by the American Psychiatric Associations Diagnostic and Statistical Manuals and the World Health Organization International Classification of Disease, are also subject to change over time. Furthermore, if risk factors vary over time and/or if cumulative exposure to risk factors influences the rates of outcome occurrence, prospective investigations have the added complication—and expense—of monitoring the exposures as well as the disease occurrence prospectively. There may also be artifactual testing effects introduced by frequent reassessment of study group.

A final, but not inconsequential, problem in prospective designs is that loss to follow-up may be significant. Certain types of high-risk populations of interest to psychiatric epidemiologists, such as residents of inner cities, are especially difficult to trace. It is essential that careful subject tracking systems be built into prospective studies at baseline. If the pattern of loss to follow-up is related to exposure or length of observation, these factors must be taken into account in analysis in order to prevent bias in estimates of association.

Retrospective Cohort Studies. The previous section highlighted some of the difficulties in gathering longitudinal data on exposure and outcomes prospectively over time. A cost-effective alternative, known as the retrospective cohort study, is sometimes available to investigators. In a retrospective cohort study, information on disease status is obtained at the time of the study, or shortly before. Information on risk factors is available from records collected in the past at the actual time of the exposure. Thus, as in a prospective cohort study, measures of exposure and disease status are collected at the point in chronologic time during which these events took place, thereby permitting cause and effect to be distinguished. This cost-effective design is not readily accessible to researchers in every situation and depends on the availability of cohorts with good, complete exposure information.

Researchers should take advantage of opportunities for conducting retrospective cohort studies because of the enormous costs associated with prospective designs. Investigators contemplating a retrospective cohort study should be aware of several common limitations associated with this type of study, however, and should attempt to minimize the impact of these potential problems in their proposed investigations. First, quality of data regarding exposure may be of lower quality than information collected in a prospective fashion because the investigator has no control over data collection and relies on extant record information. Second, the information available for potential confounding variables may be limited. A third problem resides in the difficulties in tracing cohort members, which increase as the time interval between exposure and first attempt to follow up widens. An additional problem is that the cohort membership assembled by the investigator may depend on the outcome status; in such instances the cohort that is formed for a study may not represent the total population experience, leading to bias. Last, for episodic or treatable conditions it may be necessary to gather retrospective information on past episodes of illness occurring over an extended time interval as well as the current outcome status of the study subject. As discussed previously with cross-sectional studies, the quality of data on psychiatric outcomes will be compromised if the investigation depends extensively on recall data.

One of the first epidemiological studies in psychiatry to use the application of the retrospective cohort design was the Iowa 500 study (Morrison et al., 1972; Tsuang et al., 1979a, b). The goal was to study the long-term outcomes of schizophrenia, mania, and depression. The study was conducted in the 1970s, and cohorts were identified from psychiatric hospital admission records of all patients admitted to the state psychiatric hospital in Iowa between 1934 and 1945, approximately 30–40 years before the study began. This investigation was possible because detailed symptom information had been gathered at the Iowa hospital. In addition, this hospital was the single treatment facility for all serious cases of mental disorders in the state. Using the Feigner et al. criteria (1972), records of 3,800 cases were reviewed, and subjects for three diagnostic study groups were assembled: schizophrenia (n = 200), mania (n = 100), and depression (n = 225). A nonpsychiatric surgical group was also selected using records of patients treated for appendectomy or herniorrhaphy during the same time period, matched to the psychiatric groups for sex, socioeconomic status, and age range. The members of the four study groups and their first-degree relatives were then located and interviewed between 1975 and 1979. The interview assessed the physical and psychiatric treatment history, family history, and long-term psychosocial outcomes. The principal outcomes assessed were marital, occupational, residential and psychiatric status, which included schizophrenic, affective, and neurotic symptomatologies. Interviewers were blind to the study group membership. The outcome measures, along with family data, were compared among the four different study groups.

Case–Control Studies. MacMahon and Pugh's definition of a case–control study in their classic 1970 textbook (p. 241) remains one of most concise descriptions to date of the basic procedures of this study design: "A case control study is an inquiry in which groups of individuals are selected in terms of whether they do (the cases) or do not (the controls) have the disease of which the etiology is to be studied, and the groups are then compared with respect to existing or past characteristics judged to be of possible relevance to the etiology of the disease."

Conceptually, the case–control study differs from other epidemiologic designs primarily by the approach taken in sampling study subjects, which is on the basis of disease status. Contemporary epidemiologists regard case–control studies as a method of sampling the population experience of exposures and disease onsets from closed or open cohorts (Walker, 1991). Cases are members of the population who have developed the disease outcome. Controls are sampled from the population from which the cases arise. Because the subjects are initially selected on the basis of disease status and information on exposures is subsequently obtained retrospectively, subject selection in case–control designs is often referred to as retrospective sampling.

The case–control design is advantageous for the study of rare diseases, and it is a relatively rapid and inexpensive method of inquiry. Case–control studies are usually restricted to a single outcome of interest, but they can accommodate a range of independent or interacting exposures. Case–control studies are not efficient for studying rare exposures, however, unless a rare exposure is a cause of a high proportion of cases for a particular outcome. Another limitation of many types of case–control studies is that they cannot be used to compute rates of disease occurrence in the population at risk, but only the relative rates between the exposed and unexposed (with a notable exception being the population-based case–control study). Case–control studies are also highly susceptible to bias; that is, the association between exposure and outcome occurrence measured in the study may be different from the true magnitude. Sources and control of bias are discussed in the concluding section of this chapter.

Selection of Cases. A case–control study requires a clear and reproducible set of criteria by which cases are identified, including both inclusion and exclusion rules. If diagnostic criteria for the outcome under study are controversial (which is the case for most psychiatric disorders), a case–control study should ideally be designed to include multiple case groups based on variously defined criteria. Representativeness is not the ultimate goal in a case definition. Instead, the investigator should seek to define a case group that reflects a homogeneous etiologic entity. Thus, for example, in a study of schizophrenia, an investigator would not seek to enroll a representative sample of all schizophrenics in the region under study. Instead, a subgroup believed to share a common etiologic pathway should be explicitly defined and enrolled as a case group.

Although most studies of psychiatric disorders currently focus on prevalent (i.e., existing) cases, incident (newly onset) cases are generally considered preferable in case–control studies. Prevalent cases may be enrolled at different stages of the disease process, complicating the interpretation of relationships between exposures and outcomes. Prevalent cases may also be exposed to etiologic agents both before and after the onset of disease, further clouding the interpretations of study results. An additional problem with prevalent cases is that individuals may alter their exposure levels after disease onset. For example, depressed persons may change their socialization patterns, diets, or activity levels. The relative risk measured after exposure levels have been altered in response to the disease may be different from measures based on exposure levels assessed before disease onset. This type of error in relative risk is sometimes referred to as protopathic bias. In general, use of prevalent cases can blur the distinction between factors related to onset versus course of disease, even for exposures occurring exclusively before disease incidence.

To select cases, a sampling protocol must be established. Features of this protocol should include (1) inclusion and exclusion criteria (e.g., age, sex, race); (2) the sampling frame (e.g., admissions records, registry data); and (3) sampling procedures (e.g., a total population census or random, systematic, stratified samples). The number of cases omitted by inclusion and exclusion criteria should be reported. In addition, the number of subjects who met inclusion criteria but were lost to study should be reported along with reasons for loss.

The usual sources of cases include (1) all individuals with disease onset in a specified period of time; (2) a representative subset of all population cases obtained by probability sampling; and (3) all cases seen at a particular medical care facility or group of facilities in a specified period of time. Although community-based cases (1) and (2) are preferred for studies of psychiatric conditions, they are not without limitations. A common problem associated with community-based cases concerns "caseness" definitions that incorporate history of prior treatment or diagnoses by health care professionals. Such community case series may in fact be restricted to individuals who use services, who may differ from all cases in the population in terms of socioeconomic status, education, and other potential risk factors. Also, community cases often have lower rates of cooperation than cases currently in medical care, and these refusals lead to increased bias.

Cases identified in inpatient (hospital) settings, although a cost-effective source of study subjects, are highly likely to introduce serious methodological problems in studies of psychiatric disorders. Treated cases usually differ from cases in the population on a broad range of social and demographic characteristics that may increase the difficulty of locating a comparable control group. Hospitals are often selective as to the type of patients whom they will treat (e.g., chronic cases may be served in state institutions, whereas first-admission cases may be treated in private institutions), and it is unlikely that cases identified in these centers will be comparable to all cases of disorder arising in the population either in exposure or disease characteristics. When the probability for hospitalization differs for cases, noncases, and individuals with the exposure characteristic under study (a common result of high comorbidity in hospitalized cases), a spurious association may be detected. This well-known limitation of hospital-based case–control studies was first described by Berkson (1946).

Lastly, a major impediment for psychiatric research in the United States is the virtual absence of comprehensive population registries covering a broad range of psychiatric disorders. In exceptional instances, communities may have systems of care providing comprehensive coverage of all members of the population and maintaining linked medical records of all treatment contacts. The Monroe County, New York, registry is an example of a population-wide registry for psychiatric disorders. In such instances, treatment records can be used to assemble a case series for severe disorders that are usually seen in a treatment facility at some point in time (e.g., schizophrenia). However, for other conditions in which only a small portion of cases are seen in treatment, such as depression and anxiety disorders, even a coordinated treatment system or treatment registry is an inadequate source of cases. For these disorders, a true population-based case series can only be identified through investigator-initiated population screening or assessment, which may be comparable to a population survey in total costs and level of effort.

Selection of Controls. Controls are used to evaluate whether the frequency or level of past exposures among the cases is different from that among comparable persons in the source population who do not have the disease under consideration. The selection of controls in a case–control study has been a subject of considerable controversy (Miettinen, 1985a). Nevertheless, theoretical and practical guidelines for selecting a valid control group have been proposed in the epidemiologic literature (Miettinen, 1985b). Controls should be representative of the population from which the cases arise in terms of their exposure distribution. This translates into three fundamental principles: (1) the cases and controls should come from a shared population source; (2) the selection of controls should be independent of the exposure or risk factor under study; and (3) exclusion criteria should be applied in a standardized (symmetric) fashion for both cases and controls in regard to ancillary factors (such as age), secondary diagnoses, or comorbid conditions (Schwartz and Link, 1989).

If it can be established that all cases are drawn from a defined geographic area, then controls should be selected from the same area so that their exposure distribution represents the source population for cases. Controls are frequently drawn from the same neighborhoods as cases in order to increase the likelihood that the two groups share a similar source population.

In selecting a source of controls, another consideration is the feasibility of obtaining information on study factors that can be collected in a comparable fashion as in the case group. This comparability should extend to records (quality and completeness), diagnostic procedures, response rates, and recall of exposure and knowledge of disease. Using hospitalized controls (such as surgical patients) in a case–control study in which cases are enrolled from an inpatient setting may increase comparability between groups in terms of the respondent's willingness to participate and other characteristics that may have influenced help-seeking. The interviews would also be conducted in a similar environment, which would increase comparability in terms of selective recall of health and exposure histories. However, it may be difficult to ascertain whether hospitalized controls have been selected independently of exposure so that their exposure distribution is representative of the population experience from which the cases arise.

Controls may also be selected as being similar to cases with respect to extraneous (confounding) factors, that is, variables that may lead to differences between cases and controls that do not reflect differences in risk factors under study. This procedure is referred to as matching. Usually, matching is limited to age, sex, and race. It is not cost-effective to employ matching in control selection unless information on matching factor is available before subject selection begins.

Two common forms of matching are individual (or pairwise) matching and group (or frequency) matching. In individual matching, one or more controls are selected for each case, and controls are identical to the case on the matched characteristics. In group matching, controls are selected in a manner that ensures that the proportions of the matching characteristics within the control group are the same as the case group. For continuous variables, such as age, the variable can be either categorized for purposes of matching or a "caliper" or tolerance limit for the match can be defined (e.g., age within five years of the case).

There are several limitations of matching. The costs may increase substantially as the number of matching variables increases. If individual matching involves multiple variables, it may be difficult to locate a control who matches a case on all characteristics, and many potential controls may be lost to the study because they share some, but not all, of the characteristics of a member of the case group. In addition, the pursuit of comparability between controls and cases in matching can go too far. If cases and controls are matched on a risk factor or on a measure of the disease process, no differences between cases and controls may be observed on that risk factor or some exposures or characteristics that are true causes. This problem is referred to as *overmatching*. Another potential problem can occur when supernormal controls are selected in comparison to the cases. We have illustrated this point in the selection of controls for family studies (Tsuang et al, 1988). In this study we selected two groups of controls, one which was unscreened for psychiatric symptoms and one control group which was screened for having a history of psychiatric symptoms. Since this was a family study we compared the rate of psychiatric illness in the relatives of various psychiatric disorders with the rate of illness in the two control groups previously described. The largest difference occurred with affective disorders, which were more frequent among the relatives of the unscreened controls than among relatives of the screened controls. These results suggested that gathering data on both screened and unscreened controls will yield more generalizable results than either alone. It should be noted that control of effects of confounding factors can also be handled in data analysis, and this approach to achieving a balance between case and control groups is preferred in most contemporary studies.

Cost and feasibility enter into control group selection regardless of whether matching is employed. Different sources of controls vary in cost and feasibility. Two cost-effective sources of controls discussed earlier include (1) (for a hospital-based case series) a control group consisting of patients suffering from an illness unrelated to the disease under study and (2) neighbors. Economic constraints also dictate the number of controls to be drawn from a given source. The control group is characteristically of equal or larger size than the case group and generally should not exceed the case group by more than a factor of 4 or 5 (Rothman, 1986). Controls are easier to identify than cases, and increasing the size of the control group may be an economical approach to enhancing statistical power in data analysis.

When the process of selecting control subjects is undertaken, the cases usually have already been identified. Controls may be selected in a pairwise fashion with each case (e.g., next admission with certain diagnosis, neighbor, sibling), or controls may be selected as a group according to a sampling protocol. Examples of this latter approach include a community probability sample or a systematic sample of all traffic accident admissions (or patients) in given period. As with cases, an explicit protocol for selection procedures should be prepared and adhered to. Exclusion rules for specific individuals should also be clarified (e.g., exclusion of individuals with other psychiatric disorders).

If each source of controls is not an optimal reference group for the exposure likelihood of the case series, multiple control groups can be employed. Differences in magnitude of association between exposure and disease occurrence using alternate control groups may be helpful in assessing causality and sources of bias.

Case-Crossover Study. The case-crossover study is a variation of matched case–control study that can be applied to identify potential causes ("triggers" or "triggering exposures") of acute onset of event outcomes during the time span of an individuals life (Maclure, 1991). This method does not involve external control subjects. For a series of individuals, the occurrence of an acute event (e.g., panic attack), in the person-time following a short transient exposure (e.g., intense traumatic event) is compared with the event experience of the same individual when there was no such exposure. Procedure-wise, for each individual subject, a specified time period immediately before the event is treated as the case, and a comparable, randomly sampled period without such event as the control. Statistical analysis similar to that for matched case–control study can be applied to estimate odds ratio associated with specified periods of time after exposure, and the empirical latency following exposure is identified by maximization of the odds ratio.

Case-cohort. The case-cohort design is an alternative to the case–control study nested within a cohort (Rothman and Greenland, 1998). A random sample from the original, total cohort forms the subcohort. Subcohort members ("controls") are selected without matching on time. Person-time can be calculated for each exposure profile in the subcohort and extrapolated back to the total cohort. It has a simple sampling scheme but a more complex analysis. There are several advantages of case-cohort design over a nested case–control study. The rate, (in addition to rate ratio) of an outcome event can be estimated. Without needing to match with cases, different outcome events can be studied simultaneously and control selection based on the original roster can begin before all cases are identified.

Measures of Exposure Status in a Case–Control Study. In a case–control study, disease status is determined at the time of subject selection. Therefore, measures obtained on study subjects focus on exposure histories. Measurement of exposure history in a case–control study should be made using well-defined and relevant variables. Timing of exposure, both current and past, must be ascertained. Comparable methods of collecting information on exposure must be used for cases and controls. Controls are less likely to be thinking about exposures related to disease than cases, and efforts must be made to minimize selective recall in the comparison groups. Whenever possible, records of exposure levels made before disease onset should be used, but, regardless of the types of measures that are employed, information sources must be the same for cases and controls.

Investigators gathering data on cases and controls should be blind to the case or control status. Additionally, checks on the comparability of exposure information should be made. For example, nonresponse rates for key exposure variables should be contrasted and found to be comparable for cases and controls. Frequency of reporting characteristics that are not of etiologic relevance should also be comparable between case and control groups.

Uses of Case–Control Studies in Psychiatric Research. An exemplary case–control study in psychiatric research is Brown and Harris's study of depression among women in the Camberwell district of London, described in their 1978 book, *Social Origins of Depression.* These investigators hypothesized that onset of a depressive episode was precipitated by two stages of stress: (1) a underlying susceptibility to depression induced by exposure to certain social conditions or stressors with sustained psychological sequelae (vulnerability factors) and (2) triggering of the episode among vulnerable women by a recent life stress or major difficulty (provoking agents). A third set of factors, principally including past loss, were hypothesized to influence the severity and shape of pathology and were labeled "symptom formation factors."

Brown and Harris enrolled multiple case groups in their study, including groups of both treated and community cases. Each case group was subdivided by severity and onset (incident vs. chronic prevalent cases). The first case series consisted of patients (73 inpatients, 41 outpatients) aged 18–65 who made visits to Camberwell district psychiatrists during the study period and who were given a diagnosis of primary depression without underlying alcoholism or organic causes. An urban community case series was obtained from two random samples of women aged 18–65 in the Camberwell district conducted four years apart. A rural community case series was also assembled from surveying women who lived on an island in the Outer Hebrides. Interview data were used to subdivide the case groups further on the basis of meeting borderline or full case criteria or representing onset or chronic cases.

The primary source of controls were 295 women in the Camberwell community survey who were interviewed and found to be without depression. Nondepressives in the rural survey were also available as a control series. All cases and controls were interviewed about their histories of vulnerability and provoking factors. Stresses described in the interview were rated by panels of judges to control for biased reporting of the impact of events by depressed respondents.

The principal finding of this study was that risk of depression in community women was increased when a provoking agent occurred in the presence of three vulnerability factors (loss of a mother before age 11, presence of three or more children under age 14 at home, absence of a confiding relationship with husband or boyfriend). This model was re-evaluated for different case groups (severe vs.

borderline cases, treated vs. untreated, chronic vs. recent onset cases). One important finding was that no association was observed for treated cases of depression and certain vulnerability factors, notably the presence of three or more children under 14 years at home. This vulnerability factor was observed to be negatively associated with help-seeking, possibly cancelling any observable elevated risk in treated cases. This elegant case–control study illustrates the importance of employing multiple case groups in studies of psychiatric disorders and the significance of using population-based samples to investigate the etiology of psychopathology.

Hybrid Studies. Each of the three basic observational epidemiologic study designs described thus far: cross-sectional, case–control, and cohort can be developed further by adding special design features to permit estimation of additional parameters and/or to handle complex exposure or disease courses (Zahner et al., 1995). In psychiatric epidemiology, various features of sociological studies have been invoked to handle the variable course of risk factors and disease outcomes. Using the terminology of Kleinbaum et al. (1982), we are referring to these derivative studies as hybrid designs. We do not attempt to catalog each possible hybrid design, but, rather, will select examples that illustrate some of the influential hybrid studies in psychiatric epidemiology. The interested reader is referred to the textbook by Kleinbaum et al. (1982) for a more formal presentation of these and other hybrid studies.

Repeated Cross-Sectional Survey. A hybrid study design that is based on the cross-sectional survey is the repeated cross-sectional survey. In this type of study, independent, representative samples of a target population are drawn at two or more time periods and assessed separately. It is important to note that in a repeated cross-sectional survey, unlike a cohort study, different study samples are assessed at each time period. This type of hybrid study permits analysis of changing levels of disease rates in a population over time and of changing levels of association between exposure and disease when follow-ups of a single study cohort are not feasible. This hybrid design was employed in the U.S. National Sample Surveys (Gurin et al., 1960; Veroff et al., 1981), in which two cross-sectional mental health and service use surveys involving separate national probability samples of the entire U.S. adult population were conducted in 1957 and 1976. To estimate changes in the mental health status over time, the data from the 1957 and 1976 national surveys were pooled into one database. Tests for differences in measures by year of survey were used to identify whether the mental health of Americans had changed over the decades between the surveys. Another major study in psychiatric epidemiology, the Stirling County study, included repeated cross-sectional surveys as well as cohort follow ups at each major assessment period in order to be able to examine secular population changes that would not be represented adequately in the prospective study cohort as it aged over time (Murphy et al., 1984).

Multistage Studies. A type of hybrid design known as a two (or multiple) stage study combines features of case–control and cross-sectional survey methodologies. In these studies, a cross-sectional survey employing a brief and inexpensive mental health screening instrument is conducted in the first stage of inquiry. Using the results of the screening information, a smaller sample of cases (screen positives) and controls (screen negatives) are selected with known probability from the cross-sectional survey sample. More extensive information is obtained on these case and control subjects in a second (and sometimes third) stage of data collection. Population prevalence estimates can be obtained from second-stage data by assigning weights to the study data reflecting the probability of selection at each stage and by adjusting for disease classification errors in the screening instrument. Variance adjustments may also be required to represent the underlying sampling scheme in analysis (Cain and Breslow, 1988). The accuracy of estimation in multistage studies depends on several factors, most notably on the quality of the screening instrument used in the first stage to identify cases and controls (Shrout et al., 1986; Newman et al., 1990). Also, because subjects are reinterviewed in multiple waves within a very short time span, there may be loss to follow up from subjects who consider multiple stages of assessment too burdensome. Retest practice effects may also occur if similar questions are repeated in both stages.

Two-stage studies have been used in a number of child mental health studies where data collection costs can be large because information is gathered from multiple informants. The Rutter et al. (1975) Isle of Wight and Inner London Borough studies of child psychiatric disorders in eight-year-old children and the Bird et al. (1988) Puerto Rican study of children are examples of two-stage studies in child psychiatric epidemiology. Another example of a multistage study is the Dohrenwend et al. (1992) study of socioeconomic status and psychiatric disorders in a birth cohort of 4,914 Israel-born adults of European and North African background, also described in Dohrenwend (1995).

Panel Studies. An example of a hybrid study based on a cohort design is a panel study. In a panel study, repeated measures are taken on both exposure and disease characteristics of the cohort at each follow-up period. This type of design permits flexible handling of changing exposure levels and variable disease course over the study period. The 22 year follow-up of a Midtown Manhattan study (Srole and Fisher, 1989) is an example of a major longitudinal study in psychiatric epidemiology that has utilized the panel study design. In the Midtown Manhattan study, a probability sample of 1,660 adults aged 20–59 residing in a predominantly white residential area of central Manhattan, ranging in social character from Gold Coast to Slum, was assessed by household interviews. Two decades later, a total of 858 survivors were located, and interviews were completed with 695 individuals, or panelists. This study found no significant net change in general mental health ratings over time after 22 years of exposure to residential living in or near Manhattan.

VALID GROUP COMPARISONS IN OBSERVATIONAL STUDIES

When two groups are compared in an observational study, the estimate of relative risk measuring the association between an exposure and disease outcome can be distorted by a number of factors that compromise the validity of the estimate. Factors contributing to noncomparability of groups include (1) the population composition of the groups; (2) the information obtained from each group; and (3) extraneous attributes unevenly distributed between the groups that may explain the difference in rates of disease occurrence (Miettinen, 1985a). Noncomparability from any of these sources results in a biased relative risk estimate, that is, the relative risk observed in the study data differs from the true value. The bias may be negative (i.e., the observed estimate falls closer to the null value than the true relative risk) or positive (i.e., the observed estimate is farther from the null value). There are three broad classes of biases frequently encountered in epidemiologic studies: biases of selection, information, and confounding (Monson, 1990).

Selection Bias

Selection bias is most likely to occur in studies where the outcome status is known at the start of the study and is used to select subjects, as in case–control or retrospective cohort studies. If enrollment of exposed and nonexposed individuals is influenced by the disease status, selection bias will occur. For example, in a retrospective cohort study designed to study the association between occupational exposures and onset of Alzheimer's disease, if health records of individuals with Alzheimer's have been removed for any purpose related to the outcome status, such as for processing worker compensation, the disease experience in the study group will be underestimated. Consequently, the relationships between exposure and disease outcome will be biased.

Considerable attention has been given to sources of selection bias in case–control studies. To avoid selection bias in a case–control design, the distribution of the exposures in the control group should be representative of the population at risk. The sample of individuals enrolled into the control group may be systematically nonrepresentative for a number of reasons (Lewis and Pelosi, 1990). For example, individuals may refuse to cooperate in interviews, and this noncooperation may be systematically associated with the exposure under study. In a hospital-based case–control study, admission into a hospital may be determined by factors such as comorbidity that is related to the exposures under study, a source of bias described earlier in this chapter as "Berkson's bias." If the true source population of the case group is difficult to identify, the potential for selection bias increases because control subjects may not be sampled from the true population at risk. Methods described earlier for control selection (shared population sources for cases and controls, selection of control subjects independently of exposure status, symmetric exclusion criteria for cases and controls) can effectively minimize selection bias in these studies.

Information Bias

Information bias refers to invalid estimates of the relationship between exposure and disease outcomes resulting from information obtained on study subjects. One form of information bias occurs when the data gathered for the different study groups is not comparable (observation bias). For example, observation bias can occur in a prospective cohort study when there is attrition because subjects are lost to follow-up. When subject loss occurs, incomplete information is obtained about disease development on subjects who are not followed over time. If subjects who are lost to follow-up from the exposed and unexposed cohorts have a different disease experience than the study participants in their respective cohorts, estimates of relative risk made from the available study data may be biased. Greenland (1977) provides a detailed account of the conditions in which nonresponse can lead to biased estimates in cohort studies.

Information bias can also occur when the comparison groups give information with varying levels of accuracy (recall bias). For example, mothers giving birth to mentally retarded children might recall medications taken during pregnancy with greater accuracy than mothers delivering healthy children.

Misclassification of a subject's exposure or disease status because of measurement error is another form of information bias. For dichotomous exposures and outcomes the direction of bias in the estimate of relative risk will be toward the null if misclassification is nondifferential: that is, it occurs with the same magnitude and direction within the different study groups being compared (e.g., similar exposure misclassification rates for cases and controls in a case–control study; similar disease misclassification rates for exposed and nonexposed subjects in a cohort study). However, if misclassification occurs differentially for the comparison groups, the direction of bias can be in any direction. Even small amounts of misclassification error can lead to substantial bias in estimates in relative risk (Kleinbaum et al., 1982), and it is important to use measurement methods and data collection procedures that will ensure the highest degree of accuracy in classifying study subjects. The impact of measurement error on study estimates can be examined by recomputing estimates that adjust for error rates either through sensitivity analyses or by modeling measurement error (Rosner et al., 1989; Armstrong, 1990).

Confounding Bias

Confounding bias occurs when the study samples in the comparison groups are imbalanced with respect to other characteristics that are independent determinants of the disease under study. These ancillary characteristics, known as confounders, will be found to be associated with both the exposure and the disease in the study sample. Table 2 illustrates a hypothetical situation in which confounding bias could occur in a psychiatric research context.

In Table 2, it can be observed that age is a predictor of the outcome under study because mortality density is higher among the older subjects. In addition, age is unevenly distributed between the comparison groups; the schizophrenic group has more person-years contributed by younger subjects. Even though the true mortality rate ratio should be 3.0 comparing schizophrenia with bipolar disorder, the relative risk estimated in the total study sample is only 1.5. Hence, unless adjustments are made for differences in age distributions between the study groups, the observed relative risk will be biased.

Bias from confounding variables can be handled at two stages of a study: either in the subject selection phase or in the data analysis stage. In the subject selection stage, confounding can be minimized by restriction or matching. In restriction, subject selection is limited to certain categories of a confounding variable. For example, in the example of age and mortality density, confounding by age could be controlled by restricting the age range of all subjects in the study to one age group,

TABLE 2. Confounding in a Comparative Study of the Mortality Rate (Density) of Schizophrenia and Bipolar Disorder

	Deaths	Person-Years	Mortality Rate (per 1,000 person-years)
Young subjects (< 45 years of age)			
Schizophrenia	18	6,000	3.0
Bipolar disorder	2	2,000	1.0
Relative risk = 3.0			
Old Subjects (45 + years of age)			
Schizophrenia	30	2,000	15.0
Bipolar disorder	30	6,000	5.0
Relative risk = 3.0			
All subjects (young and old)			
Schizophrenia	48	8,000	6.0
Bipolar disorder	32	8,000	4.0
Relative risk = 1.5			

such as selecting all study subjects with schizophrenia and bipolar disorder to be under age 45. Alternatively, confounding could be controlled by matching schizophrenic and bipolar study groups on age during subject selection, using the procedures described in the section on case–control studies. Matching will ensure that the groups are balanced with respect to the confounding factor. However, as discussed earlier in the overview of case–control studies, there are several drawbacks to matching. The association between age and the outcome cannot be directly estimated if matching is employed in subject selection. Also, matching can be inefficient and expensive compared with methods of controlling confounding in data analysis.

In the analysis phase, confounding is commonly controlled by use of stratified analyses or multivariable regression models. [These procedures are described in Chapter 3 (this volume) and are only briefly summarized here.] In stratified analyses, the study sample is grouped by the categories of the confounding variables. Relative risk estimates can be calculated within each group of the confounding variable. If the stratum-specific estimates do not differ from each other (usually evaluated by a chi-squared test of heterogeneity or determined a priori), a summary estimate of relative risk can be calculated by computing a weighted average of the stratum-specific relative risks. A variety of weighting schemes can be employed (Kleinbaum et al., 1982), and the most common method, suggested by Mantel and Haenzsel (1959), uses a weight that is inversely proportional to the variance in each stratum.

In the example provided in Table 2, the stratum-specific estimates of relative risk are identical to each other, equalling 3 in both older and younger patients. A summary measure of relative risk would also equal 3. However, if the relative risks differ for different levels of a confounder, interaction is said to exist between the confounder and the exposure under study with respect to the disease outcome. In this case, summary estimates of relative risk will not represent the true nature of the relationship between the exposure and the disease outcome because the value of the estimate depends on the subject's status on the confounding variable. If an interaction exists, the separate stratum-specific estimates of relative risk should be reported for separate categories of the confounding variables, for example, for older and for younger subjects.

Multivariable regression models can also be used to adjust for the influence of confounding variables on the exposure and disease outcome by introducing confounders as covariate independent terms in these models. Multivariable models can also be used to evaluate interactions. For a more detailed discussion of control of confounding, the interested reader is referred to basic texts in epidemiology (Kleinbaum et al., 1982; Monson, 1990; Rothman, 1986; Walker, 1991). Maldanado and Greenland (1993) discuss alternative analytic approaches to evaluating and controlling confounding in an epidemiologic investigation.

CONCLUSION

The ultimate goal of an epidemiological study and corresponding methodology is to establish causation for primary disease prevention. The application of screening is used to prevent disease or its consequences by identifying individuals at a point in the natural history when the disease process can be altered through intervention (Fletcher et al, 1996). There are three levels of prevention that are targeted: (1) primary prevention targets asymptomatic persons to identify early risk factors for disease in order to arrest the pathologic process before symptoms develop; (2) secondary prevention targets persons early in the disease process in order to improve prognosis and; (3) tertiary prevention targets persons who are developing complications in order to avert the sequelae of such complications. Therefore, a screening test is used to identify an early marker of disease progression so that intervention can be implemented to interrupt the disease process (Mausnerand and Bahn, 1974). Until the occurrence of death, it may be possible at each stage of the evolution of the disease process to apply appropriate measures to prevent continued progression and deterioration of the subjects condition. The different levels of prevention can be fully understood only in relation to the natural progression of disease.

ACKNOWLEDGMENTS

The methodology presented in this chapter was based on work which is funded in part by the Harvard Training Program in Psychiatric Epidemiology and Biostatistics (NIMH training grant 5-T32-MH17119).

REFERENCES

Aneshensel CS, Estrada AL, Hansell MJ, Clark VA (1987): Social psychological aspects of reporting behavior: Lifetime depressive episode reports. J Health Social Behav 28:232–246.

Armstrong BG (1990): The effects of measurement errors on relative risk regressions. Am J Epidemiol 132:1176–1184.

Berkson J (1946): Limitation of the application of fourfold table analysis to hospital data. Biom Bull 2:47–53.

Bird HR, Canino G, Rubio-Stipec M et al. (1988): Estimates of the prevalence of childhood maladjustment in a community survey in Puerto Rico. Arch Gen Psychiatry 45:1120–1126.

Brenner MH (1973): "Mental Illness and the Economy." Cambridge, Harvard University Press.

Brown GW, Harris T (1978): "Social Origins of Depression." New York: Free Press.

Cain KC, Breslow NE (1988): Logistic regression analysis and efficient design for two-stage studies. Am J Epidemiol 128:1198–1206.

Chiang CL (1968): "Introduction to Stochastic Processes in Biostatistics." New York: Wiley.

Cleary PD, Houts PS (1984): The psychological impact of the Three Mile Island accident. J Hum Stress 10:28–34.

Cobb S, Kasl SV (1977): "Termination: The Consequences of Job Loss." DHEW(NIOSH) Publication No. 77–224. Washington, DC.

Cochran WG (1977): "Sampling techniques," 3rd ed. New York: Wiley.

Decoufle P, Holmgreen P, Boyle CA, Stroup NE (1992): Self-reported health status of Vietnam veterans in relation to perceived exposure to herbicides and combat. Am J Epidemiol 135:312–323.

Dohrenwend BP (1995): "The problem of validity in field studies of psychological disorders," Revisited. In Tsuang MT, Tohen M, Zahner GEP (eds): "Textbook in Psychiatric Epidemiology." New York: Wiley.

Dohrenwend BP, Levav I, Shrout PE. et al. (1992): Socioeconomic status and psychiatric disorders: The causation–selection issue. Science 255:946–952.

Eaton WW, Kramer M, Anthony JC. et al. (1989): The incidence of specific DIS/DSM-III mental disorders: Data from the NIMH Epidemiologic Catchment Area Program. Acta Psychiatr Scand 79:163–178.

Elandt-Johnson RC (1975): Definition of rates: Some remarks on their use and misuse. Am J Epidemiol 102:267–271.

Elwood JM (1988): "Causal Relationships in Medicine: A Practical System for Critical Appraisal." New York: Oxford University Press.

Feighner JP, Robins E, Guze SM. et al. (1972): Diagnostic criteria for use in psychiatric research. Arch Gen Psychiatry 26:57–63.

Fletcher RH, Fletcher SW, Wagner EH (1996): "Clinical Epidemiology: The Essentials," 3rd ed. Baltimore: Williams and Wilkins.

Freeman J, Hutchison GB (1980): Prevalence, incidence, and duration. Am J Epidemiol 112:707–723.

Freeman J, Hutchison GB (1986): Duration of disease, duration indicators, and estimation of the risk ratio. Am J Epidemiol 124:134–149.

Funch DP, Marshall JR (1984): Measuring life stress: Factors affecting fall-off in the reporting of life events. J Health Social Behav 25:453–464.

Gibbons RD, Hedeker D, Elkin I. et al. (1993): Some conceptual and statistical issues in analysis of longitudinal psychiatric data: Application to the NIMH Treatment of Depression Collaborative Research Program Dataset. Arch Gen Psychiatry 50:739–750.

Greenland S (1977): Response and follow-up bias in cohort studies. Am J Epidemiol 106:184–187.

Gurin G, Veroff J, Feld S (1960): "Americans View Their Mental Health." New York: Basic Books.

Hagnell O, Lanke J, Rorsman B, Ojesjo L.(1982): Are we entering an age of melancholy?: Depressive illnesses in a prospective epidemiological study of over 25 years: The Lundby Study, Sweden Psychol Med 12:279–289.

Hamilton M (1960): A rating scale for depression. J Neurol Neurosurg Psychiatry 23:56–62.

Helzer J (1981): Methodological issues in the interpretations of the consequences of extreme situations. In Dohrenwend, B. S, Dohrenwend, B. P (eds): "Stressful Life Events and Their Contexts." New York: Prodist, pp 108–129.

Kasl SV (1979): Mortality and the business cycle. Some questions about research strategies when utilizing macro-social and ecological data. Am J Public Health 69:784–788.

Kasl SV, Chisholm RF, Eskenazi B (1981): The impact of the accident at the Three Mile Island on the behavior and well-being of nuclear workers. Part II. Job tension, psychophysiological symptoms, and indices of distress. Am J Public Health 71:484–495.

Kessler RC, Wethington RC (1991): The reliability of life event reports in a community survey. Psychol Med 21:723–738.

Kish L (1965): "Survey Sampling." New York: Wiley.

Kleinbaum DG, Kupper LL, Morgenstern H (1982): "Epidemiologic Research: Principles and Quantitiative Methods." Belmont CA: Lifetime Learning Publications.

Klerman GL (1988): The current age of youthful melancholia: Evidence for increase in depression among adolescents and young adults. Br J Psychiatry 152:414.

Kramer M (1957): A discussion of the concepts of incidence and prevalence as related to epidemiologic studies of mental disorders. Am J Public Health 47:826–840.

Lewis G, Pelosi AJ (1990): The case–control study in psychiatry. Br J Psychiatry 157:197–207.

Maclure M (1991): The case-crossover design: A method for studying transient effects on the risk of acute events. Am J Epidemiol 133:144–153.

MacMahon B, Pugh TF (1970): "Epidemiology: Principles and Methods." Boston: Little Brown.

Maldanado G, Greenland S (1993): Simulation study of confounder selection strategies. Am J Epidemiol 138:923–936.

Mantel N, Haenszel W (1959): Statistical aspects of the analysis of data from retrospective studies of disease. J Natl Cancer Inst 22:719–748.

Mausner JS, Bahn AK (1974): "Epidemiology: An Introductory Text." Philadelphia: W.B. Saunders Company.

Miettinen OS (1985a): "Theoretical Epidemiology." New York: Wiley.

Miettinen OS (1985b): The case–control study: Valid selection of subjects (with discussions). J Chronic Dis 38:543–558.

Monson RR (1990): "Occupational Epidemiology," 2nd ed. Boca Raton: CRC Press.

Morrison J, Clancy J, Crowe R, Winokur G (1972): The Iowa 500: I. Diagnostic validity in mania, depression and schizophrenia. Arch Gen Psychiatry 27:457–461.

Morton RF, Hebel JR, McCarter RJ (2001): "A Study Guide to Epidemiology and Biostatistics," 5th ed. Gaithersburg, MD: Aspen Publishers, Inc.

Murphy JM, Oliver DC, Monson RR et al (1988): Incidence of depression and anxiety: The Stirling County Study. Am J Public Health 78:534–540.

Murphy JM, Sobol AM, Neff RK et al (1984): Stability of prevalence: Depression and anxiety disorders. Arch Gen Psychiatry 41:990–997.

Neugebauer R (1981): The reliability of life event reports. In Dohrenwend, B. S, Dohrenwend, B. P (eds): "Stressful Life Events and Their Contexts." New York: Prodist, pp 85–107.

Newman SC, Shrout PE, Bland RC (1990): The efficiency of two-phase designs in prevalence surveys of mental disorders. Psychol Med 20:183–193.

Robins LN (1985): Epidemiology: Reflections on testing the validity of psychiatric interviews. Arch Gen Psychiatry 42:918–924.

Robins LN, Helzer JE, Weissman MM. et al. (1984): Lifetime prevalence of psychiatric disorders in three sites. Arch. Gen. Psychiatry 41:949–948.

Rosner B, Willet W, Spiegelman D (1989): Correction of logistic regression relative risk estimates and confidence intervals for systematic within-person measurement error. Stat Med 8:1051–1070.

Rothman KJ (1986): "Modern Epidemiology." Boston: Little Brown.

Rothman KJ, Greenland S (1998): "Modern Epidemiology," 2nd ed. Philadelphia: Lippincott-Raven.

Rutter M, Cox A, Tupling C, Berger M, Yule W (1975): Attainment and adjustment in two geographical areas: I. The prevalence of psychiatric disorder. Br J Psychiatry 126:493–509.

Schrader G, Davis A, Stefanovic S, Christie P (1990): The recollection of affect. Psychol Med 20:105–109.

Schwartz S, Link BG (1989): The "well control" artefact in case/control studies of specific psychiatric disorders. Psychol Med 19:737–742.

Shrout PE, Dohrenwend BP, Levav I (1986): A discriminant rule for screening cases of diverse diagnostic types: Preliminary results. J Consult Clin Psychol 54:314–319.

Srole L, Fischer AK (1989): Changing lives and well-being: The Midtown Manhattan panel study, 1954–1976. Acta Psychiatr Scand 79(Suppl 348):35–44.

Tsuang MT, Woolson RF, Fleming JA (1979a): Long term outcome of major psychoses: I Schizophrenia and affective disorders compared with psychiatrically symptom-free surgical conditions. Arch Gen Psychiatry 36:1295–1301.

Tsuang MT, Dempsey GM (1979b): Long term outcome of major psychoses: II Schizoaffective disorder compared with schizophrenia, affective disorders, and a surgical control group. Arch Gen Psychiatry 36:1302–1304.

Tsuang MT, Fleming JA, Kendler KS, Gruenberg AS (1988): Selection of controls for family studies: biases and implications. Arch Gen Psychiatry 45:1006–1008.

Veroff J, Douvan E, Kulka RA (1981): "The Inner American: A Self Portrait From 1957 to 1976." New York: Basic Books.

Walker AM (1991): Observation and Inference. An Introduction to the Methods of Epidemiology. Chestnut Hill, MA: Epidemiology Resources, Inc.

Weissman MM, Myers JK (1978): Affective disorders in a United States urban community: The use of research diagnostic criteria in an epidemiologic survey. Arch Gen Psychiatry 35:1304–1311.

Zahner GE, Hsieh C, Fleming JA (1995): "Introduction to Epidemiologic Research Methods. Textbook in Psychiatric Epidemiology," 1st ed. New York: Wiley.

CHAPTER 2

Analysis of Categorized Data:Use of the Odds Ratio as a Measure of Association

STEPHEN L. HILLIS AND ROBERT F. WOOLSON

Department of Statistics and Actuarial Science (S. L. H., R. F. W.) and Department of Biostatistics (R. F. W.), The University of Iowa College of Public Health, Iowa City, IA 52242.

INTRODUCTION

In this chapter we discuss the use of the odds ratio as a measure of association between two dichotomous variables that typically indicate the presence or absence of a specific characteristic. For instance, in a clinical trial that randomly assigns subjects with a particular disease to either a drug group or a control group, the researcher is interested in the association between the dichotomous variables outcome status (improvement or no improvement) and treatment status (drug or control).

We consider the general situation where the data can be summarized by the familiar 2×2 contingency table presented in Table 1. For example, suppose that in a randomized study designed to assess the effect of lithium on manic depression in males, 30 male patients with manic depression are treated with lithium and 40 are given a placebo. In the first 3 months, 8 of the patients treated with lithium have manic-depressive episodes while 28 of the patients given the placebo have episodes. Table 2 presents these data.

In practice, the data for Table 1 are usually generated from one of three possible sampling methods: the *cross-sectional study*, the *prospective* (or *cohort*) *study*, or *the retrospective* (or *case–control*) *study*. We now briefly discuss the methods; a more detailed discussion of the methods and their advantages and disadvantages can be found in an epidemiologic methods textbook such as that of Kleinbaum et al. (1982) or Miettinen (1986).

In a *cross-sectional study* a random sample of size N is selected from the population of interest, and then the presence or absence of the characteristics corresponding to variables 1 and 2 is determined for each subject. For example, to

Textbook in Psychiatric Epidemiology, *Second Edition*, Edited by Ming T. Tsuang and Mauricio Tohen.
ISBN 0-471-40974-X

TABLE 1. Data Layout for a 2 × 2 Contingency Table

		Variable 2: Present	Variable 2: Absent	
Variable 1	Present	O_{11}	O_{12}	R_1 (Row totals)
	Absent	O_{21}	O_{22}	R_2 (Row totals)
	Column totals	C_1	C_2	N = Grand total

TABLE 2. Data Layout for a Hypothetical Randomized Study of the Effect of Lithium on Manic Depression in Males

		Episodes within 3 months: Present	Episodes within 3 months: Absent	
Treatment	Lithium	8	22	30
	Placebo	28	12	40
		36	34	70

study the association between gender (male or female) and psychosis (present or absent) in a community, a random sample could be drawn from the community, followed by the classification of each subject with respect to gender and psychosis. Of course, the psychosis classification would be determined by an appropriate diagnostic instrument.

In prospective and retrospective studies, two random samples are selected. Let variable 1 be the *antecedent variable*—that is, the subject can be classified in terms of the presence or absence of the variable 1 characteristic before a similar classification is possible for variable 2. For example, in clinical trials, treatment status (drug or placebo) is assigned before the outcome status (improvement or no improvement) is known, and hence treatment status is the antecedent variable. In studying the association between a risk factor variable, such as family history of psychiatric disease (present or absent), and a disease, such as depression, clearly the risk factor variable is antecedent.

In a *prospective study*, random samples of size R_1 and R_2 (see Table 1) are selected from the two populations corresponding to the two possibilities (called *levels*) of variable 1. The subjects are then followed over a specified period of time, after which subjects are classified according to variable 2. The study of the effect of lithium on manic depression described earlier is a *randomized* prospective study, since the subjects are randomly assigned to the two levels of variable 1. As an example of a nonrandomized prospective study, one could study the association between family history of alcoholism and a particular psychiatric disorder by

TABLE 3. Data Layout of a Hypothetical Retrospective Study of the Association Between Family History of Alcoholism and a Particular Psychiatric Disorder

		Disorder		
		Present	Absent	
Family history of alcoholism	Yes	20	5	25
	No	30	55	85
		50	60	110

following two samples selected from populations of subjects with and without a family history of alcoholism over a period of, say, 20 years and then recording the presence or absence of the disorder.

In a *retrospective study*, two random samples of size C_1 and C_2 (see Table 1) are selected from the two populations corresponding to the two levels for variable 2. For example, in a retrospective study of the association between family history of alcoholism and a psychiatric disorder, samples would be taken from populations with and without the disorder. A determination of family history status could then be ascertained by a combination of methods, such as examining medical records and interviewing subjects and relatives. Hypothetical data for such a study are given in Table 3; here the samples are selected from subjects (called "cases") having the disorder and from a control group of subjects (called "controls") without the disorder. Since one sample is selected from cases and one from controls, this is also referred to as a *case–control study*.

Each type of study has its advantages and disadvantages in terms of possible biases, expense, time consumption, and population parameters that can be estimated; again, the reader is referred to an epidemiologic methods textbook for a discussion of the pros and cons of each study design. Our purpose is to discuss a measure of association—the odds ratio—that can be estimated from all three studies. However, before discussing the odds ratio, we first review the most frequently used statistical tests of association.

TESTS OF ASSOCIATION

For all three sampling methods, the null hypothesis of no association between variable 1 and variable 2 can be tested using the familiar *chi-squared statistic*

$$\chi^2 = \frac{(O_{11} - E_{11})^2}{E_{11}} + \frac{(O_{12} - E_{12})^2}{E_{12}} + \frac{(O_{21} - E_{21})^2}{E_{21}} + \frac{(O_{22} - E_{22})^2}{E_{22}},$$

where $E_{ij} = R_i C_j / N$ is the expected frequency for the ijth cell under the null hypothesis of no association. For the lithium study data in Table 2 we have $E_{11} = (30)(36/70) = 30(0.514) = 15.429$; that is, since 51.4% of the subjects had

TABLE 4. Data Summary for a Prospective Study

Variable 1	Sample Size	Proportion With Variable 2 Characteristic
Sample 1	R_1	$\hat{p}_1 = O_{11}/R_1$
Sample 2	R_2	$\hat{p}_2 = O_{21}/R_2$

TABLE 5. Data Summary for the Data in Table 2, Treated as a Prospective Study

Treatment	Sample Size	Proportion Having Episodes within 3 Months
Lithium	30	$\hat{p}_1 = 8/30 = 0.27$
Placebo	40	$\hat{p}_2 = 28/40 = 0.70$

episodes, then under the hypothesis of no association between episodes and treatment we expect that 51.4% of the 30 subjects assigned to the lithium group would have episodes.

If the chi-squared statistic exceeds the $(1 - \alpha)$ 100th percentile of a chi-squared distribution with 1 degree of freedom, denoted by $\chi^2_{\alpha:1}$ then the null hypothesis of no association is rejected and one concludes that there is an association between variables 1 and 2 (at a significance level equal to α). For example, at a significance level of 0.05, we conclude that there is an association if the calculated χ^2 exceeds $\chi^2_{0.005:1} = 3.84$. This test is intuitive since the chi-squared statistic increases as the observed frequencies deviate more from the expected frequencies. This test is called the *chi-squared test*.

For a prospective study, an alternative to the 2×2 contingency table for summarizing the data is a presentation of the proportion of subjects in the two samples having the variable 2 characteristic, as shown in Table 4. This format is illustrated in Table 5 for the prospective lithium study data given in Table 2. Thus we see that 27% of subjects taking lithium had episodes within the 3-month period, whereas 70% of subjects on placebo had episodes. These sample proportions estimate the corresponding population proportions; that is, for the population of male patients with manic depression from which subjects in this study were sampled, we estimate that 27% would not suffer episodes within 3 months if treated with lithium, while 70% would have episodes within 3 months if not treated with lithium, but instead given a placebo.

Similarly, for a retrospective study, we can tabulate the proportion of subjects in the two samples having the variable 1 characteristic, as shown in Table 6. This format is illustrated in Table 7 for the retrospective study data given in Table 3. We see that 40% of the subjects with the psychiatric disorder have a positive family history of alcoholism compared with only 8.3% of the control subjects. The proportions serve as estimates of the corresponding population proportions. Thus, we estimate that 40% of the disorder population has a positive family history of alcoholism compared with 8.3% of the control population.

TABLE 6. Data Summary for a Retrospective Study

Variable 2	Sample Size	Proportion With Variable 1 Characteristic
Sample 1	C_1	$\hat{p}_1 = O_{11}/C_1$
Sample 2	C_2	$\hat{p}_2 = O_{12}/C_2$

TABLE 7. Data Summary for the Data in Table 3, Treated as a Retrospective Study

Disorder	Sample Size	Proportion with Family History of Alcoholism
Present	50	$\hat{p}_1 = 20/50 = 0.40$
Absent	60	$\hat{p}_2 = 5/60 = 0.08333$

Let n_1 and n_2 denote the sample sizes (thus for a prospective study $n_1 = R_1$ and $n_2 = R_2$, while for a retrospective study $n_1 = C_1$ and $n_2 = C_2$) and define

$$\bar{p} = \frac{(n_1\hat{p}_1 + n_2\hat{p}_2)}{(n_1 + n_2)}.$$

For a prospective study, $\bar{p}$ is the overall proportion of observations in the combined samples having the variable 2 characteristic, while for a retrospective study $\bar{p}$ is the proportion of observations in the combined samples having the variable 1 characteristic.

Consider the test statistic

$$z = \frac{\hat{p}_1 - \hat{p}_2}{\hat{\sigma}_{(\hat{p}_1 - \hat{p}_2)}},$$

where

$$\hat{\sigma}_{(\hat{p}_1 - \hat{p}_2)} = \sqrt{\bar{p}(1 - \bar{p})\left(\frac{1}{n_1} + \frac{1}{n_2}\right)}$$

is the estimated standard deviation of $\hat{p}_1 - \hat{p}_2$ under the null hypothesis of no association. If $z > z_{\alpha/2}$ or if $z < -z_{\alpha/2}$, where z_α is the $(1 - \alpha)$100th percentile of the standard normal distribution, then the null hypothesis of no association is rejected at a significance level equal to α. For the usual significance level of $\alpha = 0.05$, we use $z_{0.025} = 1.96$. Under the null hypothesis of no association the population proportions are equal, and hence their difference is zero. Thus this test is intuitive, since it rejects the null hypothesis if the difference of the sample proportions is statistically different from zero. We refer to this test as the *large sample test of equal proportions*.

It can be shown that $z^2 = \chi^2$ and $(z_{\alpha/2})^2 = \chi^2_{\alpha:1}$. Since rejecting the null hypothesis of no association if $z > z_{\alpha/2}$ or $z < -z_{\alpha/2}$ is equivalent to rejecting the null hypothesis if $z^2 > (z_{\alpha/2})^2$; that is, if $\chi^2 > \chi^2_{\alpha:1}$, we see that the chi-squared test and the large sample test of equal proportions always agree in terms of rejecting or accepting the null hypothesis. Also, both tests yield the same p value.

The large sample test of equal proportions and chi-squared test should not be used unless the sample sizes are adequate. A conservative rule often given is that all of the expected cell frequencies (the E_{ij} in the chi-squared test) should be at least 5. The reason for this sample size requirement is that under the null hypothesis, the z statistic has an *approximate* normal distribution and the χ^2 statistic has an *approximate* chi-squared distribution, with the approximations improving as the sample sizes increase. For small sample sizes the approximations are not acceptable.

An alternative to the chi-squared test and large sample test of equal proportions is *Fisher's exact test*. This test can be used with any sample size. Given specific values for the row and column totals, under the assumption of no association between variables 1 and 2 it is possible to compute the exact probability for each possible 2×2 table. For an observed 2×2 table, a p value can then be calculated by summing the probabilities of all possible tables having the same row and column totals as the observed table and that deviate at least as much as the observed table from the hypothesis of no association. For a stated significance level, the null hypothesis of no association will be rejected if the p value is less than or equal to the significance level. The computations required for Fisher's exact test are such that this test is almost always performed by using either a table or computer.

Since Fisher's exact test requires considerably more computer time than the chi-squared test, especially for large samples, Fisher's exact test has generally been used for small sample sizes with the chi-squared test being used for moderate or large sample sizes. However, as computers have become increasingly faster, Fisher's exact test has been used more frequently for larger sample sizes.

Usually the two tests give similar p values for large sample sizes. In Example 1 (below) we find that the p values for the data for Table 3 resulting from Fisher's exact test and the chi-squared test are both approximately zero.

Although Fisher's exact test has the advantage of yielding exact inference results for any sample size, its disadvantage is that it requires a computer or table to use and is not based on a simple intuitive statistic. The advantage of the chi-squared test and the large sample test of equal proportions is that they are based on intuitive statistics and can easily be performed using a pocket calculator. Thus, although increasing computer speed will lead to more frequent use of Fisher's exact test for large sample sizes, we expect that the chi-squared test and the large sample test of equal proportions will remain important for historical and pedagogical reasons.

Example 1. For the data in Table 3 we perform the chi-squared test and the large sample test of equal proportions using a 0.05 significance level. For the chi-squared test the expected values are $E_{11} = 50(25)/110 = 11.3636$, $E_{12} = 60(25)/110 = 13.6364$, $E_{21} = 50(85)/110 = 38.6364$, and $E_{22} = 60(85)/110 =$

46.3636. Thus

$$\chi^2 = \frac{(20 - 11.3636)^2}{11.3636} + \frac{(5 - 13.6364)^2}{13.6364} + \frac{(30 - 38.6364)^2}{38.6364} + \frac{(55 - 46.3636)^2}{46.3636} = 15.573.$$

Since $\chi^2 = 15.573 > \chi^2_{0.05:1} = 3.84$, we reject the null hypothesis of no association and conclude that there is an association between the disorder and family history of alcoholism.

For the large sample test of equal proportions we have from Table 7 $\hat{p} = 0.4$ and $\hat{p} = 0.08333$. Thus $\bar{p} = (n_1\hat{p}_1 + n_2\hat{p}_2)/(n_1 + n_2) = [50(0.4) + 60(0.083330)]/(50 + 60) = 0.22727$. Alternatively, since $\bar{p}$is the proportion of subjects in the combined samples with a positive family history, we could have computed $\bar{p} = R_1/N = 25/110 = 0.22727$. Our test statistic is given by

$$z = \frac{\hat{p}_1 - \hat{p}_2}{\hat{\sigma}_{\hat{p}_1 - \hat{p}_2}} = \frac{0.4 - 0.08333}{\sqrt{0.22727(0.77273)\left(\dfrac{1}{50} + \dfrac{1}{60}\right)}} = 3.9463.$$

Since $z = 3.9463 > z_{0.025} = 1.96$, we reject the null hypothesis of no association and again conclude that there is an association between the disorder and family history of alcoholism.

Note that $z^2 = (3.9463)^2 = 15.573 = \chi^2$ and that $z^2_{0.025} = (1.96)^2 = 3.84 = \chi^2_{0.05:1}$, and thus these tests are equivalent.

In Table 8 is a computer program and partial output from a computer analysis of these data using the SAS (Statistical Analysis System) statistical package. The results for the chi-squared and Fisher's exact test are indicated in bold. The p value is the smallest significance level such that we can still reject the null hypothesis, given the data. Thus for the chi-squared test it is that the value of α such that $\chi^2_{\alpha:1} = 15.573$, which from the computer output is more than 0.0001 (it is in the column labeled "Prob"). Note that for Fisher's exact test there is no test statistic but just a p value, which in this case is 8.913E − 05 = 0.00008913. We see that this p value is in agreement with the p value of more than 0.0001 for the chi-squared test.

Several other measures of association are included in the SAS output: the likelihood ratio chi-squared, the continuity adjusted chi-squared, and the Mantel–Haenzel chi-squared, in addition to one-tailed p values for Fisher's exact test. The continuity adjusted chi-squared is similar to the chi-squared statistic except that it is adjusted slightly with the intent to improve the chi-squared approximation. A brief discussion with references for the likelihood ratio chi-squared and Mantel–Haenszel chi-squared is included in the *SAS/STAT User's Guide*. For large sample sizes, these statistics usually are similar.

The output under "Estimates of the Relative Risk (Row1/Row2)" in Table 8 is discussed later in Inference for the Odds Ratio for a Single 2 × 2 Table.

TABLE 8. SAS Statements and Partial SAS Output for Example 1

SAS Statements

```
data data1;
  input Family_History $ Alcoholism $ count;
  cards;
  yes present 20
  yes absent 5
  no present 30
  no absent 55
proc freq data = data1 order = data;
  weight count;
  table Family_History * Alcoholism / chisq relrisk;
  exact or;
run;
```

Partial SAS Output

Table of Family_History by Alcoholism
Family_History
Alcoholism

Frequency Percent Row Pct Col Pct	Present	Absent	Total
Yes	20	5	25
	18.18	4.55	22.73
	80.00	20.00	
	40.00	8.33	
No	30 55		85
	27.27	50.00	77.27
	35.29	64.71	
	60.00	91.67	
Total	50	60	110
	45.45	54.55	100.00

Statistics for Table of Family_History by Alcoholism

Statistic	DF	Value	Prob
Chi-square	**1**	**15.5725**	**< 0.0001**
Likelihood ratio chi-square	1	16.1897	< 0.0001
Continuity adj. chi-square	1	13.8216	0.0002
Mantel–Haenszel chi-square	1	15.4310	< 0.0001

Fisher's Exact Test

Cell (1, 1) Frequency (F)	20
Left-sided Pr ⇐ F	1.0000
Right-sided Pr > ⇐ F	8.074E-05
Table probability (P)	7.082E-05
Two-sided Pr < = P	**8.913E-05**

TABLE 8. (*Continued*)

Estimates of the Relative Risk (Row1/Row2)

Type of Study	Value	95% Confidence Limits	
Case–control (odds ratio)	**7.3333**	**2.4998**	**21.5129**
Cohort (col1 risk)	2.2667	1.6001	3.2109
Cohort (col2 risk)	0.3091	0.1389	0.6876

Odds Ratio (Case–Control Study)

Odds ratio	**7.3333**
Asymptotic conf limits	
95% lower conf limit	**2.4998**
95% upper conf limit	**21.5129**
Exact conf limits	
95% lower conf limit	**2.3180**
95% upper conf limit	**27.0680**

Sample size = 110

THE ODDS RATIO AS A MEASURE OF ASSOCIATION

Reporting the test of association result is only a first step in an analysis and by itself can be misleading. For example, in many situations one can argue that there must be some, although perhaps not much, association between the two dichotomous variables of interest. For example, males and females may respond somewhat differently to treatments. Thus what we are often interested in is not whether there is an association, but rather the degree of association.

Furthermore, the result of a hypothesis test is related to the sample size. If there is a true association, then as the sample size increases, the probability increases that the hypothesis test will reject the null hypothesis of no association; in statistical terms, the power of the test increases as the sample size increases. Since there is usually some underlying association (although perhaps of not much magnitude) we expect to have a significant test result when very large samples are used. However, finding a statistically significant association means only that we can conclude that there is some association; it does *not* imply that the degree of association is of *practical* importance, even if the p value is quite small.

Consider the data for the randomized prospective study of the effect of lithium on manic depression in males given in Tables 2 and 5. Let p_1 denote the probability (or *risk*) that a male patient with manic depression (selected from the same population as the study sample) treated with lithium will have an episode within 3 months, and let p_2 denote the probability that a male patient with manic depression given the placebo will have an episode within 3 months. Since $\hat{p}_1 = 0.27$ of the lithium patients had episodes within 3 months compared with $\hat{p} = 0.7$ of the placebo patients (see Table 5), we estimate p_1 and p_2 to be 0.27 and 0.7, respectively.

There are three common ways of estimating the magnitude of the association between the treatment and episodes variables: the *risk difference*, the *relative risk*, and the *odds ratio*. The *risk difference* is the difference of the probabilities, $p_1 - p_2$; the *relative risk* is the ratio of the probabilities, p_1/p_2; and the *odds ratio* is the ratio of the odds for each population, that is, $[p_1/(1-p_1)]/[p_2/(1-p_2)]$. These quantities can be estimated by replacing the population probabilities p_1 and p_2 by their sample estimates $\hat{p}_1$ and $\hat{p}_2$. Thus the sample estimate for the risk difference is $0.27 - 0.7 = -0.43$, the sample estimate for the relative risk is $0.27/0.7 = 0.39$, and the sample estimate for the odds ratio is $[0.27/0.73]/[0.7/0.3] = 0.37/2.33 = 0.16$.

Often it is of interest to compare the degree of association between two dichotomous variables for different populations. For example, suppose that data similar to the lithium study data given in Table 3 for male patients with manic depression have been collected for placebo and lithium groups of female patients with manic depression. Furthermore, suppose that 33% of the female placebo group subjects had episodes within 3 months. What proportion of the female lithium group would we expect to find having episodes after 3 months if the association between treatment and episodes is the same for females as it is for males?

The easy answer is that it just depends on which measure of association we are using. However, we quickly discover some problems. Since the estimated risk for the male lithium sample is 0.43 less than for the male control sample, then correspondingly the estimated risk for the female lithium sample should be 0.43 less than the estimated risk (0.33) for the female control sample using the risk difference measure, giving us an answer of $0.33 - 0.43 = -0.10$! This clearly is an unsatisfactory answer. Even if the answer had not been negative, it seems clear that the risk difference can be an unsatisfactory measure of association when comparing different populations; for example, a risk difference of 0.10 resulting from proportions of 0.01 and 0.11 intuitively represents a much stronger association than does a risk difference of 0.10 resulting from proportions of 0.50 and 0.60.

Now consider the relative risk measure. Since for the males the estimated risk for the lithium sample is $0.27/0.7 = 0.39$ of the estimated risk for the control sample, then correspondingly for the females the proportion in the lithium sample having episodes should be 0.39 times the proportion (0.33) in the control sample having episodes, giving us an answer of $0.39(0.33) = 0.13$. There is also a problem with this answer. Suppose that 13% of the females in the lithium sample had an episode. If we alternatively define the risk to be the probability of not having an episode, instead of the probability of having an episode, then for the males the estimated relative risk is $(1 - 0.27)/(1 - 0.7) = 0.73/0.3 = 2.43$, while for the females it is $(1 - 0.13)/(1 - 0.33) = 1.30$. We see that although the sample relative risks are the same for males and females if risk is defined as the probability of having an episode, the sample relative risks are quite different if we define the risk as the probability of not having an episode. For this reason the relative risk can also be problematic when comparing different populations.

Before discussing the odds ratio, let us say a few words about odds in general. If the probability for an event, such as winning a game, is denoted by p, then the odds of the event is defined as the fraction $p/(1-p)$. Thus, for example, if the probability of winning when playing a slot machine is 0.4, then the odds of winning is $0.4/0.6 = 2/3$ or 0.67. We say that the odds of winning "are 2 to 3," written as 2:3, because, on average, for every 2 wins there are 3 losses. This is a sensible measure for a gambler, because if his odds somehow double, then he is doing twice as well as before, since he is winning twice as many games for each game lost on average as before.

Similarly, the odds is a useful measure for medical data. For the lithium study data for male patients with manic depression in Table 2 the population odds of a male patient on lithium having an episode is defined by $p_1/(1 - p_1)$. An estimate for the population odds is the sample odds $\hat{p}_1/(1 - \hat{p}_1) = (8/30)/(22/30) = 8/22 = 0.37$. Thus, for the population of patients given lithium, we estimate that, on average, for every 22 patients not having episodes, 8 will have episodes. Note that the sample odds can be estimated by the number in the sample having the characteristic divided by the number not having it. The sample odds of a male patient on placebo having an episode is $28/12 = 2.67$. The sample odds ratio, $(8/22)/(28/12) = 0.37/2.33 = 0.16$, compares the odds of having an episode for the lithium sample with the odds of having an episode for the placebo sample and is an estimate of the population odds ratio $[p_1/(1 - p_1)]/[p_2/(1 - p_2)]$. No association between the treatment and episode variables implies that $p_1 = p_2$; that is, males with manic depression in the placebo and lithium populations have the same probability of having an episode within 3 months. Thus no association also implies that the population odds ratio is equal to 1.

Let us return to the question of what proportion of females on lithium we would expect to have episodes if 33% of the female placebo group had episodes and the association (measured by the odds ratio) between treatment and episodes is the same for males and females. Since the sample odds ratio for the males was 0.16 and the odds of an episode for females in the placebo sample is $0.33/0.67 = 0.49$, we expect the proportion of females in the lithium group that have episodes, denoted by $\hat{p}_{1;\,\text{fem}}$, to be such that the male and female odds ratios are equal, that is,

$$0.16 = \frac{\hat{p}_{1;\,\text{fem}}/[1 - \hat{p}_{1:\,\text{fem}}]}{0.49}.$$

Solving gives us $\hat{p}_{1;\,\text{fem}} = 0.085$.

Suppose that 8.5% of the females in the lithium group had an episode. We have just shown that for both males and females the sample odds ratio is equal to 0.16. It is easy to show that if we consider the odds of not having an episode instead of the odds of having an episode, then the odds ratios for both the males and females are also equal (they are equal to $1/0.16 = 6.25$). This demonstrates the usefulness of the odds ratio for comparing different populations.

Not only is the odds ratio useful for comparing the association between two dichotomous variables for different populations, it also has a great advantage over the relative risk and the risk difference for a single population when a retrospective sampling scheme is utilized, as shown by the following example. Consider the data for our retrospective study of the association between family history of alcoholism and a particular psychiatric disorder given in Table 3 and summarized in Table 7. From Table 7 we estimated that 40% of the disorder population has a positive family history of alcoholism compared with 8.333% of the control population. Let $p_1^{(f)}$ denote the probability of a subject with the disorder having a positive family history of alcoholism and $p_2^{(f)}$, denote the probability of a subject without the disorder having a positive family history of alcoholism. Because samples were taken from the populations with and without the disorder, the sample estimates $\hat{p}_1 = 0.4$ and $\hat{p}_2 = 0.08333$ estimate $p_1^{(f)}$ and $p^{(}f)_2$, respectively, and thus estimates for the relative difference $p_1^{(f)} - p_2^{(f)}$, the relative risk $p_1^{(f)}/p_2^{(f)}$, and the odds ratio $[p_1^{(f)}/(1 - p_1^{(f)})]/[p_2^{(f)}/(1 - p_2^{(f)})]$ can be estimated by replacing the population probabilities by the sample estimates.

However, since family history of alcoholism is the risk factor, we would like to relate family history of alcoholism to the probability of having the disorder. That is, we are more interested in measures of association that are functions of the risk of having the disorder than the risk of having a positive family history of alcoholism. Let $p_1^{(d)}$ denote the probability of a subject with a positive family history of alcoholism having the disorder and $p_2^{(d)}$ denote the probability of a subject without a positive family history of alcoholism having the disorder. Now, although the relative risk and risk difference based on $p_1^{(d)}$ and $p_2^{(d)}$ are not the same as those based on $p_1^{(f)}$ and $p_2^{(f)}$, it can be shown that the odds ratios are the same; that is,

$$\frac{p_1^{(f)}/(1 - p_1^{(f)})}{p_2^{(f)}/(1 - p_2^{(f)})} = \frac{p_1^{(d)}/(1 - p_1^{(d)})}{p_2^{(d)}/(1 - p_2^{(d)})}.$$

Hence, even though $\hat{p}_1 = 0.4$ and $\hat{p}_2 = 0.08333$ are estimates of $p_1^{(f)}$ and $p_2^{(f)}$ and do not estimate $p_1^{(d)}$ and $p_2^{(d)}$, the sample odds ratio

$$\begin{aligned}[\hat{p}_1/(1 - \hat{p}_1)]/[\hat{p}_2/(1 - \hat{p}_2)] &= [O_{11}/O_{21}]/[O_{12}/O_{22}] \\ &= [20/30]/[5/55] \\ &= 7.33\end{aligned}$$

estimates the common odds ratio. Thus we can say that (1) the odds of a subject with a positive family history of alcoholism having the disorder is 7.33 times greater than the odds of a subject without a positive family history of alcoholism having the disorder, or (2) the odds of a subject with the disorder having a family history of alcoholism is 7.33 times greater than the odds of a subject without the disorder having a family history of alcoholism. Clearly the first statement is more meaningful.

In contrast, the risk difference $p_1^{(d)} - p_2^{(d)}$ and relative risk $p_1^{(d)}/p_2^{(d)}$ cannot be estimated by replacing $p_1^{(d)}$ and $p_2^{(d)}$ by $\hat{p}_1$ and $\hat{p}_2$, since these are estimates of $p_1^{(f)}$ and $p_2^{(f)}$. Furthermore, because of the sampling scheme, sample estimates of $p_1^{(d)}$ and $p_2^{(d)}$ are not available. However, if $p_1^{(d)}$ and $p_2^{(d)}$ are small, then it can be shown that the odds ratio provides an approximation to the relative risk $p_1^{(d)}/p_2^{(d)}$, showing yet another advantage of the odds ratio.

INFERENCE FOR THE ODDS RATIO FOR A SINGLE 2 × 2 TABLE

For a retrospective study, the population and sample odds ratios are defined in the same way as for a prospective study, except with the roles of variable 1 and variable 2 reversed. Thus for a prospective study the sample odds are defined by

$$\hat{\Psi} = (O_{11}/O_{12})/(O_{21}/O_{22}), \tag{1}$$

and for a retrospective study the sample odds are defined by

$$\hat{\Psi} = (O_{11}/O_{21})/(O_{12}/O_{22}), \tag{2}$$

But Equations (1) and (2) are both equal to

$$\hat{\Psi} = \frac{O_{11}O_{22}}{O_{21}O_{12}}, \tag{3}$$

which estimates the population odds ratio and is the same regardless of whether we define the risk as the probability of a subject having the variable 1 characteristic or as the probability of a subject having the variable 2 characteristic. For a cross-sectional study the population odds ratio is defined in terms of conditional probabilities, treating one of the variables as fixed (that is, as a risk variable) and the other variable as the response variable. The sample odds ratio for a cross-sectional study is also given by Equation 3. Thus, inference using the odds ratio does not depend on which sampling design: prospective, retrospective, or cross-sectional, is employed, which is another desirable quality of the odds ratio.

A large sample 95% confidence interval for $\log \Psi$ is given by

$$\log \hat{\Psi} \pm 1.96\hat{\sigma}_{\log \hat{\Psi}}, \tag{4}$$

where

$$\hat{\sigma}^2_{\log \hat{\Psi}} = \frac{1}{O_{11}} + \frac{1}{O_{12}} + \frac{1}{O_{21}} + \frac{1}{O_{22}}$$

is the estimated variance of $\log \hat{\Psi}$. It is assumed that each $O_{ij} > 0$; if any of the 4 cell frequencies are 0, the variance estimate is not computed. A 95% confidence interval for Ψ is obtained by exponentiating the endpoints of the confidence interval for $\log \Psi$. This procedure requires a large sample size and hence is also referred to as an *asymptotic* confidence interval. More generally, a $(1 - \alpha)100\%$ confidence interval results if 1.96 is replaced by $z_{\alpha/2}$ in the confidence interval expression.

Alternatively, an *exact* 95% confidence interval can be computed iteratively, based on the distribution of the sample odds ratio, conditional on the row and column totals. This confidence interval is called an *exact* confidence interval because it is based on the *exact* conditional distribution of the sample odds ratio, in contrast to the large sample confidence interval, which is based on a normal distribution that *approximates* the unconditional distribution of the logarithm of the sample odds ratio. The advantage of the exact confidence interval method is that it is always valid, regardless of the cell sizes. For this reason, we recommend its use over the large sample interval. The disadvantages of the exact confidence interval are the same as for Fisher's exact test: it requires a computer to compute and is not based on a simple intuitive statistic. Furthermore, for very large sample sizes, it may not be feasible because of the amount of computing time involved.

Usually the interpretation of the odds ratio and its confidence interval compares the odds of the variable 2 (or outcome variable) characteristic occurring for each level of variable 1 (the antecedent or risk variable), regardless of which sampling method is used.

Example 2. Again consider the data for the retrospective study of the association between family history of alcoholism and a particular psychiatric disorder given in Table 3. We have

$$\hat{\psi} = \frac{O_{11}O_{22}}{O_{21}O_{12}} = \frac{20(55)}{30(5)} = 7.33$$

and

$$\hat{\sigma}^2_{\log \hat{\Psi}} = \frac{1}{O_{11}} + \frac{1}{O_{12}} + \frac{1}{O_{21}} + \frac{1}{O_{22}}$$

$$= \frac{1}{20} + \frac{1}{5} + \frac{1}{30} + \frac{1}{55} = 0.3015.$$

Thus $\hat{\sigma}^2_{\log \Psi} = \sqrt{0.3015} = 0.549$, and a 95% confidence interval using Equation 4 for $\log \psi$ is given by

$$\log(7.33) + 1.96(0.549) = (0.91594, 3.0680).$$

Exponentiating the endpoints gives the 95% confidence interval for ψ:

$$[\exp(0.91594), \exp(3.068)] = (2.50, 21.50).$$

Interpretation. We have 95% confidence that the odds of a subject with a positive family history of alcoholism having the disorder is between 2.50 and 21.50 times greater than the odds of a subject without a positive family history of alcoholism having the disorder.

The odds ratio estimate of 7.33 and large sample (or asymptotic) and exact confidence interval results for the population odds ratio are given in the SAS output in Table 8 under "Odds Ratio (Case–Control Study)." Our calculation of the large sample interval agrees (except for a slight rounding error) with the SAS confidence interval of (2.4998, 21.5129). For the SAS output the exact 95% confidence interval is (2.3180, 27.0680). Which interval should be reported? We favor reporting the exact confidence interval, since it is appropriate even if the sample size is not large. For large sample sizes the two methods typically give similar results.

The odds ratio estimate and large sample confidence interval can also be found in the "Estimates of the Relative Risk (Row1/Row2)" section of the output, on the line labeled "Case–Control (Odds Ratio)." in this section, the "Cohort (coll risk)" of 2.2667 = $(20/25)/(30/85)$ is an estimate of the relative risk p_1/p_2 under the assumption that this is a prospective (or cohort) study, where p_1 is the

TABLE 9. Data Layout for a Hypothetical Randomized Study of the Effect of Lithium on Manic Depression in Females

		Episodes within 3 months		
		Present	Absent	
Treatment	Lithium	15	105	120
	Placebo	43	57	100
		58	162	220

probability that a person with a positive history of alcoholism will have the psychiatric disorder. However, this estimate and its corresponding confidence interval are not valid since this is not a prospective study.

ODDS RATIO INFERENCE AND TESTS OF ASSOCIATION FOR SEVERAL 2 × 2 TABLES

Consider the data for the study of the effect of lithium on manic depression in males given in Table 2. In Table 9 are hypothetical data collected for females with manic depression.

If the probability of an episode is related to gender (that is, gender is a confounding variable), then the combined population odds ratio can be quite different from the gender-specific odds ratios, even if the gender-specific odds ratios are equal, and thus we would want to control for the gender variable. This can be done by testing the null hypothesis of no association between treatment and episodes for males and for females using the Mantel–Haenszel test (Mantel and Haenszel, 1959; Mantel, 1963) described below. If there is a significant association, then the degree of association between the treatment and episodes variables can be estimated separately for males and females. If the two odds ratios are similar, then it is also meaningful to estimate a weighted average of the odds ratios to summarize the degree of association.

More generally, in this section we consider the situation where the data have been stratified into K subgroups (or strata) with respect to one or more suspected confounding variables, in order to make the subjects within each stratum more homogeneous. The data for the kth stratum ($k = 1, \dots, K$) can be summarized in a 2×2 contingency table relating variable 1 to variable 2, as shown in Table 10. The Mantel–Haenszel test, described below, is used to test the null hypothesis of no association between variables 1 and 2 for each of the K strata.

The rationale for the Mantel–Haenszel test is as follows. Under the null hypothesis of no association for each stratum and conditional on the row and margin totals, the expected value of $O_{11}^{(k)}$, the frequency in the first cell of the kth table, is given by

$$E_{11}^{(k)} = R_1^{(k)} C_1^{(k)} / N^{(k)}$$

TABLE 10. Data Layout for a 2 X 2 Contingency Table for the kth Stratum, for $k = 1, \ldots, K$

		Variable 2		
		Present	Absent	
Variable 1	Present	$O_{11}^{(k)}$	$O_{12}^{(k)}$	$R_1^{(k)}$ (Row totals)
	Absent	$O_{21}^{(k)}$	$O_{22}^{(k)}$	$R_2^{(k)}$ (Row totals)
	Column totals	$C_1^{(k)}$	$C_1^{(k)}$	$N^{(k)}$ = Grand total

and the variance of $O_{11}^{(k)}$ is

$$V_{11}^{(k)} = \frac{C_1^{(k)} C_2^{(k)} R_1^{(k)} R_2^{(k)}}{N^{(k)} N^{(k)} [N^{(k)} - 1]}.$$

Let X denote the sum of the frequencies in the first cells of the K tables; that is,

$$X = \sum_{k=1}^{K} O_{11}^{(k)}.$$

It follows that the expected value and variance of X are

$$E(X) = \sum_{k=1}^{K} E_{11}^{(k)} \quad \text{and} \quad V(X) = \sum_{k=1}^{K} V_{11}^{(k)}.$$

The Mantel–Haenszel test is given by

$$\chi_{\text{MH}}^2 = \frac{[X - E(X)]^2}{V(X)} = \frac{\left[\Sigma_{k=1}^{K} O_{11}^{(k)} - \Sigma_{k=1}^{K} E_{11}^{(k)}\right]^2}{\Sigma_{k=1}^{K} V_{11}^{(k)}},$$

which has an approximate chi-squared distribution with one degree of freedom under the null hypothesis. Thus, for a significance level equal to α, we reject the null hypothesis of no association if $\chi_{\text{MH}}^2 > \chi_{\alpha;1}$. The Mantel–Haenszel test can be used if either the $N^{(k)}$ are large or if K is large (even if the $N^{(k)}$ are small.)

Since we have conditioned on the row and column totals in each table (that is, we have treated them as fixed), then, from knowing the frequency in the first cell of a table the other three cell frequencies can be found. Hence they do not provide any additional information concerning the association, explaining why the Mantel–Haenszel statistic is based only on one of the frequencies in each table.

Note that χ_{MH}^2 tends to be large if $O_{11}^{(k)}$ is consistently larger or consistently smaller than $E_{11}^{(k)}$, while it can be close to zero if $O_{11}^{(k)}$ is greater than $E_{11}^{(k)}$ for some strata and $O_{11}^{(k)}$ is less than $E_{11}^{(k)}$ for other strata. Thus the Mantel–Haenszel test is designed for the alternative hypothesis of a consistent association between variable 1 and variable 2 across the K strata—that is, most of the strata-specific odds ratios are greater than 1 or most of them are less than 1. The test has little power to detect an association where some of the stratum-specific odds ratios are less than 1 and some are greater than 1.

An estimate of a weighed average of the stratum-specific odds ratios is provided by the Mantel–Haenszel estimator

$$\hat{\psi}_{\mathrm{MH}} = \frac{\sum_{k=1}^{K}\left[O_{11}^{(k)}O_{22}^{(k)}/N^{(k)}\right]}{\sum_{k=1}^{K}\left[O_{21}^{(k)}O_{12}^{(k)}/N^{(k)}\right]}.$$

If the stratum-specific odds ratios are equal, then $\hat{\psi}_{\mathrm{MH}}$ estimates the common odds ratio. If the individual odds ratios differ greatly, then usually we would want to estimate them separately rather than estimate an average of them.

A 95% confidence interval for the common odds ratio (or a weighted average if stratum-specific population odds ratios are not equal) is obtained by exponentiating the endpoints of the interval

$$\log \hat{\psi}_{\mathrm{MH}} \pm 1.96\hat{\sigma}_{\log \hat{\psi}_{\mathrm{MH}}}, \tag{5}$$

where $\hat{\sigma}^2_{\log \hat{\psi}_{\mathrm{MH}}}$ is the estimated variance for $\hat{\psi}_{\mathrm{MH}}$ given by Robins, Breslow, and Greenland (1986).

Another estimate for the common odds ratio is the *logit* estimator (Woolf, 1954), defined as follows. Let

$$\hat{\psi}^{(k)} = \frac{O_{11}^{(k)}O_{22}^{(k)}}{O_{21}^{(K)}O_{12}^{(k)}}$$

denote the odds ratio estimate for the kth stratum. The logit estimator, denoted by $\hat{\psi}_{\mathrm{Logit}}$, is defined by

$$\log \hat{\psi}_{\mathrm{Logit}} = \frac{\sum_{k=1}^{K} w^{(k)} \log \hat{\psi}^{(k)}}{\sum_{k=1}^{K} w^{(k)}},$$

where

$$w^{(k)} = \left(\hat{\sigma}^2_{\log \hat{\psi}^{(k)}}\right)^{-1} = \left(\frac{1}{O_{11}} + \frac{1}{O_{12}} + \frac{1}{O_{21}} + \frac{1}{O_{22}}\right)^{-1}.$$

Thus $\hat{\psi}_{\mathrm{Logit}}$ is a weighted average of the stratum-specific log odds-ratio estimates, with each $\log \hat{\psi}^{(k)}$weighted by the inverse of its estimated variance; hence it provides an estimate of the corresponding weighted average of the population log odds ratios. A 95% confidence interval is obtained by exponentiating the endpoints of the interval

$$\log \hat{\psi}_{\mathrm{Logit}} \pm 1.96\hat{\sigma}_{\log \hat{\psi}\mathrm{Logit}}, \tag{6}$$

where

$$\hat{\sigma}^2_{\log \hat{\psi}_{\text{Logit}}} = \left[\sum_{k=1}^{K} w^{(k)} \right]^{-1}.$$

Note that the estimate $\hat{\psi}_{\text{Logit}}$ of the common odds ratio differs from the Mantel–Haenszel estimate $\hat{\psi}_{\text{MH}}$.

The Breslow–Day (1980) test can be used to test the null hypothesis of homogeneity of odds ratios, that is, that the strata-specific odds ratios are equal. Although this test is not suited for hand calculation, it is included in the SAS FREQ procedure. This test requires a large sample size within each stratum. However, even if the assumption of homogeneity of odds ratios does not hold, the two confidence interval procedures discussed are still valid procedures for estimating a weighted average of the odds ratios, although it usually will be more useful to examine confidence intervals for individual odds ratios when the odds ratios differ substantially. In addition to performing the Breslow–Day test, it is advisable to compute the stratum-specific odds ratios in order to obtain some idea of the degree of heterogeneity.

Example 3. For the data for the randomized study of the effect of lithium on manic–depression in males and females given in Tables 2 and 9: (1) estimate the gender-specific odds ratios; (2) test if the gender-specific odds ratios are equal using the Breslow–Day test; (3) test the null hypothesis of no association, controlling for gender, using the Mantel–Haenszel test; (4) estimate a weighted average of the odds ratios using the Mantel–Haenszel estimate and $\hat{\psi}_{\text{Logit}}$; and (5) give 95% confidence intervals for the weighted average of the odds ratios. In Table 11 is a partial output from a SAS analysis of these data. Pertinent results are indicated in bold.

Solutions:

1. Letting $\hat{\psi}_1$ and $\hat{\psi}_2$ denote the sample odds ratio for the males and females, respectively, we have $\hat{\psi}_1 = 8(12)/[28(22)] = 0.1558$ and $\hat{\psi}_2 = 15(57)/[43(105)] = 0.1894$. These estimates are given in the first part of the output as part of the separate analyses for the males and females. Thus we see that the two odds ratio estimates are quite close.

   Interpretation: We estimate that the odds of a male with manic depression on lithium having an episode within 3 months are 16% of the odds for a male with manic depression in the control group. For a female with manic depression on lithium, the estimated odds for the lithium group are 19% of the odds for the control group.

2. Based on the Breslow–Day test results reported at the end of the SAS output in Table 11, there is not sufficient evidence to conclude that the gender-specific odds ratios are different ($p = 0.7598$). (Note: we would have rejected the null hypothesis of homogeneity at, say, the 0.05 significance level if the p value was less than 0.05).

TABLE 11. SAS Statements and Partial Output for Example 3

SAS Statements

```
data data1;
  input Gender $ Treatment $ Episodes $ count;
cards;
  male lithium present 8
  male lithium absent 22
  male placebo present 28
  male placebo absent 12
  female lithium present 15
  female lithium absent 105
  female placebo present 43
  female placebo absent 57
proc freq data = data1 order = data;
  weight count;
  table gender*treatment*episodes/chisq   relrisk cmh;
run;
```

Partial SAS output

Table 1 of Treatment by Episodes
Controlling for Gender = male

Frequency Percent Row Pct Col Pct	Episodes Present	 Absent	 Total
Lithium	8 11.43 26.67 22.22	22 31.43 73.33 64.71	30 42.68
Placebo	28 40.00 70.00 77.78	12 17.14 30.00 35.29	40 57.14
Total	36 51.43	34 48.57	70 100.00

Statistics for Table 1 of Treatment by Episodes
Controlling Gender —male

Statistic	DF	Value	Prob
Chi-square	1	12.8867	0.0003

Estimates of the Relative Risk (Row1/Row2)

Type of Study	Value	95% Confidence	Limits
Case-control (Odds Ratio)	**0.1558**	**0.0543**	**0.4474**
Cohort (Col1 Risk)	0.3810	0.2035	0.7132
Cohort (Col2 Risk)	2.4444	1.4529	4.1126

(*Continued*)

TABLE 11 (*Continued*)

Table 2 of Treatment by Episodes
Controlling for Gender —female

Treatment	Episode		
Frequency Percent Row Pct Col Pct	Present	Absent	Total
Lithium	15 6.82 12.50 25.86	105 47.73 87.50 64.81	120 54.55
Placebo	43 19.55 43.00 74.14	57 25.91 57.00 35.19	100 45.45
Total	58 26.36	162 73.64	220 100.00

Statistics for Table 2 of Treatment by Episodes
Controlling Gender —female

Statistic	DF	Value	Prob
Chi-Square	1	26.1373	< 0.0001

Estimates of the Relative Risk (Row1/Row2)

Type of Study	Value	95% Confidence Limits	
Case-Control (Odds Ratio)	**0.1894**	**0.0969**	**0.3702**
Cohort (Col1 Risk)	0.2907	0.1721	0.4911
Cohort (Col2 Risk)	1.5351	1.2782	1.8437

Summary Statistics for Treatment by Episodes
Controlling for Gender
Cochran-Mantel-Haenszel Statistics (based on table scores)

Statistic	Alternative Hypothesis	DF	Value	Prob
1	Nonzero Correlation	1	38.6553	< 0.0001
2	Row Mean Scores Differ	1	38.6553	< 0.0001
3	**General Association**	**1**	**38.6553**	< **0.0001**

Estimates of the Common Relative Risk (Row1/Row2)

Type of Study	Method	Value	95% Confidence Limits	
Case-Control	**Mantel-Haenszel**	**0.1793**	**0.1018**	**0.3158**
(Odd Ratio)	**Logit**	**0.1790**	**0.1017**	**0.3153**
Cohort	Mantel-Haenszel	0.3212	0.2147	0.4806
(Col1 Risk)	Logit	0.3249	0.2173	0.4858
Cohort	Mantel-Haenszel	1.6642	1.3963	1.9834
(Col2 Risk)	Logit	1.6159	1.3595	1.9207

Breslow-Day Test for
Homogeneity of the Odds Ratios

Chi-Square	0.0935
DF	1
Pr > ChiSq	**0.7598**

3. Computations for the Mantel–Haenszel test statistic:

$$O_{11}^{(1)} = 8 \qquad O_{11}^{(2)} = 15 \qquad X = 8 + 15 = 23$$

$$E_{11}^{(1)} = 36(30)/70 = 15.4286 \qquad E^{(2)}O_{11} = 58(120)/220 = 31.6364$$

$$E(X) = E_{11}^{(1)} + E_{11}^{(2)} = 15.4286 + 31.6364 = 47.065$$

$$V_{11}^{(1)} = \frac{36(34)(30)40}{70(70)69} = 4.3443 \qquad V_{11}^{(2)} = \frac{58(162)(120)100}{220(220)219} = 10.6374$$

$$V(X) = V_{11}^{(1)} + V_{11}^{(2)} + 4.3443 + 10.6374 = 14.9817$$

$$X_{\text{MH}}^2 = \frac{[X - E(X)]^2}{V(X)} = \frac{(23 - 47.065)^2}{14.9817} = 38.655$$

Since $\chi_{\text{MH}}^2 = 38.655 > X_{0.05:1} = 3.84$, we reject the null hypothesis of no association and conclude that there is an association between treatment and episodes, controlling for gender ($\alpha = 0.05$). In agreement with our calculations, the SAS output (labeled "General Association") gives the same value for the Mantel–Haenszel statistic and a corresponding p value of < 0.0001.

4.

$$\hat{\psi}_{\text{MH}} = \frac{8(12)/70 + 15(57)/220}{28(22)/70 + 43(105)/220} = 0.1793$$

is the Mantel–Haenszel estimate of the weighted average of the odds ratios.

Computations for $\hat{\psi}_{\text{Logit}}$:

$$w^{(1)} = \left(\frac{1}{8} + \frac{1}{28} + \frac{1}{22} + \frac{1}{12}\right)^{-1} = 3.4542$$

$$w^{(2)} = \left(\frac{1}{15} + \frac{1}{43} + \frac{1}{105} + \frac{1}{57}\right)^{-1} = 8.5477$$

$$\log \hat{\psi}_{\text{Logit}} = \frac{w^{(1)}\log \hat{\psi}^{(1)} + w^{(2)}\log \hat{\psi}^{(2)}}{w^{(1)} + w^{(2)}}$$

$$= \frac{(3.4542)\log(0.1558) + 8.5477\log(0.1894)}{3.4542 + 8.5477} = 1.720099$$

$$\hat{\psi}_{\text{Logit}} = \exp(-1.720099) = 0.1790.$$

In this example the two estimates $\hat{\psi}_{\text{MH}} = 0.1793$ and $\hat{\psi}_{\text{Logit}} = 0.1790$ are very close. Since the Breslow–Day test is not significant, the sample sizes are large (hence the Breslow–Day test is valid), and the sample odds ratios are close, we consider that these estimates are for a common odds ratio.

Interpretation: We estimate that the odds of a patient with manic depression on lithium having an episode within 3 months is 18% of the odds of a patient with manic depression in the control group having an episode, controlling for gender.

5. Computations for a 95% confidence interval using Equation 6:

$$\hat{\sigma}^2_{\log \hat{\psi}_{\text{Logit}}} = \left[w^{(1)} + w^{(2)}\right]^{-1} = (3.4542 + 8.5477)^{-1} = 0.0833201$$

$$\hat{\sigma}_{\log \hat{\psi}_{\text{Logit}}} = \sqrt{0.0833201} = 0.2886$$

$$\log \hat{\psi}_{\text{Logit}} \pm 1.96\hat{\sigma}_{\log \hat{\psi}_{\text{Logit}}} = -1.720099 \pm 1.96(0.2886)$$

$$= (-2.285755, -1.15443)$$

95% confidence interval for $\hat{\Psi}_{\text{Logit}}$:

$$[\exp(-2.285755), \exp(-1.154443)] = (0.1017, 0.3153).$$

Interpretation: We have 95% confidence that the odds of having an episode within 3 months for a lithium patient with manic depression is between 10% and 32% of the odds for a control patient with manic depression, controlling for gender.

This confidence interval can be found in the section "Estimates of the Common Relative Risk (Row1/Row2)" in the SAS output in Table 11 and is called the "Logit" method for the case–control type of study. The first confidence interval (0.1018, 0.3158) for the case–control type of study, labeled "Mantel–Haenszel," is the 95% confidence interval using the interval given by Equation 5.

MATCHED-PAIRS ANALYSIS

A matched-pairs analysis is a stratified analysis where each stratum consists of a sample size of two, with one subject at one level of the risk variable (variable 1) and the other subject at the other level of the risk variable. For example, in a randomized prospective study comparing two treatments (drug vs. placebo), subjects are matched according to similarity of suspected confounding variables (such as age and gender), and then one member of each pair is randomly assigned to one of the treatments, with the other member receiving the other treatment. Table 12 shows how matched-pairs data are usually summarized.

Although Table 12 looks similar to the 2×2 contingency table in Table 1 for unmatched data, it is quite different in that it treats the matched pair as the basic sampling unit rather than the individual subject. For example, in Table 12, a is the number of matched pairs for which both subjects survived, while b is the number of matched pairs for which the subject assigned to treatment 1 survived while the subject assigned to treatment 2 died. Furthermore, there are N pairs, or $2(N)$ subjects.

Using the analysis methods of the previous section, it can be shown the Mantel–Haenszel test statistic for testing the null hypothesis of no association, controlling for each stratum (and hence controlling for the variables used for

TABLE 12. Data Layout for Matched-Pairs Data

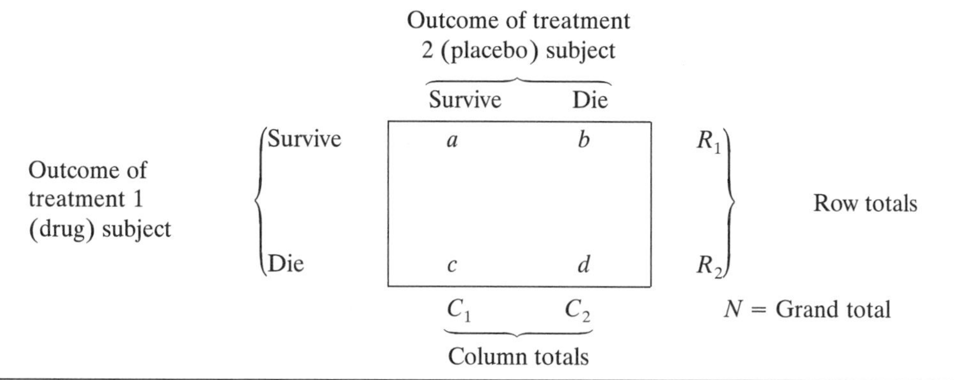

		Outcome of treatment 2 (placebo) subject		
		Survive	Die	
Outcome of treatment 1 (drug) subject	Survive	a	b	R_1 (Row totals)
	Die	c	d	R_2
		C_1	C_2	N = Grand total
		Column totals		

matching subjects), is given by

$$\chi^2_{\mathrm{MH}} = \frac{(b - c)^2}{b + c}.$$

The null hypothesis of no association is rejected if $\chi^2_{\mathrm{MH}} > \chi^2_{\alpha;1}$. The test is equivalent to McNemar's test. An estimate of the common odds ratio (odds of a treatment 1 subject surviving divided by the odds of a treatment 2 subject surviving) is

$$\hat{\psi}_{\mathrm{MH}} = b/c$$

If homogeneity of the odds ratios is not assumed, then $\hat{\psi}_{\mathrm{MH}}$ is an estimate of a weighted average of the odds ratios. A large sample 95% confidence interval for the common odds ratio (or weighted average) is given by

$$(b/c)\exp\left(\pm 1.96\sqrt{1/b + 1/c}\right),$$

where it is assumed that b and c are greater than 0.

Example 4. Consider the following randomized matched prospective study of the effect of lithium on manic depression in males. Sixty males with manic depression are matched according to age (within five years) and clinical condition (mild, moderate, or severe), resulting in 30 matched pairs. Using random assignment, one member of each pair is assigned to the lithium treatment and the other member to the placebo treatment. The data for this study are summarized in Table 13. We see, for example, that there are two matched pairs where both subjects had seizures within 3 months.

An estimate of the common odds ratio is $\hat{\psi}_{\mathrm{MH}} = 6/19 = 0.316$, and a 95% confidence interval for the common odds ratio is given by

$$(6/19)\exp\left(\pm 1.96\sqrt{1/6 + 1/19}\right) = (0.126, 0.791).$$

TABLE 13. Data Summary for a Randomized Matched-Pair Prospective Study of the Effect of Lithium on Manic Depression in Males

		Episodes within 3 months for subject on placebo		
		Present	Absent	Row totals
Episodes within 3 months for subject on lithium	Present	2	6	8
	Absent	19	3	22
	Column totals	21	9	30 = Grand total

Interpretation: We have 95% confidence that the odds of having an episode within 3 months for a male lithium patient with manic depression is between 0.126 and 0.791 times the odds for a male control patient with manic depression, controlling for age and clinical condition.

LOGISTIC REGRESSON

We conclude this chapter by showing how the ideas discussed thus far can be viewed within the more general logistic regression framework. For our discussion it is assumed that the reader is familiar with multiple linear regression analysis.

We consider the situation where we are interested in studying the relationship between a dichotomous outcome (or response or dependent) variable and several independent (or explanatory) variables; the independent variables can be either quantitative (continuous or discrete) or qualitative. The two levels of the outcome variable will be coded as 1 and 0, with 1 corresponding to the occurrence of the event of interest. For example, in our randomized prospective study of the effect of lithium on manic depression, we consider episodes (1 = presence of episodes, 0 = absence of episodes) to be the outcome variable and treatment and gender to be the independent variables. We are interested in how treatment and episodes are related after controlling for gender. Although all of these variables are qualitative, we might also want to consider controlling for quantitative variables, such as age or income. Using the Mantel–Haenszel procedure, we can control for quantitative variables only if we categorize them (for example, age: < 30, 30–50, > 50).

In least-squares regression, the mean of the outcome variable is modeled as a linear function of the independent variables. For example, for the simple linear regression model

$$E(Y/x) = \beta_0 + \beta_1 x,$$

where x is a value of the independent variable and $E(Y/x)$ is the mean (or expected value) of Y given x. In this model, each unit increase in x results in an increase equal to β_1 in the expected value of Y.

Now suppose that Y is a dichotomous variable with its levels coded as 1 and 0. Then the expected value of Y is just the probability of the event corresponding to level 1; that is, $p_x = E(Y/x)$ is the probability that $Y = 1$ given x. Thus we might consider a model similar to the one above where we model p_x as a linear function of the independent variable:

$$p_x = \beta_0 + \beta_1 x. \tag{7}$$

However, there are two problems with this model. First, p_x is bounded by 0 and 1, but the equation $\beta_0 + \beta_1 x$ is not bounded by 0 and 1; hence this model could produce absurd estimates for p_x. Second, we have already argued that an increase in p_x from, say, 0.01 to 0.10, is intuitively more of an increase than an increase from 0.50 to 0.60. Thus, although each unit increase in x results in an increase equal to β_1 in x, the practical effect of the change depends on the base value of p_x and hence on the value of x.

The *logistic regression model* models the log of the odds as a linear function of the independent variables. For example, for one independent variable we have

$$\log \frac{p_x}{1 - p_x} = \beta_0 + \beta_1 x.$$

The function $\log[p_x/(1 - p_x)]$ is called the *logit function* of p_x. This model overcomes the two problems inherent in Equation 7. Since the odds can be between 0 and ∞, then the range of the log of the odds is $(-\infty, \infty)$, which is the same as the range of the function $\beta_0 + \beta_1 x$. Furthermore, now a one unit increase in x results in a *proportionate* increase in the odds equal to $1 - \exp(\beta_1)$. For example, if an increase in x from 1 to 2 doubles the odds, similarly an increase in x from 10 to 11 will also double the odds. Hence, the practical effect of a unit increase in x on p_x does not depend on the value of x.

The logistic regression approach has two main advantages over the stratification approach described in the previous sections: (1) Quantitative independent variables do not have to be categorized and (2) the investigator can much more thoroughly investigate the relationship between the response probability and the independent variables. The advantage of the stratification approach is its conceptual simplicity. In the following example we show how the stratification approach can be viewed within the context of the logistic regression framework, but it is beyond the scope of this chapter to demonstrate the flexibility of analysis provided by the logistic regression model that is not available with the stratification approach (for a more detailed discussion, see Kleinbaum et al., 1982, Chapter 21).

Example 5. For the male manic depression data in Table 2 the outcome variable is episodes and the independent variable is treatment. Consider the logistic regression model

$$\log \frac{p_x}{1 - p_x} = \beta_0 + \beta_1 x, \tag{8}$$

where x is the treatment ($x = 1$ if lithium, $x = 0$ if placebo) and p_x is the probability of a subject given treatment x having episodes within 3 months. Thus $p_{x=1}$ is the probability of a subject on lithium having episodes within 3 months, while $p_{x=0}$ is the probability of a subject on placebo having episodes within 3 months. In Eq. (8) the log of the odds of having episodes is modeled as a function of treatment only.

TABLE 14. SAS Statements and Partial SAS Output for Three Logistic Regression Models Fitted to the Manic Depressive Data

SAS Statements

```
data data1;
  input treatment episodes n;
cards;
  1 8 30
  0 28 40
proc logistic data = data1;
  model episodes/n = treatment / expb;
  * *note: EXPB option displays exponentiated values of estimates * *;
  title "Males only";
data data2;
  input gender treatment episodes n;
  cards;
1 1 8 30
1 0 28 40
0 1 15 120
0 0 43 100
proc logistic data = data2;
  model episodes/n = gender treatment /expb;
  title "Males and females - main effects model";
proc logistic data = data2;
  model episodes/n = gender treatment gender*treatment/expb;
  title "Males and females  full model";
run;
```

Partial SAS Output

Males only
The LOGISTIC Procedure

Response Profile

Ordered Value	Binary Outcome	Total Frequency
1	Event	36
2	Nonevent	34

Analysis of Maximum Likelihood Estimates

Parameter	DF	Estimate	Standard Error	Chi-Square	Pr > ChiSq	Exp(Est)
Intercept	1	**0.8473**	0.3450	6.0305	0.0141	2.333
Treatment	1	**−1.8589**	0.5381	11.9360	**0.0006**	**0.156**

Odds Ratio Estimates

Effect	Point Estimate	95% Wald Confidence Limits	
treatment	**0.156**	**0.054**	**0.447**

TABLE 14. (*Continued*)

Males and females—main effects model

The LOGISTIC Procedure

Response Profile

Ordered Value	Binary Outcome	Total Frequency
1	Event	94
2	Nonevent	196

Analysis of Maximum Likelihood Estimates

Parameter	DF	Estimate	Standard Error	Chi-Square	Pr > ChiSq	Exp(Est)
Intercept	1	−0.2621	0.1912	1.8801	0.1703	0.769
gender	1	1.0525	0.3088	11.6135	**0.0007**	2.865
treatment	**1**	**−1.7210**	**0.2891**	35.4258	**< 0.0001**	**0.179**

Odds Ratio Estimates

Effect	Point Estimate	95% Wald Confidence Limits	
gender	2.865	1.564	5.248
treatment	**0.179**	**0.102**	**0.315**

Males and females—full model

The LOGISTIC Procedure

Response Profile

Ordered Value	Binary Outcome	Total Frequency
1	Event	94
2	Nonevent	196

Analysis of Maximum Likelihood Estimates

Parameter	DF	Estimate	Standard Error	Chi-Square	Pr > ChiSq	Exp(Est)
Intercept	1	−0.2819	0.2020	1.9471	0.1629	0.754
gender	1	1.1291	0.3998	7.9762	0.0047	3.093
treatment	1	−1.6637	0.3420	23.6639	< 0.0001	0.189
gender * treatment	1	−0.1952	−0.6376	0.0937	**0.7595**	0.823

In Table 14 are the SAS statements and output for fitting the Equation 8 model and two other logistic regression models using the method of maximum likelihood estimation. The output for the Equation 8 model is titled "Males only." We see that the treatment variable is statistically significant (p value = 0.0006) from the "Analysis of Maximum Likelihood Estimates" section of the SAS output, and thus we conclude that there is an association between treatment and episodes. The parameter estimates are $\hat{\beta}_0 = 0.8473$ and $\hat{\beta}_1 = -1.8589$. Since the odds ratio (the odds of a lithium group subject having an episode divided by the odds of a control group subject having an episode) is given by

$$\psi = \frac{\dfrac{p_{x=1}}{1 - p_{x=1}}}{\dfrac{p_{x=0}}{1 - p_{x=0}}}$$

it follows from Equation 8 that $\psi = \exp(\beta_1)$. Hence the maximum likelihood estimate of ψ is $\hat{\psi} = \exp(\hat{\beta}_1) = \exp(-1.8589) = 0.156$, which is the same as $\hat{\psi} = 8(12)/[28(22)]$, as calculated using Eq. (3). This estimate ($\hat{\psi} = 0.156$) is displayed in the "Analysis of Maximum Likelihood Estimates" output (in the "Exp(Est)" column) and also in the "Odds Ratio Estimates" output (in the "Point Estimate" column.)

In the second model we use the male and female manic-depression data from Tables 2 and 9 and model the log of the odds of having an episode as a function of treatment and gender by fitting the model

$$\log \frac{p_{x_1, x_2}}{1 - p_{x_1, x_2}} = \beta_0 + \beta_1 x_1 + \beta_2 x_2. \tag{9}$$

In this model x_1 is the treatment variable (1 = lithium, 0 = placebo), x_2 is the gender variable (1 = male, 0 = female), and p_{x_1, x_2} is the probability of an episode for a subject with treatment $= x_1$ and gender $= x_2$. It can be shown that this model assumes a common odds ratio—that is, the odds of a lithium group subject having an episode divided by the odds of a control group subject having an episode is the same for each gender. From the SAS output (titled "Males and females—main effects model") we see that treatment ($p < 0.0001$) and gender ($p = 0.0007$) are each significant. Since treatment is significant, we conclude that there is a significant association between treatment episodes, controlling for gender ($p < 0.0001$). Note that this was the same conclusion reached in Example 3 using the Mantel–Haenszel test ($p < 0.0001$). Similarly, since gender is significant, we can conclude that there is a significant association between gender and episodes, controlling for treatment ($p = 0.0007$).

We can compute an estimate for the common odds ratio by noting that, for a given value of x_2, the common odds ratio is given by

$$\psi = \frac{\dfrac{p_{x_1=1, x_2}}{1 - p_{x_1=1, x_2}}}{\dfrac{p_{x_1=0, x_2}}{1 - p_{x_1=0, x_2}}}$$

and hence it follows from (9) that $\psi = \exp(\beta_1)$. Thus the maximum likelihood estimate of ψ is $\hat{\psi} = \exp(\hat{\beta}_1) = \exp(-1.7211) = 0.1789$, which agrees with $\hat{\psi}_{\text{MH}}$ and $\hat{\psi}_{\text{Logit}}$ computed in Example 3. This estimate ($\hat{\psi} = 0.179$) is displayed in the

"Analysis of Maximum Likelihood Estimates" output in the "Exp(Est)" column and also in the "Odds Ratio Estimates" output (in the "Point Estimate" column.)

A 95% confidence interval for the common odds ratio is given by the interval $\exp(\hat{\beta}_1 \pm 1.96\hat{\sigma}_{\hat{\beta}_1})$, where $\hat{\sigma}_{\hat{\beta}_1}$ is the estimated standard deviation of $\hat{\beta}_1$. From the SAS output we have $\hat{\sigma}_{\beta 1} = 0.2891$. Thus our 95% confidence interval is $(0.1015, 0.3153)$, which agrees very closely with the intervals given in Example 3. This confidence interval, rounded to $(0.102, 0.315)$, is displayed in the section labeled "Odds Ratio Estimates" (in the "95% Wald Confidence Limits" columns).

The third model is

$$\log\frac{p_x}{1 - p_x} = \beta_0 + \beta_1 x_1 + \beta_2 x_2 + \beta_3 x_1 x_2. \tag{10}$$

The output for this model is titled "Males and females—full model." In this model we have included the interaction term $x_1 x_2$, which represents the interaction between treatment and gender. It can be shown that this third model does not assume a common odds ratio, unless $\beta_3 = 0$. From the output we see that the p value for the interaction term is 0.7595. Thus there is not sufficient evidence to conclude that $\beta_3 \neq 0$; that is, there is not sufficient evidence to conclude that the odds ratios are different. Note that this p value agrees with the Breslow–Day p value of 0.7598 in Example 3.

ACKNOWLEDGMENTS

This work was partially supported by The University of Iowa Psychiatric Epidemiology/Biostatistics Training Program, NIMH grant MH15168.

REFERENCES

Breslow N, Day NE (1980): "Statistical Methods in Cancer Research," vol I, "The Analysis of Case–Control Studies." Lyon: IARC.

Kleinbaum DG, Kupper LL, Morgenstern H (1982): "Epidemiologic Research: Principles and Quantitative Methods." Belmont, CA: Wadsworth.

Mantel N (1963): Chi-square tests with one degree of freedom: Extensions of the Mantel–Haenszel procedure. J Am Stat Assoc 58:690–700.

Mantel N, Haenszel W (1959): Statistical aspects of the analysis of the analysis of data from retrospective studies of disease. J Natl Cancer Inst 22:719–748.

Miettinen OS (1976): Estimability and estimation in case-referrent studies. Am J Epidemiol 103:226–235.

Robins J, Breslow N, Greenland S (1986). Estimators of the Mantel–Haenszel variance consistent in both sparse data and large-strata limiting models. 42:311–323.

Rosner B (1990): "Fundamentals of Biostatistics." Boston, MA: PWS-Kent.

Woolf B (1954): On estimating the relation between blood group and disease. Annals of Human Genetics 19, 251– 253.

CHAPTER 3

Methods in Psychiatric Genetics

STEPHEN V. FARAONE, DEBBY TSUANG, and MING T. TSUANG

Harvard Medical School, Department of Psychiatry at Massachusetts Mental Health Center, Harvard Institute of Psychiatric Epidemiology and Genetics, Pediatric Psychopharmacology Unit, Psychiatry Service, Massachusetts General Hospital (S.V.F) Department of Psychiatry and Behavioral Sciences, Department of Epidemiology, School of Public Health, University of Washington, Seattle, WA, Mental Illness, Research, Education and Clinical Center, VA Puget Sound Health Care System, Seattle Division (D.T.), Harvard Medical School, Department of Psychiatry at Massachusetts Mental Health Center, Harvard Institute of Psychiatric Epidemiology and Genetics, VA Cooperative Research Project on Genetics of Schizophrenia, Brockton-West Roxbury Veterans Affairs Medical Center, Department of Epidemiology, Harvard School of Public Health, Psychiatry Service, Massachusetts General Hospital (M.T.T.).

INTRODUCTION

Psychiatric genetics is a multidisciplinary field with roots in human genetics, psychiatry, molecular biology, statistics, and epidemiology. Thus, students of psychiatric genetics face a difficult challenge: to acquaint themselves with diverse methodologies and specialize in those needed to achieve their scientific goals. In this chapter we introduce these methods and provide references for more advanced studies of particular issues.

Some readers may be surprised to find discussions of genetics in a textbook of psychiatric epidemiology. After all, epidemiologists usually concern themselves with describing the distribution and determinants of disease as a function of exposure to some environmental variable. This leads naturally to the goal of finding *environmental* risk factors that cause illness. In contrast, classical genetics focuses on genetic mechanisms and, in experimental studies, may even seek to strictly control the environment and eliminate environmental variance. Put simply, epidemiologic research often treats genetic determinants as noise and environmental agents as the signal; genetic studies reverse the roles of genes and environment.

Psychiatric genetics favors neither extreme and adopts the position of genetic epidemiology, which has been defined as, "a science that deals with etiology, distribution, and control of disease in groups of relatives and with inherited causes of disease in populations" (Morton, 1982). Genetic epidemiologists examine the distribution of illness within families with the goal of finding genetic *and* environmental causes of illness. Thus, psychiatric genetics considers both environmental and genetic risk factors—and their interaction—to be on an equal footing. In this

Textbook in Psychiatric Epidemiology, Second Edition, Edited by Ming T. Tsuang and Mauricio Tohen.
ISBN 0-471-40974-X

paradigm the epidemiologists' concept of "exposure" must extend to genes and family relationships.

It is crucial to recognize the importance of environmental factors to psychiatric genetics because genetic epidemiologists have been accused (incorrectly) of ignoring the environment. Of course, much of the literature in psychiatric genetics does sounds purely genetic. Studies seek to demonstrate familiality, find genes, and estimate heritability. However, in many of these studies, the role of environment is always implicit, even when not mentioned directly. Our point is simple. Although psychiatric genetics seeks to clarify how genes lead to psychiatric illness, most researchers agree that the pathway from **genotype**[1] to **phenotype** cannot be understood without reference to environmental agents that trigger illness in susceptible individuals.

Ironically, psychiatric genetics has provided the strongest evidence supporting the idea that nongenetic factors play a causal role in the expression of psychiatric illness. Most notable in this regard are twin studies. These show that both members of a pair of **monozygotic** (MZ) twins will be affected with schizophrenia or mood disorder only between 50% and 70% of the time, depending on the disorder. By revealing that 30–50% of MZ co-twins are unaffected, despite sharing 100% of their genes in common, the twin method clearly points to the influence of environmental factors in the etiology of these disorders.

THE CHAIN OF PSYCHIATRIC GENETIC RESEARCH

Work in psychiatric genetics tends to follow a series of questions in a logical progression (Table 1). This sequence, which has been called the "chain of genetic epidemiologic research" (Faraone et al., 1999). is as follows: First, we ask "Is the disorder familial?" In other words, does it run in families? Second, "What is the relative magnitude of genetic and environmental contributions to disease etiology and expression?" Third, "How is the disease transmitted from generation to generation?" Fourth, "If genes mediate this transmission, where are they located?" Fifth, "What are the genetic and environmental mechanisms of disease?"

Is the Disorder Familial?

Since this question is the easiest to answer it frequently is the first to be asked. For example, observations of disorders "running in families" may come from clinicians

TABLE 1. Chain of Psychiatric Genetic Research

Questions	Methods
Is disorder familial?	Family study
What are the relative contributions of genes and environment?	Twin and adoption studies
What is the mode of transmission?	Segregation analysis
Where is the gene (or genes) located?	Linkage and association studies

[1]Genetic and statistical terms are defined in the Appendix to this chapter.

who often treat patients from the same family. Of course, once familiality is informally established in a clinical setting, it remains to be confirmed with a rigorous research design, known as the family study method.

Selection of Probands. Ideally, a family study should use the blind case–control paradigm, a staple of epidemiology and behavioral science. The cases and controls used in genetic studies are known as **probands**. We usually select probands with the disorder from a source that is "enriched" with the diagnosis of interest. For example, patients in psychiatric clinics are more likely to have bipolar disorder than patients in a family practice clinic. Furthermore, patients in a bipolar specialty clinic are more likely to have bipolar disorder than patients in a general psychiatric clinic.

Selection from clinics instead of the general population is useful for two reasons. First, to achieve an adequate number of cases from the general population we would need to screen many individuals. This is costly and of dubious benefit. Second, multiple stages of ascertainment increase the probabilities of ill probands being "true cases" and of normal probands not having the disorder under study. Individuals who seek treatment and are given a clinical diagnosis are more likely to have experienced the level of distress and disability that the diagnostic nosology requires for psychiatric illness. This combined with the fact that individuals free of illness are rarely referred means that psychiatric clinic populations have a higher base rate of all psychiatric illnesses than does the general population.

The positive predictive power of a diagnosis (the proportion of those with the disorder among all patients receiving the diagnosis) increases with increases in the base rate of the disorder being diagnosed (Meehl and Rosen, 1955). Thus, multiple stage ascertainment increases the positive predictive power by using clinic status to increase the proportion of "true cases" in the sample that is assessed by the research protocol. Unavoidably, this method of increasing the positive predictive power will increase the false negative rate. In this context, false negatives are those who have a disorder but are (1) not referred to a clinic or (2) referred but do not receive a clinical diagnosis. Thus, the generalizability of results will be limited to the degree that these false negatives differ from the probands enrolled in our study. Treatment is, of course, the most notable factor that will differentiate these groups.

Likewise, multistage screening of controls decreases the probability of misclassifying someone with the disorder as a control. Of course, since screened controls are selected for absence of the disorder of interest, they cannot be considered representative of the general population. However, work in psychiatric epidemiology indicates that screened controls are very effective when the goal of a project is to delineate factors that differentiate controls from cases (Tsuang et al., 1988). Furthermore, unscreened controls frequently have rates of psychopathology and its correlates that are above the population expectation (Gibbons et al., 1990; Kruesi et al., 1990; Shtasel et al., 1991). Thus, unscreened controls are often heavily contaminated with cases, thereby obscuring the effects of the variable of interest.

We emphasize that controls should be screened only for the disorder being studied, not for other psychiatric disorders or conditions. When controls are screened for additional disorders, the results can spuriously indicate a familial relationship between the disorder used to select cases and the disorders that were screened from controls (Kendler, 1990). For example, we know that alcoholism and anxiety disorders both run in families. Consider a family study of alcoholism that screens control, but not alcoholic, probands for anxiety disorders. Since anxiety is familial, the rates of anxiety among relatives of controls will be decreased by the screening process. In contrast, the rates in relatives of alcoholics will not be decreased. Thus, anxiety disorders will be more prevalent among the relatives of alcoholics due to the choice of control group.

The selection of controls should satisfy the comparability principles required for meaningful inferences in case–control epidemiological studies (Miettinen, 1985; Wacholder, 1992 a–c). It is usually not possible to establish a primary study base with a geographically defined population. This is so because the clinics from which probands are selected may serve a broad geographic region that is difficult to delineate. This is especially true for specialty clinics at universities. In many cases the reputation of the clinic attracts patients from great distances.

The usual approach is to establish a secondary study base defined by the ascertainment source. The use of secondary study bases limits generalizability and does not produce a representative sample from a geographical population. Nevertheless, it does allow for meaningful case–control comparisons if the controls are individuals who could have been cases had they developed the disorder of interest during the time of investigation (Miettinen, 1985; Wacholder, 1992 a–c). When sampling from a clinic, this requires that if the control subjects had needed treatment for the disorder, they would have been referred to the clinics that provided the case probands. For example, in a general hospital outpatient setting, it is likely that patients who seek treatment for medical disorders in medical clinics would go to the same hospital's psychiatric clinic for the treatment of a psychiatric disorder.

Of course, instead of establishing a secondary study base, it is possible to match cases and controls on "relevant" variables. One problem here is defining what is and is not a "relevant" variable. Age, sex and socioeconomic status are usually considered, but others may be appropriate. However, matching should be used cautiously so as to avoid the "matching fallacy" (Meehl, 1970) and "overmatching" (Miettinen, 1985; Greenland and Morgenstern, 1990). As discussed by Meehl (1970), matching on specific variables often unmatches on others. In addition to creating unusual samples, this also leads to reduced statistical efficiency and biased estimates (Wacholder et al., 1992c). These problems are most severe when the matching variable is strongly associated with the disorder under study.

An obvious example of the matching fallacy is as follows. Numerous studies find that attention deficit hyperactivity disorder (ADHD) interferes with school achievement (Faraone et al., 1993). Thus, matching controls to ADHD subjects on school achievement would create an unusually high functioning ADHD sample or an unusually low functioning control sample. It may be difficult to draw meaningful inferences from such samples. Instead of matching, we use statistical methods to examine and control for the effects of potentially confounding variables.

Following the selection of cases and controls, the study attempts to assess the diagnostic status of as many of the relatives of cases and controls as possible. The aim is to compare rates of illness in relatives of cases to rates in the relatives of controls. To estimate these rates of illness accurately, care must be taken to assess as many relatives as possible. However, psychiatric disorders affect emotions, thinking, and interpersonal relationships. Thus, nonparticipation may not be random with respect to illness status; family members who are ill may be more likely to refuse participation than those who are well. Paranoid schizophrenia provides a good example of this problem. Paranoia leads to distrusts of strangers, friends, and family. This makes it difficult for a paranoid person to agree to answer the many questions required by psychiatric interviews.

If a disorder has a genetic etiology, then relatives of ill probands should carry a greater risk for the illness than relatives of controls. In addition, the risk to relatives of probands should be correlated with their degree of relationship to the proband, or the amount of genes they share in common. First-degree relatives such as parents, siblings, and children, share 50% of their genes, on average, with the proband. They should be at greater risk for the disorder than second-degree relatives (grandparents, uncles, aunts, nephews, nieces, and half-siblings) because second-degree relatives share only 25% of their genes with the proband.

A genetic hypothesis predicts that the risk to relatives of ill probands is higher than that for relatives of controls and that the risk to relatives of probands increases as the amount of genes shared increases. In practice, however, it is rare that a family study will have the resources to diagnose second- or third-degree relatives. Most studies assess only first-degree relatives. Table 2 displays the familial pattern of risk found in the families of schizophrenic probands. These risk figures come from many of the earlier European family studies and conform to the

TABLE 2. Rates of Schizophrenia Among Relatives of Schizophrenic Patients

Type of Relative	Percent at Risk
First-degree relatives	
Parents	4.4
Children	12.3
Both parents schizophrenic	36.6
Brothers and Sisters	8.5
Neither parent schizophrenic	8.2
One parent schizophrenic	13.8
Fraternal twins of opposite sex	5.6
Fraternal twins of same sex	12.0
Identical Twins	57.7
Second-degree relatives	
Uncles and Aunts	2.0
Nephews and Nieces	2.2
Grandchildren	2.8
Half brothers or half sisters	3.2
Third-degree relatives	
First cousins	2.9
General population	0.86

Source: Based on Slater and Cowie (1971) with the exception of twin data from Shields and Slater (1975). Adapted, with permission from Tsuang, Faraone, and Johnson (1997)

expectation that first-degree relatives are at highest risk, followed by second- and then third-degree relatives.

Family Study versus Family History. In planning a family study of psychiatric illness we must choose between two approaches for the evaluation of family members: the **family history** and **family study** methods (Faraone et al., 1999). The family history method collects diagnostic information about all family members by interviewing only one or several informants per family. This method uses a specialized instrument such as the interview for Family History Research Diagnostic Criteria (FH-RDC; (Andreasen et al.,1977)) or the Family Interview for Genetic Studies (FIGS; (NIMH Genetic Initiative, 1992)).

In contrast, the family study method determines diagnoses by interviewing all family members directly. Several excellent structured psychiatric interviews are available but only one was designed specifically for genetic studies: the Diagnostic Interview for Genetic Studies (DIGS; Faraone et al., 1996; Nurnberger et al., 1994).

An obvious advantage of the family history method is its low cost; interviewing a few family members is less costly then interviewing all family members. However, several researchers have shown that family history data underestimate true rates of many psychiatric disorders. The overall strategy of these studies has been to collect family history data on the same subjects who have also been diagnosed by the family study method. By using the family study method as the "gold standard" they can estimate the accuracy of the family history method.

Mendlewicz et al. (1975) examined the accuracy of the family history method in the context of a family study of mood disorders. The probands were 140 patients with either bipolar disorder or major depressive disorder. When the probands were used as informants for the family history method, the rates of mood disorders in the family were underestimated. The family history method was most accurate when the informant was the child or spouse of the person being diagnosed.

Similar results were reported by Andreasen et al. (1977). They determined the specificity and sensitivity of family history diagnoses using an adaptation of the Research Diagnostic Criteria they termed the Family History Research Diagnostic Criteria. *Specificity* is the probability of correctly classifying a subject as well by the family history method if that subject is assessed as well by the family study method. *Sensitivity* is the probability that the subject is diagnosed ill by family history if they are diagnosed ill by the family study method. In their application to mood disorders, the specificity was high but the sensitivity was low. For example, among family members classified as having a mood disorder by direct interview, only 59% were so classified by the family history method.

It is possible to improve the sensitivity of the family history method by using several informants to provide information about the subject being diagnosed. In the Andreasen et al. (1977) study, when only probands were interviewed via the FH-RDC, the lifetime prevalence of mood disorders among relative's was 11%. This rate increased to 17% when other relatives were interviewed along with the proband. However, both rates underestimated the 25% rate obtained by the family study method.

Orvaschel et al. (1982) found that the family history method was better for some types of relatives than for others. For example, in their study, the sensitivity of the family history method was lower when the subject being diagnosed was male. Sensitivity was higher if the relative being diagnosed was ill at the time of the family history interview. This latter finding makes intuitive sense; we are more likely to know of a relative's problems if, for example, they are in a psychiatric hospital at the time we are asked about their condition.

Other studies have shown that the accuracy of family history assessments varies by diagnosis. Thompson et al. (1982) found that sensitivities for major depression and alcoholism were much higher than for generalized anxiety, drug abuse, phobic disorder, and depressive personality. Moreover, diagnoses based on spouse or offspring reports were more sensitive than those based on parent or sibling reports.

In the family study of mood disorders by Gershon and Guroff (1984), the family history method was most sensitive (96%) when the informant was being asked about a proband. It was halved to 48% when the relative being diagnosed was not a proband. Notably, there was a positive linear relationship between sensitivity and the number of informants. The sensitivity was only 15% with one informant, but increased to 67% when five informants were used. Specificity decreased only a little, from 99% to 92%, when the number of informants was increased from one to five.

In a relatively large study of 609 mood-disordered probands and 2,216 first-degree relatives, Andreasen et al. (1986) confirmed the results from previous validity studies of the family history method. Relative to the family study method, rates of illness in relatives were always underestimated by the family history method using the FH-RDC. One key exception was the diagnosis of antisocial personality: The family history rate of this disorder was three times greater than the direct interview estimate. Thus, it may be that the family history method is more valid than direct interview when the disorder in question has a pejorative connotation.

In Andreasen et al.'s (1986) study the sensitivities and specificities of the family history method were consistent with previous reports. The sensitivities were low. They ranged from 31% for schizophrenia to 69% for "psychotic disorder." As expected, the specificities were higher. These ranged from 84% for probable depressive disorder to 100% for schizophrenia and schizoaffective disorder. The sensitivity of the family history method was best when the informant was a parent of the subject being asked about. For depression the sensitivities were 62% for parent informants, 51% for sibling informants and 37% for child informants.

Ideally, the diagnoses of subjects should use three sources of information: direct interviews with the subject, family history interviews with informants who are familiar with the subject, and medical records when available. All sources of information about a given individual, are then combined into a consensus diagnosis (Gershon and Guroff, 1984; Leckman et al., 1982). As suggested by the research reviewed previously, the direct interview and medical record usually provide more useful information than the family history assessment. In fact, two studies find that diagnoses based on direct interviews alone closely approximate best estimate diagnoses (Gershon and Guroff, 1984; Leckman et al., 1982). However, a diagnosis based only on medical records is often a suitable proxy to the best estimate diagnosis (Gershon and Guroff, 1984).

Silverman and colleagues (1986) evaluated the reliability of the family history method for dementing illnesses such as Alzheimers disease. When rating the same individual, different informants had high levels of agreement on the presence of dementia and its age at onset. The rates of dementia found in this family history study were similar to what had been found in previous family studies using direct methods of assessment. The authors concluded that multiple informants would likely increase the validity of the family history method but, because they did not directly evaluate relatives, inferences about validity were limited.

Kosten, Anton, and Rounsaville (1992) examined the validity of the family history method for five diagnoses used in a family study of opiate addiction: depression, anxiety, antisocial personality, alcoholism, and drug abuse. For diagnosing family members, the sensitivities were uniformly low, ranging from 6% to 39%. Specificities were greater than 95%, with the exception of depression, which had a specificity of 54%.

The authors also provided data about the type and number of informants. Spouses and children were better informants than parents or siblings. For alcoholism and drug abuse, females were better informants than males. Increasing the number of informants improved the accuracy of the family history method for depression, antisocial personality, and alcoholism, but not for anxiety disorders or drug abuse.

Collection of data using the family history method may be influenced by the presence of psychiatric illness in the informant. Kendler and colleagues (1991) asked **discordant** twins about depression, anxiety, and alcoholism in their parents. Twins are discordant if only one has the disease being studied. Compared with the unaffected twin, those with a history of major depression or generalized anxiety were more likely to report the same disorder in their parents. This effect was not observed for alcoholism. However, since direct interview data had not been collected on the parents, it is not certain if the affected twin was over reporting psychopathology or the unaffected twin was underreporting it. Nevertheless, this study underscores the need for more methodological work to clarify the utility of the family history method for specific disorders.

Table 3 outlines the advantages and disadvantages of the family history and family study methods. The choice between the two requires a trade-off between data quality and the expense of data collection. The family history method is the method of choice when there are not sufficient data to justify the expense of a family study. Thus, it is a good choice for initial pilot phases of a genetic investigation. However, after the family history method demonstrates familiality, the family study is the tool of choice for examining the details of familial transmission.

If the question at hand dictates the use of the family history method, the following recommendations should be considered: (1) use the FH-RDC, FIGS or some other semistructured method for eliciting the family history; (2) because the family history method has low sensitivity, use less stringent diagnostic criteria than

TABLE 3. Family Study versus Family History Method

Method	Pros	Cons
Family history	Practical, high specificity	Low sensitivity
Family study	High quality data	Expensive

that used for direct interview data; (3) use multiple informants for each person to be diagnosed; (4) seek out informants who have had substantial contact with the person to be diagnosed; (5) remember that the method is most valid when the person to be diagnosed is ill at the time of interviewing the informant. These "rules of thumb" provide a rough guide for planning a family history study. The papers discussed in this chapter should be consulted for information about specific disorders.

Caveats. The family study is a practical and robust tool for psychiatric genetics. In many cases, it has provided the initial hint that a disorder might have a genetic component. However, we must be cautious in concluding that a disorder is caused by genes after we observe that it is familial. Disorders can "run in families" for nongenetic reasons such as shared environmental adversity, viral transmission, and social learning. Also, since the culture and environment shared by family members tends to increase as the degree of relationship decreases, the pattern of risk due to environmental factors may mimic the pattern expected for genetic relationships.

Family data on tuberculosis provide a good example of such confounding. Data collected in the 1940s showed that the risk to family members related to probands who had tuberculosis increased with the degree of genetic relationship. That is, first-degree relatives had higher rates of tuberculosis than second-degree relatives. McGue et al., (1985) pointed out that the distribution of familial risk for schizophrenia and that for tuberculosis both showed that the risk to relatives of ill probands increased with the amount of genes shared with the proband. However, the patterns differed in a few subtle ways that allowed them to show that the risk for schizophrenia was transmitted genetically whereas tuberculosis was transmitted through the environment.

Our point is straightforward: The finding of familial transmission cannot be unambiguously interpreted. Although family studies are indispensable for establishing the familiality of disorders, they cannot, by themselves, establish what type of transmission. All mechanisms that could lead to a familial clustering of disease should be considered.

What are the Relative Contributions of Genes and Environment?

Genes, environment and their interaction: these are the ingredients of the pathophysiological brew that engenders psychopathology. Psychiatric genetics seeks to assay these ingredients and determine their relative proportions. The tools for this venture are twin and adoption studies Faraone et al. (1999).

Unfortunately, twin and adoption studies are fairly difficult to implement because of the difficulty in finding and collecting large enough samples that are informative for the disorder to be studied. Twin births are rare and twins with psychopathology are even rarer. Adoption is relatively common, but laws in most countries make it impossible to study the biological relatives of adopted children.

However, valuable resources for twin and adoption studies do exist and these have fueled work in this area for many decades. For example, countries like Denmark have extensive adoption and twin registries in addition to psychiatric registries. By recording all twin births, adoptions, and psychiatric contacts in a specified geographical region, these registries have allowed researchers to proceed with genetic studies of gene–environment relationships. Linkage of the psychiatric registries with the twin and adoption registries has created unique opportunities for genetic epidemiologic investigations of some psychiatric disorders.

Twin Studies. The biological process of twinning creates a natural experiment in psychiatric genetics. Identical or **monozygotic** (MZ) twins inherit identical **chromosomes** and thereby have 100% of their genes in common. In contrast, the genetic similarity of fraternal or **dizygotic** (DZ) twins is no different than that of siblings. On average, DZ twins share 50% of their genes. Thus, MZ and DZ twins are markedly different with regard to their genetic similarity. However, if twin pairs are reared in the same household then the degree of environmental similarity between MZ twins should be no different than that between DZ twins. The astute reader will note that our comments regarding genetic similarity are *facts* of inheritance, but our comments about the environment are *assumptions*. The correctness of these assumptions is key to the valid use of the twin method.

Since MZ twins are genetic copies of one another, any differences between a pair of MZ twins are assumed to be due primarily to environmental influences. In contrast, differences between DZ twins could be due to either genetic or environmental influences. Thus, comparing the co-occurrence of a psychiatric disorder in the two types of twins provides information about the relative contributions of genetic and environmental factors in the etiology of the disorder. The co-occurrence of a disorder in both twins is called concordance; if one twin has the disorder and the other does not, the twins are discordant for the disorder.

Twin data for psychiatric disorders are usually expressed as concordance rates. Because we assume the same environmental similarity for both types of twins, a higher concordance rate for MZ compared with DZ twins indicates the operation of genetic mechanisms. We can use pairwise or probandwise concordance rates, depending on the method of sampling the twins. The **pairwise concordance** rate is defined as the proportion of twin pairs in which both twins are ill. To compute this, count the number of twin pairs **concordant** for the disorder and divide the result by the total number of pairs. We use this method of computing concordance when the probability of sampling any specific ill individual is so low that two ill co-twins are never independently sampled as probands.

However, when the sampling probability is higher, the probandwise concordance rate is the method of choice. **Probandwise concordance** is the proportion of proband twins that have an ill co-twin. Thus, it is the number of concordant pairs plus the number of concordant pairs in which both the twins are probands, divided by the total number of pairs.

Frequently, twin data are used to estimate the **heritability** of a disorder. Heritability measures the degree to which genetic factors influence variability in the manifestation of the disorder (the phenotype) . We divide phenotypic variability (V_p) into two pieces: genetic variability (V_g) and environmental variability (V_e). This partitioning of phenotypic variability assumes that genetic and environmental factors are statistically independent (i.e., $V_p = V_g + V_e$). Heritability in the broad sense (h_2) is the ratio of genetic and phenotypic variances (i.e., $h_2 = V_g/V_p$).

As these formulas show, a heritability of one indicates that variability in the phenotype is due to genetic factors alone. In contrast, a heritability of zero attributes all phenotypic variation to environmental factors. However, a key point

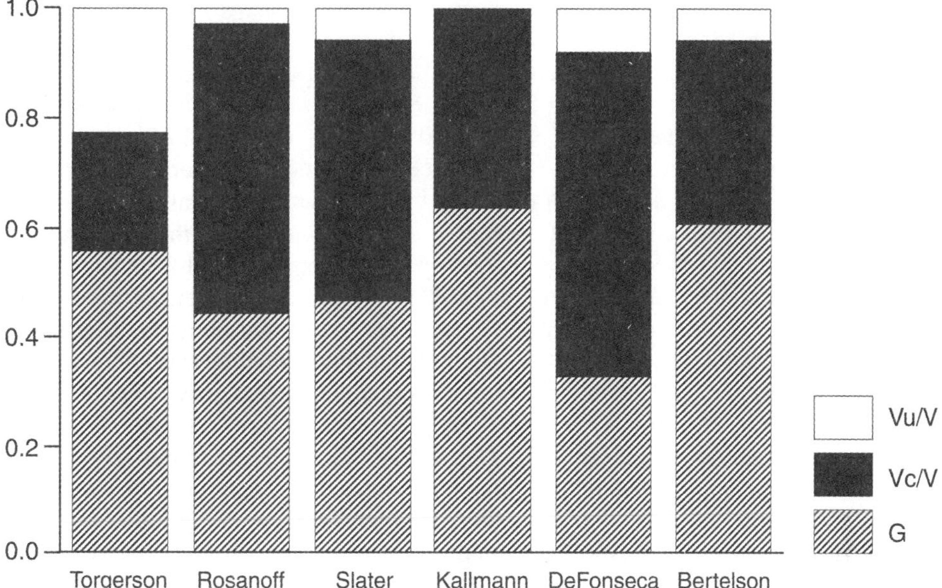

Figure 1. The relative contributions of genetic (G), common environmental (Vc/V), and unique environmental (Vu/V) variance to the liability to mood disorders.

here is that a zero heritability does not mean that the etiology of the phenotype can be explained solely by environmental influence. Retardation due to phenylketonuria (PKU), is a classic case for demonstrating this point.

PKU is caused by a **recessive** gene. Infants who inherit two copies of this gene (they are **homozygous**) suffer from a complete deficiency of the enzyme required to metabolize phenylalanine. These children will become retarded only if they ingest phenylalanine. Heritability estimated on a sample of individuals who have the pathogenic genotype will be zero simply because there is no genetic variability in the sample. In this case, any variability in the PKU trait must be due to the environment.

The details of methods for calculating heritability are beyond the scope of this chapter. Smith (1974) and Plomin et al. (1990) provide information about the calculation and interpretation of this measure. Also see LaBuda et al. (1993).

Figure 1 gives an example of how twin data can shed light on the etiology of psychiatric illnesses. The figure presents results from six different twin studies of broadly defined mood disorders, or "manic-depressive disorder" (Tsuang and Faraone, 1990). Each bar on the graph represents a single study. The cross-hatched part of each bar indicates what percentage of the disorder could be attributed to genetic factors. The black part of the bar indicates what percentage could be attributed to common or shared environmental factors. The white part of the bar indicates the proportion of variance due to unique environmental factors or events experienced by one twin but not the other. This pattern of results attributes approximately 60% of the variance in mood disorders to genetic factors; it attributes 30–40% of the variance to common environmental factors. Unique environmental effects appear to have accounted for less than 10% of the variance in these six studies.

This is a relatively simple analysis of twin data. Twin methodology can become mathematically sophisticated. If we have data from parents and siblings of twins or indices of the environment, then specialized methods can provide information about gene–environment interaction and gene–environment correlation. An excellent reference for these methods is the book by Neale and Cardon (1992).

Two additional twin study designs deserve special mention. When monozygotic twins are reared apart, we have a unique—but rare—opportunity to study the relative importance of genes and environment. Since MZ twins reared apart do not share a common environment, any phenotypic similarity must be due to genetic factors. We cannot invoke shared environment as a cause of phenotypic concordance. However, MZ twins with psychiatric illness are rare, and cases of such twins reared apart are even rarer. Thus, this design cannot be routinely used.

A second twin study design uses the children of discordant MZ twins. The logic of this design is straightforward. If a disorder is caused by a genotype in combination with environmental factors, then the well member of a discordant MZ twin pair should carry the genotype. Presumably, they did not develop the disorder because they had not been exposed to a relevant environmental cause. If so, then the children of the well twin should have the same risk for the disorder as the children of the ill twin.

A good example of this design is a Danish study by Fischer (1971). She examined 71 offspring of MZ twin pairs who were discordant for schizophrenia. The offspring of the schizophrenic twins had a 9.6% rate of schizophrenia; the rate among offspring of the nonschizophrenic twins was 12.9%. These two rates were not significantly different. Thus, the risk to the children of these MZ twins did not depend on the presence of schizophrenia in the twin. From this we infer that the twins who did not have schizophrenia did have the genetic susceptibility to schizophrenia and passed it on to their children in the same manner as did the ill twins. Since Gottesman and Bertelsen (1989) confirmed these results in an 18-year follow-up of Fischer's sample, the finding constitutes strong evidence that environmental factors may prevent gene expression in the unaffected twin.

Adoption Studies. Like twinning, adoption creates a useful paradigm for psychiatric genetic studies. Children adopted at an early age have a genetic relationship to their biological parents and an environmental relationship to their adopted parents. Thus, adoption studies can determine if biological or adoptive relationships account for the familial transmission of disorders. If genes are important, then the familial transmission of illness should occur in the biological, but not the adoptive, family. In contrast, if culture, social learning, or other sources of environmental transmission cause illness, then familial transmission of illness should occur in the adoptive, but not the biological, family.

There are three major adoption study designs. The parent-as-proband design compares rates of illness in the adopted offspring of parents with and without the disorder. If genetic factors mediate the disorder then rates of illness should be greater in the adopted away children of ill parents compared with the adopted children of well parents.

As its name suggests, the adoptee-as-proband design starts with ill and well adoptees and examines rates of illness in both biological and adoptive relatives. If the biological relatives of ill adoptees have higher rates of illness than the adoptive relatives of ill adoptees, then a genetic hypothesis is supported. In contrast, if the adoptive relatives show higher rates of illness then an environmental hypothesis gains support.

The third design is the cross-fostering design. This approach compares rates of illness for two groups of adoptees: one has well biological parents and is raised by ill adoptive parents and the other has ill biological parents and is raised by well adoptive parents. Higher rates of illness in the former group of adoptees compared with the latter group would imply a primarily nongenetic mode of illness transmission.

Although they are difficult to execute, adoption studies have provided extensive data for both mood disorders (Tsuang and Faraone, 1990; Cadoret, 1978; Cadoret et al., 1985; Mendlewicz and Rainer, 1977; Wender et al., 1986) and schizophrenia (Heston, 1966; Kety et al., 1968, 1978). Taken as a group, these studies support the hypothesis that the familial transmission of these disorders is due to genetic, not environmental factors.

Despite their power to disentangle genetic and environmental factors, adoption studies must be viewed with some caution due to potential methodological problems that cloud their unambiguous interpretation. First, adoptees and their families are not representative of the general population. This may limit the generalizability of results. Furthermore, adoptees are at greater risk for psychiatric illness compared with nonadopted children (Kotsopoulos et al., 1988; Deutsch et al., 1982). Although the reasons for this are not clear, this increased risk for psychiatric disorders requires that we use an adoptee control group. For example, in the adoptee-as-proband design, the relatives of ill adoptees must be compared with the relatives of well adoptees. Some other control group cannot be used, even if it is matched to the ill adoptee group on demographic measures.

Another potential problem is that it may be difficult to find a sample of adoptees who were all separated from their parents at birth. If the child has lived with a parent for even a short period of time prior to adoption, the biological relationship will have been "contaminated" by environmental factors. Some might even argue that the childs contact with the mother immediately after birth creates a residue of environmental influence that effects subsequent psychopathology.

Kety et al. (1968; 1978) presented a compelling design that deals with this problem. Their method requires a sample of biological paternal half-siblings of ill and well adoptees. Paternal half-siblings share a common father yet have different mothers. Therefore, they do not share prenatal, perinatal, or neonatal environmental exposure to the same mother. Thus, this design rules out confounding by *in utero* influences, birth traumas, and early mothering experience. In the work of Kety and colleagues, the biological paternal half-siblings of schizophrenic adoptees were at greater risk for schizophrenia than the biological paternal half-siblings of control adoptees. Such a finding clearly bolsters the hypothesis that schizophrenia is caused, at least in part, by genetic factors.

Of course, there are some environmental correlates of the biological parents that cannot be handled by the paternal half-sibling design. For example, children born to fathers of the lowest social class may share toxic environmental factors such as poor pre- and perinatal care, poor nutrition, and an adverse social environment; these may confound the genetic parent–child relationship.

Despite these potential confounds and the difficulty of ascertaining appropriate cases and controls, the adoption study remains a valuable tool for disentangling genetic and environmental contributions to the familial aggregation of psychiatric disorders. The problems we note serve to underscore a basic tenet of psychiatric genetic research: Any assertion that a disorder is caused by genetic factors must refer, not to a single study but to a series of studies using different paradigms.

What is the Mode of Transmission?

After demonstrating that a disorder is influenced by genetic factors, the next logical task is to determine the mechanism of transmission from parent to child (Faraone et al., 1999). In clinical practice, knowledge of the mode of inheritance is important for genetic counseling. This information is useful from two perspectives. Showing that the transmission of a disorder corresponds to a known mode of transmission provides clues for subsequent research steps. For example, if the transmission is clearly due to a single gene, the next step might be linkage analysis, which uses family psychiatric data and samples of **DNA** to find mutant genes (see the following discussion). In contrast, if environmental factors are implicated, then a search for such factors would be warranted.

Moreover, the mode of transmission has implications for genetic counseling. Genetic counseling is the process whereby clinical professionals inform people about either their probability of developing a genetic disorder or that of children they are planning to conceive. Ideally, in the absence of genetic linkage data, such counseling should be based on risk figures from a known model of genetic transmission. This model can be applied to an individual's pedigree to determine that individual's risk for a disorder. Morton et al. (1979) demonstrated that the degree of risk predicted depends on the model of transmission. They also found that clinically important errors in risk prediction were made when they used the wrong genetic model to make predictions.

A model of familial transmission translates assumptions about genetic and environmental causes into mathematical equations. These equations are then used to predict the distribution of a disorder that we observe in pedigrees or twin pairs. If the pattern of disorder predicted by the model is close to what we observe we say that the model fits the data. This provides evidence in favor of the model being tested. In contrast, if the predicted pattern of disorder differs from what is observed we reject the model and seek another mechanism of transmission. The term **segregation analysis** is used to describe analyses that assess the mode of disease transmission.

As the reader might suspect, the methods we discuss in this section require a good deal of mathematical and statistical expertise to be understood and correctly implemented. In the short space of this chapter we cannot present these mathematical details but instead provide an overview of the different classes of methods used to test hypotheses about genetic and environmental transmission. (However, a detailed discussion of two segregation analysis algorithms is given in a subsequent section.) Several excellent texts, review articles, and computer program documentation provide a detailed guide to these methods (Morton, 1982; Lalouel, 1983; Elston and Stewart, 1971; Bailey-Wilson and Elston, 1989).

Mathematical Modeling of Genetic and Environmental Transmission. A genetic model comprises two major components. First, we must describe how the disorder is transmitted. For example, if we believe the disorder is due to a single dominant gene, our model must include the frequency of the gene in the population. It must also require that the transmission of the gene from parent to child follow the laws of genetic transmission. For example, if a mother carries one pathogenic gene the probability that she transmits this gene to a child must be 50%. Genetic models can specify environmental effects in several ways. Consider some simple examples. In a single gene model we can specify the **penetrance** of each genotype. Penetrance indicates the probability that each genotype causes disease. If we believe that disease occurs when an environmental event (e.g., head injury) occurs in someone carrying the pathogenic gene, then our model should allow some gene carriers to be well. Another possibility is that other causes for the disease exist. If so, then people who do not carry the gene will have some probability of becoming ill. That is, the penetrance is greater than zero for those who do not carry the hypothetical disease gene.

The second component of a genetic model is a procedure for determining whether the predictions made by the model adequately describe the pattern of illness observed in families. One modeling approach attempts to predict rates of illness in various classes of relatives. The pedigree data is reduced to a table of numbers indicating the rate of illness in these classes (e.g., mothers, fathers, brothers, sisters, sons, daughters, and more distant relatives). The mathematical model is then estimated by choosing values for the model parameters (e.g., gene frequency and penetrance) that most accurately reproduce the observed rates. The observed and predicted rates can then be compared with a chi-square test to determine if any deviation between predicted and observed rates is large enough to warrant rejecting the model.

Modeling rates of illness does not capitalize on all the information available in pedigree data. By lumping all families together within one data table, we cannot directly model the transmission of genes from one generation to the next. In contrast, pedigree analysis computes the **likelihood** of the pattern of illness in each family. For this approach the raw data is not summarized into a table. Instead, the analysis uses the status of each person and their relationship to others in the pedigree who are and are not affected. An algorithm then computes the probability or likelihood that the assumed model is correct given the pedigree data and the value of model parameters. Those parameter values yielding the most likely model are used as final estimates. With this approach we establish the model's **goodness of fit** with a likelihood ratio chi-square test.

For example, when we estimate parameters for a single gene model we assume that a pair of genes at a single location or **locus** on a chromosome is responsible for the transmission of a disorder. If b represents the pathogenic version of the gene (or **allele**) and B represents the normal allele at the same locus, then there are three possible genotypes: BB, Bb, and bb. Under a Mendelian genetic model, the probability that a BB father transmits the b gene to his daughter must be zero. Likewise, the transmission probability that a parent of each genotype transmits B or b is fixed by the laws of Mendelian inheritance. This leads to a straightforward statistical test: Compute the likelihood of a Mendelian model and compare this with a model that allows the transmission probabilities to deviate from their Mendelian values. A significant difference would indicate that the single gene model could be rejected.

Types of Transmission Models. Single gene Mendelian transmission is only one of many transmission mechanisms that we use to describe family and twin data. There are three broad classes of transmission mechanisms: genes, environment, and their interaction. We find it useful to classify the genetic mechanisms into three types of models: single major gene, **oligogenic** and **multifactorial polygenic**. The word "major" indicates that one gene can account for most of the genetic transmission of a disorder. Other genes and environmental conditions may play minor roles in modifying the expression of the disease or determining its age of onset. In contrast, an oligogenic model assumes that the combined actions of several genes cause illness. These genes may combine in an additive fashion such that the probability of illness is a function of the number of pathogenic genes. Alternatively, the mechanism may be interactive. For example, three abnormal alleles at different chromosomal locations may be needed for disease to occur. Of course, a combination of additive and interactive mechanisms can also be considered.

One difficulty in testing oligogenic models is that there are many ways in which several genes might combine to cause a disorder. For example, there are 100 possible two-locus models that can describe a dichotomous trait. If the trait is trichotomous, there are 2,634 possible models (Elston and Namboodiri, 1977). A plausible argument can be made for excluding many of these possibilities because they either do not fit hypotheses about the disorder or they are biologically meaningless. Nevertheless, the number of models that remain to be tested is daunting.

The multifactorial polygenic (MFP) model proposes that a large, unspecified number of genes and environmental factors combine in an additive fashion to cause disease. The difference between oligogenic and polygenic models is one of degree. The former contain "several" genes (e.g., less than 10) whereas the latter include a "large number" of genes (e.g., 100). Geneticists originally developed polygenic models to describe quantitative traits such as height and intelligence. By specifying a "large number" of genes, these models could explain how discrete genes could cause traits that were continuously distributed in the population.

Since many diseases are qualitative categories—not quantitative dimensions—geneticists developed the concept of liability (Falconer, 1965). Liability describes an unobservable trait: the predisposition to onset with disease. As liability increases so does the probability of disease onset. Alternatively, we might assume that disease occurs when ones liability crosses a specific threshold.

In some ways, the MFP model is easier to handle statistically than oligogenic inheritance, despite the large number of components involved. Although the MFP model posits that many genes and environmental factors contribute additively to disease causation, these individual factors are not directly modeled. According to the model, liability is normally distributed. Individuals above a certain threshold on

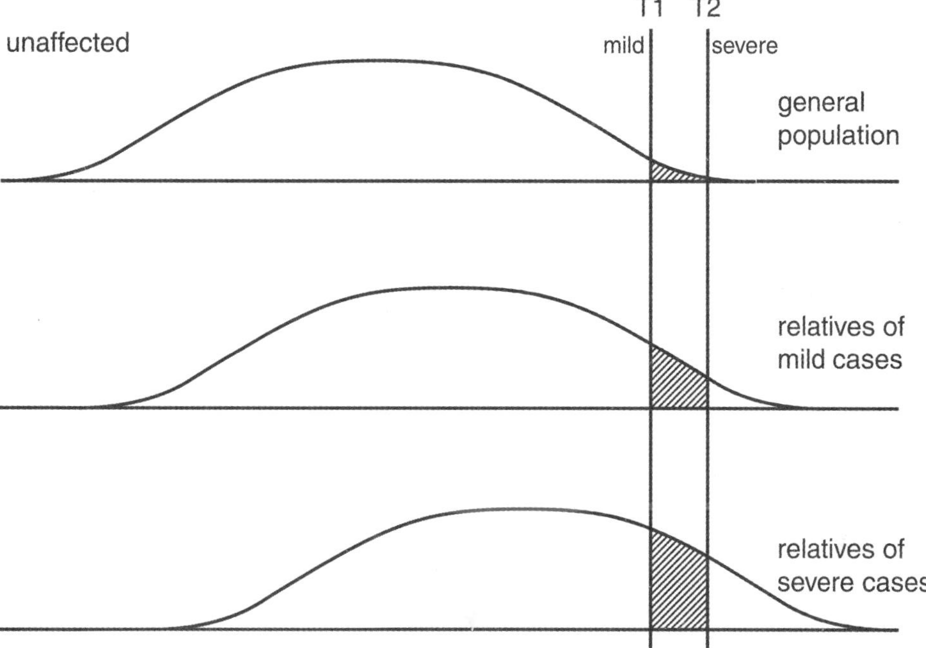

Figure 2. Multifactorial polygenic liability threshold model. The two thresholds delimit mild and severe forms of the disorder.

the liability scale manifest the disorder. More than one threshold may be placed along the liability continuum, representing varying degrees of severity, as illustrated in Figure 2. Individuals to the right of the right-hand threshold will develop a severe form of the disorder. Those to the left of the left-hand threshold may have minor problems or be unaffected, while those whose liability falls between the two thresholds would have an intermediate form of the disorder.

For example, some researchers have suggested that bipolar and unipolar disorders might be severe and mild variants of mood disorders. In this case, individuals above the highest threshold develop bipolar disorder, those below the lowest threshold are normal and those in between have unipolar disorder.

Using the statistical method of path analysis, the MFP model has been generalized to evaluate the relative contributions of genetic and environmental effects. Path analysis models partition the observed covariances or correlations between family members (with regard to a trait or disorder) into several components. Examples of such components are: (1) the effect of transmissible environment on phenotype (the cultural heritability); (2) the effect of genotype on phenotype (the genetic heritability); (3) the effect on phenotype of environmental factors unique to twins or siblings; (4) the effect of transmissible parental environment on the transmissible environment of a child raised by the parent; (5) the correlation between transmissible parental environments (i.e., nonrandom mating); (6) interactions between genes and environment; and (7) correlations between genes and environment.

McGue and colleagues (1985) applied a path analytic model to analyze family data on schizophrenia and tuberculosis. Like schizophrenia, tuberculosis aggregates in families. Unlike schizophrenia, the etiology of tuberculosis is known: originally thought to be a genetic disease, it is now known to be transmitted through a bacterial infection. The parameter estimates obtained from the path analysis of schizophrenia family data indicate a high and significant genetic heritability (0.67) along with a low and non-significant cultural heritability (0.19). For tuberculosis these estimates were reversed: genetic heritability was estimated to be 0.06, while the estimate for cultural heritability was 0.62. The familial aggregation of tuberculosis was correctly attributed to environmentally transmitted factors. This validation of the path analytic MFP model on a disorder with a known mode of transmission further validates the results of the analysis of the schizophrenia data in this study.

The **mixed model** posits that both MFP and single gene components may be involved in disease etiology. Statistical analysis of the mixed model can determine if either component alone can provide an adequate fit to the data, or if the null hypothesis of no single gene effect and no MFP effect fits best. For example, one report of a mixed model analysis of data on 79 chronic schizophrenic probands and their families (Risch and Baron, 1984) concluded that although a polygenic model also fit, these family data were consistent with a mixed model in which the major gene was recessive, had a high gene frequency and a very low penetrance.

Unfortunately, segregation analysis techniques have not yet been successful in demonstrating a definitive mode of transmission for most psychiatric disorders. There are many such studies of families with mood disorders (Tsuang and Faraone, 1990; Faraone et al., 1990) and schizophrenia (Faraone and Tsuang, 1985). One exception may be Tourette's Syndrome, a neuropsychiatric disorder characterized by multiple vocal and motor tics. Some data show the transmission of this disorder to be autosomal dominant with incomplete and sex-specific penetrance and variable expression (Pauls and Leckman, 1986).

Where is the Gene (or Genes) Located

Eventually, psychiatric genetic research leads to questions such as, "Where is the gene located?" and "What are the genetic and environmental mechanisms of disease?" This stage of inquiry requires colleagues from molecular genetics, because they can provide the methods for tracking the inheritance of these disorders through families (Faraone et al., 1999). Linkage analysis is a more powerful method of establishing genetic etiology for the psychiatric disorders than the statistical methods of segregation analysis. Segregation analysis can only show that the pattern of disease is consistent with a specific genetic model. Linkage analysis can actually determine where the gene is located on the human genome.

The search for disease genes faces formidable obstacles. Paramount among these is the number of potential disease genes. Each of us has over 50,000 genes. Moreover, only 10% of our chromosomal material (DNA) contains the coding sequences (i.e., instructions) for these genes. The average gene is made up of 3,000 base pairs (the building blocks of DNA). But the entire set of chromosomes (the **genome**) contains 3 billion base pairs. Thus, searching for disease genes might seem as difficult as looking for a needle in a haystack.

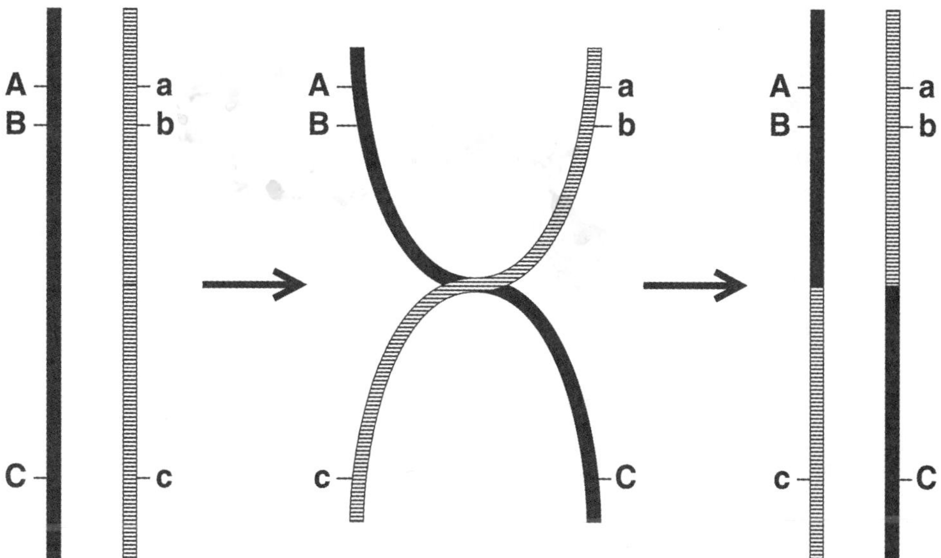

Figure 3. Schematic representation of a single crossover.

Fortunately, geneticists and statisticians have solved this genetic needle in a haystack problem. Today, there is no question that current molecular genetic and statistical technologies can find the genes that cause genetic disorders. In fact, the list of diseases with known disease genes grows each year. Examples include Huntington's disease, Alzheimer's disease, cystic fibrosis, Duchenne's muscular dystrophy, myotonic dystrophy, familial colon cancer, von Recklinhausen neurofibromatosis, and a form of mental retardation due to the fragile X syndrome. The methodology for finding genes, known as linkage analysis, is now fairly routine.

Background for Linkage Analysis. Linkage analysis is made possible by the **crossing over** that takes place between two **homologous** chromosomes during **meiosis**, the process whereby gametes are created. Genetic transmission occurs because we inherit one member of each pair of chromosomes from our mother and one from our father. However, these inherited chromosomes are not identical to any of the original parental chromosomes. During meiosis, the original chromosomes in a pair cross over each other and exchange portions of their DNA. After multiple crossovers, the resulting two chromosomes each consist of a new and unique combination of genes.

Figure 3 schematically demonstrates the result of a single crossover. In the figure, the original pair of chromosomes is represented as one dark and one light strand. Three different genes are represented with uppercase and lowercase letters signifying different alleles at the same locus.

Figure 4 represents the new chromosome pair produced by multiple crossovers. When meiosis is complete, each gamete will contain one chromosome from each of the newly formed pairs. As the figure indicates, the probability that two genes on the same chromosome will recombine during meiosis is a function of their physical

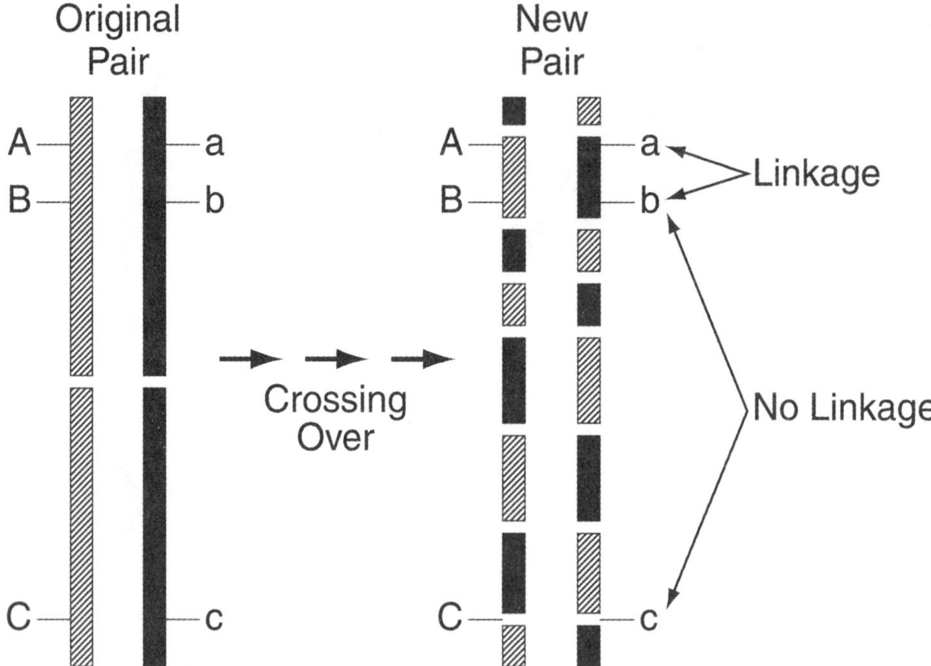

Figure 4. The new pair of chromosomes created by many crossovers.

distance from one another. We say that two loci on the same chromosome are "linked" when they are so close to one another that crossing over rarely or never occurs between them. Closely linked genes usually remain together on the same chromosome after meiosis is complete. The greater the distance between loci on the same chromosome, the more likely it is that they will recombine. This biological fact makes it possible to locate genes that are risk factors for disease.

In addition to the physical distance between loci, the number of crossovers that occur between them will determine whether or not they will recombine. An odd number will result in recombination, whereas an even number will not. If two loci are very far apart, the probability of an odd number of crossovers between them is equal to the probability of an even number. As a result, the probability of recombination is 50%. Therefore, genes on the same chromosome that are very far apart from one another are transmitted independently, as are genes on different chromosomes.

Genetic Markers for Linkage Analysis. Linkage analysis determines if a putative disease gene is closely linked to a known **genetic marker**. A genetic marker is a measurable human trait controlled by a single gene with a known chromosomal location. The marker must be **polymorphic** (i.e., more than one version of the gene exists with high frequency), and its mode of inheritance must be known. Early linkage studies used genetically controlled traits as genetic markers. Examples include color blindness, blood groups, enzymes, proteins, and systems such as human leukocyte antigen (HLA) that control immune response.

The use of genetically determined traits as genetic markers greatly restricted the use of linkage analysis because, compared with the size of the genome, relatively few markers were available. Because of their rarity, the *a priori* probability that a trait or disorder might be mapped to a known chromosomal location was low. Moreover, although these markers were polymorphic they were not remarkably so. As we discuss later, highly polymorphic markers are best because they increase the statistical power of linkage analyses. Fortunately, molecular geneticists developed laboratory methods that directly characterize DNA samples. Because of this, it is now possible to have genetic markers useful for testing linkage to all portions of the genome.

An early example of a DNA marker is the Restriction Fragment Length Polymorphism or RFLP (Botstein et al., 1980). Restriction endonucleases cut DNA into pieces. The locations of the cuts are determined by the sequence of the **nucleotides** in the DNA. There are four nucleotides: adenine (A), guanine (G), cytosine (C) and thymine (T). For example, the restriction endonuclease known as Alu I cuts DNA between the nucleotides guanine and cytosine wherever the nucleotide sequence AGCT occurs. The size of the resulting fragments is determined by the particular sequence of base pairs in the gene. Since these fragments can be measured in the laboratory, family members can be classified according to the length of the fragment that results from cutting their DNA with Alu I.

The more polymorphic the marker locus is, the higher will be the frequency of heterozygotes and therefore the more useful or informative the locus in linkage analysis. This feature of the marker is called the **polymorphism information content** (PIC) (Botstein et al., 1980). PIC is a probability that an individual will be heterozygous at the marker locus, because homozygous individuals are not informative. An ordinary RFLP can only have two forms; either the cleavage site is present or absent; therefore, the maximum possible frequency of a heterozygote in a two-allele system is 0.5. If we designate the presence of a restriction site as "present" and its absence as "negative," then the probability of a heterozygote ("present"/"absent") would be $0.5 \times 0.5 = 0.25$, and the probability of an "absent"/"present" heterozygote would be $0.5 \times 0.5 = 0.25$. In sum, the probability of a heterozygote would be $0.25 + 0.25 = 0.50$.

To increase the informative nature of an allelic locus, it is important to find marker loci that have more than two alleles. Occasionally, more than two RFLP sites may occur close enough together to be detected by a single probe. Then the variants can be treated as **haplotypes**. A haplotype is a set of alleles at more than two closely linked loci on a single DNA molecule. In general, the concept of the haplotype is only applied to a small region of a chromosome that will not be disrupted by recombination.

Much higher levels of heterozygosity are associated with a more common class of polymorphisms that occurs in repeated sequences. These are called **minisatellites** (Jeffreys and Wilson, 1985) or **variable number of tandem repeats** (VNTRs). These hypervariable loci consists of tandem repeats of oligonucleotides ranging from 10 to 60 base pairs long. The variability results in the number of repetitions of the unit sequence. Another class of tandem repeats involve dinuclotides, such as CA or TG, where the dinucleotides might be repeated 15 to 60 times. These are called **microsatellites**. It has been estimated that there are 50,000–100,000 CA or

TG repeats, or about 1 every 30–60,000 bp. However, these polymorphisms do not have definite associated phenotypes.

The newest types of markers are **single nucleotide polymorphisms** (SNPs), which are the most common type of sequence variations. Single nucleotide polymorphism (SNP) results from a single base change in which one nucleotide substitutes for another. Some SNPs create a restriction enzyme site, while others do not. SNPs are abundant and are found throughtout the genome (e.g., in exons, introns, promoters). It is anticipated that during the next two years, the SNP Consortium will generate approximately 300,000 SNPs (Marshall, 1999). It is estimated that SNPs occur, on average, every 1000 bp and have low mutation rates. However, as biallelic markers (e.g., two alternative bases), SNPs are generally less informative than microsatellite markers.

However, some current problems regarding SNPs' use limit the wide application of the SNPs in gene identification (Schork, 2000). For example, detection of an association between a specific SNP and a complex disease involves the selection of an SNP sufficiently close to the disease gene (e.g., in linkage disequilibrium or nonrandom association of alleles). The use of a greater density of markers may increase the chance of finding markers with significant association with the disease. Alternatively, haplotype analysis (e.g., using two- and three-locus halotypes rather than single locus) to investigate the association between disease loci and multiple markers may improve finding positive associations. Future uses of SNPs not only include gene discovery and mapping, but also association-based candidate polymorphism testing in diagnostics and risk profiling. However, as SNP maps and technologies develop, additional clarifications regarding their use in clinical and research arenas will be necessary.

DNA Biosensors and Gene Chips. The newest efforts in DNA analysis include DNA biosensors, gene chips and miniatruized DNA analyzers (Wang, 2000). DNA biosensors and gene chips acquire sequence specific information faster, simpler, and cheaper than traditional DNA hybridization assays. DNA biosensors use biological reactions to recognize the different nucleic acids. Multiple biosensors in connection with DNA microarrays are the newest techniques for analysis of complex DNA samples. The strengths of these devices are in the miniaturization, speed. and accuracy of the analysis. DNA microchip technology offers enormous potential for rapid multiplex analysis of nucleic acid samples. In addition, this technology offers great promise for monitoring gene expression. For example, current technology can identify differential gene-expression arrays between diseased and nondiseased samples. Hybridization studies using different colored fluorescent tags enable researchers to quantify gene expression changes in healthy versus diseased samples. This technology has not yet been widely applied to research in psychiatric disorders. While the application of DNA biosensors and gene chip technology remains in its infancy, we anticipate that such devices will impact future human genetics research.

Statistical Methods for Linkage Analysis. The statistical methods of linkage analysis capitalize on both the occurrence of crossing over and the availability of polymorphic genetic markers. They seek to compute a statistic indicating the probability that the cosegregation of genetic markers and disease within pedigrees exceeds what we would expect from the play of chance alone. Thus, linkage analysis assesses the association of disease and marker *within* families.

Linkage methods must be distinguished from the association method (discussed in a later section). This latter method assesses the association of disease and marker in individuals from different families. As an example, we would say that a population association exists between a gene and schizophrenia if schizophrenics are more likely than suitable controls to have a specific version of the gene. For example, if 80% of unrelated schizophrenics had the A version of the gene compared with only 10% of unrelated controls, we would conclude that the gene is associated with schizophrenia.

In contrast, a linkage study attempts to show that within pedigrees, schizophrenic family members tend to have the same version of the gene. For example, consider a finding of linkage between schizophrenia and a DNA marker that is expressed as one of two alleles, A or B. This means that in some families the schizophrenic members would be more likely to carry the A allele at the marker locus. If they transmitted the schizophrenia gene to offspring they would also be very likely to transmit the A allele at the marker locus. However, in other schizophrenia families, the schizophrenic patients might be more likely to carry the B version of the marker allele. If they transmitted the schizophrenia gene to offspring they would be very likely to transmit the B allele at the marker locus. The key point is that ill members from the *same* family tend to carry the same marker allele near the disease locus. If this seems confusing it may be helpful to note that the marker gene is not the disease gene; it is only physically close to the disease gene. By chance, different families will have different versions of the marker gene linked to the disease gene.

The Affected Relative Pair Method. The affected relative pair method of linkage analysis evolved from the affected sib-pair method (Weeks and Lange, 1988; Ward, 1993). The original "identity by descent" affected sibpair method worked with pairs of ill siblings having parents with four different alleles at the marker locus. That is, the father carried two versions of the gene and the mother carried two versions that differed from the father's. For example, the father might have allele A and B and the mother might have C and D. Under the null hypothesis of no linkage, the distribution of alleles shared by siblings at the locus is well defined. For example, consider any of the alleles, say A. The probability that the father transmitted it to the first child is 0.50. The probability of transmitting it to the second child is also 0.50. Therefore, the probability that he transmits A to both children is 0.50 times 0.50 or 0.25.

Now assume that the marker locus is close to a disease locus and that the two children have the disease. Because both have the disease gene, both share a segment of DNA that contains the gene and surrounding loci. The size of this segment is not fixed (it depends upon where crossovers occurred). However, the probability that the marker locus is on this segment increases with the proximity of the marker to the disease locus. If the marker and disease loci are contiguous, then the children who inherited the disease gene should also have inherited the same allele at the marker locus. We say that the shared marker allele is "identical by descent" to indicate that the alleles observed in the children are copies of the same parental allele. We know this is so only because the sibling pair method requires parents to have four different alleles at the marker locus. For example, suppose the father has allele *A* and *B* and the marker locus and the mother has *C* and *D*. If two of their children each have allele C at the marker locus then (ignoring the very small probability of mutation), we know that their *C* alleles are copies of their mother's *C* allele. Thus their *C* alleles are identical by descent.

Thus, a statistical test was developed to determine whether the observed distribution of marker alleles differed significantly from what was expected under the hypothesis of no linkage. The method was later generalized to the case in which the parental marker alleles were not all unique. In this situation we can determine if alleles are "identical by state" but not if they are "identical by descent." Identity by state means that the two alleles are the same but we cannot be certain if they are copies of the same parental gene. For example, suppose the father has allele *A* and *B* and the marker locus and the mother has *A* and *C*. If two of their children each have allele *A* at the marker locus, then we cannot determine if both received it from the father, both from the mother or one from the mother and the other from the father. Identity by state methods are needed when the marker is not polymorphic enough to result in four different alleles in the parents. Unfortunately, the loss of identity by descent information reduces statistical power (Bishop and Williamson, 1990).

The affected relative pair method is a general form of the sibling pair method. It allows all ill relative pairs to be included in the analysis. As is the case with siblings, linkage between a marker and a disorder increases the probability that any pair of ill relatives will share the same version of the DNA marker. The major advantage of the affected relative pair method is that we can use it without knowing the mode of inheritance of the disease. This makes it very appealing for studies of psychiatric disorders: As we discussed earlier, segregation studies have not been able to confirm specific modes of inheritance for these disorders. Thus, we can detect linkage with no *a priori* knowledge of the genetic and environmental parameters that mediate familial transmission. However, by eliminated information about the mode of inheritance, the method sacrifices some statistical power.

The Lod Score Method. In contrast to affected relative pair methods, the lod score method requires knowledge of the mode of inheritance. Although it is possible to estimate the mode of inheritance and test for linkage simultaneously, the usual practice is to test for linkage under an assumed genetic model. We do so by estimating the **recombination fraction**: the probability that the disease and marker genes will recombine during meiosis. The lower the probability, the greater the likelihood of linkage. The most widely used method is to compute a maximum likelihood estimate of the recombination fraction. Then a likelihood ratio test compares the odds of the data occurring given that estimate with the odds of the data if the true recombination fraction is 0.5 (this is our null hypothesis because unlinked loci recombine with a probability of 0.5).

This likelihood ratio is an odds ratio comparing the probability that linkage is present with the probability of no linkage. Since we usually examine the base 10 logarithm of the odds ratio, the test statistic is known as the lod score (log of the odds ratio). Lod scores can be summed over pedigrees. Lod scores greater than 3 are considered to be evidence in favor of linkage, while lod scores less than -2

constitute evidence against linkage. Thus, a linkage analysis will support the hypothesis of linkage if the odds favoring linkage are 1,000 to 1 (i.e., log[1000/1] = 3).

As noted above, the main drawback of the lod score method is that we must specify parameters that describe the mode of genetic transmission. However, there is a way around this problem. Greenberg (1989) showed that if we analyze our data several times under different modes of inheritance, the lod score will be greatest for the model that is closest to the true mode of inheritance. For example, we might choose to examine two dominant models and two recessive models. We might also vary the assumed frequency of the gene in the population.

So far, we have been discussing linkage analyses that involve only two loci: one marker locus and one disease locus. Since a disease gene will be surrounded by many potential marker loci, these "two point" analyses will not have optimal power to detect linkage and locate the gene. Multipoint analyses use several markers simultaneously during the linkage analysis. Multipoint mapping improves statistical power by using all available marker information in the area of the putative disease locus (Spence, 1987). Lander and Botstein (1986a, b; Lander, 1988) proposed "interval mapping" which assesses linkage, not to a single marker, but to an interval flanked by a pair of markers. Xu et al. (1998) evaluated interval mapping with statistical simulations. Compared with single point analyses, interval mapping was much more powerful, requiring 30% fewer families to detect linkage. Moreover, interval mapping was more robust to misclassification of penetrances, diagnoses, and phenocopies. Although these considerations favor a multipoint approach, the method must be used with caution. Risch and Guiffra (1992) showed that, if the mode of transmission is complex , multipoint analyses can spuriously reject linkage. However, they also show that this problem is mitigated when using high estimates of the disease allele frequency.

The lod score method has been generalized for the detection of linkage heterogeneity. That is, we can test the null hypothesis that all families are linked in favor of an alternative hypothesis that only a proportion are linked. Ott (1983) demonstrated that the Admixture test of linkage heterogeneity had better statistical properties than the Predivided Sample test. Risch (1988) developed a Bayesian procedure (the B-Test) and compared it to the Admixture and Predivided Sample tests. He concluded that the Predivided Sample test was the least suitable and that the B-test and Admixture test were similar in power. The Admixture test also has the advantage of providing estimates of (1) the recombination fraction for the linked form and (2) the proportion of linked families in the sample.

In lod score analyses, the statistical test for linkage is the lod score obtained at the maximum likelihood estimate of the recombination fraction. As this lod score increases, the evidence favoring linkage also increases. Traditionally, a lod score of three or more had been considered to be statistically significant evidence of linkage. As Ott (1991) showed, this corresponds, asymptotically, to a type I error rate of 0.0001 with 0.001 as an upper bound. This rather stringent significance level is necessary due to the low prior probability of linkage.

However, the lod score criterion of three (LOD3) may not be appropriate for complex genetic diseases like schizophrenia. A number of concerns that have been raised in the literature are worth noting. First, the LOD3 criterion was originally designed by Morton (1955) for Mendelian diseases for which it was reasonable to compute a prior probability of linkage. For nonmendelian diseases the prior probability is unknown (Clerget-Darpoux et al., 1990; Green, 1990). Morton also assumed that the test was carried out sequentially as pedigrees were collected. Thus, LOD3 does not apply to analyses of fixed sample sizes (Clerget-Derpoux et al., 1990).

The LOD3 criterion must also be adjusted for the effects of testing multiple markers. This includes both the assessment of linkage at multiple loci and the use of multiple markers to assess linkage at a single locus (Clerget-Darpoux et al., 1990; Edwards, 1990; Edwards and Watt, 1989). When there is a meaningful prior probability of linkage, Ott (1991) demonstrated that the critical alpha level should be no greater than 0.001 for as many as 100 markers but should be no greater than $1/1000 \times [g - 100]$ when the number of markers, g, is greater than 100. For the nonmendelian case there is no simple analytical solution because the prior probability of linkage is unknown (Green, 1990).

Another procedure that inflates the type I error rate is the use of multiple disease definitions in sequential linkage analyses (Goldin, 1990). For a Mendelian disease assessed with m different phenotype definitions, Green (1990) suggested adding $\log_{10}\{m\}$ to the lod score criterion. Although this is a relatively small effect, the simulation study of Clerget-Darpoux et al. (1990) showed that the error rate at LOD3 may be greater for complex diseases. Moreover, by maximizing the lod score over different modes of inheritance we are also inflating the type I error rate. Both Green (1990) and Ott (1990a) suggested that simulation methodology may be the only means of effectively controlling the type I error rate when studying nonmendelian disorders.

Guidelines for interpreting linkage results for complex genetic disorders have adjusted the usual 5% probability of false positives since linkage analysis typically consists of multiple statistical tests. For example, a genome-wide scan may initially genotype 400 markers, followed by 100 additional markers. Thus, Lander and Kruglyak (1995) proposed three levels of statistical significance for use in the interpretation of genome-wide linkage results. Suggestive linkage would occur by chance once during a genome-wide scan. For the lod score method, the p-value would be less than 0.0017 and for the sib-pair method, $p < 0.0007$. Significant linkage refers to a chance event of 0.05 times during a genome-wide scan. For this level of significance, they defined the lod score $p < 0.000049$ and for the sib-pair method, $p < 0.00002$. "Confirmed linkage" refers to the finding of a significant linkage in an initial scan, and independently confirmed in another sample.

The use of computer simulation methods to determine the appropriate lod score criterion was demonstrated by Weeks et al. (1990b). Briefly, the procedure is as follows. First, the linkage analysis is performed on real data by maximizing the lod score over genetic models and phenotype definitions. After a high lod score is found, a second analysis is performed on the same pedigrees. The only difference between the two analyses is that the first analysis uses the real marker data and the second uses simulated marker data. In the second analysis, the markers are simulated under the assumption that the disease and marker are not linked. In the simulation, marker genotypes are assigned to subjects whose parents were not studied based on the marker gene frequencies used in the first analysis and the assumption of **Hardy-Weinberg equilibrium**. Marker genotypes are assigned to other pedigree members by simulating Mendelian laws of transmission on the pedigree. The simulation step is replicated many times and, for each replicate, we record the maximum lod score attained. This provides us with the distribution of maximum lod scores expected under the null hypothesis of no linkage. To set a type I error rate of α, we choose the lod score corresponding to the $1 - \alpha$ point on the cumulative maximum lod score distribution computed by the simulation. To estimate probabilities in the upper tail of the maximum lod score distribution accurately many replications are necessary.

When the observed maximum lod score from the actual linkage analysis exceeds all of the simulated maximum lod scores, the estimated type I error rate is 0. In this case, to ensure that the true type I error rate is no greater than 0.001 with $100(1 - \phi)\%$ confidence, Weeks et al. showed that the number of simulation replicates should be greater than $\log\{\phi\}/\log\{0.999\}$. Thus, for a 95% confidence interval, 2,995 replicates are required. By maintaining a comprehensive and systematic record of all linkage analyses performed, we can generate accurate rules for declaring the statistical significance of lod scores.

Another concern in assessing the statistical significance of a linkage finding is the fact that all individuals in the sample do not contribute equally to the lod score. For example, although several factors led to the reversal of Egeland et al. (1987) highly significant linkage finding for bipolar disorder, one of these was a change in affection status of several pedigree members (Kelsoe et al., 1989). Clearly, a significant linkage finding will be more compelling if we can demonstrate that it would not lose significance if a followup study of the sample were to find a few changes in diagnosis. The computer program VaryPhen determines the degree to which the magnitude of lod scores depends on each individual in the pedigree. A final caution in the use of linkage methods is the specification of marker allele frequencies. Linkage analysis algorithms require the user to specify the population frequencies of the different alleles at the DNA marker locus. Freimer, Sandkuiji and Blower (1993) provided a discussion of this issue. They pointed out that, for some markers, it may be difficult to get correct allele frequencies because these can vary dramatically between ethnic subgroups. They note that this problem is relevant when the linkage analysis must reconstruct marker genotypes, a situation that is not unusual. Their simulations show that misspecification of allele frequencies does not affect statistical power, but can lead to both false negative and false positive linkage results. Thus, they suggest that linkage analysts determine how sensitive their results are to changes in marker allele frequencies by running several analyses.

Statistical Power. In planning and conducting a linkage study, it is important to consider the number of pedigrees (or ill relative pairs) needed to show linkage. Although the detection of heterogeneity is also of interest, it requires a much larger sample size than does the detection of linkage under heterogeneity (Cavalli-Sforza and King, 1986; Ott, 1986; Clerget-Darpoux et al., 1987; Martinez and Goldin, 1989, 1990).

Goldin and Gershon (1988) calculated the number of schizophrenic sib-pairs needed to detect linkage. Their autosomal dominant model assumed a population prevalence of 1% and no **phenocopies** (subjects without the pathogenic gene who develop the disease). The probability of persons becoming schizophrenic was 0.5 if they had one or two copies of the disease allele. They also assumed that (1) the identity by descent (IBD) of marker alleles is known exactly, that is, the marker was highly polymorphic, and (2) 50% of sibships were linked. They examined results for two values of the recombination fraction: 0.01 (which indicates very close linkage) and 0.1 (which indicates linkage, but at a ten-fold greater distance). Under these conditions, 50 pairs achieved 80% power for a recombination fraction of 0.01; while 120 pairs achieved the same level of power for a value of 0.10. Since, given the degree of polymorphism of most DNA markers, the sib-pair method usually needs information from parents, this would require data from 200 and 440 people (2 siblings and 2 parents per family), respectively, for recombination fractions of 0.01 and 0.1.

Bishop and Williamson (1990) investigated the power to detect linkage by using identity-by-state (IBS) methods. For a rare dominant disease, they found that pairs of affected grandparent–grandchild or affected first cousins were more informative for linkage analysis than pairs of affected siblings. Assuming that a marker of four alleles with equal frequency is used and that all affected relative pairs were linked with the marker, they calculated the sample size needed to detect linkage for pairs of affected grandparent–grandchild or affected first cousins. For example, for a dominant disease gene with a frequency of 0.022 and no phenocopies, 50 pairs of first cousins had 80% power to detect linkage if the recombination fraction was 0.05; the power was 20% if it was 0.20. The sample size needed increased when heterogeneity and phenocopies are allowed. Unlike the determination of IBD scores, the determination of the IBS distribution does not require information from other relatives. Thus, although in principle the power to detect linkage per pair is lower for the IBS method compared with the IBD method, the number of individuals needed for genotyping of the marker may not differ greatly between these two methods.

As pointed out by Goldin and Gershon (1988) and Bishop and Williamson (1990), the power calculations for affected sib-pairs or affected relative pairs are usually based on a 0.05 significance level; this is much less stringent than the traditional lod score significance cutoff of 3, which is approximately equal to 0.001. If the 0.001 significance level is used, the number of affected sib-pairs needed increases about 1.7 fold (88). Thus 200 sib-pairs (400 individuals) rather than 120 pairs (240 individuals) would be needed to achieve 80% power for a recombination fraction of 0.1. To make the affected relative pair significance level comparable to the traditional lod score method, Risch (1990b) proposed a maximum lod score criterion of 3 to assess the significance of linkage for relative pairs.

Risch (1990c) parameterized the IBD distribution for various relative pairs in terms of a risk ratio λ_R, which is the risk to type R relatives divided by the population prevalence. He demonstrated that λ_R is the critical parameter in determining the power to detect linkage using affected relative pairs. Based on data of McGue et al. (1983), Risch (1990b) estimated that λ_R is approximately 10 for schizophrenia. Assuming that there is no genetic heterogeneity and that a fully informative and tightly linked marker (recombination fraction = 0.0) is used, approximately 50 affected sib pairs would have 80% power to detect linkage. If the recombination fraction is 0.10, approximately 170 pairs are needed to achieve 80% power. Risch (1990d) also showed that the power of relative pairs is very sensitive to the polymorphism of the marker. For example, although 40 sib pairs have 70%

power when the marker is fully informative (i.e., very polymorphic), the power falls to 10% when the informativeness decreases by 30%.

The work of Cavalli-Sforza and King (1986) shows that it is relatively easy to achieve high power to detect linkage by using the lod score method if the disease has clear mendelian modes of transmission. For a fully penetrant dominant disease without phenocopies, 14 nuclear families each comprising two parents and three children would achieve a 50% power of detecting linkage for a recombination fraction of 0.1. This assumes that the affected parent is **heterozygous** at the marker locus, and that all families are linked. If only 50% or 30% of the families were linked, then the number of families required would be 52 and 138, respectively. These figures are optimistic for psychiatric genetics since psychiatric disorders are unlikely to be fully penetrant; **phenocopies** probably exist and genetic heterogeneity is likely.

Martinez and Goldin (1989) used a more complex model of disease in their assessment of the sample size needed for the detection of linkage. In their study, the disease prevalence was fixed to be 2%. For a dominant disease with a penetrance of 0.9 and a phenocopy rate of 5%, the average number of nuclear families (three siblings with at least one affected) needed to achieve 50% power at a recombination fraction of 0.01 was 28; this assumed that 50% of the families were linked to a fully informative marker (Martinez and Goldin, 1989). If the penetrance decreased to 0.5 then the number of families needed to maintain 50% power increased to 101. When analyses were limited to families having sibships of three with at least two affected, the power increased substantially. Using the same marker and assuming the penetrances of 0.9 and 0.5, the number of families (three siblings with at least two affected) needed to achieve a 50% power were 25 and 53, respectively.

Chen, Faraone, and Tsuang (1992b) assessed the statistical power for linkage studies of schizophrenia by simulating schizophrenia pedigrees. These simulations used the known demographic, epidemiologic, and familial features of the disorder to create pedigrees that one would expect to ascertain in a linkage study of schizophrenia. They then evaluated the power of the pedigrees using simulation methodology. They assumed that penetrance was incomplete (0.189) and age-dependent, 16% of cases were phenocopies and markers were moderately informative. Compared with Martinez and Goldin (1989), they assumed a much lower penetrance (0.189 vs. 0.5), a higher phenocopy rate (16% vs. 5%), and a 30% less informative marker. Nevertheless, for a given level of power, the sample size needed under their assumptions was not much greater than that reported by Martinez and Goldin.

For example, consider the sample size needed to attain 50% power when the recombination fraction is approximately 0.01 and 50% of families are linked with the marker. For a penetrance of 0.5, Martinez and Goldin (1989) showed that any one of the following three types of families were needed: (1) 101 nuclear family of sibship size three with at least one affected child (202 of 505 individuals affected); (2) 53 nuclear family of sibship size three but with at least two affected children (146 of 265 individuals affected); or (3) 41 nuclear families of sibship size four with at least two affected children (117 of 246 individuals affected). In these nuclear families, about one-half of the obligatory gene-carrying parents would also be affected. In the simulations by Chen et al. (1992b), 50 multigeneration pedigrees with at least 3 affected individuals were needed to achieve the same level of power. These pedigrees contained approximately 150 affected individuals and 500 subjects in total. This total is nearly identical to that in (1) above but the proportion affected is lower (30% vs. 40%). The total number of subjects is about twice that in (2) and (3) above but these latter methods require approximately half the sample to be affected. Although cases (2) and (3) require only half the sample needed, this difference is not that dramatic given that, compared with Chen et al.s findings, the results for (1), (2) and (3) assume a much higher penetrance and a much lower phenocopy rate.

What is perhaps most notable in this comparison is that the number of *affected* individuals required to achieve the same power is very similar. This suggests that the contribution of unaffected individuals to the linkage analysis is limited. Indeed, Goldin and Martinez (1989) demonstrated that ignoring marker and disease loci information of unaffected individuals results in only a small increase in the average sample size needed to detect linkage. This is intuitively reasonable. Because models of psychiatric disorders assume low penetrance, unaffected individuals are ambiguous. They may be gene carriers—who do not express the gene—or they may not carry the gene. This conceptual ambiguity translates into a loss of statistical power for the unaffected cases.

We can refer to the above referenced papers on power analysis for a general idea of how to plan for a linkage study (See also Levinson, 1993a, b). However, once the diagnostic data are collected, we can use simulation methods to estimate the power for a specific sample. Boehnke (1986) proposed using statistical simulations to evaluate the power of known pedigrees. The method now handles reduced penetrance, phenocopies, and heterogeneity (Ploughman and Boehnke, 1989; Ott, 1989a). Specialized computer programs such as SIMLINK (Ploughman and Boehnke, 1989) accomplish this purpose.

SIMLINK needs only information about phenotype, age, and pedigree structure from generated pedigrees. Genotypes must be simulated in the power analysis. To simulate genotypes, SIMLINK requires the genetic parameters of the disease locus, including the gene frequency, penetrance of each genotype, and the diseases age at onset distribution.

After generating trait genotypes, SIMLINK generates marker genotypes according to a given marker allele frequency, mendelian transmission, and the recombination fraction between trait and marker. To compute the statistical power under genetic heterogeneity, SIMLINK allows us to specify that only a proportion of pedigrees are linked to the marker. After simulating trait and marker genotypes, a maximum likelihood algorithm estimates the recombination fraction and the proportion of pedigrees linked to the marker.

For a user-specified number of replications, SIMLINK simulates the cosegregation of the disease locus with a marker locus under the assumption of a true recombination fraction r. For each replication, SIMLINK computes lod scores for several test recombination fractions (e.g., 0.01, 0.05, 0.10, 0.20, 0.30, 0.40, 0.50). For each replication, SIMLINK determines the maximum lod score for that replication. After the user-specified number of replications, say N, we are left with a distribution of N maximum summed lod scores. For a specified lod score threshold of declaring linkage, the relative frequency that the maximum summed lod score exceeds the threshold is the power of the linkage test.

Alternatives to Linkage Analysis. Linkage analysis has been extremely successful for diseases with well-defined modes of inheritance. However, it has not yet gleaned genes for psychiatric disorders. Because of this, some investigators have turned to association studies and related techniques.

Association Studies. As we discussed above, the process of crossing over during meiosis shuffles the parental genes so that the chromosomes we receive from our fathers and mothers are not identical to any of their original chromosomes. Thus, through the generations, genes are constantly shifting from one chromosome to another. As a result, we should expect no association between alleles of genes on the same chromosome. For example, assume that locus 1 can have allele a or A and locus 2 can have allele b or B. If the two loci are on the same chromosome then the probability that any chromosome contains the pair Ab, $P(Ab)$, should be equal to the probability of A, $P(A)$, times the probability of b, $P(b)$. That is, $P(Ab) = P(A) \times P(b)$. Similarly, $P(AB) = P(A) \times P(b)$ and so on. Put simply, if we know that a chromosome contains allele A at locus 1, this tells us nothing about the probability of locus 2 containing allele B or b.

This random distribution of alleles at different loci on the same chromosome is only partially true. It is an empirical fact that some loci are associated with one another so that $P(Ab)\ P(A) \times P(b)$ (100). For example, it may be that chromosomes with allele A at locus 1 are more likely to have allele b at locus 2 than we would expect by chance (i.e., than we would expect from the frequency of allele b in the population). Now, assume that locus 1 is a disease locus and that A is a dominant pathogenic allele. Also assume that locus 2 is a DNA marker locus. If the two loci are associated as indicated above, then people with the disease should be more likely to have marker allele b than people without the disease.

This nonrandom association of alleles at different loci is called linkage disequilibrium. Knowledge of its causes is essential if it is to be a tool for finding disease genes. One cause of linkage disequilibrium is the fact that the reshuffling of genes on chromosomes depends on genetic distance. If two genes are very close to one another, then they will rarely be separated by crossing over and will usually be transmitted together. Thus, due to close linkage, the alleles at two loci will tend to be transmitted together. We say "tend to" because eventually crossing over will separate them.

Fortunately, the reshuffling of linked genes can take many thousands of years. This means that, theoretically, we should be able to detect associations between diseases and DNA markers if the marker locus is *very close* to the disease locus. Compared with a linkage study, the design and analysis of an association study is straightforward. We do not require pedigrees with multiple ill members. Samples of unrelated patients and controls will suffice. Instead of a complex linkage analysis, all we need do is compare the rates of marker alleles (or genotypes) in patients and controls with standard statistical tests (Vogel and Motulsky, 1986).

A major disadvantage of association studies is that the DNA marker must be tightly linked to the disease gene. This is in contrast with the linkage method which can detect linkage over relatively large distances. Thus, with linkage analysis it is possible to "scan the genome," which is a shorthand way of saying that, if we use many markers, we can test for linkage to all chromosomal loci. In contrast, for an association study to succeed we need to know where to look for the gene. But, the reason for doing linkage and association studies is to find the gene. So how do we know where to look?

Since we do not know where to look, we can make some educated guesses. When we make such a guess we are specifying a *candidate gene*. Once we have a candidate gene we find a DNA marker that is very close to that gene and proceed with our association study. Ideally, a candidate gene would have a known pathophysiological significance. For example, Alzheimer's disease leaves a clear pathophysiological signature on the brain (senile plaques containing β-amyloid). Since the production of β-amyloid requires the amyloid precursor protein (APP), the APP gene was a logical candidate gene for Alzheimer's disease. The examination of APP as a candidate gene was further motivated by symptomatic and pathophysiological correspondences between Alzheimer's disease and Down's syndrome (Schweber, 1985). The latter syndrome was known to be caused by a trisomy of chromosome 21 and the APP gene had been mapped to chromosome 21 (Korenberg et al., 1988). Thus, APP was clearly a candidate gene for Alzheimer's disease and, eventually, studies of the APP gene among Alzheimer's disease patients found unequivocal mutations (Goate et al., 1991; Chartier-Harlin et al., 1991; Naruse et al., 1991; van Duijn et al., 1991).

Unlike Alzheimer's disease, most psychiatric disorders do not have a known pathophysiology that points to an obvious candidate gene. For example, although schizophrenia is undoubtedly a disease of the brain, the pathophysiological details have eluded careful investigation. There are many genes that *might* be relevant to schizophrenia, but none of these are credible candidate genes in the sense that the APP gene was a credible candidate for Alzheimer's disease. For example, neurotransmitter systems are dysregulated in many psychiatric disorders and the location of relevant genes is now known. Examples include genes for monoamine oxidase (Bach et al., 1988; Hsu et al., 1988a, b), dopamine-β-hydroxylase (Kobayashi et al., 1989; Lamouroux et al., 1987), tyrosine hydroxylase (Grima et al., 1987), dopamine receptor subtypes (Bunzow et al., 1988; Dearry et al., 1990; Grandy et al., 1989; Sunahara et al., 1990; Zander et al., 1981) and many others.

Psychiatric geneticists have tried to capitalize on plausible links between such genes and psychiatric illness (Blum et al., 1990; Gelernter et al., 1991; Nothen et al., 1992; Schwartz and Moises, 1993), but not without controversy (Conneally, 1991; Kidd, 1993; Pato et al., 1993). The failure of association studies to produce consistently reproducible results supports Crowe's (1993, p 76) contention that "candidate genes in psychiatry are lottery tickets." As Crowe discussed, there are approximately 30,000 genes expressed in the human brain. Any of these could be a "candidate" for psychiatric disease, yet none are well justified to the same degree that the APP gene was a credible candidate for Alzheimer's disease. As a result, the *a priori* probability is low that any one of these is associated with a specific disease.

Crowe computed that the likelihood of a false-positive result is so high that one would have to set a statistical significance level of 0.00001 to achieve a false-positive rate of 5%. If we were to use a significance level of 0.001, 80% of positive findings would be false. The traditional α level of 0.05 would yield 99.5% false-positive results.

The problem of false positive results is exacerbated by the fact that close linkage is not the only cause of disease-marker associations (Vogel and Motulsky, 1986;

Kidd, 1993; Crowe, 1993). The frequencies of DNA marker alleles varies among ethnic groups. Thus, if patient and control groups are not carefully matched for ethnicity, spurious differences in allele frequencies between groups will emerge. Also, closely linked loci can exhibit linkage disequilibrium—but this is not a necessity. Kidd (1993) gave the example of phenylketonuria (PKU), a single gene disorder of amino acid metabolism. Although the PKU gene is close to several DNA markers, none of these show linkage disequilibrium.

Because of the problems discussed above, association studies must be used and interpreted with caution. Kidd (1993) suggested that consistent replication would be the best evidence for a true association. However, he also cautioned that, to be a true replication, a subsequent study should use methods that are similar if not identical to the methods of the original study. Crowe (1993) also emphasized the importance of standardized research methods and suggested selecting probands from multiplex pedigrees to ensure that we are studying a genetic form of the illness.

Because it may be difficult to find patient and control groups that are suitably matched for ethnicity, several investigators have developed tests of linkage disequilibrium that use the parents of ill individuals as controls (Rubinstein et al., 1981; Falk and Rubinstein, 1987; Spielman et al., 1993; Ott, 1989b; Knapp et al., 1993). For example, the **transmission test for linkage** disequilibrium (TDT) uses families having at least one affected offspring and one parent who is heterozygous for the DNA marker to be tested (Spielman et al., 1993). The TDT compares the number of times heterozygous parents transmit the associated marker allele to affected offspring with the number of times they transmit the other marker allele. If these probabilities differ from what is expected by chance, then we can conclude that linkage disequilibrium exists. Although the TDT solves the problem of ethnicity matching, it still faces the problem of false positives and must be cautiously interpreted in the absence of a credible candidate gene.

Family-based association methods help to overcome some of the problems posed by ethnicity and population admixture. In these methods, such as the transmission disequilibrium test (TDT), parents or siblings of patients are used as controls. Since each parent transmits only one allele to a child, the allele that is not transmitted to the child is used as the control allele. The statistical test involves comparisons of the transmitted versus the nontransmitted allele. Because both alleles come from the same parent, there are no differences in ethnicity.

For example, consider the following table, which demonstrates a hypothetical example of dopamine D_2 receptor alleles in 50 schizophrenia families, including the affected proband and his or her parents:

Nontransmitted Alleles		D_2-1	D_2-2
Transmitted Alleles	D_2-1	25	5
	D_2-2	65	5

The most useful information gleaned from these 50 families is the 70 heterozygous parents; 65 of them transmitted the D_2-2 allele and did not transmit the D_2-1 allele. Only 5% of the parents transmitted the D_2-1 allele and not the D_2-2 allele. Thus, these data suggest that the D_2-2 allele is preferentially transmitted to the affected offspring. The TDT compares the probability that the heterozygous parents transmit the associated marker versus the other marker. If these probabilities differ by chance, then linkage disequilibrium likely exists. The weakness of these methods is that only one candidate gene can be tested at a time and that the gene is either the disease gene or is one very close to the disease gene. Methods for using single nucleotide polymorphisms in association studies to scan the genome are currently under development.

Mutation Screening. Since psychiatry has few (some would say no) good candidate genes, some investigators have suggested that, instead of demonstrating associations with polymorphic DNA markers, we should demonstrate associations with mutations that have pathophysiological significance. As we discussed previously, DNA markers are often selected because many variants exist. These markers are usually in "noncoding" portions of the genome.

Linkage studies value the high level of polymorphism of junk DNA because it increases statistical power. The physiological function of the marker is irrelevant. However, in the absence of a candidate gene, associations with junk DNA can be meaningless because such DNA could not cause the disease being studied. Because of this, several investigators have suggested that we search directly for mutations that have pathophysiological significance (Crowe, 1993; Sobell et al., 1992). In short, the goal of these methods is to find an association between an allele and a disease, not because the two are closely linked but because the allele causes the disease. Several variants of this approach have been proposed.

One approach identifies a candidate gene that is known to have two or more alleles that are of functional significance. For example, the D_4 dopamine receptor gene has several allelic forms that differ in their ability to bind the neuroleptic drugs that treat schizophrenia (Sommer et al., 1993). Thus, Sommer and colleagues compared the D_4 dopamine alleles of schizophrenics with those of controls. Although they found no differences, their work illustrates an important point: Group differences in the D_4 dopamine gene would have been more compelling than differences in a DNA marker that is next to the D_4 dopamine gene.

This first approach is useful but lacks a key ingredient: it is possible for a gene to have several different "normal" alleles of no pathophysiological significance. Thus, investigators have sought methods that identify clear mutations. For example, Crowe (1993) noted that the nature and location of apparent mutations provide information about the probability of their being pathological. He also discussed how laboratory methods can be used to demonstrate the effects of an apparently mutant gene.

A second approach to finding mutations comprises several methods that have been described as "mutation screening." Gejman and Gelernter (1993) describe the strengths and weaknesses of four types of mutation screening: **single stranded conformational polymorphisms** (SSCP), denaturing gradient gel electrophoresis, mismatch cleavage, and DNA sequencing. The epidemiologist need not know the details of each method. The key point to remember is that each method searches candidate genes for allelic variants that should have pathophysiological significance.

Methods of mutation screening represent a major advance in the application of the case–control association study. However, these methods are only a beginning. Replicating the finding and demonstrating linkage will be necessary before any "plausible mutation" can be seriously considered as a cause of disease. Replication may be difficult because, like the traditional association study, these methods are subject to the problem of false positives created by case–control differences in ethnicity and the absence of credible candidate genes.

Cytogenetic Abnormalities in Psychiatric Disorder. Cytogenetic studies examine the chromosomes under a microscope. Different human chromosomes are different sizes and have different patterns of banding when stained by various dyes. Different types of cytogenetic stains allow identification of duplications (e.g., extra segments of a part of a chromosome) or deletions (e.g., missing segments in a part of a chromosome). A routine cytogenetic study of all chromosomes or **karyotype** would screen for obvious abnormalities in chromosomal numbers, arrangement and shape.

Although cytogenetic abnormalities associated with psychiatric disorders are rare, they can facilitate gene discovery. Consider the example of Duchenne's muscular dystrophy. One patient had a small deletion on the X chromosome, which eventually led to the identification of the causative gene. Several such examples exist in families with schizophrenia, one includes chromosome 22q11.2 deletions. This deletion syndrome includes patients with velocardiofacial syndrome (VCFS), DiGeroge syndrome, and conotruncal anomaly face syndrome. The deletion is typically detected using a commercially available **fluorescent in situ hybridization** (FISH) probes. The prevalence of psychiatric disorders is high in 22q deletion syndromes. One group of investigators reported that about 26% of 50 adults with 22q deletions had schizophrenia or schizoaffective disorder (Murphy et al., 1999). Although no other single chromosomal abnormality approaches the apparent association between 22q deletions and schizophrenia, cytogenetic abnormalities on multiple other chromosomes may have associated psychiatric disturbances. Chromosomal abnormalities that have associated positive genetic linkage findings provide additional support for regions that may harbor susceptibility genes.

SAMPLING, DESIGN AND STATISTICAL ISSUES

This section contains a discussion of some of the methodological issues facing the genetic epidemiologist working in psychiatry. For further details see Faraone et al. (1999).

Ascertainment

Ascertainment or sampling is critical to an accurate assessment of the mode of inheritance. In epidemiology, sampling bias occurs when the sampling procedure creates a sample that systematically differs from the population it purports to represent. For example, we know that people who volunteer to be part of a "normal" control group have rates of psychopathology and its correlates that exceed the population expectation (Gibbons et al., 1990; Kruesi et al., 1990; Shtasel et al., 1991; Buckley et al., 1992; Risch et al., 1990; Thaker et al., 1990). Another type of bias occurs when we want to generalize our results to all people with a disorder but sample patients from a psychiatric clinic. Clearly, people who seek treatment will differ systematically from those in the community who do not.

There are many ways for a sample to be biased. However, in genetic epidemiology we use the term "ascertainment bias" to refer only to biases that affect the distribution of illness in the family. By distribution we mean the number of ill family members and the pattern of illness in the family. For example, if we design a project that recruits families having one ill parent and one ill child, we will create a sample that appears to have a dominantly transmitted disorder (because unlike recessive disorders these are usually seen in both generations of a nuclear family).

Ascertainment bias occurs when we do not sample families randomly. It is a ubiquitous problem for genetic epidemiology because the low prevalence of most genetic disorders makes it impractical to randomly sample families. For example, in a study of schizophrenia, which has a base rate of about 1% in the population, we would have to screen many hundreds of families before obtaining a sufficient sample size. Since random sampling is not feasible, we must resort to proband sampling.

A proband is a person with the illness under study who brings the family to the attention of the investigator. We say that a family has multiple probands if we independently ascertain more than one family member with the disease from the sampling frame. This will occur, for example, when we are sampling from a clinic if ill family members use the same clinic.

The literature on ascertainment problems and their remediation is complex. We will restrict our comments to the "classical" model of ascertainment, developed by Weinberg (1925) and Fisher (1934).[2] There are two types of ascertainment: complete and incomplete. **Complete ascertainment**, is difficult to attain. It refers to a simple random sampling of families to find those which have one or more members with the disease of interest. With proband sampling we have incomplete ascertainment. There are three types of incomplete ascertainment. In **truncate ascertainment**, the probability of an ill individual's being sampled (represented as π) is high. Therefore, all ill members of a family will be probands and everyone in the population with the disorder is sampled. From the point of view of statistics, this is the most desirable method of accomplishing incomplete ascertainment since, as Weinberg (1925) and Fisher (1934) demonstrated, it is not necessary to adjust data analyses statistically for this type of sampling. The estimation of genetic parameters under truncate ascertainment produces essentially the same result as under random sampling. This is so because the probability that a family is ascertained is not dependent on family size. Thus, we are not biasing families to have unusually high (or low) rates of illness. Unfortunately, truncate ascertainment is very difficult to carry out. It is only feasible for rare disorders treated in a tertiary care setting, where it is fairly certain that every ill person in a defined population will eventually be seen.

[2]The classical model may not always be appropriate, for a variety of reasons. See Ewens and Shute, 1986; Greenberg, 1986; Shute and Ewens, 1988a, b for a discussion of relevant issues.

The other extreme of sampling is **single ascertainment**. In this case, π, the probability of sampling any one person who is ill, is very low. Because of this there will be only one proband per family. In other words, assume we are sampling bipolar patients from the Boston metropolitan area. Under single ascertainment the likelihood that any specific bipolar patient in Boston will be in our sample will be very low (e.g., 0.01). Because of this, the likelihood of sampling two bipolar patients from the same family is extremely low.

Single ascertainment creates a very specific type of bias: Families with many ill members are more likely to enter a given sample. For instance, if, in a family of ten, there are six people with bipolar disorder, whereas only one of a family of three has the disorder, then the first family has six chances to be ascertained but the second family has only one chance. Thus, under single ascertainment, the probability of sampling a family is proportional to the number of ill members. This means that our estimate of the proportion of ill siblings in any sibship will be too high.

The goal of genetic modeling is to correct for this sampling bias. Fortunately, it is easy to correct our estimate of the proportion of ill siblings: We merely exclude the proband from the analysis. Thus, the proportion of ill siblings of the probands estimates the proportion of ill siblings (among sibships expressing the disorder) that we would have found had we used random sampling.

Sometimes, a proband sampling procedure is neither single nor truncate ascertainment. We call this intermediate case **multiple ascertainment**. As its name suggests, under multiple ascertainment more than one family member is independently sampled as a proband but not all ill family members are probands. Thus, π, the probability of sampling any given person who is ill, is between zero and one. In this situation, we correct our estimate of the proportion of ill siblings by weighting multiple proband families by the number of probands in the family.

As discussed in a prior section, correction for ascertainment is necessary for segregation analysis if we are to estimate correctly the parameters of genetic transmission. Thus, it is of paramount importance, in genetic epidemiologic studies, to specify the ascertainment scheme as precisely as possible before data collection begins. If the ascertainment is uncertain, an investigator cannot accurately estimate genetic parameters. If the ascertainment scheme is misspecified, then inferences drawn from the data may be false. Sometimes, investigators who have collected family data without intending to estimate genetic parameters as one of their original goals will decide later that they are interested in doing just that. Then when these investigators consult a genetic epidemiologist about carrying out segregation analyses, they are disappointed to learn that their data are unsuitable for such analyses simply because the ascertainment scheme was either not clearly specified or was nonsystematic.

The distinction between sampling procedures that are ill specified and those that are nonsystematic deserves some comment. An ill-specified sampling plan is one that cannot be reproduced because the methods of ascertainment were never recorded. We call ascertainment nonsystematic if we cannot determine which ill family members brought the family to the attention of the study. In other words we cannot be certain who the probands are. For example, if we use advertisements soliciting families with "two or more cases of schizophrenia" we are often not certain which patients in, say, a family with four schizophrenic siblings "caused" the family to be sampled. Because of this, if we ascertain families nonsystematically they cannot be used for segregation analysis to estimate genetic parameters. A second problem is that we often cannot define the population base from which we nonsystematically sampled families. This hinders our ability to generalize results.

Although these last two points argue against nonsystematic approaches to sampling, other factors must be considered as well. Paramount among these are issues of cost and efficiency. For example, families with more than one case of schizophrenia are rare (McGue and Gottesman, 1989, 1991; Pulver and Bale, 1989); systematic surveys can find such families but only at a very high cost. Since linkage studies do not *require* prior segregation analyses, it is reasonable to argue that the costs of systematic ascertainment cannot be justified. This argument gains more strength by the observation that, in the past, segregation analyses of psychiatric disorders have sometimes led to conflicting results (Tsuang and Faraone, 1990; Faraone et al., 1990).

Before leaving our discussion of ascertainment bias, we must emphasize that although investigators can choose to ascertain systematically or not, they do not have complete control over the type of systematic ascertainment (i.e., single, multiple, truncate, complete). For example, in planning a family study of a common disorder we may decide to sample from a hospital clinic. Although characteristics of the disorder may lead us to expect single ascertainment, it is always possible for us to learn that some of our probands come from the same family. Thus, it is necessary for genetic epidemiologic investigations to keep track of who is and is not a proband so that multiple ascertainment can be detected—and corrected for—should it occur.

Estimating Risk to Relatives

The simplest and perhaps most common means of analyzing genetic epidemiological data is to compute the rate of illness among relatives of ill probands and compare this with the rate observed among relatives of suitable control probands. As we discussed in the previous section, to be meaningful, these rates must be corrected for ascertainment bias. In this section we discuss two other issues that must be considered: the correlation in risk among relatives and the variable age at onset of most psychiatric disorders.

Lack of Statistical Independence Among Family Members. When comparing a group of relatives of bipolar patients with relatives of normal controls on the presence or absence of bipolar disorder, one of the many statistics available for assessing association in a 2×2 contingency table would seem to be suitable. The rows of the table would be formed by the probands diagnosis (bipolar or not) and the columns by the relatives diagnosis (bipolar or not). This would be fine if we had sampled only one relative from each family.

However, it is usually more cost effective (and genetically interesting) to sample as many relatives from a specified class (e.g., siblings) as possible. In this case, the outcomes of the relatives are not necessarily statistically independent of one another. That is, the probability of one relative being bipolar may vary with the number and pattern of bipolar relatives in the family. Since this would be true under a variety of models of genetic and/or environmental transmission, it is a priori unreasonable to assume statistical independence when analyzing such data (Weissman et al., 1986).

The statistical dependence among relatives is *theoretically* a problem. However, we know of no available statistical research that indicates to what extent this problem invalidates inferences made from statistical tests that ignore it. It seems unlikely that the estimate of rates would be biased, but the p-values from statistical tests will probably not be accurate. The degree and direction of this inaccuracy are unknown, but it is reasonable to speculate that the increased similarity of relatives (compared with unrelated subjects) would decrease the variance of estimates and increase the type I error rate.

Fortunately, there are several statistical approaches that can handle this problem. The most straightforward way to compute an accurate significance level is to use the proportion of probands having at least one ill relative as the index of familiaty. Thus, the unit of analysis becomes the proband. Since the sampling design can assure that the probands are statistically independent, we can proceed with traditional statistics (e.g., the chi-square test, logistic regression). If we are assessing a quantitative outcome (e.g., the intelligence scores among siblings of probands), we can use the mean of all relatives from a class (e.g., compute the mean intelligence score for each sibship). These means can then be analyzed with traditional statistics (if other assumptions are not violated).

Another approach is to use statistical models that do not assume independence of observations. The problem of nonindependence can be handled with the regressive models developed by Bonney (1984, 1986, 1987; Borecki et al., 1990). These models can use either categorical or continuous traits as dependent variables. They flexibly expand the well-known linear regression and logistic regression models to incorporate situations of nonindependence. The regressive logistic framework is particularly suitable for genetic work because in controlling for nonindependence due to familial correlations it allows for the estimation of parameters of genetic and environmental transmission (see the following discussion). The major drawback to this approach is that it sets the data analyst along the path of segregation analysis, which can be very time-consuming and may not be in the statistical repertoire of many investigators doing family studies.

Variable Age at Onset. Most psychiatric disorders have a variable age at onset. In some cases the range of age at onset is very wide. For example, although most patients with schizophrenia experience their first symptoms in their twenties or early thirties, some cases can begin in childhood and others after fifty. Variable age at onset hinders any interpretation of simple rates of illness because these will depend on the age of the sample. For example, say that the rate of schizophrenia was 10% in a sample of addolescents and 10% in a sample of 50 year olds. We ought to have some means of adjusting these rates to reflect our intuitive sense that the rate among adolescents—who have only just entered the period of risk—indicates a greater risk for schizophrenia than the rate among the fifty year olds—who have lived through most of the period of risk.

We achieve this adjustment by computing the **morbidity risk**: the probability that the subjects being studied are susceptible to the illness of interest (Vogel and Motulsky, 1986). An individual who is susceptible may not have onset at the time of examination, or may have died due to an unrelated cause. Thus, the morbidity risk is a probability, not a rate. It is the probability that a person will manifest the disorder if he or she lives (or had lived) long enough. For this reason, the morbidity risk is sometimes called the **lifetime risk.** Methods to estimate morbidity risk adjust the raw rate of illness in a sample to account for the well subjects who have not lived through the risk period.

If n is the total number of subjects, and m is the total number of affected then the raw rate of illness is simply m/n . Since some of the n subjects who are well may eventually onset with the disorder, the raw rate will always underestimate the morbidity risk. Thus, one approach to morbidity risk estimation has been to adjust the denominator downward. The adjusted denominator has traditionally been called the **Bezugsziffer (BZ).**

The BZ is a sum of weights reflecting each subject's length of exposure to risk up to the age of examination. If w_i is the weight for ith individual, then the morbidity risk, MR, is estimated by

$$\widehat{\text{MR}} = \frac{m}{\sum_{i=1}^{n} w_i}.$$

To assign w_i, Weinberg (1925) suggested that we empirically define a risk interval from the lowest to highest possible age at onset. For the ith individual whose age at examination is y_i, we assign $w_i = 0$ if y_i is less than the lowest age at onset, $w_i = \frac{1}{2}$ if y_i is within the risk period, and $w_i = 1$ if y_i is greater than the oldest age at onset. This method is easy to use, but limited because it assumes that the risk for onset is uniform from the lowest to highest age at onset. Chase and Kramer (1986) demonstrated that these problems could lead to a biased estimation of the true morbidity risk.

Strömgren (1935) proposed a method that assumes we know the age at onset distribution of the disease. He suggested we use the cumulative distribution, F, function of age "y" at time "i" (y_i) to create weights (w_i), that is, $w_i = F(y_i)$. For example, if the 50th percentile of the age at onset distribution was at age 25, then 25-year-olds would be given a weight of 0.50 because they have lived through only half the period of risk. If the 90th percentile were at age 60, then 60-year-olds would have a weight of 0.90.

With this approach, the estimated morbidity risk is unbiased (Larsson and Sjögren, 1954; Risch, 1983). Strömgren (1938) realized that his original method would estimate the morbidity risk to be greater than 1 under some conditions (e.g., when every subject in the sample is affected). Thus, he modified the formula such that the affected cases contribute 1 to the denominator and are thereby not weighted by their age at examination. However, several researchers have shown that this modified estimator is biased and have advised against its use (Larsson and Sjögren, 1954; Risch, 1983; Thompson and Weissman, 1981).

For computing confidence intervals or testing hypotheses, we must calculate the variance of the estimated morbidity risk. In a simplified form, the variance of the morbidity risk is a modification of the variance of a proportion, with the sample size replaced by the BZ,

$$\text{Var}(\widehat{\text{MR}}) = \frac{\widehat{\text{MR}}(1 - \widehat{\text{MR}})}{\sum_{i=1}^{n} w_i}.$$

This equation is sufficient for an approximate estimate of the MR such as Weinberg's shorter method. However, for Strömgrens estimator, a more exact form should be used (Larsson and Sjögren, 1954; Risch, 1983):

$$\text{Var}(\widehat{\text{MR}}) = \frac{\widehat{\text{MR}}}{\sum_{i=1}^{n} w_i}\left(1 - \frac{\widehat{\text{MR}}\sum_{i=1}^{n} w_i^2}{\sum_{i=1}^{n} w_i}\right).$$

Given that a prior age at onset distribution is available, Risch (1983) derived a maximum likelihood estimate (MLE) of the morbidity risk. The MLE estimate of the morbidity risk has a smaller variance than Strömgrens estimator and, for small samples, is less biased (Risch, 1983). Moreover, the MLE method can estimate the age at onset distribution simultaneously with the morbidity risk (Risch, 1983). This is useful when the age at onset distribution is unknown. Also, other methods assume that the age at onset distribution is known without error. However it has always been estimated from a sample. By simultaneously estimating the morbidity risk and the age at onset distribution, the MLE method computes a more accurate estimate of the variance of the morbidity risk. However, with simultaneous estimation, other factors, such as missing data and the form of the age at onset distribution must be considered. (For a more detailed discussion, see Cupples, Risch, Farrer, and Myers (1991) and Chen, Faraone, and Tsuang (1992a)).

To compute unbiased estimates of risk, Strömgren's method and the maximum likelihood approach must either assume or estimate the correct age at onset distribution. In practice, the required age at onset distribution is usually estimated from the observed ages at onset observed among the proband sample. However, the observed age at onset is biased toward younger ages by the underlying age structure of the susceptible population (Chen et al., 1992a; Heimbuch et al., 1980; Baron et al., 1983; Chen et al., 1993). Using the observed age at onset distribution from prevalent cases can lead to a nonnegligible bias in samples of young subjects (Chen et al., 1993). Thus, it is important to obtain an age at onset distribution corrected for the underlying population age structure rather than relying on the observed distribution.

Morbidity risk estimation must address the differential probability of disappearance from observation at any particular age between susceptible and nonsusceptible groups (Sturt, 1985). In practice, one main cause of disappearance is mortality; others include loss of follow-up or refusal of participation. Both may be increased in samples of psychiatric patients. Strömgren's method is biased by such effects but Risch's (1983) maximum likelihood method is not.

A second approach to estimating morbidity risk uses concepts from survival analysis (Lee, 1980). Statisticians developed this method to model the time to a specific outcome (e.g., the death of a patient or the failure of a machine). The survival function is the cumulative probability that the outcome does not occur as a function of time. A key feature of survival analysis is that it handles censored data; a censored datum comes from a subject who does not die, but is not observed for the entire study period.

For morbidity risk estimation, the outcome of interest is onset of illness, and the survival function presents the cumulative probability of being free from illness as a function of age. Censored cases are subjects who are unaffected at the time of examination. Thus, to apply this approach we need to know the subject's age at onset (if they have the disorder) or their age at examination (if they do not).

An early survival analysis approach to morbidity risk estimation was the Weinberg morbidity table (Slater, 1971). This was an approximation of the life table approach to survival analysis (Lee, 1980). Both methods have been superseded by the Kaplan–Meier approach (Kaplan and Meier, 1958). This latter method is approximately unbiased in large samples; the other methods are not (Breslow and Crowley, 1974). Since the information needed to compute LTR for both the actuarial and Kaplan–Meier methods is the same, the latter is the method of choice.

The Kaplan–Meier method is as follows. Suppose there are n individuals whose survival times, $t_{(i)}$, $i = 1$ to n, are available. First, we sort the n survival times in increasing order such that $t_{(1)} \le t_{(2)} \cdots t_{(n)}$. If there are tied survival times, censored ones are put before uncensored ones. Then the survival function at time t, $S(t)$, is:

$$\hat{S}(t) = \prod_{t_{(r)} \le t} \left(\frac{n - r}{n - r + 1} \right),$$

where r runs through those positive integers for which $t_{(r)} \le t$ and $t_{(r)}$ is uncensored. The morbidity risk to time t, MR(t), equals $1 - S(t)$. The variance of the Kaplan–Meier estimate of $S(t)$ is given by Greenwood's formula,

$$\mathrm{Var}\left[\hat{S}(t)\right] = \left[\hat{S}(t)\right]^2 \prod_{t_{(r)} \le t} \frac{1}{(n - r)(n - r + 1)}.$$

Survival analysis method uses the age at onset of ill relatives to compute the morbidity risk MR(t) up to the largest age in the sample. In contrast, Strömgren's method using the age at onset distribution in probands computes the full lifetime risk. Since the available data dictates the maximum age at which we can compute MR(t), the risk to ages greater than those observed is undefined. This creates some problems in application. First, if the largest observed onset is well below the upper boundary of a known risk interval, then it is difficult to justify the MR(t) as a morbidity risk estimate. Second, comparisons of morbidity risks between groups are meaningful only when the MR(t) in each group is computed at a similar age. Third, since the number of subjects still at risk usually becomes small at large ages, the variance for MR(t) may be large.

In summary, morbidity risk estimation is needed to determine the risk for manifesting disorders having a variable age at onset. Two sets of methods are available. One uses a known age at onset distribution as a weighting system; the other uses methods from survival analysis. Strömgren's estimator or Risch's maximum likelihood estimate are the method of choice among weighting methods; the

Kaplan–Meier estimator is preferable when using the survival analysis approach. Further work is needed to choose between weighting and survival analysis methods.

Family-Study Designs

The Familial–Sporadic Design. It is likely that many psychiatric disorders are etiologically heterogeneous. That is, there may be different genetic and nongenetic forms of the disease. The familial–sporadic design seeks to develop diagnostic rules that discriminate between genetic and nongenetic forms of an illness. We say that a patient has a familial form of disease if at least one relative also has the disease (or a genetically related disorder). Otherwise, we say that the patient has a sporadic form. Thus, the familial–sporadic strategy attempts to distinguish cases of illness that are more likely to be of the genetic type from those that are more likely to be of the sporadic type. Some day, when we know which mutations cause psychiatric disorders, it may be possible to specify exact diagnostic criteria for genetic and nongenetic subforms. In the meanwhile, we must use the distinction as a "proxy" for the genetic–nongenetic distinction.

The familial–sporadic method assumes that patients having one or more ill relatives are more likely to have a genetic form of the disorder; these are designated as familial cases. Patients having no ill relatives are assumed to be more likely to have an environmental form of the disorder; they are designated as sporadic cases. The designations "familial" and "sporadic" are imperfect indicators of the probability of membership in the latent, unobservable categories of "genetic" and "environmental."

As Lewis et al. (1987) pointed out, the classification of cases as familial or sporadic is a research strategy—not an etiological model. If clinical or neurobiological measures discriminate these groups, we can learn something about the relative importance of genetic and environmental factors in subgroups defined by these factors. Also, comparisons between familial and sporadic subgroups can help us develop criteria that identify a more homogeneously familial form of the illness. The familial–sporadic strategy cannot determine the mechanism of familial aggregation (e.g., single gene vs. multigene vs. environmental transmission). We must base such inferences on other information (e.g., twin, segregation analysis, and linkage studies).

A powerful version of the familial–sporadic strategy involves the comparison of concordant and discordant MZ twins. Because MZ twins share identical genotypes, an illness having complete genetic determination should be observed in both twins. Thus, it is useful to separate MZ twin pairs that both have the disease (concordant pairs) from pairs where only one has the disease (discordant pairs). Clearly, genetic factors should be more prominent in the concordant than the discordant pairs.

The success of the familial–sporadic relies on its ability to correctly assign "true genetic" cases to the familial category and "true environmental" cases to the sporadic category. We cannot do this without error. Notably, the method is insensitive to differences in the size and age structure of families (Kendler and Hays, 1982). For example, a patient with ten relatives available for study is more likely to have an ill relative than a patient with only one relative. Therefore, the availability of relatives for study will influence the accuracy of classification.

Lyons, Faraone, Kremen and Tsuang (1989a) suggested that under some conditions even a modest relationship between the familial–sporadic and genetic–nongenetic distinctions might be useful. They conducted a power analysis employing a Monte Carlo simulation procedure based on the rates of misclassification determined by Kendler (1987). They concluded that for a sample size of 175, statistical power was moderate-to-good for effect sizes greater than or equal to one standard deviation unit. Put simply, the utility of the familial–sporadic strategy depends on the size of the samples studied (the larger the better) and the size of the true, unobservable differences between the genetic and nongenetic forms of illness.

The analysis conducted by Lyons et al. (1989a) assumed that the genetic form of the disorder was caused by a single major genetic locus. Eaves, Kendler and Schulz (1986) conducted a power analysis of the familial–sporadic distinction assuming a multifactorial polygenic process in which there is a normally distributed liability to illness that is due to numerous genes and environmental factors acting in an additive fashion. They concluded that large sample sizes of probands and relatives are required to detect etiological heterogeneity with "substantial probability" when using first-degree relatives. However, these authors calculated that use of MZ twins is a much more powerful approach; when MZ twins are used as probands compared to singletons with three first-degree relatives for each proband, there is an 85% reduction in the number of probands required for equal statistical power. For example, to achieve comparable power to a family study using one first-degree relative per proband with 1,026 relatives and probands, a study of MZ twins would require 65 subjects.

Since power analyses show that the familial–sporadic strategy has low statistical power, it is notable that—even with small sample sizes—this method has produced positive results. For example, sporadic cases of schizophrenia are more likely to have had perinatal complications and brain abnormalities by computed tomography. Familial cases are more likely to have attentional deficits (Lyons et al., 1989b). We are far from having diagnostic criteria for "familial" schizophrenia, but the available data suggest that this is a possibility.

The High-Risk Design. The high risk design has two major goals: (1) to identify risk factors that increase the probability of onset in susceptible individuals and (2) to define manifestations of psychiatric genotypes that are expressed in the absence of frank illness.

To achieve the first goal, the investigator must select a sample of subjects at high risk for the disorder who have not already onset with symptoms. Ideally, these should be as young as possible so that many risk factors can be studies. This has led to the children-at-risk paradigm in which the investigator finds parents with the disease of interest and studies their children. This design has been successfully employed in studies of schizophrenia (Erlenmeyer-Kimling, 1975; Mednick et al., 1971; Fish et al., 1992) and mood disorders (Biederman et al., 1991; Orvaschel, 1990).

The cited studies (and many others) show that the children-at-risk design yields valuable information about the early signs of illness and risk factors for onset. However, such studies are difficult to perform for two reasons. First, to define "at risk" we must use parental illness. This is reasonable, but we should be aware that not all of our "at risk" sample is truly susceptible to the illness. For example, we know from family studies that approximately 10% of the children of schizophrenic patients will eventually experience schizophrenia or some other psychotic disorder (Tsuang et al., 1993). Thus, if we start with a sample of 100 children of schizophrenic patients, only 10 will eventually become psychotic. Clearly, large samples are needed if we are to be able to observe many onsets of illness.

A second burden of the children-at-risk study is the need for longitudinal follow-up. In order to predict who does and does not become schizophrenic, the children need to be followed for many years, into adolescence and adulthood. Since some subjects will be lost to follow-up, we need to plan our initial sample size accordingly. We should also plan our assessments so that we can determine if there are meaningful differences between subjects lost versus those not lost to follow-up.

The second goal of the high risk study is to define manifestations of psychiatric genotypes that are expressed in the absence of frank illness. Such phenomena are of interest because they may provide clues to the etiology or pathophysiology of disease. They may also facilitate the discovery of genes by linkage analysis. Since this type of high risk study does not seek to predict which susceptible people develop disease, it is easier to implement than the children-at-risk design. The basic design is straightforward. We compare the biological relatives of patients with the biological relatives of controls using some indicator that we believe to measure the unobservable liability to disease.

Guidelines for validating such indicators have periodically been presented in the literature. These provide some guidance for choosing measures with which to design phenotypes for linkage analysis. A summary of these is as follows.

Specificity requires that the indicator be more strongly associated with the disease of interest than with other psychiatric conditions. Putative genotype indicators should exhibit *state independence*. The measure should be stable over time and should not be an epiphenomena of the illness or its treatment. The putative indicator should be *heritable*. An indicator that does not show familial transmission will not be helpful for linkage analyses.

We should be able to demonstrate a *familial association* between the illness and the indicator. Relatives of ill probands should express the indicator to a greater degree than an appropriate control group. The illness and the indicator should also show *cosegregation* within families. The prevalence of illness among relatives who manifest the indicator should be higher than among relatives who do not.

Finally, an indicator should have *biological and clinical plausibility*: even if shoe size met other criteria, it would be suspect as a valid indicator due to its lack of biological or clinical plausibility. Clinical plausibility might be demonstrated by showing that the indicator resembles the clinical phenomenology of the illness. For example, negative symptoms are a prominent feature of schizophrenia that may be an expression of the genotype among relatives of schizophrenic patients (Tsuang et al., 1991). Neurodiagnostic indicators will have some biological plausibility if they assess brain regions believed to be impaired by the disorder.

Examples of Algorithms for Segregation Analysis

This section provides some detailed information on two popular segregation analysis models, the unified model as implemented in POINTER (Morton et al.,

1983) and the regressive logistic model (Bonney, 1984, 1986, 1987) as implemented in REGTL (Sorant and Elston 1989a) of the Statistical Analysis for Genetic Epidemiology computer programs (Bailey-Wilson and Elston, 1989). In discussing these methods, we will focus on how the algorithms deal with issues that are particularly relevant to the genetic epidemiology of psychiatric disorders.

POINTER was originally based on the mixed model proposed by Morton and MacLean (1974). In this model, a genetic trait is assumed to be due to the influence of a major locus with Mendelian transmission, a polygenic component, and random environmental effects. For qualitative traits like psychiatric disorders, the model assumes an underlying "liability" or predisposition to illness, x, that is normally distributed, $N(u, V)$. Illness occurs only in those individuals who exceed a threshold on the liability continuum. The liability is composed of three components: (1) a major locus effect, g, with two alleles A and B; (2) a multifactorial transmissible effect, c, with normal distribution $N(0, C)$, and (3) a random, nontransmitted environmental component e, also normally distributed $N(0, E)$, with $x = g + c + e$ and $V = G + C + E$. For qualitative traits such as diagnoses, the mean (u) and variance (V) of liability are assumed to be 0 and 1, respectively.

At the major locus, the "A" allele is responsible for the increase of liability, that is, it is the disease gene. The three genotypes AA, AB, and BB have mean liabilities of μ_{AA}, μ_{AB} and μ_{BB}. The frequency of "A" is q. The displacement between the two homozygotes (AA and BB) on the scale of x is t, and the degree of dominance of the "A" allele is indexed by $d = (\mu_{AB} - \mu_{AA})/(\mu_{BB} - \mu_{AA})$. For dominant traits, $\mu_{AB} = \mu_{BB}$ and $d = 1$; for recessive traits, $\mu_{AB} = \mu_{AA}$ and $d = 0$.

The unified model extends the mixed model by including parameters to model the probabilities that individuals with the genotypes AA, AB, and BB transmit the "B" allele to offspring (Lalouel et al., 1983; Elston and Stewart, 1971). We use τ_{AA}, τ_{AB}, and τ_{BB} to denote these probabilities. The multifactorial polygenic component is indexed by the heritability parameter, h. Heritability is the ratio of the variance of the multifactorial effect to the total variance of the trait. It ranges from a low of 0, indicating no multifactorial effect, to a high of 1, indicating that the trait being modeled can be completely accounted for by multifactorial polygenic factors. POINTER can correct for variable age at onset by specifying age specific liability classes. However, this approach assumes that risk to relatives is associated with the age at onset of the proband. Unfortunately, Iselius and Morton (1991) indicated that genetic transmission probabilities are not correctly implemented in POINTER. As a result, nonmendelian transmission probabilities are not interpretable when families are selected through probands.

In the REGTL logistic regressive model, the likelihood of the data is modeled as function of the following parameters: (1) each person can be one of three types, AA, AB or BB, with the following population frequencies: ψ_{AA}, ψ_{AB}, or ψ_{BB}. For a genetic model, "A" refers to the gene that predisposes to illness and AA, AB, and BB are genotypes; (2) each type is associated with a probability that expresses the susceptibility to become ill: γ_{AA}, γ_{AB}, and γ_{BB}. Under a genetic model these are termed the "penetrances" of each genotype; (3) for disorders having a variable age at onset, the probability of becoming ill is also a function of two age distribution parameters: β (the baseline effect) and α (the age adjustment coefficient). These parameters determine the mean and variance of the logistic distribution of age at onset; (4) each type (AA, AB, or BB) is also associated with a probability that an individual of the type will transmit the "A" factor to a child. These are the transmission probabilities: τ_{AA}, τ_{AB}, and τ_{BB}.

POINTER computes the maximum likelihood estimates of parameters using the numerical maximization algorithm GEMENI (Morton et al., 1983). REGTL uses MAXFUN of the Statistical Analysis for Genetic Epidemiology computer programs (Sorant and Elston, 1989b). The likelihood ratio statistic for a test of two nested models is twice the difference of loglikelihoods, $-2\{\ln[L_1] - \ln[L_2]\}$; L_1 is the likelihood of the restricted model and L_2 is the likelihood of the general model. The restricted model is defined by placing restrictions on the parameters of the general model. A significant chisquare test statistic indicates that the restricted model provides a significantly poorer fit to the data than does the general model.

For example, under the most general model, all three transmission probabilities are estimated; in contrast, the genetic model restricts these probabilities to follow the laws of mendelian transmission (i.e., $\tau_{AA} = 1$, $\tau_{AB} = 0.5$, and $\tau_{BB} = 0.0$). Comparing this restricted model to the general model, a significant test would indicate that the genetic model could be rejected. The degrees of freedom of the chi-square test statistic are equal to the difference in the number of estimated parameters between the two models. When a parameter is estimated to equal its minimum or maximum possible value (i.e., the estimate went to a bound), the parameter is usually not counted as an estimated parameter for the purposes of computing degrees of freedom.

The likelihood ratio statistic is only appropriate when the parameters of the restricted model are a proper subset of the parameters of the general model. To test genetic and nongenetic hypotheses, a variety of restricted models can be compared to more general models. Nonnested models can be compared using Akaikes Information Theoretic Criterion (AIC), (Akaike, 1974).

$$\text{AIC} = -2\ln[\text{likelihood}] + 2[\text{number of estimated parameters}].$$

Although tests of statistical significance are not possible, smaller AICs correspond to better fitting models.

To be certain that the maximization routines converge at the true maximum, it is a good idea to estimate each model several times using different sets of starting parameter values. For POINTER, a strategy for hypothesis testing is as follows: (1) for the *Mixed* model, estimate the polygenic heritability parameter (h) along with three single gene parameters: the gene frequency (q), the degree of dominance (d) and the displacement (t). The transmission probabilities, τ_{AA}, τ_{AB}, and τ_{BB} should be fixed mendelian values (i.e., $\tau_{AA} = 1$, $\tau_{AB} = 0.5$, and $\tau_{BB} = 0.0$). (2) for the *Generic Mendelian* model fix the polygenic heritability parameter to zero. (3) for the *Dominant*, *Codominant, and Recessive Mendelian* models restrict the generic Mendelian model by fixing the dominance parameter, d, to 1.0, 0.5 and 0.0, respectively. (4) for the *Multifactorial Polygenic* model restrict the mixed model by estimating only the heritability parameter, h.

For REGTL, the strategy for hypothesis testing was as follows: (1) for the *General* model, the type frequencies must sum to 1 and each must be greater than or equal to 0 and less than or equal to 1. The transmission probabilities and the susceptibilities should be free to vary between zero and one; the susceptibilities can be different for males and females; (2) for the *Hardy–Weinberg* model restrict the general model by estimating a gene frequency (q_A) and using the genetic principle of Hardy–Weinberg to compute the type frequencies from the gene frequency; (3) for the *Sex Independent* model require males and females to have equal susceptibilities for each type (i.e., $\gamma_{ij(\text{female})} = \gamma_{ij(\text{male})}$). This tests whether the effect of type varies with gender; (4) for the *Environmental Transmission* model restrict the three transmission probabilities to be equal to one another (i.e., $\tau_{AA} = \tau_{AB} = \tau_{BB}$). By setting the transmission probabilities equal to one another, this model assumes that the type of the parent does not determine the type of the child. This tests whether the hypothesized pathogenic factor (the "A" factor) is transmitted from parent to offspring. The acceptance of this model would imply that the distribution of illness in families can be accounted for by *nonfamilial* attributes of the environment; (5) for the *Cultural Transmission* model set the transmission probabilities as follows: $\tau_{AA} = \tau_{AB} = 1$, and $\tau_{BB} = 0$. That is, individuals with the pathogenic "*A*" factor always transmit the factor, regardless of the presence of a possible second dose of that factor. Those without the pathogenic factor cannot transmit the factor. The acceptance of this model would implicate, as etiological agents, environmental factors transmitted from ill parents to their children; (6) for the "τ_{AB}-*Free* model, set the τ_{AB} parameter equal to its mendelian value of 0.5. This is a frequently used test of mendelian transmission.; (7) for the generic mendelian model set the transmission probabilities to mendelian values (i.e., $\tau_{AA} = 1$, $\tau_{AB} = 0.5$, and $\tau_{BB} = 0.0$). The susceptibilities (i.e., the penetrances for each genotype) should be allowed to vary freely between 0 and 1; (8) for the *Dominant*, *Codominant and Recessive Mendelian* models set the transmission probabilities to Mendelian values. Model dominance by requiring the penetrance of the *AB* genotype to equal that of the *AA* genotype (i.e.,$\gamma_{AA} = \gamma_{AB}$). For the recessive model, set the penetrance of the *AB* genotype to be equal to that of the *BB* genotype (i.e., $\gamma_{BB} = \gamma_{AB}$). For codominance, require the penetrance of the *AB* genotype to be midway between the penetrances of the *AA* and *BB* genotypes (i.e., $\gamma_{AB} = 5\{\gamma_{AA} + \gamma_{BB}\}$).

POINTER and REGTL use different methods to correct for the ascertainment (i.e., sampling) bias caused by the nonrandom sampling of families through probands. POINTER uses the classical approach to ascertainment correction by requiring the specification of π, the probability that an ill individual is ascertained as a proband. It is a good idea to test the robustness of POINTER's results by performing analyses with π equal to 0.1, 0.5, and 0.9. REGTL takes a conditional likelihood approach in which the likelihood one would compute for a random sample is divided by the likelihood of a conditioned subset (in our cases the probands). In REGTL analyses, all probands from each family should be included in the conditioned subset. The nonparametric approach taken by REGTL frees one from making strong assumptions regarding ascertainment which, if incorrect, could bias parameter estimation.

The population prevalence used for the calculation of likelihoods also differs between the two models. POINTER requires the user to specify the population prevalence based on prior knowledge of the epidemiology of the disease. Genetic parameters may be biased if the prevalence is specified incorrectly. In contrast, REGTL can estimate the gene frequency from the family data used for the segregation analysis. Since the method of ascertainment used by REGTL allows us to use normal control families in the segregation analysis, we can obtain a reasonably precise estimate of population prevalence because the ascertainment method corrects for the fact that the control probands were selected on basis of not having the disease. Although the control families provide little statistical information about the segregation of illness, they provide much information about the population prevalence. Since this information influences the likelihood function, it influences the final maximum likelihood estimate of prevalence.

The two algorithms take different approaches to modeling gender differences, which are common in psychiatric illness (DeLisi et al., 1989; Goldstein et al., 1989; Faraone et al., 1991; Pauls, 1979; Harris et al., 1991; Cloninger et al., 1978; Berney, 1989). In REGTL, we can test for a significant sex effect by comparing a model with sex specific penetrances for each genotype to a model in which penetrance is not sex dependent. In POINTER, we cannot test for a sex effect but must model sex differences by specifying sex specific prevalences prior to the analysis. To do this we must assume sex specific liability classes. POINTER models these classes by estimating sex specific thresholds on the liability continuum. The threshold for expressing the disorder would be higher for the sex that has the lower population prevalence of the disorder.

Disease Genes and Environmental Mechanisms. In addition to assessing the role of a specific susceptibility gene associated with disease, it is also important to consider the possible impact of other genetic and environmental factors that could interact with the gene of interest. Discovery of genes that influence the susceptibility to mental illnesses will promote further investigation of the effects of environmental risk factors. One strategy that might be used to study this interaction includes the following: a CYP2A6 polymorphism leading to altered nicotine metabolism has been shown to correlate with cigarette smoking. Persons with one variant are less likely to develop lung cancer, even if they smoked, compared to persons who have another genetic variant, even if they did not smoke. This is an example of the potential interactions between genes and environment and is a field called **ecogenetics**. In the absence of genetic information, studies of environmental risk factors may erroneously dismiss the effect of the environment. Discovery of disease-associated genotypes will enable more accurate estimates of the environmental factors of interest.

Four of the simplest gene-environmental interaction patterns described by Khoury et al. (1993) and Ottman et al. (1990) are described below. These patterns are simplistic because they only consider one single-gene locus and one environmental factor without regard to dose of exposure. Both exposures are considered dichotomous (present or absent). However, they help to illustrate the complexity of interpreting the associations between genotype and environment. It is assumed that all individuals have a background risk of I. Exposed individuals without the genotype have a disease risk $I \times Re$ (Re refers to the risk due to the environmental factor in the absence of the target genotype compared to unexposed individuals without the genotype). Therefore, if $Re = 1$, then the exposure is not a risk factor in the absence of the genotype. If $Re > 1$, then the exposure has an effect even in the absence of the genotype. Also, unexposed individuals with the susceptible genotype have a risk of $I \times Rg$ (Rg refers to the risk due to the genotype in the absence of the environmental factor). If $Rg = 1$, then the genotype requires an environmental exposure to increase disease risk. If $Rg > 1$, then the genotype alone produces excess risk. If $Rg < 1$, then in the absence of the environmental risk factor, the genotype protects against the disease. Individuals with both the genotype and environmental risk factor have a disease risk of $I \times Rge$ (where Rge is the ratio of disease risk in exposed individuals with the genotype to disease risk in unexposed individuals without the genotype; reflects the strength of the interaction). Rg, Re, and Rge are relative risks estimated in case–control studies from the corresponding odds ratios.

In epidemiologic studies, two commonly considered statistical models are the additive model, where $Rge = Rg + Re - 1$ and the multiplicative model, where $Rge = Rg \times Re$. Each of these patterns assumes that both genes and environment play a role in pathogens and the combination of adverse environment and the pathogenetic gene always leads to increased risk for adverse outcomes.

Pattern 1 assumes that neither the pathogenic gene or the adverse environment alone results in excess risk ($Rg = 1$ and $Re = 1$). The classic example is phenylalanine hydroxylase deficiency responsible for phenylketonuria (PKU). In this condition, neither genotype alone nor exposure alone produces the disease. Only the combination results in increased risk for the disease. A gene carrier cannot metabolize phenylalanine, which is an essential amino acid widely found in all diets. When this type of gene–environmental interaction occurs, the effect of the environment is only observed in individuals with the PKU gene mutation.

Pattern 2 assumes that the pathogenic genotype exacerbates the effects of the environmental risk factor but no effect in its absence ($Rg = 1$, $Re > 1$). An example of this type of interaction is sunlight exposure on skin cancer. Individuals exposed to excessive sunlight are at increased risk of developing skin cancer, but this increased risk is much greater in persons with a condition called xeroderma pigmentosa (XP). In this case, $Rg = 1$ because the genotype requires an environmental exposure to manifest clinically. However, $Re > 1$ because sunlight is a general risk factor for skin cancer even amongst individuals without XP.

Pattern 3 is the converse of pattern 2 in that having a certain genotype alone is associated with the risk, regardless of the environmental exposures. The environmental risk factor may exacerbate the outcome of the pathogenic genotype but does not affect the outcome in the absence of the genotype. In this case, $Rg > 1$, and $Re = 1$. An example may be glucose-6-phosphate dehydrogenase (G6PD) deficiency and fava beans. Eating fava beans alone does not produce anemia; whereas individuals with G6PD deficiency may develop anemia, even in the absence of fava beans in their diet.

Pattern 4 is the combination of both genetic and environmental risk factors, and the risk is the greatest in the presence of both. An example is the interaction between cigarette smoking and the inheritance of α-1 antitrypsin deficiency. Individuals with α-1 antitrypsin deficiency have a high risk of emphysema, even if they don't smoke ($Rg > 1$). Smokers have a high risk even if they don't have α-1 antitrypsin deficiency ($Re > 1$). Both conditions independently increase the risk for the development of emphysema, but the risk is the greatest in individuals with both risk factors.

The effect of genetic–environmental interactions are further complicated by the number of genetic loci involved, the nonadditivity of the genetic effects, the dose of the environmental exposure, and the presence of etiologic heterogeneity. Epidemiological studies can be useful in the initial evaluation of genetic–environmental interactions; failure to consider both components of disease may lead to erroneous inferences concerning the role of genes in disease etiology.

PSYCHIATRIC GENETICS AND PSYCHIATRIC EPIDEMIOLOGY

As this chapter shows, psychiatric genetics is a multidisciplinary endeavor. It combines the methodological talents of the epidemiologist, the mathematical proficiency of the statistician and the laboratory wizardry of the molecular geneticist. It is notable that the great pioneers of psychiatric genetics—Weinberg, Strömgren, Rudin, Slater, Essen-Möller and others—used epidemiologic methods to show that major psychiatric disorders were heritable. This set the stage for the biological revolution in psychiatry.

Although we now look toward molecular genetics and neuroscience to clarify the etiological and pathophysiological details of psychiatric illness, these are unlikely to succeed without a continued partnership with epidemiology. Indeed, with the exception of Alzheimer's disease, attempts to find genes for psychiatric illness have been disappointing (Tsuang et al., 1993).

Because of this, there has been a growing methodological literature pertaining to the linkage analysis of complex diseases such as schizophrenia (Ott, 1990a, b; Risch, 1990a–d; Lander, 1988; Merikanges et al., 1989; Weeks et al., 1990a). In this context "complex" is a shorthand way of saying that the disease is not transmitted in a simple mendelian fashion.

Many complexities plague psychiatric genetics and many solutions have been proposed in the above referenced articles. We have summarized them in ten key points as follows: (1) use standardized diagnostic criteria; (2) define diagnoses that will be included as affected cases before the data collection; (3) use assessment and diagnostic procedures that minimize false positive diagnoses; (4) ascertain pedigrees and collect data in a manner that can be reproduced by other investigators; (5) collect detailed clinical and demographic data to allow comparisons with other samples; (6) maintain complete blindness between the psychiatric diagnoses and marker statuses of all subjects; (7) implement procedures to facilitate the follow-up of pedigree members; (8) implement procedures to minimize laboratory errors; (9) use a threshold of statistical significance that takes into account the data analytic issues unique to complex nonmendelian disorders; (10) allow other investigators access to complete pedigree and clinical information relevant to any publications of linkage results.

It is instructive to note that most of these points are directly relevant to the epidemiologic foundation of a linkage study. This suggests to us that advances in psychiatric epidemiology may be needed to expedite work in psychiatric genetics.

APPENDIX

The following is a brief glossary of some of the genetic and statistical terms used in this chapter. It is based, in part on Pato, Lander, and Schulz (1989), Faraone and Santangelo (1992) and Faraone et al. (1999):

Allele: One of several alternative forms of a gene.

Autosome: A chromosome that does not determine sex; there are 22 homologous pairs of autosomes in humans.

Bezugsziffer (BZ): The adjusted denominator used in morbidity risk calculations.

CA repeat: A DNA marker evaluated with polymerase chain reaction (PCR) methodology; the method uses the fact that sequences of cytosine (C) and adenine (A) are repeated a variable number of times at many chromosomal loci. These are highly polymorphic and therefore very useful for linkage analysis.

Centimorgan: A measure of genetic distance over which the probability of recombination occurring is approximately 1%.

Chromosome: A rodlike structure present in the cell nucleus containing genes. The chromosome is made up of a long double helix of DNA and associated proteins.

Complete ascertainment: Random sampling of families from a population.

Concordant twin pair: A twin pair is concordant if both have (or both do not have) the disorder being studied. The pair is discordant otherwise.

Crossing over: The biological mechanism whereby chromosomes exchange DNA during meiosis.

Cytogenetics: The study of the number and structure of chromosomes under a microscope.

Discordant twin pair: A twin pair is discordant if one has the disorder being studied and the other does not. The pair is concordant otherwise.

Dizygotic twins: Twins who are no more genetically alike than siblings. Also called fraternal twins. (See "monozygotic twins").

DNA biosensors: Devices that utilize biological reactions to recognize the different nucleic acids.

DNA marker: A DNA marker is said to exist at a chromosomal locus when laboratory procedures can differentiate individuals on the composition of the DNA at that locus.

DNA: Deoxyribonucleic acid, a complex molecule formed by two strands of linearly arranged nucleotides. Each DNA molecule contains many genes.

Dominant: A phenotype caused by one allele is said to be dominant with respect to a phenotype caused by a second allele if an individual carrying both alleles shows the former (not the latter) phenotype.

Ecogenetics: A field that studies potential interactions between genes and environment.

Expressivity: The extent to which a given phenotype is manifest in an individual.

Family history method: The collection of diagnostic data using informants.

Family study method: The collection of diagnostic data by direct interview.

FISH, fluorescent *in situ* hybridization: A laboratory method that uses fluorescent tags to identify deletions in chromosomal segments.

Gene chips: This newest technology offers enormous potential for rapid automation of multiplex analysis of nucleic acid samples.

Gene: An inherited sequence of DNA which serves some biological function.

Genetic marker: Any measurable human trait controlled by a single gene with a known chromosomal location.

Genome: The complete set of gene loci on an organism's chromosomes.

Genotype: An individual's genetic composition at a specified chromosomal location.

Goodness of fit: The ability of a statistical model to describe data. We say a model has a good fit if it accurately predicts the observed data.

Haplotype: A set of alleles at two or more closely linked loci on a small segment of DNA.

Hardy–Weinberg equilibrium: The conditions under which gene and genotype frequencies remain constant from one generation to another. Under Hardy–Weinberg equilibrium, if the frequency of allele A is p and that of allele B is q, then the probabilities of the three genotypes are as follows: $AA{:}p^2$; AB: $2pq$; BB: q^2.

Heritability: The degree to which variability in the manifestation of the disorder (the phenotype) is influenced by genetic factors. We divide phenotypic variability (V_p) into two pieces: genetic variability (V_g) and environmental variability (V_e). Heritability in the broad sense (h^2) is the ratio of genetic and phenotypic variances (i.e., $h^2 = V_g/V_p$).

Heterozygous: A genotype is heterozygous if the two alleles at its locus are different.

Homologous chromosomes: Chromosomes that pair during meiosis. One was contributed by the father, the other by the mother.

Homozygous: A genotype is said to be homozygous if the two alleles at its locus are identical.

Karyotype: The collective features of a set of condensed chromosomes. The human karyotype consists of 23 pairs of chromosomes.

Karyotyping: A laboratory procedure that finds gross structural abnormalities in chromosomes.

Lifetime risk: The probability that individuals will onset with the illness of interest at some time during their lifetime. Also called morbidity risk.

Likelihood: The result of a computation that indexes the probability of having observed a set of data if a specific model of genetic transmission were true.

Linkage: The tendency of two alleles at different loci on the same chromosome to be inherited together. The greater the physical proximity, the smaller the probability of genetic recombination occurring between them and therefore the greater the probability they will be coinherited.

Locus: A position on a chromosome occupied by a gene or marker.

Lod score: The logarithm to the base 10 of the likelihood that a given set of data about genetic recombination arises by virtue of two loci being linked at a specified recombination fraction divided by the likelihood that the data would arise by nonlinkage. A lod score of 3 or greater has traditionally been considered strong evidence for linkage between a marker and a disease. A lod score of -2 or less is considered strong evidence for excluding linkage between a marker and a disease.

Meiosis: The process whereby gametes (sperm and egg) are created.

Microsatellites: A type of variable number of tandem repeats which typically involve dinucleotides, such as CA or TG, where they might be repeated 15 to 60 times. These types of markers are very useful in linkage analysis because they are highly polymorphic.

Minisatellites or variable number tandem repeats: A class of hypervariable loci consisting of tandem repeats of oligonucleotides ranging from 10 to 60 base pairs long. This is a class of highly polymorphic genetic markers.

Mixed model: A model of inheritance that includes both single gene and multifactorial polygenic parameters.

Mode of inheritance: The pattern of inheritance (e.g., dominant, recessive, polygenic) of a particular allele.

Monozygotic twins: Twins who share all of their genes in common. Also known as identical twins (see "dizygotic twins").

Morbidity risk: The probability that individuals will onset with the illness of interest at some time during their lifetime. Also called lifetime risk.

Multifactorial polygenic inheritance: When a large, unspecified number of genes and environmental factors combine in an additive fashion to cause disease.

Multiple ascertainment: Indicates that more than one proband is independently sampled as a proband but not all ill family members are probands. Thus, the probability of sampling any given person who is ill is between 0 and 1.

Nucleotides: The molecular building blocks of DNA: adenine (A), guanine (G), cytosine (C) and thymine (T).

Oligogenic inheritance: When several genes acting additively or interactively combine to produce a phenotype.

Pairwise concordance rate: The proportion of twin pairs in which both twins are ill. To compute this, count the number of twin pairs concordant for the disorder and divide by the total number of pairs. Use this when the probability of ascertaining any specific ill individual is so low that two ill co-twins are never independently sampled as probands

Penetrance: The proportion of individuals with a given genotype that actually manifest a particular phenotype.

Phenocopy: An individual who exhibits a trait without carrying the gene that causes the trait.

Phenotype: An observable trait.

PIC, polymorphism information content: A measure describing how useful a particular DNA marker is for genetic linkage. The information content increases with the number of different alleles of a marker.

Polymerase chain reaction (PCR): A method which creates many copies of a piece of DNA.

Polymorphic: Indicates the existence of two or more genetically different classes in a population (as in "polymorphic marker"). A DNA marker locus is said to be highly polymorphic if many different alleles exist at that locus. Markers with a high degree of polymorphism allow one to distinguish the maternal and paternal derivation of alleles observed in a sibship. High levels of polymorphism are associated with increasing levels of statistical power in linkage analysis.

Proband: Any member of a family who causes the family to be ascertained (sampled).

Probandwise concordance: The proportion of proband twins that have an ill co-twin: the number of concordant pairs plus the number of concordant pairs in which both the twins are probands, divided by the total number of pairs.

Recessive: Opposite of dominant.

Recombination fraction: The probability that the disease and marker genes will recombine during meiosis. The recombination fraction is proportional to the physical distance between the disease and marker genes. It ranges from 0 (they are "right next to one another") to 0.50 (they are on opposite ends of the same chromosome or on different chromosomes).

Recombination: Process by which a pair of homologous chromosomes physically exchanges sections yielding a new combination of genes.

RFLP, Restriction fragment length polymorphism: When a restriction enzyme is used to digest DNA, chromosomal regions are cut into fragments. Some of these fragment lengths are variable in the population. Loci where this is the case are RFLPs; they provide convenient DNA markers for linkage analysis.

Segregation analysis: A mathematical modeling procedure applied to family study data with the goal of determining the mode of genetic transmission.

Single ascertainment: Indicates that the probability of sampling any one person who is ill is very low. Because of this there will be only one proband per family.

SNP, single nucleotide polymorphisms: A type of genetic markers resulting from a single base change in which one nucleotide substitutes for another. It is the most common type of sequence variations.

SSCP, single strand conformational polymorphisms: Technique useful in the detection of nucleotide changes, including those as small as a single basepair change.

TDT, transmission test for linkage disequilibrium: Family-based association study analysis using nonshared alleles of the parents or siblings of patients as the control alleles.

Truncate ascertainment: Indicates that the probability of an ill individual's being sampled is high. Therefore, all ill members of a family will be probands and everyone in the population with the disorder is sampled.

VNTR, Variable number of tandem repeats: An RFLP which is highly polymorphic (i.e., there are many variants) because of a single DNA sequence which is tandemly repeated a different number of times for different individuals, hence the name. These are highly polymorphic and therefore very useful for linkage analysis.

ACKNOWLEDGMENTS

Preparation of this article was supported in part by the National Institute of Health Grants MH57934, HD37694, HD37999 to Dr. Faraone and MH43518 and MH46318 to Dr. M. Tsuang.

REFERENCES

Akaike H (1974): A new look at statistical model identification. IEEE Trans Auto Con AC-19:716–723.

Andreasen NC (1986): The family history approach to diagnosis: How useful is it? Arch Gen Psychiatry 43:421–429.

Andreasen NC, Endicott J, Spitzer RL, Winokur G (1977): The family history method using diagnostic criteria. Reliability and validity. Arch Gen Psychiatry; 34:1229–1235.

Bach AWJ, Lan NC, Johnson DL, Abell CW, Bembenek ME, Kwan S-W, Seeburg PH, Shih JC (1988): cDNA cloning of human liver monoamine oxidase A and B: molecular basis of differences in enzymatic properties. Proc Nat Acad Sci 85:4934–4938.

Bailey-Wilson JE and Elston RC (1989): Statistical Analysis for Genetic Epidemiology. New Orleans, Dept. of Biometry and Genetics, LSU Medical Center.

Baron M, Risch N, Mendlewicz J (1983): Age at onset in bipolar-related major affective illness: Clinical genetic implications. J. Psychiatric Res 17:5–18.

Berney TP (1989): Fragile X syndrome and disorders of the sex chromosome. Curr Opin Psychiatry 2:593–598.

Biederman J, Rosenbaum JF, Bolduc EA, Faraone SV, Hirshfeld DR (1991): A high risk study of young children of parents with panic disorder and agoraphobia with and without comorbid major depression. Psychiatry Res 37:333–348.

Bishop DT and Williamson JA (1990): The power of identity-by-tate methods for linkage analysis. J Am Hum Genet 46:254–265.

Blum K, Noble EP, Sheridan PJ, Montgomery A, Ritchie T, Jagadeeswaran P, Nogami H, Briggs AH, Cohn JB (1990): Allelic association of human dopamine D2 receptor gene in alcoholism. JAMA 263:2055–2060.

Boehnke M (1986): Estimating the power of a proposed linkage study: A practical computer simulation approach. J Am Hum Genet 39:513–527.

Bonney GE (1984): On the statistical determination of major gene mechanisms in continuous human traits: Regressive models. J Am Hum Genet 18:731–749

Bonney GE (1986): Regressive logistic models for familial disease and other binary traits. Biometrics 42:611–625

Bonney GE (1987): Logistic regression for dependent binary observations. Biometrics 43:951–973.

Borecki IB, Lathrop GM, Bonney GE, Yaouanq J, Rao DC (1990): Combined segregation and linkage of genetic hemochromatosis using affection status, serum iron, and HLA. Am J Hum Genet 47:542–550.

Botstein D, White RL, Skolnick M, Davis RW (1980): Construction of a genetic linkage map in man using restriction fragment length polymorphisms. J Am Hum Genet 32:314–331.

Breslow N and Crowley J (1974): A large sample study of the life table and product limit estimates under random censorship. Ann Stat 2:437–453.

Buckley P, O'Callaghan E, Larkin C, Waddington JL (1992): Schizophrenia research: The problem of controls. Biol Psychiatry 32:215–217.

Bunzow R, Van TH, Grandy DK, Albert P, Salon J, Christie M, Machida CA, Neve KA, Civelli O (1988): Cloning and expression of a rat D2 dopamine receptor cDNA. Nature 336:783–787.

Cadoret RJ (1978): Evidence for genetic inheritance of primary affective disorder in adoptees. Am J Psychiatry 135:463–466.

Cadoret R J, O'Gorman TW, Heywood E, Troughton E (1985): Genetic and environmental factors in major depression. J Affect Disord 9:155–164.

Cavalli-Sforza LL and King M-C (1986): Detecting linkage for genetically heterogeneous diseases and detecting heterogeneity with linkage data. Am J Hum Genet 38:599–616.

Chartier-Harlin M-C, Crawford F, Houlden H, Warren A, Hughes D, Fidani L, Goate A, Rossor M, Roques P, Hardy J, Mullan M (1991): Early-onset Alzheimer's disease caused by mutations at codon 717 of the b-amyloid precursor protein gene. Nature 353:844–846.

Chase GA and Kramer M (1986): The abridged census method as an estimator of lifetime risk. Psychol Med 16:865–871.

Chen WJ, Faraone SV, Orav EJ, Tsuang MT (1993): Estimating age at onset distributions: The bias from prevalent cases and its impact on risk estimation. Genet Epidemiol 10:43–60.

Chen WJ, Faraone SV, Tsuang MT (1992a): Estimating age at onset distributions: A review of methods and issues. Psychiat Genet 2:219–238.

Chen WJ, Faraone SV, Tsuang MT (1992b): Linkage studies of schizophrenia: A simulation study of statistical power. Genet Epidemiol 9:123–139.

Clerget-Darpoux F, Babron M-C, Bonaïti-Pellié C (1987): Power and robustness of the linkage homogeneity test in genetic analysis of common disorders. J Psychiatr Res 21:625–630.

Clerget-Darpoux F, Babron M-C, Bonaïti-Pellié C (1990): Assessing the effect of multiple linkage tests in complex diseases. Genet Epidemiol. 7:245–253.

Cloninger CR, Christiansen KO, Reich T, Gottesman II (1978): Implications of sex differences in the prevalences of antisocial personality, alcoholism, and criminality for familial transmission. Arch Gen Psychiatry 35:941–951.

Conneally PM (1991): Association between the D_2 dopamine receptor gene and alcoholism. A continuing controversy. Arch Gen Psychiatry 48:757–759.

Crowe RR (1993): Candidate genes in psychiatry: An epidemiological perspective. Am J Med Genet Neuropsychiatric Genet 48:74–77.

Cupples LA, Risch N, Farrer LA, Myers RH (1991): Estimation of morbid risk and age at onset with missing information. Am J Hum Genet 49:76–87.

Dearry A, Gingrich JA, Falardeau P, Fremeau RT. J, Bates MD, Caron MG (1990): Molecular cloning and expression of the gene for a human D1 dopamine receptor. Nature 347:72–76.

DeLisi LE, Dauphinais ID, Hauser P (1989): Gender differences in the brain: Are they relevant to the pathogenesis of schizophrenia? Comp Psychiatry 30:197–208.

Deutsch CK, Swanson JM, Bruell JH, Cantwell DP, Weinberg F, Baren M (1982): Short Communication: Overrepresentation of adoptees in children with attention deficit disorder. Behav Genet 12:231–238.

Eaves LJ, Kendler KS, Schulz SC (1986): The familial sporadic classification: Its power for the resolution of genetic and environmental etiological factors. J Psychiatric Res 20:115–130.

Edwards JH (1990): The linkage detection problem. Ann Hum Genet 54:253–275.

Edwards JH and Watt DC (1989): Caution in locating the gene(s) for affective disorder. Psychol Med 19:273–275.

Egeland JA, Gerhard DS, Pauls DL, Sussex JN, Kidd KK, Allen CR, Hostetter AM, Housman DE (1987): Bipolar affective disorders linked to DNA markers on chromosome 11. Nature 325:783–787.

Elston RC and Namboodiri KK (1977): Family studies of schizophrenia. Bull Int Stat Inst 47:683–697.

Elston RC and Stewart J (1971): A general model for the genetic analysis of pedigree data. Hum Hered 21:523–542.

Erlenmeyer-Kimling L (1975): A prospective study of children at risk for schizophrenia: Methodological considerations and some preliminary findings, in Wirt R, Winokur G, Ross M (eds.): "Life History Research in Psychopathology." Minneapolis, MN, University of Minnesota Press, pp 22–46.

Ewens WJ and Shute NCE (1986); A resolution of the ascertainment sampling problem. Theoretical Population Biology 30:388–412.

Falconer DS (1965): The inheritance of liability to certain diseases, estimated from the incidence among relatives. Ann Hum Genet 29:51–71.

Falk CT and Rubinstein P (1987): Haplotype relative risks: An east reliable way to construct a proper control sample for risk calculations. Ann Hum Genet 51:227–233.

Faraone SV, Biederman J, Keenan K, Tsuang MT (1991): A family-genetic study of girls with DSM-III attention deficit disorder. J Am Psychiatry 148:112–117.

Faraone SV, Biederman J, Krifcher B, Keenan K, Moore C, Sprich S, Ugaglia K, Jellinek MS, Spencer T, Norman D, Seidman L, Kolodny R, Benjamin J, Kraus I, Perrin J, Chen W, Tsuang MT (1993): Evidence for independent transmission in families for Attention Deficit Hyperactivity Disorder (ADHD) and learning disability: Results from a family-genetic study of ADHD. Am J Psychiatry 150:891–895.

Faraone SV, Blehar M, Pepple J, Moldin S, Norton J, Tsuang MT, Nurnberger JI, Malaspina D, Kaufmann CA, Reich T, Cloninger CR, DePaulo JR, Berg K, Gershon ES, Kirch DG, Tsuang MT (1996): Diagnostic accuracy and confusability analysis: An application to the Diagnostic Interview for Genetic Studies. Psychol Med 26:401–410.

Faraone SV, Kremen WS, Tsuang MT (1990): Genetic transmission of major affective disorders: Quantitative models and linkage analyses. Psychol Bull 108:109–127.

Faraone SV and Santangelo S (1992): Methods in Genetic Epidemiology. In Fava M, Rosenbaum JF (eds.): "Research Designs and Methods in Psychiatry." Amsterdam, The Netherlands, Elsevier, pp 87–105.

Faraone SV and Tsuang MT (1985): Quantitative models of the genetic transmission of schizophrenia. Psychol Bull 98:41–66.

Faraone SV, Tsuang D, Tsuang MT (1999): "Genetics of Mental Disorders: A Guide for Students, Clinicians, and Researchers." New York: Guilford.

Fischer M (1971): Psychosis in the offspring of schizophrenic monozygotic twins and their normal co-twins. Br J Psychiatry 118:43–52.

Fish B, Marcus J, Hans SL, Auerbach JG, Perdue S (1992): Infants at risk for schizophrenia: Sequelae of a genetic neurointegrative defect. A review and replication analysis of pandysmaturation in the Jerusalem infant development study. Arch Gen Psychiatry 49:221–235.

Fisher RA (1934): The effect of methods of ascertainment upon the estimation of frequencies. Ann Eugen 6:13–25.

Freimer NB, Sandkuiji LA, Blower SM (1993): Incorrect specification of marker allele frequencies: Effects on linkage analysis. Am J Hum Genet 52:1102–1110.

Gejman PV and Gelernter J (1993): Mutational analysis of candidate genes in psychiatric disorders. Am J Med Genet Neuropsychiatric Genet 48:184–191.

Gelernter J, O'Malley S, Risch N, Kranzler HR, Krystal J, Merikangas K, Kennedy JL, Kidd KK (1991): No association between an allele at the D_2 dopamine receptor gene (DRD2) and alcoholism. JAMA 266:1801–1807.

Gershon ES and Guroff JJ (1984): Information from relatives. Diagnosis of affective disorders. Arch Gen Psychiatry 41:173–180.

Gibbons RD, Davis JM, Hedeker DR (1990): A comment on the selection of "healthy controls" for psychiatric experiments. Arch Gen Psychiatry 47:785–786.

Goate A, Chartier-Harlin M-C, Mullan M, Brown J, Crawford F, Fidani L, Giuffra L, Haynes A, Irving N, James L, Mant R, Newton P, Rooke K, Roques P, Talbot C, Pericak-Vance M, Roses A, Williamson R, Rossor M, Owen M, Hardy J (1991):

Segregation of a missense mutation in the amyloid precursor protein gene with familial Alzheimer's disease. Nature 349:704–706.

Goldin LR (1990): The increase in type I error rates in linkage studies when multiple analyses are carried out on the same data: A simulation study. (Abstract). Am J Hum Genet 47:A180.

Goldin LR and Gershon ES (1988): Power of the affected-sib-pair method for heterogeneous disorders. Genet Epidemiol 5:35–42.

Goldin LR and Martinez MM (1989): The detection of linkage and heterogeneity in nuclear families when unaffected individuals are considered unknown. In Elston RC, Spence MA, Hodge SE, MacCluer JW (eds.): "Multipoint Mapping and Linkage Based upon Affected Pedigree Members." New York: Alan R. Liss pp 195–200.

Goldstein JM, Tsuang MT, Faraone SV (1989): Gender and schizophrenia: Implications for understanding the heterogeneity of the illness. Psychiatry Res 28:243–253.

Gottesman II and Bertelsen A (1989): Confirming unexpressed genotypes for schizophrenia. Risks in the offspring of Fischer's Danish identical and fraternal discordant twins. Arch Gen Psychiatry 46:867–872.

Grandy DK, Litt M, Allen L, Bunzow JR, Marchionni M, Makam H, Reed L, Magenis RE, Civelli O (1989): The human dopamine D2 receptor gene is located on chromosome 11 at q22-q23 and identifies a TaqI RFLP. Am J Hum Genet 45:778–785.

Green P (1990): Genetic linkage and complex diseases: A comment. Genet Epidemiol 7:25–27.

Greenberg DA (1986); The effect of proband designation on segregation analysis. Am J Hum Genet 39:329–339.

Greenberg DA (1989): Inferring mode of inheritance by comparison of lod scores. Am J Med Genet 34:480–486.

Greenland S and Morgenstern H (1990): Matching and efficiency in cohort studies. Am J Epidemiol 131:151–159.

Grima B, Lamouroux A, Boni C, Julien J-F, Javoy-Agid F, Mallet J (1987): A single human gene encoding multiple tyrosine hydroxylases with different predicted functional characteristics. Nature 326:707–711.

Harris T, Surtees P, Bancroft J (1991): Is sex necessarily a risk factor to depression? Br J Psychiatry 158:708–712.

Heimbuch RC, Matthysse S, Kidd KK (1980): Estimating age-of-onset distributions for disorders with variable onset. Am J Hum Genet 32:564–574.

Heston LL (1966): Psychiatric disorders in foster home-reared children of schizophrenic mothers. Br J Psychiatry 112:819–825.

Hsu Y-PP, Powell JF, Chen S, Weyler W, Ozelius L, Bruns G, Utterback M, Mallet J, Gusella JF, Breakefield XO (1988a): Molecular genetic studies of MAO genes. In Dalstrom A, Belmaker H, Sandler M. (eds.): "Progress in Catecholamine Research: Part A. Basic and Peripheral Mechanisms." New York, Alan Liss, pp 89–95.

Hsu Y-PP, Weyler W, Chen S, Sims KB, Rinehart WB, Utterback MC, Powell JF, Breakefield XO (1988b): Structural features of human monoamine oxidase A elucidated from cDNA and peptide sequences. J Neurochemistry 51:1321–1324.

Iselius L and Morton NE (1991): Transmission probabilities are not correctly implemented in the computer program POINTER. Am J Hum Genet 49:459.

Jeffreys AJ, Wilson T, Thein SL (1985): Hypervariable "minisatellite" regions in human DNA. Nature 314:67–73.

Kaplan EL and Meier P (1958): Nonparametric estimation from incomplete observations. Am Stat Assoc 53:457–481.

Kelsoe JR, Ginns EI, Egeland JA, Gerhard DS, Goldstein AM, Bale SJ, Pauls DL, Long RT, Kidd KK, Conte G, Housman DE, Paul SM (1989): Re-evaluation of the linkage relationship between chromosome 11p loci and the gene for bipolar affective disorder in the old order Amish. Nature 342:238–243.

Kendler KS (1987): Sporadic vs familial classification given etiologic heterogeneity: Sensitivity, specificity, and positive and negative predictive power. Genet Epidemiol 4:313–330.

Kendler KS (1990): The super-normal control group in psychiatric genetics: Possible artifactual evidence for coaggregation. J Psychiat Genet 1:45–53.

Kendler KS and Hays P (1982): Familial and sporadic schizophrenia: A symptomatic, prognostic and EEG comparison. Am Psychiatry 139:1557–1562.

Kendler KS, Silberg JL, Neale MC, Kessler RC, Heath, AC, Eaves LJ (1991): The family history method: Whose psychiatric history is measured? Am J Psychiatry 148:1501–1504.

Kety SS, Rosenthal D, Wender PH, Schulsinger F (1968): The types and prevalence of mental illness in the biological and adoptive families of adopted schizophrenics. J Psychiat Res 1:345–362.

Kety SS, Rosenthal D, Wender PH, Schulsinger F, Jacobson B (1978): The biologic and adoptive families of adopted individuals who became schizophrenic: Prevalence of mental illness and other characteristics. In Wynne LC, Cromwell RL, Matthysse S (eds.) "The Nature of Schizophrenia: New Approaches to Research and Treatment." New York: Wiley, pp 25–37.

Khoury MJ, Beaty TH, Cohen BH (1993): "Fundamentals of Genetic Epidemiology". New York: Oxford University Press.

Kidd KK (1993): Associations of disease with genetic markers: Deja vu all over again. Am J Med Genet Neuropsychiatric Genet 48:71–73.

Knapp M, Seuchter SA, Baur MP (1993): The haplotype-relative-risk (HRR) method for analysis of association in nuclear families. Am J Hum Genet 52:1085–1093.

Kobayashi K, Kurosawa Y, Fujita K, Nagatsu T (1989): Human dopamine-beta hydroxylase gene: two mRNA types having different 3′-terminal regions are produced through alternative polyadenylation. Nucleic Acids Res 17:1089–1102.

Korenberg J, West R, Pulst S (1988): The amyloid protein precursor gene maps to chromosome 21 sub-bands q21.15-q21.1. Neurology 38:265.

Kosten TA, Anton SF, Rounsaville BJ (1992): Ascertaining psychiatric diagnoses with the family history method in a substance abuse population. J Psychiatr Res 26:135–147.

Kotsopoulos S, Côte A, Joseph L, Pentland N, Stavrakaki C, Sheahan P, Oke L (1988): Psychiatric disorders in adopted children: A controlled study. Am. J Orthopsychiatry 58:608–612.

Kruesi MJP, Lenane MC, Hibbs ED, Major J (1990): Normal controls and biological reference values in child psychiatry: Defining normal. J Am Acad Child Adolesc Psychiatry 29:449–452.

LaBuda MC, Gottesman II, Pauls DL (1993): Usefulness of twin studies for exploring the etiology of childhood and adolescent psychiatric disorders. Am J Med Genet Neuropsychiatric Genet 48:47–59.

Lalouel JM, Rao DC, Morton NE, Elston RC (1983): A unified model for complex segregation analysis. Am J Hum Genet 35:816–826.

Lamouroux A, Vigny A, Faucon BN, Darmon MC, Franck R, Henry JP, Mallet J (1987): The primary structure of human dopamine-beta-hydroxylase: insights into the relationship between the soluble and the membrane-bound forms of the enzyme. Eur Mol Biol 6:3931–3937.

Lander ES (1988): Splitting schizophrenia. Nature 336:105–106.

Lander ES and Botstein D (1986a): Mapping complex genetic traits in humans: New methods using a complete RFLP linkage map. Paper presented at the Cold Springs Harbor Symposium on Quantitative Molecular Biology.

Lander ES and Botstein D (1986b): Strategies for studying heterogeneous genetic traits in humans by using a linkage map of restriction fragment length polymorphisms. Proceedings of the National Academy of Science 83:7353–7357..

Lander E, Kruglyak L (1995): Genetic dissection of complex traits. Nature Genetics Nov.: 241–247.

Larsson T, Sjögren T (1954): A methodological, psychiatric and statistical study of a large Swedish rural population. Acta Psychiatr Neurol Scand (Suppl) 89:40–54.

Leckman JF, Sholomska D, Thompson WD, Belanger A, Weissman MM (1982): Best estimate of lifetime diagnosis: A methodological study. Arch Gen Psychiatry 39:879–883.

Lee EL (1980): "Statistical Methods for Survival Data Analysis." Belmont, Lifetime Learning.

Levinson DF (1993a): Linkage information in small family structures: Comparison of pedigrees with three to five affected members. Psychiatric Genet 3:45–57.

Levinson DF (1993b): Power to detect linkage with heterogeneity in samples of small nuclear families. Am J Med Genet Neuropsychiatric Genet 48:94–102.

Lewis SW, Reveley AM, Reveley MA, Chitkara B, Murray RM (1987): The familial/sporadic distinction as a strategy in schizophrenia research. Br J Psychiatry 151:306–313.

Lyons MJ, Faraone SV, Kremen WS, Tsuang MT (1989a): Familial and sporadic schizophrenia: A simulation study of statistical power. Schiz Res 2:345–353.

Lyons MJ, Kremen WS, Tsuang MT, Faraone SV (1989b): Investigating putative genetic and environmental forms of schizophrenia: Methods and findings. Int Rev Psychiatry 1:259–276.

Marshall E (1999): Genomics: drug firms to create public database of genetic mutations. Science 284:406–407.

Martinez MM and Goldin LR (1989): The detection of linkage and heterogeneity in nuclear families for complex disorders: One versus two major loci. Am J Hum Genet 44:552–559.

Martinez MM and Goldin LR (1990): Power of the linkage test for a heterogeneous disorder due to independent inherited causes: A simulation study. Genet Epidemiol 7:219–230.

McGue M and Gottesman II (1989) Genetic linkage in schizophrenia: Perspectives from genetic epidemiology. Schiz. Bull. 15:453–464.

McGue M and Gottesman II (1991): The genetic epideminology of schizophrenia and the degree of linkage studies. Eur Arch Psychiatr Clin Neuro Sci 240:174–181.

McGue M, Gottesman II, Rao DC (1983): The transmission of schizophrenia under a multifactorial threshold model. AM J Hum Genet 35:1161–1178.

McGue M, Gottesman II, Rao DC (1985): Resolving genetic models for the transmission of schizophrenia. Genet Epidemiol 2:99–110.

Mednick SA, Mura E, Schulsinger F, Mednick B (1971): Perinatal conditions and infant development in children with schizophrenic parents. Soc Biol (Suppl) 18:103.

Meehl P and Rosen A (1955): Antecedent probability and the efficiency of psychometric signs, patterns, or cutting scores. Psychol Bull 52:194–216.

Meehl PE (1970): Nuisance variables and the ex post facto design. In Radner M, Winokur S. (eds.): "Minnesota Studies in the Philosophy of Science." Minneapolis, MN, University of Minnesota Press, pp 373–402.

Mendlewicz J, Fleiss JL, Cataldo M, Rainer JD (1975): Accuracy of the family history method in affective illness. Arch Gen Psychiatry 32:309–314.

Mendlewicz J and Rainer JD (1977): Adoption study supporting genetic transmission in manic-depressive illness. Nature 268:327–329.

Merikangas KR, Spence A, Kupfer DJ (1989): Linkage studies of bipolar disorder: Methodologic and analytic issues. Report of MacArthur foundation workshop on linkage and clinical features in affective disorders. Arch Gen Psychiatry 46:1137–1141.

Miettinen OS (1985): "Theoretical Epidemiology." New York, Wiley.

Morton LA, Kidd KK, Matthysse SW, Richards RL (1979): Recurrence risks in schizophrenia: Are they model dependent? Behav Genet 9:389–406.

Morton NE (1955): Sequential tests for the detection of linkage. Am J Hum Genet 7:277–318.

Morton NE (1982): "Outline of Genetic Epidemiology." Basel, Karger.

Morton NE and MacLean CJ (1974): Analysis of family resemblance. III. Complex segregation analysis of quantitative traits. Am J Hum Genet 26:489–503.

Morton NE, Rao DC, Lalouel J-M (1983): "Methods in Genetic Epidemiology." New York, Karger.

Murphy KC, Jones AL, Owen MJ (1999): High rates of schizophrenia in velo-cardio-facial syndrome. Arch Gen Psychiatry 56:940–945.

Naruse S, Igarashi S, Kobayashi H, Aoki K, Inuzuka T, Kaneko K, Shimizu T, Iihara K, Kojima T, Miyatake T, Tsuji S (1991): Mis-sense mutation Val-lle in exon 17 of amyloid precursor protein gene in Japanese familial Alzheimer's disease. Lancet 337:978–979.

Neale MC and Cardon LR (1992): "Methodology for genetic studies of twins and families." The Netherlands, Kluwer Academic Publishers.

NIMH Genetics Initiative (1992): "Family Interview for Genetic Studies." Rockville, MD: National Institute of Mental Health.

Nothen MM, Erdmann J, Korner J, Lanczik M, Fritzer J, Fimmers R, Grandy DK, O'Dowd B, Propping P (1992): Lack of association between dopamine D_1 and D_2 receptor genes and bipolar affective disorder. Am J Psychiatry 149:199–201.

Nurnberger JI, Jr, Blehar MC, Kaufmann CA, York-Cooler C, Simpson SG, Harkavy-Friedman J, Severe JB, Malaspina D, Reich T, Miller M, Bowman ES, DePaulo JR, Cloninger CR, Robinson G, Moldin S, Gershon ES, Maxwell E, Guroff JJ, Kirch D, Wynne D, Berg K, Tsuang MT, Faraone S.V, Pepple JR, Ritz AL (1994): Diagnostic Interview for Genetic Studies. Rationale, unique features, and training. Arch Gen Psychiatry 51:849–859.

Orvaschel H (1990): Early onset psychiatric disorder in high risk children and increased familial morbidity. J Am Acad Child and Adolesc Psychiatry 29:184–188.

Orvaschel H, Thompson WD, Belanger A, Prusoff BA, Kidd KK (1982): Comparison of the family history method to direct interview: Factors affecting the diagnosis of depression. J Affect Disord 4:49–59.

Ott J (1983): Linkage analysis and family classification under heterogeneity. Ann Hum Genet 47:311–320.

Ott J (1986): The number of families required to detect or exclude linkage heterogeneity. Am J Hum Genet 39:159–165.

Ott J (1989a): Computer-simulation methods in human linkage analysis Proc Nat Acad Sci, U.S.A. 86:4175–4178.

Ott J (1989b): Statistical properties of the haplotype relative risk. Genet Epidemiol; 6:127–130.

Ott J (1990a): Genetic linkage and complex diseases: A comment. Genet Epidemiol 7:35–36.

Ott J (1990b): Invited editorial: Cutting a Gordian knot in the linkage analysis of complex human traits. Am J Hum Genet 46:219–221.

Ott J (1991): "Analysis of Human Genetic Linkage." Baltimore, Johns Hopkins University Press.

Ottman R (1990): An epidemiologic approach to gene-environment interaction. Genet Epidemiol 7:177–185.

Pato CN, Lander ES, Schulz SC (1989): Prospects for the genetic analysis of schizophrenia. Schiz Bull 15:365–372.

Pato CN, Macciardi F, Pato MT, Verga M, Kennedy JL (1993): Review of the putative association of dopamine D2 receptor and alcoholism: A meta-analysis. Am J Med Genet Neuropsychiatric Genet 48:78–82.

Pauls DL (1979): Sex effect on the risk of mental retardation. Behav Genet 9:289–295.

Pauls DL and Leckman JF (1986): The inheritance of Gilles De La Tourette's syndrome and associated behaviors. Evidence for autosomal dominant transmission. N Engl J Med 315:993–997.

Plomin R, Defries JC, McLearn GE (1990): "Behavioral Genetics. A primer." New York, Freeman.

Ploughman LM and Boehnke M (1989): Estimating the power of a proposed linkage study for a complex genetic trait. Am J Hum Genet 44:543–551.

Pulver AE and Bale SJ (1989): Availability of schizophrenic patients and their families for genetic linkage studies: Findings from the Maryland epidemiology sample. Genet Epidemiol 6:671–680.

Risch N (1983): Estimating morbidity risks with variable age of onset: Review of methods and a maximum likelihood approach. Biometrics 39:929–939.

Risch N (1988): A new statistical test for linkage heterogeneity. Am J Hum Genet 42:353–364.

Risch N (1990a): Genetic linkage and complex diseases, with special reference to psychiatric disorders. Genet Epidemiol 7:3–7.

Risch N (1990b): Linkage strategies for genetically complex traits. I. Multilocus models. Am J Hum Genet 46:222–228.

Risch N (1990c): Linkage strategies for genetically complex traits. II. The power of affected relative pairs. Am J Hum Genet 46:229–241.

Risch N (1990d): Linkage strategies for genetically complex traits. III. The effect of marker polymorphism on analysis of affected relative pairs. Am J Hum Genet 46:242–253.

Risch N and Baron M (1984): Segregation analysis of schizophrenia and related disorders. Am J Hum Genet 36:1039–1059.

Risch N and Giuffra L (1992): Model misspecification and multipoint linkage analysis. Hum Her 42:77–92.

Risch SC, Lewine RJ, Jewart RD, Eccard MB, McDaniel JS, Risby ED (1990): Ensuring the normalcy of "normal" volunteers. Am J Psychiatry 147:682–683.

Rubinstein P, Walker M, Carpenter C, Carrier C, Krassner J, Falk C, Ginsberg F (1981): Genetics of HLA disease associations: The use of the haplotype relative risk (HRR) and the "haplo-delta" (Dh) estimates in juvenile diabetes from three racial groups. Hum Immunol 3:384.

Schork NJ, Fallin D, Lanchbury, S (2000): Single nucleotide polymorphisms and the future of genetic epidemiology. Clinic Genet 58:250–264.

Schwartz XL and Moises HW (1993): No association between schizophrenia and homozygosity at the D_3 dopamine receptor gene. Am J Med Genet Neuropsychiatric Genet 48:83–86.

Schweber MA (1985): A possible unitary genetic hypothesis for Alzheimer's disease and Down's syndrome. Ann NY Acad Sci 450:223–238.

Shields J and Slater E (1975): Genetic aspects of schizophrenia. Br J Psychiatry (Spec Pub) 9:32–40.

Shtasel DL, Gur RE, Mozley D, Richards J, Taleff MM, Heimberg C, Gallacher F, Gur RC (1991): Volunteers for biomedical research. Recruitment and screening of normal controls. Arch Gen Psychiatry 48:1022–1025.

Shute NCE and Ewers WJ (1988a): A resolution of the ascertainment sampling problem. II. Generalizations and numerical results. Am J Hum Genet 43:374–386.

Shute NCE and Ewers WJ (1988b): A resolution of the ascertainment sampling problem. III. Pedigrees. Am J Hum Genet 43:387–395.

Silverman JM, Breitner JCS, Mohs RC, Davis KL (1986): Reliability of the family history method in genetic studies of Alzheimer's disease and related dementias. Am J Psychiatry 143:1279–1282.

Slater E and Cowie V (1971): "The Genetics of Mental Disorder." London, Oxford University Press.

Smith C (1974): Concordance in twins: Methods and interpretation. Am J Hum Genet 26:454–466.

Sobell JL, Heston LL, Sommer SS (1992): Delineation of genetic predisposition to multifactorial disease: A general approach on the threshold of feasibility. Genomics 12:1–6.

Sommer SS, Lind TJ, Heston LJ, Sobell JL (1993): Dopamine D_4 receptor variants in unrelated schizophrenic cases and controls. Am J Med Genet Neuropsychiatric Genet 48:90–93.

Sorant AJM and Elston RC (1989a): Segregation analysis of a truncated (censored) trait with logistic P.D.F. (REGTL version 1.0). In Bailey-Wilson JE, Elston RC (eds.): "Statistical Analysis for Genetic Epidemiology." New Orleans: Department of Biometry and Genetics, LSU Medical Center.

Sorant AJM and Elston RC (1989b): A subroutine package for function maximization (A users guide to MAXFUN version 5.0). In Bailey-Wilson JE, Elston RC (eds.): "Statistical Analysis for Genetic Epidemiology." New Orleans, Dept. of Biometry and Genetics, LSU Medical Center.

Spence MA (1987): Genetic Linkage: Sampling issues and multipoint mapping. J Psychiatr Res 21:631–637.

Spielman RS, McGinnis RE, Ewens WJ (1993): Transmission test for linkage disequilibrium: The insulin gene region and insulin-dependent diabetes mellitus (IDDM). Am J Hum Genet 52:506–516.

Strömgren E (1935): Zum ersatz des Weinbergschen 'abgekurzten verfahrens' zugleich ein beitrag zur Frage von der Erblichkeit des Erkrankungsalters bei der Schizophrenie. Z Ges Neurol Psychiatrie 153:784–797.

Strömgren E (1938): Beitrage zur psychiatrischen erblehre auf grund von Untersuchungen an einer Inselbevolkerung. Acta Psychiatr Neurol Scan (Suppl) 19:1–257.

Sturt E (1985): Estimating morbidity risks with variable age of onset (correspondence). Biometrics 41:311–313.

Sunahara RK, Niznik HB, Weiner DM, Stormann TM, Brann MR, Kennedy JL, Gelernter E, Rozmahel R, Yang Y, Israel Y, Seeman P, O'Dowd BF (1990): Human dopamine D1 receptor encoded by an intronless gene on chromosome 5. Nature 347:80–83.

Thaker GK, Moran M, Lahti A, Adami H, Tamminga C (1990): Psychiatric morbidity in research volunteers. Arch Gen Psychiatry 47:980.

Thompson WD, Orvaschel H, Prusoff BA, Kidd KK (1982): An evaluation of the family history method for ascertaining psychiatric disorders. Arch Gen Psychiatry 39:53–58.

Thompson WD and Weissman MM (1981): Quantifying lifetime risk of psychiatric disorder. J Psychiatric Res 16:113–126.

Tsuang MT and Faraone SV (1990): "The Genetics of Mood Disorders." Baltimore, Johns Hopkins.

Tsuang MT, Faraone SV, Johnson P (1997): "Schizophrenia: The Facts." Oxford, UK, Oxford University Press.

Tsuang MT, Faraone SV, Lyons MJ (1993): Advances in psychiatric genetics. In Costa e Silva JA, Nadelson CC, Andreasen NC, Sato M. (eds.): "International Review of Psychiatry," Vol I. Washington, D.C, American Psychiatric Press, pp 395-440.

Tsuang MT, Fleming JA, Kendler KS, Gruenberg AM (1988): Selection of controls for family studies: Biases and implications. Arch Gen Psychiatry 45:1006–1008.

Tsuang MT, Gilbertson MW, Faraone SV (1991): Genetic transmission of negative and positive symptoms in the biological relatives of schizophrenics. In Marneros A, Tsuang MT, Andreasen N (eds.): "Positive vs. Negative Schizophrenia." New York: Springer, pp 265–291.

Tsuang MT and Vandermey R (1980): "Genes and the Mind: Inheritance of Mental Illness." London: Oxford University Press.

van Duijn CM, Hendriks L, Cruts M, Hardy JA, Hofman A, Van Broeckhoven C (1991): Amyloid precursor protein gene mutation in early-onset Alzheimer's disease. Lancet 337:978.

Vogel F and Motulsky AG (1986): "Human Genetics: Problems and Approaches." Berlin, Springer.

Wacholder S, McLaughlin JK, Silverman DT, Mandel JS (1992a): Selection of controls in case–control studies. I. Principles. Am Epidemiol 135:1019–1028.

Wacholder S, Silverman DT, McLaughlin K, Mandel S (1992b): Selection of controls in case-control studies. II. Types of controls. Am Epidemiol 135:1029–1041.

Wacholder S, Silverman DT, McLaughlin K, Mandel S (1992c): Selection of controls in case-control studies. III. Design options. Am Epidemiol 135:1042–1050.

Wang J (2000): From DNA biosensors to gene chips. Nuc Acids Res 28:3011–3016.

Ward P (1993): Some developments on the affected-pedigree-member method of linkage analysis. Am Hum Genet 52:1200–1215.

Weeks DE, Brustowicz L, Squires-Wheeler E, Cornblatt B, Lehner T, Stefanovich M, Bassett A, Gilliam TC, Ott J, Erlenmeyer-Kimling L (1990a): Report of a workshop on genetic linkage studies in schizophrenia. Schiz Bull 16:673–686.

Weeks DE and Lange K (1988): The affected-pedigree-member method of linkage analysis. Am Hum Genet 42:315–326.

Weeks DE, Lehner T, Squires-Wheeler E, Kaufmann C, Ott J (1990b): Measuring the inflation of the lod score due to its maximization over model parameter values in human linkage analysis. Genet Epidemiol 7:237–243.

Weinberg W (1925): Methoden und Technik der Statistik mit besonderer Bercksichtigun der Sozialbiologie. In Gottstein A, Schlossmann A, Teleky L (eds.): "Handbuch der sozialen Hygiene und Gesundheitsfrsorge 1. Grundlagen und methoden." Berlin, Verlag von Julius Springer, pp 71–148.

Weissman MM, Merikangas KR, John K, Wickramaratne P, Prusoff BA, Kidd KK (1986): Family-genetic studies of psychiatric disorders. Developing technologies. Arch Gen Psychiatry 43:1104–1116.

Wender PH, Kety SS, Rosenthal D, Schulsinger F, Ortmann J, Lunde I (1986): Psychiatric disorders in the biological and adoptive families of adopted individuals with affective disorders. Arch Gen Psychiatry 43:923–929.

Xu J and Weisch DG, Meyers DA. (1998): Genetics of complex human diseases: genome screening, association studies and fine mapping. Clin Experimental Allergy 28:1–5.

Zander KJ, Fischer B, Zimmer R, Ackenheil M (1981): Long-term neuroleptic treatment of chronic schizophrenic patients: Clinical and biochemical effects of withdrawal. Psychopharmacology 73:43–47.

CHAPTER 4

Reliability

PATRICK E. SHROUT

Department of Psychology, New York University, New York, NY 10003.

INTRODUCTION

In psychiatric epidemiology, assessment of mental conditions and of risks for psychiatric disorder relies heavily on information provided by patients (or survey respondents) and by informants who are close to the patient or respondent. How good is the information provided by these people, and how good are the assessment inferences that we make on the basis of this information? The quality of the assessment in psychiatry and epidemiology is typically characterized by the reliability and validity of the measure. *Reliability* is the degree to which a measurement is reproducible and not affected by transient assessment noise. *Validity* is the degree to which the measurement is useful. Although validity is the ultimate criterion by which to judge a measure, we know that a measure will not be useful if it is dominated by measurement noise. This means that reliability is a necessary condition for validity, but it is not sufficient to guarantee validity.

Even though reliability is only an intermediate step toward quality measurement, it is often methodologically interesting because it is a problem that can usually be fixed. Reliability can be improved by structuring and standardizing the assessment procedure, by improving the training of both the respondents and those carrying out the assessment, and by averaging replicate measurements. If problems of unreliability are not addressed, then subsequent problems of validity are intractable. This is why reliability was given so much attention in developing the Versions III and IV of the *Diagnostic and Statistical Manual* of the American Psychiatric Association (American Psychiatric Association, 1980, 1994).

Epidemiologists must attend both to the reliability of diagnostic measures and risk measures. Two features of psychiatric epidemiology make reliability more of an enduring problem in this field than in others. One feature is the previously mentioned dependence on information provided by respondents or informants. Respondent reports present many opportunities for noise to enter the recorded data: the understanding of the question, the recall and reporting of the answer, and the coding and entry of the data. The other feature is the epidemiologists' search for novel populations and risk groups that might provide clues to the

Textbook in Psychiatric Epidemiology, Second Edition, Edited by Ming T. Tsuang and Mauricio Tohen.
ISBN 0-471-40974-X

etiology of mental disorders. New populations require new assessments of reliability, since populations vary in language, literacy and cultural expression of disorders. As we will see, the variability of the trait under study in the new population also affects the reliability of measures.

In this chapter we examine methods for evaluating reliability of measures used in psychiatric epidemiology. We first review the classic psychometric theory of reliability. We then survey the methods used to study reliability, both for measures of psychopathology and epidemiological risk. In this survey we distinguish quantitative measures and those that classify respondents into categories. We incorporate a set of numerical examples that illustrate the most important measures. We also provide references to some recent methodological work that tells us about the precision of reliability estimates themselves.

THE RELIABILITY COEFFICIENT

Consider a single measurement procedure. Respondents are sampled from a specific population, measured in some way, and assigned a numerical value that is represented by the variable X. If the characteristic being measured is qualitative, such as having a certain diagnosis, then the variable X might be defined to be binary, that is, $X = 1$ if the respondent has the characteristic, and $X = 0$ otherwise. If the characteristic is quantitative, such as severity of illness or exposure, then X might be defined to take some well-specified numerical score.

The variance of X, σ_X^2, is a population parameter that describes how much the measurements differ from person to person in the population being studied. In some populations σ_X^2 might be relatively small, while in other populations the variance might be large. Small variance implies that the measurement distinction is subtle in the population, while large variation implies the opposite. In populations with small overall variation in X, any measurement error may be quite serious.

According to classic reliability theory, it is useful to decompose σ_X^2 into two components, $\sigma_X^2 = \sigma_E^2 + \sigma_T^2$ where σ_E^2 is variance due to measurement noise and σ_T^2 is variance due to systematic differences between persons being measured. We will discuss how these two components are estimated later. This decomposition implies that random measurement noise increases the total measurement variation. If measurement errors can be eliminated, then the error variance, σ_E^2, goes to zero and the total variance shrinks to σ_T^2. If errors dominate the measurement, then the majority of σ_X^2 may be attributable to σ_E^2, even if there is systematic variation between persons that is of interest.

In its purest form, the reliability coefficient, R_X, is a ratio of the population parameters, σ_T^2 and σ_X^2,

$$R_X = \frac{\sigma_T^2}{\sigma_X^2} = \frac{\sigma_T^2}{\left[\sigma_T^2 + \sigma_E^2\right]}. \tag{1}$$

R_X varies from zero (X is due entirely to unsystematic stochastic processes) to unity (X is due entirely to systematic individual differences). It can be thought of as the proportion of σ_X^2 that represents genuine, replicable differences in subjects.

It turns out to be a useful quantity in statistical analyses as well. For example, it can be shown that the correlation between X and another variable Y will get smaller as the reliability coefficient of either variable gets smaller (Cochran, 1968; Snedecor and Cochran, 1967).

How do we evaluate different values of R_X? If we know that a measure truly has a reliability of 0.50, then we know that only half its variance is systematic. That may not be what we hope for, but it might be good enough for some preliminary studies. For more definitive studies, we should aim to have reliability above 0.80. To provide some interpretive guidelines, Shrout (1998) recommends the following characterizations of reliability values: (0.00, 0.10), *virtually no reliability*; (0.11, 0.40), *slight*; (0.41, 0.60), *fair*; (0.61, 0.80), *moderate*; (0.81, 1.0), *substantial reliability*.[1] For a complete development of R_X and its implications, see Lord and Novick (1968) or Dunn (1989).

DESIGNS FOR ESTIMATING RELIABILITY

To estimate R_X we need to define what is meant by systematic variation of X. Classical psychometric theory defines this hypothetically. Suppose that a subject is selected and is measured once to produce the score X_1. Now suppose that it is possible to make the measurement over and over again without affecting the subject, and without recall of the previous X_j values (where j indexes each replicate measure). Classical measurement theory defines the systematic part of X to be the average of all of these hypothetically infinite measurements of the selected subject. This systematic component of the measurement is written as $T = E(X)$, which is interpreted as the expected average of the many replications of X. Note that if the measurement were height or weight, then it would actually be possible to take many repeated measurements of this sort.

In psychiatric epidemiology, reliability is estimated by approaching the hypothetical ideal with approximately replicate measurements. If there is virtually no variation across replications of X, then we infer that σ_E^2 is small in magnitude and that reliability is very good. If variation across replications is observed, then the magnitude of the within-subject variation is compared to that of the between-subject variation using the definition of R_X in Equation (1) above.

The most common replication design calls for making the X measurement at two points in time (the *test–retest design*). Variation in the X values across replications and across respondents is used to estimate σ_E^2, σ_T^2, and σ_X^2, and these can be used to estimate R_X. The formal equations for these estimates are presented in a later section.

Although theoretically and intuitively appealing, the test–retest design falls short of the hypothetical ideal in several ways. On one hand, the second measurement is often affected by systematic biological, psychological, and social changes in the respondent. These systematic changes make the estimate of σ_E^2 appear larger than it would have been at a single measurement instance. When legitimate change is included with error, the estimate of the reliability of the first assessment is too

[1] In setting standards for reliability, however, we must be aware that *estimates of reliability* may be smaller than the *actual reliability* because of systematic bias, which is discussed later.

small. On the other hand, if the respondents remember their original responses, and then try to be "good" by reporting the same thing, then the reliability estimate may be too large. Methodologists who address these opposing biases recommend that the second assessments be carried out after a long enough period to reduce memory artifacts, but promptly enough to reduce the probability of systematic changes. Recommendations of how long the period should be are more products of opinion than science.

Test–retest designs can be used with the whole range of measures made in psychiatric epidemiology. Interviews, questionnaires, ratings, and physical measurements can all be repeated after an appropriate time. It is not always necessary, however, to wait to obtain a replicate measurement. When the measurement is a judgment, such as the Global Assessment Scale (Endicott, Spitzer, Fleiss, et al., 1976), it is possible to have two independent ratings made at the same time. Moreover, time can be frozen by video-recording the structured interview so that ratings can be obtained from those viewing the recording. Although these alternatives to traditional test–retest designs overcome the confounding of unreliability with genuine growth or development, they bring with them their own problems. These have been discussed by several authors, including Spitzer (1983). Insofar as the respondent's idiosyncratic responses contribute to unreliability, then estimates based on a single recorded interview may underestimate the level of random variation in the actual ratings obtained in the field. For this reason, interrater reliability studies using recorded interviews are expected to overestimate true reliability.

When the measurement procedure under study is a questionnaire that includes several items pertaining to a single underlying psychological trait or symptom dimension, it is also possible to obtain some information about reliability from a single assessment time. The items that relate to the same underlying concept are considered to be replications of each other. The degree to which the patterns of responses suggest that they are empirically related is used as evidence of reliability. This inference is made on the basis of the *internal consistency* of the questionnaire responses.

Internal consistency measures of reliability are affected by some biases that make them underestimate actual reliability, and others that make them overestimate reliability (Raykov, 1997). They will underestimate reliability if the items within the set are not close replications of each other. For example, a scale of depression symptoms may contain some items on mood, others on psychophysiological complaints, and yet others on cognitive beliefs. Although these are all expected to be related to depression, they are not exact replications of each other. To the degree that the correlations among the items is due to the different item content rather than error, the overall reliability estimate will be smaller than it should be.

Reliability may be overestimated by the internal consistency design if the whole interview is affected by irrelevant global response patterns, such as mood or response biases. For instance, some respondents may perceive that acknowledging symptoms is socially undesirable and may systematically underreport more bizarre problems. Others may fall into a pattern of denying everything. These so-called *response biases* inflate internal consistency reliability estimates. They are often addressed by mixing the items across many conceptual domains, editing the items so that half are keyed as a symptom when the respondent says "no" and half are keyed the opposite way. Scales of Yea-saying, and Need-for-approval are also sometimes constructed to identify those respondents who are susceptible to response biases. The validity of these scales, however, is a subject of open discussion.

Given the possibility of opposing biases, how should we evaluate internal consistency results? If the results appear to indicate high reliability, look for response artifacts that might have inflated the estimate. If provisions have been taken to address response biases, then the high level of reliability might be real. If the results indicate that there is low reliability, then look to see if the items included within the internal consistency analysis are heterogeneous in content. It is possible that a set of items that are heterogeneous might have adequate test–retest reliability even though the internal consistency estimate is low.

Because various reliability designs have different strengths and weaknesses, it is always helpful to incorporate multiple designs into a reliability program. By systematically studying the kinds of replication, one can gain an insight into sources of measurement variation. This is what is recommended by Cronbach and colleagues (1972) in their comprehensive extension of classical test theory known as *Generalizability Theory*. This theory encompasses both reliability and validity by asking about the extent to which a measurement procedure works in different populations, at different times, with different raters, who may have different training. This broad perspective easily included designs such as those on the Diagnostic Interview Schedule (Anthony et al., 1985; Helzer et al., 1985) that compared results from interviews done by "lay" interviewers to those done by mental health professionals. To the extent that the trained lay interviewers performed like the professionals, the results might be interpreted as test–retest reliability of the DIS. If the level of training actually made a difference, then the results might be interpreted as the validity of using lay interviewers (assuming that the professionals are the ideal interviewers for this structured measure). From the generalizability perspective, it is neither a reliability or validity study, but rather a study of the generalizability of DIS results across time and interviewer type. For more information about generalizability theory at an accessible level, see the text by Shavelson (1991)

THE EFFECT OF POPULATION VARIANCE ON RELIABILITY

In all of the reliability designs reviewed above we assumed that respondents were sampled from the population that is to be studied. By randomly sampling from the population, we can obtain an unbiased estimate of σ_X^2. Note that any bias that is introduced in estimating σ_X^2 can have serious effects on the estimate of R_X. Epidemiologists should be especially sensitive to the fact that samples of patients should not be used in a reliability study if the ultimate survey is to be carried out in the general population. Relative to the variance in community surveys, the variance of most psychiatric measures will be too large in treated samples. The bias is usually concentrated in the σ_T^2 term of $\sigma_X^2 = \sigma_T^2 + \sigma_E^2$, and thus the reliability often appears to be better in the treated population than in a community population. When the reliability study sample has been constructed using stratified samples of cases and noncases, then it is often possible to undo the bias through weighting (e.g., Jannarone et al., 1987).

STATISTICAL REMEDIES FOR LOW RELIABILITY

If an investigator discovers that a quantitative measure is not sufficiently reproducible, there are several remedies that have been mentioned briefly before. The measure itself can be changed, the training of those administering it can be improved, or perhaps some special instructions can be developed for the respondents that improve the purity of the measurement outcome. These are examples of procedural remedies that are often effective. There is also a statistical remedy: Obtain several independent replicate measurements and average their results. The idea is simple: Averages of replicate measures are by definition more systematic than the individual measures themselves, so the reliability of the sum or average of items or ratings will be consistently higher than that of the components. The degree to which reliability is expected to improve in the composites is described mathematically by Spearman (1910) and Brown (1910). Let the sum of k ratings or items $(X_1, X_2, X_3, \ldots, X_k)$ be called $W(k)$. Then the expected reliability of $W(k)$ can be written as a function of k and the reliability of the typical measurement, R_X, according to the Spearman–Brown formula,

$$R_{W(k)} = \frac{kR_X}{1 + (k-1)R_X}. \tag{2}$$

Equation 2 is based on assumptions about the comparability of the measurements that are averaged or summed into $W(k)$, not on the form or distribution of the individual measurements. Because the result is not limited by the distribution of the X measures, the formula is even useful in calculating the expected reliability of a scale composed of k binary (0,1) items as well scales composed of quantitative ratings or items. Note that averaging measures only is a remedy for low reliability if there is some evidence of replicability. It is clear that R_W will be zero if R_X is zero, regardless of the magnitude of k.

The Spearman–Brown formula is especially useful for internal consistency reliability studies. When multiple items are available as replicate measures, it is usually the reliability of the scale score (the sum or average of items) that is of interest. While we could use the internal consistency design to calculate the average item reliability, and then using that result in Equation 2 to calculate the expected scale reliability, these steps are combined when one uses certain estimation formulas, such as the classic *coefficient alpha* of Cronbach (1951).

The relationship described in the Spearman–Brown formula can also be used in studies of interrater reliability to determine how many independent ratings need to be averaged to obtain an ideal level of reliability, say C_R. If the obtained level of reliability for a single rater is R_X, then the number of raters that are needed to produce an averaged-rater reliability of C_R is

$$k = \frac{C_R(1 - R_X)}{R_X(1 - C_R)}. \tag{3}$$

For example, if each rater only has a reliability of $R_X = 0.40$ and one wants a reliability of $C_R = 0.75$, then Equation 3 gives $k = 4.5$. This means that averages of four raters would be expected to have less than 0.75 reliability, while averages of 5 raters would exceed the target reliability of 0.75.

RELIABILITY THEORY AND BINARY JUDGMENTS

The reliability theory just reviewed does not make strong assumptions about the kind of measurement embodied in X, and indeed many of the results hold for binary variables such as ones that might represent specific psychiatric diagnoses (e.g., $X = 1$ when the respondent is thought to have current major depression, $X = 0$ otherwise). Kraemer (1979) has shown explicitly how the results work with binary judgments. From her mathematical analysis of the problem it can be seen that the systematic component of X that I have called $T = E(X)$ will end up as a proportion falling between the extremes of 0 and 1. It represents the expected proportion of diagnosticians who would give the diagnosis to the respondent being evaluated. If T is close to 1, then most diagnosticians would say that the respondent is a case, and if T is close to 0, then most would say that the respondent is not a case. Note that while X itself is binary, T is quantitative in the range $(0, 1)$.

Because averages are quantitative (at least as n gets large), the psychometric results from the Spearman–Brown formula are applicable only when the composite of interest is quantitative. This is often the case when X represents binary items in a symptom scale. Of interest is the count of symptoms, which is closely related to the average of symptom items. However, if we really want a binary variable as the outcome, then the Spearman–Brown result does not apply. For example, diagnoses of several independent judges are sometimes combined into a "consensus diagnosis" that is itself binary. If the consensus rule is one that requires that all judges make the diagnosis before the diagnosis is applied, the result might be less reliable than some of the individual diagnosticians! (See Fleiss and Shrout, 1989). The total consensus rule is as weak as the least reliable diagnostician, because each has veto power regarding whether the consensual diagnosis is made.

Many of the classic psychometric results depend on the assumed symmetry of errors. Because T is defined as an average, by definition about half the errors go in one direction and half in the other. For diagnoses, however, the errors that attract attention are those that seem to cause clinically relevant discrepancies. For example, if we know that a certain set of presentation facts are viewed by 90% of trained clinicians as indicating schizophrenia, then the clinically relevant discrepancies are those diagnosticians who argue that the diagnosis of schizophrenia is inappropriate. Persons who insist that schizophrenia should be diagnosed with more than 90% certainty are not usually considered in practical terms to be outliers.

The interest in the asymmetry of errors in diagnoses prompts some researchers to decompose interrater discrepancies into ones that are consistent with problems of sensitivity and specificity. From this perspective it can be shown that the reliability coefficient of Equation 1 is a function of both kinds of errors. If we focus on one kind of error only, such as sensitivity, the classic relation between reliability and validity no longer holds necessarily. There are some examples in which different levels of reliability are consistent with the same level of sensitivity. (One usually finds that the assumed specificity or prevalence varies with the reliability in examples such as this.) (See Carey and Gottesman, 1978). When asymmetric errors are of central interest, the results reviewed in this chapter may not be totally applicable.

The role of asymmetric errors in binary ratings is only one special aspect of such data. Another is the relation of the expected mean of a binary variable and the expected variance of that variable. For variables that are normally distributed, the mean contains no information about the variance of the variable, but for variables that are binomial (a very common distribution for binary variables), the variance is necessarily small for variables with means near zero or one. This fact has implications in the interpretation of Equation 1, the definition of the reliability coefficient. If the prevalence of a diagnosis is low in a population, then σ_T^2 will be small. If the level of error variance is held constant, but σ_T^2 is made smaller, then R_X will be smaller. One way to interpret this result is that the level of error must be reduced to study disorders that have smaller base rates in the population. Any randomly false positive diagnosis makes the diagnostic system seem unreliable for rare disorders. In this case the diagnostic system is unreliable because the precious few true positives are swamped by the random false positives. Nevertheless, the fact that reliability is empirically related to prevalence has caused some commentators to question the utility of reliability measures in binary variables (Grove et al., 1981; Guggenmoos-Holzmann, 1993; Spitznagel and Helzer, 1985). Others of us have argued that dropping the statistic because of the challenge of measuring rare disorders is misguided (Shrout, 1998; Shrout et al., 1987) because the reliability statistic is useful in describing the effects of measurement error on statistical analyses. Kraemer (1992) lucidly reviewed the rationale of reliability studies and showed how the challenge of establishing reliability of categorical data is affected by various features of the measurement situation and the design of the reliability study.

In the next section I present a survey of reliability statistics that can be used to evaluate data from reliability studies. One of these statistics is Cohen's kappa (Cohen, 1960). It is especially designed for categorical outcomes, but it shares with the quantitative statistics its interpretation as estimators of the reliability coefficient in Equation 1. Although the special features of binary data require a careful consideration of the effects of errors in epidemiological analyses, the general concerns for the concept of reliability as reviewed in the preceding sections are usually relevant for multivariate analyses that treat binary distinctions as dummy variables.

RELIABILITY STATISTICS: GENERAL

As we have seen, the reliability coefficient of Equation 1 is defined in terms of variances: variances of systematic person characteristics σ_T^2, and variances of measurements across replications for a single person, σ_E^2. There are several ways to estimate the variance ratio shown in Equation 1 (Dunn, 1989), but one direct method is simply to estimate the separate variance components and then combine them in the form of Equation 1. Estimates of this sort are called *intraclass correlations*.

Intraclass correlation is not a single statistic but rather a family of statistics that can be used for estimating reliability. In this section we will review several versions that can be used with a wide variety of variables. We focus here on the easiest part of reliability analysis, "point estimation" of the statistic that summarizes the reliability results. Although it is important, we do not have the space to present the methods that must be used to estimate 95% confidence intervals for the study results. The form of the interval estimators depends on the nature and distribution of the data, and new methods are being actively developed in the literature. For reviews of methods for confidence intervals see Dunn (1989), Shrout (1998), and Blackman and Koval (2000). It is important to note, however, that estimates of reliability are often less precise than we would like (Walter et al., 1998), and that this fact is made clear by the use of confidence intervals.

The intraclass correlation point estimates are derived from information summarized in the Analysis of Variance (ANOVA) of the data from the reliability study. The ANOVA treats each subject as a level of the SUBJECTS factor. Usually subjects are considered to be a *random factor*, because they are selected to be representative of a population of interest.

If the replicate measurements of the subjects are systematically obtained using a certain set of k raters or measuring devices, then the ANOVA might involve a two-way SUBJECTS by MEASURES design. If, on the other hand, the replicate measurements of each subject are obtained by randomly sampling k measures, then the analysis would use a one-way ANOVA.

One-way ANOVA Analyses

Table 1 illustrates data that might be collected in reliability study of relative informants. Each of $N = 10$ probands is rated by $k = 3$ distinct relatives. Between-subject variation can be estimated using all k ratings, and within-subject variation is used to estimate the magnitude of the error variation. When the relationships of the relatives vary from proband to probands (e.g., siblings for one proband, parents for another, cousins for a third), these data do not have a data analytic structure for informant. If there had been such a structure, we might have considered a proband-by-relationship two-way ANOVA. In our analysis we will

TABLE 1. Hypothetical Data on Functioning of Ten Probands by Three of Their Relatives

Proband	Relative 1	Relative 2	Relative 3
1	29	32	17
2	23	33	28
3	19	17	18
4	6	10	5
5	13	20	20
6	0	0	2
7	10	11	15
8	5	1	15
9	31	26	19
10	15	17	18

assume that the informants are essentially a random sample of possible informants for a given respondent.

Table 2 shows the layout of the one-way ANOVA, along with the numerical estimates obtained from the data in Table 1. The actual computation of the ANOVA results can be obtained from standard computer software, such as SPSS RELIABILITY (SPSS, 2001). The numerical example illustrates a pattern in which the between-subjects (probands) mean squares is substantially larger than the within-subjects mean squares. Consistent with an informal examination of the hypothetical data in Table 1, this pattern suggests that the differences between subjects' mean ratings are larger than the disagreements among relatives regarding the subjects' scores.

The reliability estimate for the one-way ANOVA is calculated using the first formula in Part A of Table 3. This form of the intraclass correlation was called

TABLE 2. Analysis of Variance When Replications are Nested within Subjects: One-way ANOVA

Source of Variation	*df*	Sums of Squares	Mean Squares (MS)	Table 1 Example: MS on *df*
Between subjects	$n - 1$	BSS	$\text{BMS} = \text{BSS}/(n-1)$	BMS = 251.0 on 9 *df*
Within Subjects	$n(k-1)$	WSS	$\text{WMS} = \text{WSS}/[n(k-1)]$	WMS = 22.2 on 20 *df*

TABLE 3. Versions of Intraclass Correlation Statistics Useful for Various Reliability Designs

Type of Reliability Study Design	Raters fixed or Random	Version of Intraclass Correlation[a]
		Part A: Reliability of single rater
Nested *n* subjects rated by *k* different raters	Random	$\text{ICR}(1,1) = \dfrac{\text{BMS} - \text{WMS}}{\text{BMS} + (k-1)\text{WMS}}$
Subject by rater crossed design	Random	$\text{ICR}(2,1) = \dfrac{\text{TMS} - \text{EMS}}{\text{TMS} + (k-1)\text{EMS} + k(\text{JMS} - \text{EMS})/n}$
Subject by rater crossed design	Fixed	$\text{ICR}(3,1) = \dfrac{\text{TMS} - \text{EMS}}{\text{TMS} + (k-1)\text{EMS}}$
		Part B: Reliability of the average of k ratings
Nested: *n* subjects rated by *k* different raters	Random	$\text{ICR}(1,k) = \dfrac{\text{BMS} - \text{WMS}}{\text{BMS}}$
Subject by rater crossed design	Random	$\text{ICR}(2,k) = \dfrac{\text{TMS} - \text{EMS}}{\text{TMS} + (\text{JMS} - \text{EMS})/n}$
Subject by rater crossed design	Fixed	$\text{ICR}(3,k) = \dfrac{\text{TMS} - \text{EMS}}{\text{TMS}}$

[a]BMS and WMS refer to between-subject and within-subject mean squares from a one-way ANOVA. TMS, JMS, and EMS refer to between-subjects (targets), between measures (judges) and error mean squares from two-way ANOVA based on *n* target-subjects and *k* raters.

TABLE 4. Hypothetical Data on Assessment of Depression and Functioning[a]

Respondent	$X1$	$X2$	$Z1$	$Z2$
1	0	1	17	11
2	1	1	17	15
3	0	0	26	25
4	0	0	24	22
5	0	0	19	14
6	0	0	22	16
7	0	0	17	18
8	0	0	23	19
9	1	0	19	16
10	0	1	18	12
11	0	0	21	18
12	1	1	13	11
13	0	0	21	23
14	0	0	22	17
15	0	0	15	12
16	0	0	20	18
17	0	0	21	20

[a] $X1$ and $X2$ represent test–retest diagnoses of major depression ($X = 1$, present; $X = 0$, not present), and $Z1$ and $Z2$ represent ratings of adaptive functioning.

ICR(1, 1) by Shrout and Fleiss (1979), and we retain that designation. To illustrate the calculation with the numerical example from Table 1, we find,

$$\text{ICR}(1, 1) = (251.0 - 22.2)/(251.0 + 2^{*}22.2) = 0.77.$$

This result describes the reliability of a single randomly selected informant. About 77% of the variance of a single informant's ratings is attributable to systematic differences between subjects. Although the stability of the result might be questioned because of the limited sample size, the result is encouraging that *this rating*, in *this population* appears to be made fairly reliably by a single informant.

Suppose that it is possible to obtain three informant ratings for each subject in the survey. How much more reliable would the average of the three ratings be than an individual informant? The answer can be calculated using the Spearman–Brown formula (Equation 2), with $k = 3$ and $R_X = 0.77$. Alternatively, one can use the formula for ICR(1, k) shown in Part B of Table 3. This formula is obtained by algebraically combining the expression for ICR(1, 1) with the Spearman–Brown formula. In this case the answer is ICR(1, k) = 0.91. About 91% of the variance of the average of three randomly chosen informants is attributable to systematic differences between subjects.

Two-way ANOVA Analyses.

Table 4 illustrates data that might be collected in a reliability study of two professional raters or interviewers. As a result of the interview by Interviewer 1 we have both a binary diagnosis [disorder present ($X = 1$) vs. disorder absent ($X = 0$)] and a quantitative score such as a total functioning score (called Z in the table). Replicate scores and diagnoses are obtained by a second interviewer, called

TABLE 5. Analysis of Variance When Replications Have Structure: Two-Way ANO

Source of Variation	*df*	Sums of Squares	Mean Squares (MS)	Table 4 Examples: MS on *df*
Between subjects (targets)	$n-1$	TSS	TMS = TSS/$(n-1)$	Variable X: 0.254 on 16 *df* Variable Z: 25.7 on 16 *df*
Between measures (judges)	$(k-1)$	JSS	JMS = JSS/$(k-1)$	Variable X: 0.029 on 1 *df* Variable Z: 67.8 on 1 *df*
Residual (error)	$(n-1)(k-1)$	ESS	$\text{EMS} = \dfrac{\text{ESS}}{(n-1)(k-1)}$	Variable X: 0.092 on 16 *df* Variable Z: 2.67 on 16 *df*

Interviewer 2. The hypothetical data on $X1$, $X2$, $Z1$, and $Z2$ are shown for seventeen respondents. The layout of the two-way ANOVA is shown in Table 5, along with numerical results from the Table 4 examples.

Only two interviewers were used in the reliability study illustrated in Table 4, but we might consider the two to be a random sample from all possible interviewers from the study. If so, then they must *not* be selected on the basis of their special skills as interviewers, but rather should be selected to be representative. When interviewers who are employed in the reliability study represent the population of potential interviewers, we say that they are *random* effects.

In some cases we are interested in the ratings of specific interviewers rather than a population of interviewers. Suppose Interviewer 1 is a doctoral candidate who carried out her own data collection, and that Interviewer 2 is a colleague who is hired to document that the ratings are systematic. In this case we simply wish to describe the quality of data collected by the doctoral candidate, and we say that the interviewers are *fixed* effects.

Depending on whether the raters are considered to be random or fixed, we use different versions of the intraclass correlation to estimate reliability. When we wish to estimate the reliability of a randomly sampled interviewer, we use the expression for ICR(2, 1) shown in Part A of Table 3. This intraclass correlation is not only a function of the between-subjects mean squares and the error mean squares, but also the between-measure (judge) mean squares. If different raters are more or less liberal in assigning high scores, then the final variability of the ratings will be affected. ICR(2, 1) takes this extra variation into account in estimating reliability.

In the two examples of Table 4, one reveals a large between-measure effect and the other does not. From the numbers in Table 4 it can be seen that the $Z2$ ratings are usually smaller than the $Z1$ ratings. Rater 2 seems to believe that most subjects are functioning somewhat worse than perceived by Rater 1. Even with this rater difference, the reliability of Z is higher than the reliability of X, according to the data in Table 4. The ICR(2, 1) for Z is calculated as

$$(25.7 - 2.67)/(25.7 + (1)^*2.67 + 2^*(67.8 - 2.67)/17) = 0.64.$$

The ICR(2, 1) for X is calculated as

$$(0.254 - 0.092)/(0.254 + (1)*0.092 + 2*(0.029 - 0.092)/17) = 0.48.$$

For the rating of adaptive functioning we could consider averaging both individual Z ratings to obtain a more reliable score. We can use either the Spearman–Brown formula, or the expression ICR(2, k) to calculate the reliability of the mean of two such ratings. In this case, the result is 0.78 rather than 0.64.

Although the reliability of the binary X variable is worse than that of the quantitative Z variable, it would not usually be meaningful to rely on an average diagnosis instead of a truly binary rating. For this reason the ICR(2, k) form of the intraclass correlation would not be applied to X in Table 4.

The calculations carried out so far have assumed that the two sets of ratings in Table 4 are representative of a host of possible interviewers. Now we turn our attention to the situation in which the two raters can be considered to be fixed. In this case we can either ignore systematic rater differences in mean ratings, or we can adjust for them.

The expression for ICR(3, 1) in Part A of Table 3 is appropriate when we wish to describe the reliability of a single fixed rater. Unlike ICR(2, 1), this version of the intraclass correlation is not affected by the between-rater mean squares. On the average, ICR(3, 1) will be larger in magnitude than ICR(2, 1). By fixing the raters to certain persons, the extraneous variation due to sampling of raters is eliminated and the resulting reliability is usually higher.

This effect is especially obvious for Z, which had a large between-rater effect. The ICR(3, 1) for Z is calculated as

$$(25.7 - 2.67)/(25.7 + (1)*2.67) = 0.81.$$

ICR(3, 1) for X is not much different than ICR(2, 1), as the rater effects were small:

$$(0.254 - 0.092)/(0.254 + (1)*0.092) = 0.47.$$

The Reliability of the Average of k Fixed Measures: Cronbach's α

Just as ICR(1, 1) and ICR(2, 1) can be used in the Spearman–Brown formula to determine how much reliability improves by using an average score, so can ICR(3, 1) be used when an average measurement is of interest. In this case the reliability of the averaged measurement can be computed directly using ICR(3, k) from Table 3. For the quantitative Z variable, the reliability of the average is expected to be 0.90.

One common application of ICR(3, k) is to internal consistency analyses of psychometric scales. Items in self-report questionnaires are usually fixed in that the same items are used with all respondents. Suppose that n subjects are administered k scale items, and the results are analyzed using the two-way ANOVA layout of Table 5. The estimate of the reliability of the sum or average of the k fixed items can be computed using ICR(3, k). The result is identical to the internal consistency estimate known as Cronbach's α (Cronbach, 1951). α is computed directly by computer programs such as SPSS RELIABILITY (SPSS, 2001).

OTHER RELIABILITY STATISTICS

Cohen's κ

When binary data such as that for variable X in Table 4 are collected, reliability can be estimated directly using Cohen's κ (Cohen, 1960). Fleiss and Cohen (1973) showed that κ is conceptually equivalent to ICR(2, 1) in Table 3. It can be calculated simply using the entries of a two-by-two table showing the diagnostic agreement. In general, this agreement table might be laid out as follows:

	Rater 1: +	Rater 2: −	Total
Rater 2: +	a	b	$a + b$
Rater 2: −	c	d	$c + d$
Total	$a + c$	$b + d$	n

Cohen (1960) pointed out that while cells a and d represent agreement, it is not sufficient to evaluate reliability by reporting the overall proportion of agreement, $P_o = (a + d)/n$. This statistic may be large even if raters assigned diagnoses by flipping coins or rolling dice. His κ statistic adjusts for simple chance mechanisms,

$$\kappa = \frac{P_o - P_c}{1 - P_c},$$

where P_o is the observed agreement, $[(a + d)/n]$, and P_c is the expected agreement due to chance:

$$P_c = [(a + c)(a + b) + (b + d)(c + d)]/n^2.$$

When computing κ by hand, it is sometimes more convenient to use the following equivalent expression:

$$\kappa = \frac{ad - bc}{ad - bc + n(b + c)/2}.$$

When the X data in Table 4 are tabulated into a two-by-two table like that shown above, we get $a = 2$, $b = 2$, $c = 1$, and $d = 12$. The observed agreement, $P_o = 0.82$, but the expected agreement by chance is $P_c = 0.67$. Using either of the expressions for κ, we find the reliability to be 0.46. As expected, this is quite close to the value of 0.48 obtained using ICR(2, 1).

One advantage of calculating the reliability of binary judgments using κ instead of intraclass correlation methods is that the expressions for κ's standard error and confidence bounds are explicitly suited to binary data. κ can also be generalized to describe the overall reliability of classifications into multiple categories. Fleiss (1981) provides an overview of many forms of κ, and Donner and colleagues (Donner, 1998; Donner and Eliasziw, 1992, 1994, 1997; Donner et al., 1996, 2000) have done much to describe the sampling variation of κ statistics.

Product moment correlation

If the reliability study yields two measurements, and if the raters are considered to be fixed (rather than representative of a pool of raters), then reliability can be estimated by computing the product moment correlation between the two measures. This is the usual correlation statistic built into most computer programs and calculators. When the ratings are quantitative, the correlation is known as the *Pearson correlation*, and when the ratings are binary it is known as the *phi coefficient*. Regardless of what they are called, they are comparable to the ICR(3, 1) version of the intraclass correlation described above. For the Z variables the Pearson correlation is $r_P = 0.83$ and for the X variables in Table 4 the phi coefficient is $r_P = 0.47$. These are very close to the ICR(3, 1) values of 0.81 and 0.47 obtained on the same data.

SUMMARY AND CONCLUSIONS

Unreliability is a measurement problem that can often be rectified by improving interview procedures, or by using statistical sums or averages of replicate measures. Determining the extent to which unreliability is a problem, however, can be challenging. There are various designs for estimating reliability, but virtually all have some biases and shortcomings. Studies of sampling variability of reliability statistics (Donner, 1998; Dunn, 1989; Cantor, 1996) have suggested that sample sizes in pilot studies are often not adequate to give stable estimates about the reliability of key measurement procedures. It is important that reliability studies be considered critically in search for ways to improve measurement procedures. Specifically, if the reliability of a measure appears to be very good, ask whether there are biases in the reliability design that might bias the results optimistically. Were the respondents sampled in the same way in the reliability study that they will be in the field study? Was the respondent given the chance to be inconsistent, or did the replication make use of archived information? If serious biases are not found, and the reliability study produced stable estimates, then one can put the issue of reliability behind, at least for the population at hand.

If the reliability of a measure appears to be poor, one should also look for biases in the reliability design. How similar were the replications? Could the poor reliability results be an artifact of legitimate changes over time, heterogeneous items within a scale, or artificially different measurement conditions? Was the sample size large enough to be sure that reliability is in fact bad? Be especially suspicious if you have evidence of validity of a measure that is purported to be unreliable. Rather than dismissing a measure with apparently poor reliability, ask whether it can be improved to eliminate noise.

REFERENCES

American Psychiatric Association AP (1980): "Diagnostic and Statistical Manual of Mental Disorders." 3rd ed: Washington, DC: American Psychiatric Association.

American Psychiatric Association AP (1994): "Diagnostic and Statistical Manual of Mental Disorders" 4th ed: Washington, DC: American Psychiatric Association.

Anthony JC, Folstein M, Romanoski AJ, Von Korff MR, Newstadt GR, Chahal R, Merchant A, Brown CH, Shapiro S, Kramer M, Gruenberg EM (1985): Comparison of the lay Diagnostic Interview Schedule and a standardized psychiatric diagnosis. Arch Gen Psychiatry, 42:667–675.

Blackman NJ-M and Koval JJ (2000): Interval estimation for Cohen's kappa as a measure of agreement. Stat Med 19:723–741.

Brown W (1910): Some experimental results in the correlation of mental abilities. Br J Psychol, 3, 296–322.

Cantor AB (1996): Sample-size calculations for Cohen's kappa. Psycholol Methods 1:150–155.

Carey G and Gottesman II (1978): Reliability and validity in binary ratings: Areas of common misunderstanding in diagnosis and symptom ratings. Arch Gen Psychiatry 35:1454–1459.

Cochran, WG (1968): Errors in measurement in statistics. Technometrics 10:637–666.

Cohen J (1960): A coefficient of agreement for nominal scales. Educ Psychol Measurement 20:37–46.

Cronbach LJ (1951): Coefficient alpha and the internal structure of tests. Psychometrika 16:297–334.

Cronbach LJ, Gleser GC, Nanda H. Rajaratnam N (1972): "The Dependability of Behavioral Measurements: Theory of Generalizability for Scores and Profiles." New York: Wiley.

Donner A (1998): Sample size requirements for the comparison of two or more coefficients of inter-observer agreement. Stat Med 17:1157–1168.

Donner A and Eliasziw M (1992): A goodness-of-fit approach to inference procedures for the kappa statistic: confidence interval construction, significance-testing and sample size estimation. Stat Med 11:1511–1519.

Donner A and Eliasziw M (1994): Statistical implications of the choice between a dichotomous or continuous trait in studies of interobserver agreement. Biometrics 50:550–555.

Donner A and Eliasziw M (1997): A hierarchical approach to inferences concerning interobserver agreement for multinomial data. Stat Med 16:1097–1106.

Donner A, Eliasziw M, Klar N (1996): Testing the homogeneity of kappa statistics. Biometrics 52:176–183.

Donner A, Shoukri MM, Klar N, Bartfay E (2000): Testing the equality of two dependent kappa statistics. Stat Med 19:373–387.

Dunn G (1989): "Design and Analysis of Reliability Studies." New York: Oxford University Press.

Endicott J, Spitzer RL, Fleiss JL, et al. (1976): The Global Assessment Scale: A procedure for measuring overall severity of psychiatric disturbance. Arch Gen Psychiatry 33:766–771.

Fleiss JL (1981): "Statistical Methods for Rates and Proportions." 2nd ed. New York: Wiley.

Fleiss JL, Cohen J (1973): The equivalence of weighted kappa and the intraclass correlation coefficient as measured on reliability. Educ Psychol Measurement 33:613–619.

Fleiss JL, Shrout PE (1989): Reliability considerations in planning diagnostic validity studies. In Robins l (ed): "The Validity of Psychiatric Diagnoses" New York: Guilford, pp 279–329.

Grove WM, Andreason NC, McDonald-Scott P, Keller MB, Shapiro RW (1981): Reliability studies of psychiatric diagnosis: Theory and practice. Arch Gen Psychiatry 38:408–413.

Guggenmoos-Holzmann I (1993): How reliable are chance-corrected measures of agreement? Stat Medicine 12:2191–2205.

Helzer JE, Robins LN, McEvoy LT, Spitznagel EL, Stoltzman RK, Farmer A, Brockington IF (1985): A comparison of clinical and Diagnostic Interview Schedule diagnosis: Physician reexamination of lay-interviewed cases in the general population. Arch Gen Psychiatry 42:657–666.

Jannarone RJ, Macera CA, Garrison CZ (1987): Evaluating interrater agreement through "case–control" sampling. Biometrics 43:433–437.

Kraemer HC (1979): Ramifications of a population model for kappa as a coefficient of reliability. Psychometrika 44:461–472.

Kraemer HC (1992): Measurement of reliability for categorical data in medical research. Stat Methods Med Research 1:183–199.

Lord FM and Novick MR (1968): "Statistical Theories of Mental Test Scores." Reading, MA: Addison-Wesley.

Raykov T (1997): Estimating composite reliability for congeneric measures. Applied Psychol Measurement 21:173–184.

Raykov T (1997): Scale reliability, Cronbach's coefficient alpha, and violations of essential tau-equivalence with fixed congeneric components. Multivariate Behavioral Res 32:329–353.

Shavelson RJ and Webb NM (1991): "Generalizability Theory: A Primer. Newbury Park, CA: Sage.

Shrout PE (1998): Measurement reliability and agreement in psychiatry. Stat Methods Med Res 7:301–317.

Shrout PE and Fleiss JL (1979): Intraclass correlations: Uses in assessing rater reliability. Psychol Bull 86:420–428.

Shrout PE and Fleiss JL (1981): Reliability and case detection. In Wing J, Bebbington P, RLN (eds): "What is a Case? The Problem of Definition in Psychiatric Community Surveys." London: Grant, McIntyre, pp 117–128.

Shrout PE and Newman S (1989): Design of two-phase prevalence surveys of rare disorders. Biometrics 45:549–555.

Shrout PE, Skodol AE, Dohrenwend BP (1986): A multimethod approach for case identification and diagnosis: First stage instruments. In J. E. Barrett (Ed.), "Mental disorders in the community: Progress and Challenge." New York. Guilford Press. pp. 286–303.

Shrout PE, Spitzer RL, Fleiss JL (1987): Quantification of agreement in psychiatric diagnosis revisited. Arch Gen Psychiatry 44:172–177.

Shrout PE, Yager T (1989): Reliability and validity of screening scales: Effects of reducing scale length. J Clin Epidemi 42:69–78.

Snedecor GW, Cochran WG (1967): "Statistical Methods," 6th ed. Ames, IA: Iowa State University Press.

Spearman C (1910): Correlation calculated from faulty data. Br. J. Psychol 3:271–295.

Spitzer RL (1983): Psychiatric diagnosis: Are clinicians still necessary? Comprehensive Psychiatry 24:399–411.

Spitzer RL, Endicott J, Robins E (1975): Clinical criteria and DSM-III. Amer. J. Psychiatry 132:1187–1192.

Spitznagel EL, Helzer JE (1985) A proposed solution to the base rate problem in the kappa statistic. Arch Gen Psychiatry 42:725–728.

SPSS I (2001): SPSS for Windows (10th ed.). Chicago: SPSS Inc.

Walter SD, Eliasziw M, Donner A (1998): Sample size and optimal designs for reliability studies. Stat Med 17:101–110.

CHAPTER 5

Validity: Definitions and Applications to Psychiatric Research

JILL M. GOLDSTEIN and JOHN C.SIMPSON

Harvard Medical School Department of Psychiatry, Harvard Institute of Psychiatric Epidemiology and Genetics, Massachusetts Mental Health Center, Boston, MA 02115 and VA Boston Healthcare System, Mental Health Careline, Boston, MA

INTRODUCTION

Measurement is a process of linking unobservable theoretical concepts to empirical indicators (Carmines and Zeller, 1979). There are two basic properties of measurement that ensure the strength of this linkage: reliability and validity. In this chapter, we discuss the concept and usage of validity. Reliability was discussed fully in a previous chapter, but, for convenience, we define it here simply as the reproducibility of an empirical measure (e.g., internal consistency of the items in a scale, reproducibility of a measurement on different occasions, or agreement between raters). For an empirical indicator to be valid it must first be reliable, but indicators can be reliable without also being valid.

There are a number of ways to assess validity, not all of which are used for every measure of interest. In fact, validity has a number of meanings in different contexts and is perhaps one of the most overused words in the scientific literature. In this chapter, we discuss validity as it applies to the measurement of a construct, that is, the process of "construct validity." We also discuss validity as it applies to relationships between constructs, that is, to the internal validity and external validity of a presumed causal relationship. We provide examples of how validity is applied and statistically evaluated in psychiatric research.

VALIDITY OF A CONSTRUCT

An essential feature of scientific research is often the measurement of abstract concepts and relationships between abstract concepts. *Validity* can be defined as the extent to which an empirical indicator of a concept actually represents the concept of interest (Cronbach and Meehl, 1955; Anastasi, 1976; Nunnally, 1978). For example, if one used a particular symptom checklist to measure "major

Textbook in Psychiatric Epidemiology, Second Edition, Edited by Ming T. Tsuang and Mauricio Tohen. ISBN 0-471-40974-X

depressive disorder," validity asks the question, how accurate is this empirical indicator for diagnosing major depressive disorder? Thus, validity refers to the question: "For what purpose is the indicator being used?" (e.g., to diagnose major depressive disorder) and "How accurate is it for that purpose?" In fact, an indicator (e.g., an instrument such as a test, a rating, or an interview) can be valid for one purpose, but not for another (Cronbach, 1971). Thus, one validates the instrument *in relation to its intended purpose* (Cronbach, 1971; Nunnally, 1978; Carmines and Zeller, 1979). If an instrument is to be scientifically useful, it must be both reliable (i.e., result in consistent findings over repeated measurements) and valid (i.e., represent the concept it is intended to represent).

Unlike reliability, validity is an unending process (Nunnally, 1978) in which one attempts to capture the essence of the concept of interest as accurately as possible. It therefore involves a theoretical understanding of the concept of interest in order to measure it accurately. It also involves an assessment of the empirical relationships between an instrument and criteria chosen to evaluate whether the instrument assesses what it is intended to assess. There are three basic ways in which validity is assessed: content validity, criterion validity, and construct validity.

Content Validity

For every abstract concept, there is a universe of items that one might sample in order to measure the concept operationally. *Content validity* involves the adequacy with which one samples the domain of items (Nunnally, 1978). Content validity is ensured by the procedures used to construct items for a test (Nunnally, 1978). One must first specify the universe of items that one hypothesizes will accurately measure the concept of interest. Second, items are then sampled from this domain. If certain kinds of items are central to understanding the concept, one may decide to oversample these types. Finally, selected items are put into a testable form (Carmines and Zeller, 1979).

For example, if one were interested in measuring (diagnosing) "schizophrenia," one would choose, among other things, items such as bizarre delusions or other types of delusions, various kinds of hallucinations, formal thought disorder, and flat affect. An instrument would then be constructed in order to assess these items. Different types of diagnostic instruments have been constructed that are based on certain assumptions about how to acquire accurate assessments of the items.

For example, the Diagnostic Interview Schedule (DIS) (Robins et al., 1981) was designed to allow lay interviewers to assess symptom items in a dichotomous form, as present or absent, and was wholly dependent on the patient's response to each item. That is, there was an assumption that clinical judgement was unnecessary to assess symptomatology. In contrast, the Schedule for Affective Disorders and Schizophrenia (SADS) (Endicott and Spitzer, 1978) was designed to allow for clinical questioning to assess symptom items. Clinical/diagnostic knowledge was required in order to use the SADS instrument. In addition, ratings of SADS items consisted of a severity scale rather than present versus absent, as in the DIS. As one can see, these two instruments are based on different assumptions regarding how to assess a similar domain of symptom items. One can then assess the content validity of these two approaches, even though the evaluation of content validity alone would provide an incomplete assessment of the validity of these instruments.

There are two standards by which content validity is assessed: the representativeness of the collection of items chosen and the type of test construction used to measure the concept. There are, however, no statistical means of assessing content validity. Essentially, content validity is dependent on appeals to reason regarding the accuracy of the content sampled, or a consensus among experts, and the adequacy with which the items are put into a testable form (Cronbach and Meehl, 1955; Nunnally, 1978).

Examples of Assessment of Content Validity

Streiner (1993) recommended the use of a "content validity matrix" as a means of ensuring that items in a scale are appropriately tapping the intended domains. In such a matrix, each column represents a distinct domain within the general domain of interest, and each row represents a single item. As a means of improving reliability, each domain is represented by several items (i.e., in terms of the content validity matrix, each column should have check marks in several rows). On the other hand, to minimize ambiguity of interpretation, each item should tap only one domain (i.e., each row should have only a single check mark).

As an example of the relevance of domains and items to content validity, we can make use of a study by Schwartz et al., (1975) who devised the Social Adjustment Interview Schedule to investigate outcome in schizophrenia. Within this general domain, the authors conceptually identified eight role areas (i.e., domains) and devised multiple questions (i.e., items) within each role area to address performance and subjective feelings. The different domains included work role (18 items), household role (15 items), marital role (9 items), and social and leisure roles (54 items). Typical items within the work domain included the questions "Are you employed now?" and "Are you confident about your ability to do the job?" Within the marital domain, typical items included "In general, how do you and your spouse get along?" and "Have you been able to talk about feelings and problems with your spouse recently?" There would probably be little disagreement about content validity in this example. In other words, most would agree that these four questions comprise two sets of items, that the first two items are related to work roles, whereas the latter two concern marital roles, and furthermore that there is little if any overlap between the content of these specific items.

Not all applications of content validity will be as straightforward, particularly if the concepts being measured are abstract, that is, not directly observable. For example, Cloninger (1987) devised an 80-item self-report inventory called the Tridimensional Personality Questionnaire (TPQ) to investigate three hypothesized dimensions of personality: harm avoidance, novelty seeking, and reward dependence. Cloninger's approach to content validity is apparent in his description of how the items were devised (p 580): "To quantify behavioral variation on each dimension separately, questions were specified that were theoretically expected to involve minimal interaction among the dimensions. In practice, this meant that questions were chosen to evaluate the behaviors that were thought to be characteristic of individuals deviant on one dimension and average on the others." As evidence that this standard was achieved, Cloninger reported that the intercorrelations among the three major TPQ scales (calculated using the Pearson product-moment correlation coefficient) were "negligible or weak" and low relative to the reported index of internal consistency (Cronbachs α coefficient; see Chapter 9 for a discussion in the context of reliability). However, the interpretation of these results is complicated because weak intercorrelations were expected in some cases for theoretical reasons (e.g., a weak negative correlation between novelty seeking and harm avoidance).

A somewhat different perspective was presented by Takeuchi et al. (1993), who translated the TPQ into Japanese and replicated Cloninger's (1987) study using a large sample of Japanese university students. Like Cloninger (1987), Takeuchi et al. (1993) reported negligible or weak intercorrelations between the three major scales. However, they also reported results from a factor analysis that were not completely consistent with the theoretical model. (Factor analysis is a multivariate statistical procedure that is used to explain covariation among a set of observed variables in terms of a reduced number of unobserved, latent variables; (e.g., see Kim and Mueller, 1978 for an introductory explanation). Within the framework of Streiner's content validity matrix (Streiner, 1993), for example, if each derived factor was considered to define a separate domain (i.e., column) in the matrix, then the harm avoidance, novelty seeking, and reward dependence items should have loaded on different factors. While this was by and large the result for harm avoidance and reward dependence, "the novelty seeking scale showed a scattering factor structure, with several equivocal items loaded on two or more factors; reduction or reorganization of items might be required here" (Takeuchi et al., 1993, p 277). On the other hand, all reported items had factor loadings above the cutoff of 0.4 on only one of the six factors, and this was consistent with Streiner's ideal (1993) of only one check mark per item in the content validity matrix.

Criterion Validity

The second type of validity is referred to as *criterion validity* (*or predictive validity*). It is concerned with measuring something that is *external* to the measurement of the concept itself, called the *criterion* (Cronbach and Meehl, 1955; Nunnally, 1978). For example, one dimension of predictive criterion validity for psychiatric diagnoses is to relate them to predictions of outcome. (Examples of this are discussed in detail later in this chapter.) Unlike content validity, which essentially depends on a consensus among experts, predictive validity is dependent on empirical results. *Predictive validity* refers to the empirical relationships between the instrument under study and external events or behaviors that can occur at three points in time: before, during, or after the instrument is used. In many studies, the empirical relationship is statistically estimated by a correlation if continuous data are used.

Post-dictive validity refers to correlating events or behaviors that have occurred in the past with the instrument one is presently using. These assessments are referred to as *retrospective*. For example, one might have a specific prediction about the early developmental history of patients, with a particular diagnosis that is being currently assessed with an instrument. Post-dictive validity entails correlating early history information with the diagnostic assessment currently obtained using the instrument under study.

Concurrent validity refers to correlating a measure and some criterion *at the same point in time*. This involves what are known as *cross-sectional assessments*. Thus, for example, if there were a laboratory test for diagnosing major depressive disorder, one could correlate the instrument used to diagnose the disorder with a laboratory test taken when the patient was interviewed.

The form of predictive validity most commonly referred to correlates a measure with a criterion that is assessed at some *future point in time*. This form of validity entails prospective assessments. A common use of predictive validity in psychiatry is to assess outcomes of a specific diagnostic group under study, under the assumption that certain diagnostic groups have worse or better outcomes than others (see examples below).

A fourth form of criterion validity is referred to as *discriminant validity*. Discriminant validity assesses whether certain external criteria (i.e., events or behaviors) are uncorrelated with the measure of interest compared with other criteria that are hypothesized to be related to the measure of interest. That is, is the measure of interest uncorrelated with events or behavior with which one expects it would be independent? This has also been referred to as *assessing the specificity* of the relationship between the measure of the concept of interest and the external criteria chosen to relate to the concept.

It is important to mention here that criterion validity is often assessed using correlations (when continuous data are involved). The strength of the correlation is often interpreted as the strength of the validity of the measure. However, the strength of the correlation depends not only on the variability and other characteristics of the measure of interest, including its reliability, but also on the choice, measurement, and reliability of the criterion.

Examples of Criterion Validity

For examples of applications of criterion validity, we turn to two recent studies in the psychiatric literature. The first study (Addington et al., 1993) provides a fairly typical example of the use of correlational techniques. At issue was whether a self-report instrument can be used in populations of patients with schizophrenia to obtain valid ratings of depression. To examine this question, the authors compared self-report ratings obtained using the Beck Depression Inventory (BDI) with ratings of the Calgary Depression Scale (CDS), a semistructured interview designed to assess depression in schizophrenics. In this study, the CDS is the criterion because it makes use of informed judgements by trained clinicians, which form the current "gold standard" for identifying depression in clinical populations. BDI and CDS scores were compared by calculating the Pearson product-moment correlation coefficient (e.g., see Woolson, 1987), after creating scatterplots to examine the joint distribution of BDI and CDS scores as well as identifying any outliers. The latter step was essential because the presence of even a single outlier (i.e., an extreme and atypical value) could easily distort the product-moment correlation (e.g., see Simpson 1982).

Another important methodologic step employed by Addington et al., (1993) was to compare correlations between the BDI and CDS in clinically distinct subgroups of schizophrenic patients: inpatients versus outpatients, and (within these subgroups) patients who either did or did not require assistance in completing the self-report instrument. In this particular study, the correlation between the BDI and CDS was stronger among inpatients than outpatients, regardless of whether the patients required assistance ($r = 0.84$ vs. $r = 0.96$). However, the substantially greater percentage of inpatients requiring assistance (34% of inpatients vs. 12% of the outpatients) led the authors to conclude that "depressed affect can be assessed in patients with schizophrenia by both self-report and structured interview, but the Beck Depression Inventory poses difficulties in use with inpatients" (Addington et al., 1993, p. 561).

For our purposes, however, the substantive findings of this study were less important than the fact that this study admirably illustrated the critical importance of selecting and describing validation samples that are clinically meaningful in the context of the measurement instrument of interest (Streiner, 1993). In particular, users of such instruments need to be aware that published validation studies might have used "samples of convenience" (e.g., university students) that do not approximate the clinical population the user has in mind and that the results of such studies do not necessarily generalize to other samples.

Our second example of criterion validity in psychiatric research (Somervell et al., 1993) also illustrates the critical importance of the validation sample. In this study, the validity of using a questionnaire (the Center for Epidemiologic Studies Depression Scale, or CES-D) (Radloff, 1977) as a case identification tool in studies of mood disorders among Native Americans was investigated. CES-D scores were compared with DSM-III-R diagnoses (American Psychiatric Association, 1987) based on a structured psychiatric interview (the Lifetime Version of the Schedule for Affective Disorders and Schizophrenia, Endicott and Spitzer, 1978). The authors had concerns about the cross-cultural applicability not only of the screening instrument but also of the criterion itself (e.g., DSM-III-R diagnoses of affective disorders). For purposes of the study, however, it was assumed that DSM-III-R diagnoses would be relevant among Native Americans.

Although the CES-D, like the BDI in the above example, yields a numerical score, its proposed use as a screening instrument for depression was for the purpose of identifying not the degree of depression, but the presence of a particular clinical syndrome, namely, DSM-III-R major depression. The criterion was therefore a categorical (i.e., qualitative) rating rather than a numerical (i.e., quantitative) rating, making it inappropriate to use correlational procedures. Instead, to evaluate the validity of the instrument for case identification, the authors employed statistical methods that have been expressly developed for qualitative data, including sensitivity, specificity, and receiver operating characteristic (ROC) analysis.

Sensitivity and specificity are both calculated using data that have been summarized in a 2×2 table of frequencies (see Table 1 for definitions and computational formulas). In the example at hand, a 2×2 table was used to cross-classify the numbers of screened persons with and without the criterion (e.g., a DSM-III-R diagnosis of major depression) who either did or did not score above the cutoff for depression in the screening instrument, the CES-D. (ROC analysis was used to determine the optimal cutoff value for the CES-D.) As an illustrative finding, the sensitivity for DSM-III-R major depression was 100% (i.e., all three persons in the sample with a diagnosis of major depression scored above the cutoff on the CES-D). The corresponding value of specificity was 82% (i.e., 82% of those persons in the sample who did not have diagnoses of major depression scored below the CES-D cutoff for depression). It follows directly from the reported specificity value of 82% that 18% (100% − 82%) of the persons in the sample with

TABLE 1. 1. Computation of Indices of Criterion Validity and Predictive Value[a]

a	Criterion		
Rating	Present	Absent	Total
Positive	a	b	$a + b$
Negative	c	d	$c + d$
Total	$a + c$	$b + d$	N

[a] a, b, c, d, and N are frequencies (e.g., numbers of persons rated). Sensitivity = $a/(a + c)$; the probability of a positive rating among those possessing the criterion. Specificity = $d/(b + d)$; the probability of a negative rating among those lacking the criterion. Positive predictive value = $a/(a + b)$; the probability of having the criterion among those with positive ratings. Negative predictive value = $d/(c + d)$; the probability that those with negative ratings will not have the criterion. Prevalence = $(a + c)/N$; the base rate of the criterion in the validation sample.

no psychiatric diagnoses or with DSM-III-R diagnoses other than major depression scored above the CES-D cutoff and would have been classified as depressed by that screening instrument.

Whether or not this degree of misclassification error (or invalidity) is considered to be an unacceptably high "false-positive" rate depends on the proposed use of the instrument and on the comparable "operating characteristics" of alternative instruments. For example, a higher CES-D cutoff value could be expected to decrease the false-positive rate (via increased specificity), but at the expense of sensitivity. In this particular study, a higher CES-D cutoff actually increased specificity without decreasing sensitivity, but this was probably attributable to the small number of cases with DSM-III-R diagnoses of major depression. In most studies there is a systematic trade-off between sensitivity and specificity, and for that reason both of these indices of criterion validity must be considered together in determining whether a particular instrument is more valid than the available alternatives. ROC analysis provides a useful framework for making such comparisons (e.g., see Murphy et al., 1987). In the present example, the non-negligible false-positive rate was consistent with the investigators concerns (based on previous research by a number of researchers using other samples) that the CES-D might be reflecting symptoms of not only major depression but also increased levels of anxiety, demoralization, or even physical ill health (Somervell et al., 1993).

The study by Somervell et al. (1993) also illustrates the difference between criterion validity and the related, but nevertheless distinct, concept of predictive value. *Positive predictive value* is literally the predictive value of a positive rating, that is, the probability of having the criterion of interest *given* a positive rating on the instrument under investigation. (Formulas for calculating positive predictive value, and the related index, negative predictive value, are given in Table 1.) Since the criterion (e.g., DSM-III-R major depression) is frequently of more direct clinical importance than the rating (e.g., a particular CES-D score), positive and negative predictive values are often more clinically meaningful than sensitivity and specificity. For example, most clinicians would probably be more interested in the usefulness of the CES-D for predicting major depression than the other way around. However, positive predictive value is a joint function of sensitivity, specificity, and prevalence, such that low prevalence values can severely constrain the values of positive predictive value that can be realistically attained, even with very high sensitivity and specificity values (Baldessarini et al., 1983; Glaros and Kline, 1988). (Negative predictive value is similarly constrained by high prevalence values.)

In the study by Somervell et al. (1993), the prevalence of major depression can be estimated from the rate of major depression in the sample as $3/120 = 0.025$. Using a cutoff value of 16 on the CES-D, the reported specificity value of 82.1% therefore corresponds to a positive predictive value of 0.125. In other words, even though sensitivity was perfect (100%) and specificity was very high, only one of every eight persons who scored above the CES-D cutoff of 16 would be expected actually to have major depression. Even increasing the CES-D cutoff to improve specificity would not dramatically change this result. Again, this is due to the constraint imposed by the low estimated prevalence of major depression in the study population. (With the CES-D cut-off set at 28, the reported specificity value of 96.6% corresponds to a positive predictive value of 0.429.) In conclusion, this example shows that even though an instrument may have excellent criterion validity as assessed using standard indices (namely, sensitivity and specificity), the actual predictive value of the instrument could be much more limited, depending on the prevalence of the disorder of interest, which in turn may vary with the composition of the validation sample.

Construct Validity

Of the three basic types of validity, *construct validity* involves the most complex process. Content validity and criterion validity used alone are limited in contributing to understanding the relationship between the theoretical (unobserved) concept and the empirical measure used to indicate it. In fact, content and criterion validity are considered part of the process of assessing construct validity. As first pointed out by Cronbach and Meehl (1955), construct validity is essential for all abstract concepts, since there is no criterion or entire content of a domain that is wholly adequate to define the concept of interest. Construct validity is thus defined in a theoretical context. It is the extent to which one's measure of interest is related to other theoretically related concepts that are also measured (Nunnally, 1978).

There are three steps to assessing construct validity (Carmines and Zeller, 1979). First, one must have an understanding of the theoretical relationships between related concepts. Second, one must estimate the empirical relationships between operational measures of these concepts. Finally, the empirical evidence must be interpreted within the theoretical context in which the concept of interest is embedded. In addition, findings from other studies must be related to one's current findings regarding the measure and the concept it is intended to indicate. The theoretical context allows one to make theoretical predictions that then lead to empirical tests using the operational measure of the concept of interest. One study cannot wholly validate a measure of a concept. Construct validity requires a pattern of consistent findings across studies involving different samples and different settings.

Cronbach and Meehl (1955) refer to the theoretical context as the *nomologic network*. The use of the nomologic network requires relating theoretical constructs to each other, theoretical constructs to empirical indicators, and empirical indicators to each other. The construct is not reduced to the empirical indicators. It is combined with other constructs in the nomological net that allow for predictions using the empirical indicators (Cronbach and Meehl, 1955, p. 290).

Application of Construct Validity to Psychiatric Diagnosis

In psychiatry, there are no known laboratory tests for wholly identifying a psychiatric case. In 1972, Robins and Guze established five criteria that have become standards for validating a diagnosis. Kendler (1990) recently reviewed these standards for psychiatric diagnoses and pointed out a number of potential limitations to this approach. For example, he discusses the frequent need to take "fundamentally nonempirical" matters into consideration in formulating and using psychiatric diagnoses. Such matters can include, for example, various clinical, historical, and administrative issues, needs, and imperatives. For purposes of this discussion, however, we consider only the empirical criteria originally proposed by Robins and Guze (1970).

The first criterion of Robins and Guze (1970) consists of establishing the clinical description of the disorder. This involves specifying the phenomenology or symptomatology, premorbid history, age at onset, sociodemographic distribution, and precipitating factors. The clinical description criterion thus involves issues of content validity. For example, what is the domain of symptoms chosen to represent the diagnosis? "On the face of it," do these symptoms reasonably represent the domain of interest? Furthermore, how would one construct an instrument to assess these symptoms? The clinical description criterion also involves criterion validity. For example, post-dictive validity would be relating premorbid history, age at onset, or precipitating factors to the measure of diagnosis.

The second criterion refers to the relationship of the diagnostic measure to laboratory tests. As mentioned earlier, this is a form of concurrent validity. Laboratory tests may include chemical, anatomic, physiologic, or psychological tests (Robins and Guze, 1970). In psychiatry, however, at present there are no laboratory "gold standards" for validating diagnoses.

The third criterion involves the use of family history to contribute to validation. The assumption behind the use of family history is that many psychiatric disorders run in families. Thus, an increased prevalence of the same disorder in family members can be used as an indicator that the diagnosis is a valid entity. Family history can be thought of as a concurrent validator (in reference to ill relatives who are currently alive) or as a postdictive validator (in reference to relatives who were ill but who are now deceased).

The fourth criterion, commonly thought of as predictive validity in psychiatric research, relates the diagnosis of interest to outcomes, including treatment response. The assumption behind using this criterion is that individuals with the same diagnosis will have similar outcomes. Furthermore, it is sometimes assumed that certain diagnostic groups have particularly poor or good outcomes compared with other diagnostic groups. However, the use of outcome as a validating criterion is problematic because many psychiatric disorders have heterogeneous outcomes. This validating criterion will remain controversial unless more definitive knowledge regarding the specific outcomes of diagnostic groups can be elaborated.

The final criterion for validating a diagnosis involves assessing the specificity of the other criteria for a particular diagnosis. This can be referred to as *discriminant validity.* Although different diagnoses may share, for example, certain symptoms, laboratory test results, or outcomes, it is the role of discriminant validity to specify how a particular disorder is differentiated from other disorders. If it cannot be differentiated from other disorders, this becomes support for rejecting the validity of this particular diagnosis as a separate entity.

In summary, the assessment of the validity of a diagnosis cannot be accomplished in one study. As discussed with construct validity, it is an ongoing process that requires multiple studies, using different samples, across different settings. One must relate empirical evidence regarding the five criteria to each other, driven by a theory of how and why these findings "fit together" in predicted ways. The theory is the basis for developing appropriate empirical measures. The relationships between empirical measures of one's concepts of interest will contribute to testing empirically one's theory about the concept.

Threats to Construct Validity

There are a number of threats to construct validity. We will briefly mention three of the most important that are discussed in detail by Cook and Campbell (1979): inadequate theoretical conceptualization, mono-operations bias, and monomethods bias. Inadequate theoretical conceptualization leads to the development of empirical measures that do not adequately assess one's concept of interest. An inadequate representation of the concept of interest may also result from the other two threats to construct validity. *Mono-operations bias* refers to an inadequate number of empirical items used to measure a particular concept, for example, if only one question was asked to measure the concept. *Monomethods* bias refers to the inadequate use of methods to obtain empirical information on the criterion of interest. That is, the use of different methods to obtain empirical information on the same criterion will increase the reliability of that information and thus contribute to the validity of the use of that empirical data to measure the concept of interest. For example, to assess a research psychiatric diagnosis, the use of a standardized structured interview in combination with medical record review and informed clinical judgement may provide the most valid assessment of the diagnosis.

VALIDITY OF THE RELATIONSHIPS BETWEEN VARIABLES

The second use of the term *validity* that we discuss in this chapter refers to the "internal and external validity" of the empirical relationships between measures used to assess abstract concepts. Internal and external validity are discussed thoroughly by Cook and Campbell (1979) in relation to quasi-experimental design studies. They are also discussed in basic textbooks on epidemiology (MacMahon and Pugh, 1970; Susser, 1973).

Internal validity refers to the extent to which a relationship found to be statistically significant is a causal relationship. Internal validity is an empirical issue. That is, do the empirical measures used to assess concepts of interest relate to each other in a causal way? It is also a theoretical issue in that the presumed causal association between variables must be coherent with other empirical evidence and theory.

In epidemiology, there are five "criteria of judgement" that are used to aid in establishing a causal relationship Susser (1973): (1) the temporal (time) sequence of variables, (2) the consistency of associations on replication, (3) the strength of the association, (4) the specificity of association, and (5) the coherency of the explanation of the association. The *time sequence* refers to the temporal order of the variables of interest. The *consistency of the association* refers to its reliability. The strength of the association is measured empirically using relative risk, correlational or nonparametric statistics. *Specificity* refers to what we previously discussed as discriminant validity. Finally, the *coherence criterion* refers to a more theoretical question of whether the explanation of the association between the variables of interest "fits" with pre-existing theory and evidence. These five criteria are then used to make judgments regarding whether the empirical association between variables has internal validity or causal plausibility.

The causal plausibility of a relationship may in part be dependent on the type of study design used to assess one's variables of interest. In a controlled experimental study, one may specifically manipulate the time order of variables and experimentally control for confounding factors that may be threats to internal invalidity. However, many epidemiologic studies are not experimental, but rather are observational and what has been called *quasi-experimental* (Cook and Campbell, 1979). In these types of studies, it may be more difficult to establish the internal validity of the relationship between variables. There are a number of threats to internal validity that may arise in using nonexperimental designs. They are discussed in detail by Cook and Campbell (1979, p 5159) and briefly described here.

Suppose that in a treatment study one found that treatment "a" was significantly better for a specific diagnostic group than treatment "b," as measured by pre- and post-treatment measurements of symptomatology. However, suppose there was no random assignment to treatment; thus the study was not an experimental design. The following threats to the "internal validity" of the effect of treatment "a" may be operating and should be addressed. In general, threats to internal validity have to do with the possibility of *differential* effects of events on the treatment versus the control groups that are not due to the treatment of interest per se.

History effects refer to the influence of events outside of the control of the study that may differentially affect the outcomes of the groups being studied but have little relationship to the treatment of interest. *Maturation* involves the differential development of participants in each group that is not due to treatment effects. *Testing and instrumentation effects* refer, respectively, to the number of times a test is given resulting in differential learning effects and changes in instrumentation over time that differentially affects one's groups unrelated to treatment effects.

Statistical regression artifacts are especially difficult to control for. They can occur if the groups at pretreatment time are not equivalent, that is, do not come from the same population. In a nonrandomized study, one attempts to match groups on certain pretreatment variables. However, the matching variables may be unreliable themselves, resulting in unmatched groups at pretreatment assessment time. Respondents with high scores on unreliable pretreatment variables may score lower at posttreatment time, and the reverse may be true for respondents with low scores on unreliable pretreatment variables. The expected direction of the change in unreliable scores from pre- to posttreatment is always toward the population mean (Cook and Campbell, 1979). This is referred to as *regression to the mean*. Thus, the change in one's treatment groups would not be due to treatment, but rather to these regression artifacts. One way to control for these artifacts is to ensure that pretreatment matching variables are as reliable as possible. It is often difficult to make one's groups completely comparable, and therefore using experimental designs in treatment studies is preferable, although not always possible.

A classic example of how regression artifacts can adversely affect results was the Westinghouse–Ohio University study of Head Start (preschool education) (Campbell and Elebacher, 1970). In this study, the cases and controls were undermatched for socioeconomic status, resulting in making Head Start look damaging to children. This occurred because controls were selected from a more able population than Head Starters. That is, the pretreatment or pretest matching variable, socioeconomic status, which includes educational status, was unreliable. When cognitive measures were assessed post-Head Start, the control groups cognitive scores regressed to their population mean, which were higher than those in the Head Start group. The population means of the two groups were different, because the controls were originally selected from a population that was educationally and cognitively more advanced than the Head Start group (Campbell and Elebacher, 1970). When controls were appropriately selected for comparison with the Head Start children, the Head Start program was shown to have a significant impact on the cognitive functioning of the children who experienced the program.

Selection effects are related to regression artifacts. Selection becomes a threat to internal validity when the characteristics of one's groups are different, and this results in differential changes from pre- to posttreatment assessment between groups. For example, *mortality* can result in selection artifacts. *Mortality effects* refer to the differential dropout or refusal rates between the groups that may affect the group's posttreatment mean. For example, if the more severely ill patients dropped out of treatment "a," then post-treatment assessment of symptoms among the treatment a group may look better due to the differential dropout of severely ill patients in that group rather than to effects of treatment "a" on symptomatology.

Other threats to internal validity discussed by Cook and Campbell (1979, pp. 53–55) include differential social influences on the groups being compared. For example, communication between patients in the treatment and control groups about the treatment of interest may result in rivalry between the groups, "resentful demoralization" of the group receiving a less desirable treatment, or imitation of one group by the other.

The *external validity* of a significant result refers to the extent to which a finding is generalizable to and across persons, time periods, and settings (Cook and Campbell, 1979). Random sampling of ones groups from the population of interest contributes to the ability to "generalize to" the population of interest. *Generalizing across* populations refers to the identification of those populations to which the findings can be applied. That is, it refers to the extent of the generalization of findings to other populations aside from those that were directly studied or subpopulations among those studied. For example, most readers would be cautious about generalizing across males and females from a study of health services utilization based solely on a sample of males.

The threats to external validity can be thought of as interaction effects with the treatment of interest (Cook and Campbell, 1979). For example, differences in treatment response between the sexes or socioeconomic statuses will lower the generalizability across the population as a whole. There are three types of interaction effects that are threats to external validity: interactions of selection, setting, and history with treatment (Cook and Campbell, 1979, pp. 73–74). For example, selection interactions, or systematic recruitment artifacts, may result in findings being attributable only to those recruited into the study. The same can be said for interactions of treatment with setting and history. For example, using a university setting may limit ones generalizability across other settings. Conducting the treatment study during a particular historical period may not allow generalizability to future time periods. To minimize both of these threats, multiple studies would need to be implemented using different populations at different historical time periods.

SUMMARY

In summary, *validity* can have different meanings depending on the context in which it is used. It is applied to the measurement of concepts, called *construct validity*, and to the relationship between operational measures, called the *internal and external validity of a presumed causal relationship.* As applied to construct validity, it is an unending process in which one attempts to measure a concept of interest as accurately as possible. Thus, as discussed, validity involves a theoretical understanding of the concept as well as an empirical assessment of the criteria chosen to operationalize the concept. This chapter discussed three basic ways in which validity is assessed: content validity, criterion validity, and construct validity. Content and criterion validity can be thought of as part of the process of assessing construct validity. One study cannot wholly validate a measure of a concept. It requires a pattern of consistent findings across studies involving different samples and different settings.

The other way in which validity has been discussed in this chapter refers to the "internal and external validity" of empirical relationships between operational measures of the concepts of interest. *Internal validity* refers to the extent that a statistically significant relationship is a causal one. There are a number of ways in which causal plausibility is assessed, for example, the five criteria of judgement used in epidemiologic studies (Susser, 1973). In addition, causal plausibility is dependent on the type of study design employed. As discussed, quasi-experimental designs are open to a number of threats to internal validity, for example, regression artifacts, history, and selection effects. Experimental study designs, in which one manipulates the time order of variables and controls for confounding factors, are less vulnerable to threats to internal validity. Finally, *external validity* refers to the extent that one can generalize the study findings to and across persons, time periods, and settings. To minimize threats to external validity, multiple studies are needed in which the study populations, the historical time periods, and the setting are varied.

ACKNOWLEDGMENTS

This chapter was written while Dr. Goldstein was supported by NIMH RO1 MH56956. The authors thank Nicole Cullen for help in manuscript preparation.

REFERENCES

Addington D, Addington J, Maticka-Tyndale E (1993): Rating depression in schizophrenia: A comparison of a self-report and an observer scale. J Nerv Ment Dis 181:561–565.

American Psychiatric Association (1987) DSM-III-R: "Diagnostic and Statistical Manual of Mental Disorders." Washington, DC: American Psychiatric Press.

Anastasi A (1976): "Psychological Testing." London: Macmillan.

Baldessarini RJ, Finkelstein S, Arana GW (1983): The predictive power of diagnostic tests and the effect of prevalence of illness. Arch Gen Psychiatry 40:569–573.

Campbell DT, Elebacher A (1970): How regression artifacts in quasi-experimental evaluations can mistakenly make compensatory education look harmful. In Helmuth J (ed): Compensatory Education: A National Debate, Vol 3. "Disadvantaged Child." New York: Brunner/Mazel.

Carmines EG, Zeller RA (1979): "Reliability and Validity Assessment. Series Quantitative Applications in the Social Sciences." Beverly Hills, CA: Sage University Press.

Cloninger CR (1987): A systematic method for clinical description and classification of personality variants. A proposal. Arch Gen Psychiatry 44:573–588.

Cook TD, Campbell DT (1979): Quasi-experimentation design and analysis issues for field settings. Chicago: Rand McNally College Publishing.

Cronbach LJ (1971): Educational Measurement. In Thorndike RL (ed): "Test Validation." Washington, DC: American Council on Education.

Cronbach LJ, Meehl PE (1955): Construct validity in psychological tests. Psychol Bull 52:281-302.

Endicott J, Spitzer RL (1978): A diagnostic interview: The Schedule for Affective Disorders and Schizophrenia. Arch Gen Psychiatry 35:837–844.

Glaros AG, Kline RB (1988): Understanding the accuracy of tests with cutting scores: The sensitivity, specificity, and predictive value model. J Clin Psychol 44:1013–1023.

Kendler KS (1990): Toward a scientific psychiatric nosology. Strengths and limitations. Arch Gen Psychiatry 47:969–973.

Kim JO, Mueller CW (1978): Factor analysis: statistical methods and practical issues. Beverly Hills: Sage Publications.

MacMahon B, Pugh TF (1970): "Epidemiology: Principles and Methods." Boston: Little, Brown.

Murphy JM, Berwick DM, Weinstein MC et al. (1987): Performance of screening and diagnostic tests: application of receiver operating characteristics analysis. Arch Gen Psychiatry 44:550–555.

Nunnally JC (1978): "Psychometric Theory." New York: McGraw-Hill.

Radloff LS (1977): The CES-D Scale: a self-report depression scale for research in the general population. Applied Psychol Measurement 1:385–401.

Robins E, Guze SB (1970): Establishment of diagnostic validity in psychiatric illness: Its application to schizophrenia. Am J Psychiatry 126:983–987.

Robins LN, Helzer JE, Croughan J et al. (1981): The NIMH diagnostic interview schedule: its history, characteristics, and validity. Arch Gen Psychiatry 38:381–389.

Schwartz CC, Myers JK, Astrachan BM (1975): Concordance of multiple assessments of outcome in schizophrenia: On defining the dependent variables in outcome studies. Arch Gen Psychiatry 32:1221–1227.

Simpson JC (1982): Amino acid levels in schizophrenia and Celiac disease: Another look. Biol Psychiatry 17:1353–1357.

Somervell PD, Beals J, Boehnlein J et al. (1993): Criterion validity of the Center for Epidemiologic Studies Depression Scale in a population sample from an American Indian village. Psychiatry Res 47:255–266.

Streiner DL (1993): A checklist for evaluating the usefulness of rating scales. Can J Psychiatry 38:140–148.

Susser M (1973): Causal thinking in the health sciences. Concepts and strategies of epidemiology. London: Oxford University Press.

Takeuchi M, Yoshino A, Kato M et al. (1993): Reliability and validity of the Japanese version of the Tridimensional Personality Questionnaire among university students. Comp Psychiatry 34:273–279.

Woolson RF (1987): Statistical Methods for the Analysis of Biomedical Data. New York: Wiley.

CHAPTER 6

Mental Health Services Research

JACK D. BURKE, JR.

Department of Psychiatry, Harvard Medical School, and The Cambridge Hospital, Cambridge, MA 02139

INTRODUCTION

One aim of epidemiology is to understand the functioning of health services (Morris, 1957). Research on mental health services is undertaken on several levels of investigation, including the clinical, program, and systems levels (National Advisory Mental Health Council, 1991). Major questions about the delivery of health services can be summarized with four terms (Teh-wei Hu and Charles E. Windle, personal communication, November 11, 1988):

Equity: Access to health services for the general population can be influenced by socioeconomic, geographic, and cultural factors. In the United States, access to health services appears to be a major problem for disadvantaged groups, such as the working poor who have no health insurance, residents of sparsely populated rural areas, or minority groups who are alienated from established health care institutions. In addition to access, another problem identified has been the influence of socioeconomic and ethnocultural factors on provision of care, through the diagnostic process as well as choice of treatment.

Efficiency: Providing the right mix of services and delivering the highest level of care possible with a given level of resources have become increasingly important issues as health care expenditures have risen as a proportion of the gross domestic product.

Economy: To some extent, in the United States questions about health economics have been reduced to simple policy questions about how to pay for health care. But questions such as the influence that any particular payment or reimbursement scheme has on the delivery of health care services and the influence of payment systems on provider behavior have become increasingly important.

Effectiveness: Ensuring the highest quality of care, and presumably through that care ensuring the highest level of health for the population, have become

Textbook in Psychiatric Epidemiology, Second Edition, Edited by Ming T. Tsuang and Mauricio Tohen.
ISBN 0-471-40974-X

increasingly urgent. While a great deal of research has been supported to study the fundamental mechanisms of nature and to translate the findings into efficacious therapies, too little is known about the way that treatment is provided in everyday clinical practice or how well commonly accepted therapeutic practices work.

Since all four of these topics deal with assessment within populations, with attention to variation across groups, and usually have an integral relationship to questions of type of disease and level of impairment, they are intrinsically based on epidemiologic findings and methods. While health services research is a multidisciplinary field, epidemiology provides the basis for assessing the health needs of a population, and its research methods provide a tool to test ways to improve the level of health (Baasher et al., 1982).

In mental health research, the rapid developments in epidemiologic methods have made it possible to begin addressing some of the key questions about delivery of mental health services. In particular, as the distribution of mental illnesses in the population, and the resulting impairment from them, have been clarified through epidemiologic studies, and as clinical research has shown the benefit of treatment, mental health services have become a growing focus of both research and policy interest. This progress in related fields has helped to overcome the tendency researchers and policy makers have had in the past to dismiss mental health service delivery as an unwieldy or unapproachable subject.

DESCRIPTIVE STUDIES OF MENTAL HEALTH SERVICES

Two of the most important issues from a public health perspective are to determine the need for mental health care in a population and to assess the extent of "unmet need." This concept of unmet need raises consideration of *equity*, *efficiency*, and *economy* in delivering mental health services. But uncertainty about effectiveness of treatment, at the clinical, program, and systems levels, has led to controversy about how to determine when mental health services are needed (Klerman et al., 1992). This controversy leads some policymakers to discuss "demand" for services, to emphasize the consumer's role, rather than "need," which might emphasize the provider's view.

To address these issues, studies of services actually provided help to describe the service delivery system and level of care available. These studies of people seen within treatment settings provide information about the nature of services provided and the characteristics of patients who use them. Studies of a community population allow a more direct comparison of individual diagnostic status and use of mental health services.

Surveys of Institutions

Until the late 1970s, when epidemiologic methods in psychiatry became more powerful, information on the distribution of mental disorders from most populations in the world came from surveys of the patients in mental institutions. In the United States, these surveys have been sponsored by the U.S. Public Health

Service. In the past they have focused on state and county hospitals; with the evolving service delivery system, the periodic census of patients has expanded to include private hospitals, free-standing units (like community mental health centers), general hospitals, and federal hospitals, including veterans' medical centers.

For the last day of 1969, the National Reporting Program of NIMH found that 471,451 patients were in psychiatric inpatient units; by 1992, the number had fallen to 214,714. The principal location of that care changed as well, with 78.4% in state and county hospitals in 1969 and 38.7% in state and county hospitals by 1992. Another striking finding was the growth in outpatient services, especially in the 1970s. The estimate of people receiving outpatient services rose from 1.1 million in 1969 to 2.6 million in 1979 (Taube and Barrett, 1985) and 2.8 million in 1992 (Center for Mental Health Services, 1996). However, one shortcoming of these data is the lack of comparable information on office visits to individual practitioners, such as psychiatrists, psychologists, and social workers.

Minority Groups. One of the most difficult tasks facing services researchers is understanding the relative overrepresentation among inpatients of individuals who are African-American or Native American. While the admission rate might be partly explained by socioeconomic factors, the predominance of diagnoses of schizophrenia rather than bipolar disorder among African-Americans has raised questions about possible bias in the diagnostic practices for different groups. At the same time, minority groups such as African-Americans or Native Americans are underrepresented in many outpatient settings, especially when patients with Medicaid are excluded, and have low rates of services use (Snowden and Cheung, 1990; Surgeon General, 1999; Snowden and Thomas, 2000; Novins DK et al., 2000).

Jails and Prisons. Studies of special institutions have also been conducted. One of the most important sites to explore has been correctional institutions. A study of male detainees in Cook County (Chicago) jails showed that the prevalence of mental disorders among a random sample of 728 males charged with misdemeanors or felonies was two to three times higher than among individuals from the same demographic groups in the general population (Teplin, 1990). Results such as these have suggested that the largest mental institution in the United States is apparently the Los Angeles County jail (Torrey et al., 1990). Efforts to address the treatment needs of these inmates involve such initiatives as diversion programs, to keep mentally ill offenders from being incarcerated (Steadman et al., 1999; 2001a); acceptability of telepsychiatry for evaluation of jail inmates (Brodey et al., 2000); and development of treatment algorithms specifically for the prison setting (Buscema et al., 2000).

Surveys of Populations

While data from the NIMH Epidemiologic Catchment Area (ECA) program have been useful in estimating prevalence of mental disorders in the general population (Robins et al., 1984; Myers et al., 1984; Regier et al., 1988a, b), they also provide a basis for estimating use of services by the population. Each respondent in the five-site sample reported on use of mental health services on an inpatient and outpatient basis, with extensive information on the type of provider used.

Initial reports from the ECA demonstrated that about 6 to 7% of the adult population reported an ambulatory visit for mental health reasons to a health provider in the 6 month period before the first interview. Of these respondents reporting visits, about half saw a general medical provider only, and half saw a mental health specialist at least once. For all 9,543 respondents in the first three sites, about 16 to 25% of all ambulatory health care visits in a 6-month period were reportedly made for mental health problems (Shapiro et al., 1984).

From 14 to 18% of the respondents reported at least one admission for general medical conditions during the year prior to the first ECA interview. For mental health reasons, from 2 to 6% of respondents reported an inpatient admission. This figure was variable across sites, as the community with the highest rate of admissions had the largest number of psychiatric beds available. A similar association was shown for rates of ambulatory mental health visits. The explanation for these associations of higher use with higher supply of services is uncertain. Associations between services use and supply could result from better effort at reducing unmet need, from providing better geographic, financial, or other means to access services, or from inducing demand through increased supply (Shapiro et al., 1984).

Subsequent analyses of these data have projected estimates of services use to the adult U.S. population for a one-year period by combining data from the first ECA interview with the follow-up interview conducted approximately one-year later. These new estimates suggested that the one-year prevalence of DSM-III disorders covered by the Diagnostic Interview Schedule (DIS) was 28.1%, or about 44.7 million people aged 18 years or over. About 1% of the population had an inpatient stay for mental health reasons and about 10.7% had an outpatient visit in this same one-year period. For outpatient visits, about 5.6% of the population was seen in the mental health specialty sector and about 6.4% in the general medical sector, with some individuals being seen in both. About 64% of individuals with an active diagnosis of schizophrenia received any mental health service in a one-year period, and about 54% of those with major depression did (Regier et al., 1993).

With newer data derived from the National Comorbidity Survey (NCS) as well as the ECA, composite estimates suggest that about 8% of adults have a diagnosable DSM-III-R disorder and also use mental health services in a given year. Since about 28% of adults have been found to have a mental or substance use disorder in a one-year time frame, the Surgeon General estimates that the remainder, about 20% of adults in the United States, have a diagnosable disorder and do not receive any mental health services during a one-year period (Regier et al., 1993; Kessler et al., 1994; Surgeon General, 1999).

Minority Groups. National estimates are helpful in determining services use overall and demonstrate that the majority of individuals with mental disorders do not receive mental health treatment. Concerns about *equity* in access and *efficiency* in providing services make it important to examine variations in services use. Another study examining services use in the ECA data demonstrated that individual characteristics associated with using mental health services included being white, female, and aged 25 to 65 years. This study carefully controlled for diagnostic status, so it provides important confirmation that being young or old, nonwhite, or male make people with mental disorders less likely to receive treatment for their disorders (Leaf et al., 1988; Klerman et al., 1992). These findings reinforce the impression gained from the National Reporting Program and studies of specific populations that minority populations are under-served by the treatment system.

Primary Care Populations. Epidemiologic data from studies of general populations suggest that many people with mental disorders are seen primarily or exclusively in general medical settings. Studies assessing the presence of these disorders in patients seen in primary care settings in this country and abroad have verified a high prevalence of serious mental disorders in patient populations: from 15 to 28% of patients have a current mental disorder in a range of studies. The prevalence figure is even higher when more inclusive, but less precise instruments (such as self-report questionnaires rather than research diagnostic interviews) are used as case identification measures (Shepherd et al., 1981; Regier et al., 1988a, b; Katon and Shulberg, 1992). At least one study using a research interview and measures of duration and disability showed that a significant proportion of these conditions are serious and chronic in nature (Regier et al., 1985).

These findings of the importance of primary care in the *de facto* mental health services system (Regier et al., 1978, 1993) become even more significant when the *effectiveness* of care is examined. A range of studies comparing the primary care clinician's recognition of mental disorders in patients whose interview indicates presence of at least one mental disorder show that only 10 to 50% of patients are detected as having a diagnosable disorder (Regier et al., 1988a,b; Kessler et al., 1985). Efforts to improve detection and diagnosis have not been shown to improve outcomes, a goal that has been difficult to achieve (Tiemens et al., 1999; Simon GE 1998; Rost et al., 1998; Burns et al., 2000).

Overview of Services Use. Efforts to compare services use estimates based on surveys of institutional providers with estimates based on surveys of the population have shown reasonable agreement, especially for inpatient care. For example, the ECA estimate for patients receiving care in a state or county mental hospital was 338,000 adults, and the NIMH National Reporting Program estimate was 351,000. For general hospitals, the estimates were 606,000 and 609,000, respectively. However, the ECA estimates for some forms of treatment, such as number of persons with visits to mental health center outpatient clinics, was much lower than reported to the National Reporting Program (Manderscheid et al., 1993). Discrepancies could be accounted for by the fact that the ECA was not designed to provide a nationally representative sample (Regier et al., 1988a). Also, self-reported data on ambulatory health care visits, as used in the ECA, often suffer from inaccuracies in number of visits, time frame, or place of service (Shapiro et al., 1984; Manderscheid et al., 1993).

ANALYTIC STUDIES OF MENTAL HEALTH SERVICES

Epidemiologic data show that the burden of mental disorders in the population is a large one. Even with only about one in five individuals with a diagnosable disorder using services in any one-year period, the cost of providing treatment is large as well. Mental health services research has been increasingly concerned with *economic* issues, including the cost associated with these disorders, as well as the effect of different payment systems on the way that care is delivered. Data showing that access is uneven, that the general medical system is important in providing care, and that some nonmedical institutions like jails have populations with need for service have also made it increasingly important to examine the interactions between parts of the health care and human service system to see if *efficiency* and *economy* can be improved.

Costs of Mental Disorders

With the data on prevalence in the population and use of mental health services, it has been possible to estimate the costs of providing care to people with mental disorder. Initial estimates were made for the year 1985. The direct costs, in terms of payment for treatment and related services, were estimated as $51.4 billion. More important than this figure for direct costs of treatment is the cost to society resulting from impairment in the individuals with mental disorders through absence from work, unemployment, and need for social services. This core component of indirect costs was estimated at $116.6 billion. Additional costs of $47.5 billion reflected society's costs in terms of dealing with related accidents, crime, and other problems related to mental disorders. Overall, mental disorders cost $218.1 billion in 1985.

With inflation and increases in the population since that time, the figure today is even higher. Corrected to 1988, for example, the total costs to society were estimated at $273.3 billion (Rice et al., 1991). The Surgeon General has estimated that by 1996, direct costs of treating mental disorders in the United States had reached $99 billion, compared to the estimate of $51.4 billion for 1985. (Surgeon General, 1999)

Another way of measuring cost of illness has been developed by the World Bank and World Health Organization, in terms of "disability adjusted life years" (DALYs). This measure estimates the burden of disability and early death, which is high for disorders that have young onset, low mortality, and reduced productivity, as is true for the major mental disorders. This report suggested that 15% of the burden of disease across the world's population is caused by mental disorders. (Murray and Lopez, 1996).

Paying for Mental Health Services

About 16% of the U.S. population has no health insurance (Surgeon General, 1999). For people with mental disorders, the figure is even higher, estimated at 18% (NAMHC, 1993). Even for those people with health insurance, from a private source or a government program, the coverage for mental health services is less than for general medical services. Typically, insurance plans require the covered individual to assume a higher copayment for each mental health service or a higher deductible than for general medical services. This type of cost-sharing is termed a *demand-side* limit since it serves to reduce the patient's demand for services (Frank et al., 1992). One reason for this discrepancy in copayment and deductibles is that insurers suspect that some services, such as psychotherapy, may have less clearly defined indications or less certain effectiveness than other types of medical services. The higher demand-side limits on mental health services provide a disincentive for use in case covered patients would over-use them without this disincentive.

Evidence exists to show that use of some psychiatric services, notably psychotherapy, may be more sensitive to price than other medical services (Sharfstein et al., 1993). In a large, randomized trial conducted in the 1970s, health insurance benefits with different levels of coverage were provided to residents of six communities across the country. At one extreme, some participants received care that required no copayment, that is, was "free"; at the other extreme, participants paid 95% of the costs of care. Participants with free care were about twice as likely as those with 95% cost-sharing to use any psychotherapy services. However, the use of services was low even for those in the free care plan, as the total amount was only about $32 per enrollee (in 1984 dollars) (Manning et al., 1986). As health care expenditures have risen over the past 15 years, insurers have sometimes used any available measure to reduce their direct costs. In this study, outcome was not measured, so the findings could be interpreted simply as an endorsement of limiting mental health benefits (Borus, 1986). However, studies of the impact of state laws requiring "parity" in coverage of mental and physical disorders has demonstrated that costs did not increase much, and in some cases may have fallen. These findings, and other similar results from cases studies of individual plans, led the Surgeon General to conclude that "evidence of the effects of parity laws shows that their costs are minimal." (Surgeon General, 1999, p 428).

Another method of controlling health care use and the corresponding costs of care has also been developed. It involves the relationship between the insurer and the provider of care rather than the consumer. These limits can be called *supply-side* measures, since they introduce a disincentive to the provider to offer services. The simplest of these methods is to pay the provider a set amount for each covered individual at the beginning of the policy year; under this kind of capitated system, the provider must manage treatment resources to avoid losing money (Frank et al., 1992). Prepaid health plans represent an example of this payment system, which is intended to encourage cost-effective care and avoid overuse of services. For example, use of partial hospitalization programs may reduce the need for admission to a full-time inpatient unit.

In general medical practice, the type of payment system may not influence a clinician's decision making beyond efforts to reduce hospitalization (Greenfield et al., 1992). However, some evidence suggests that general medical clinicians in a health maintenance organization (HMO) are less likely to diagnose depression in their patients than corresponding clinicians in a fee-for-service arrangement (Wells et al., 1988). Evidence from one of the communities studied in the ECA program demonstrates that, for a given severity of illness, patients seen in an HMO received less intensive care than patients in fee-for-service settings (Norquist and Wells, 1991). Psychiatrists have begun to consider what represents a legitimate constriction on services offered to patients in a prepaid health plan, where the provider shares the risks of "overuse" of services compared with the "optimal" treatment that would be offered in a more traditional fee-for-service arrangement (Sabin, 1991). Without more guidance from studies of effectiveness and patient outcomes, these issues will likely be decided on the basis of cost containment rather than on improving public mental health (Sharfstein et al., 1993).

Interactions Between Sectors of the Health Care System

Little is known about the pathways taken by patients through the various components of the mental health system. While the components have been identified and services use has been measured, patients have not yet been tracked over time to determine the relative importance of specialty mental health care, general medical care, or other human services and voluntary care (Regier et al., 1993). Jails have been identified as an important institutional residence of individuals with mental disorders, but little is known of how services are provided in penal institutions or how these services supplement or replace other types of mental health services (NAMHC, 1991).

One interaction that has been studied is the relationship of the general medical sector with the specialty mental health sector. For some time, research has shown that people with identified mental disorders have a higher rate of using general medical services than people without a diagnosed mental disorder (Hankin and Oktay, 1979). This finding from a variety of medical settings has been generally confirmed by results from the population-based ECA study (Shapiro et al., 1984; Narrow et al., 1993) and the RAND Health Insurance Experiment (Manning and Wells, 1992). Of most interest, however, is the finding from a variety of studies that for people with mental disorders who have higher rates of medical services use, there is a reduction of this use once some mental health treatment has been obtained. This "offset effect" for services also results at times in a reduction of overall health care expenditures (Jones and Vischi, 1979; Borus et al., 1985; Mumford et al., 1984; Mumford and Schlesinger's, 1987).

At present, the offset effect is still poorly understood, and has been challenged (Sturm, 2001). Without a randomized trial, which would be very hard to conduct in most treatment settings, the methodologic limits of retrospective studies may make it difficult for policy makers to bank on any cost-offset effect. The growing focus on measuring outcome and assessing effectiveness of care is likely to receive more research attention in the immediate future.

EXPERIMENTAL STUDIES OF MENTAL HEALTH SERVICES

Finding ways to improve the quality of care offered to people with mental disorders is one of the fundamental goals of an applied research area like mental health services research. Studying "what works, for whom, under what circumstances" is a goal set by the National Institute of Mental Health and its Advisory Council (NAMHC, 1991). Once more is known about ways to maximize the *effectiveness* of mental health services, some of the controversial issues about delivery of services can be addressed. For example, it would be useful to know what impact the limited mental health benefits of most insurance programs have on patient outcome or how to provide the best mix of services to the whole population for a given level of mental health care expenditures.

Formal experimental studies to determine effectiveness of alternative treatment approaches and programs are difficult to undertake. They must be introduced into ongoing systems of care and they require extraordinary efforts at maintaining the intervention, reducing attrition, and assessing outcome in both individual and system terms. Unlike studies of new pharmacologic agents, they must enroll a wide range of patients and follow them for long periods of time, much longer than the six or eight weeks that might satisfy studies of new medications. Outcome measures must include assessment of quality of life and not just symptom reduction (NAMHC, 1991). For all of these reasons, studies of mental health treatment effectiveness in day-to-day clinical practice have been difficult to start. Their absence has been felt in recent discussion of policy options in the United States (NAMHC, 1991, 1993; Ginzberg, 1991; Goldman et al., 1993; Sharfstein et al., 1993), but notable progress is being made in selected areas.

Effectiveness Studies in Primary Care Settings

One of the first efforts to improve quality of care was to introduce self-report questionnaires to screen for mental disorders in primary care settings. If primary care clinicians could be alerted to the presence of a disorder, the diagnosis and subsequent management could presumably be improved. While early pilot studies were encouraging, a formal clinical trial using random assignment into control and experimental groups failed to find a significant improvement in overall detection of illness. Improved recognition was noted for patients who were elderly, black, or male, but overall, clinicians tended to ignore the results of the questionnaire, apparently because of the pressure of conducting routine assessment of general medical problems (Shapiro et al., 1987).

Other efforts at improving outcomes of patients in primary care included a series of projects to introduce outpatient psychiatric consultation-liaison services in primary care. In general, randomized trials of these efforts showed an improvement in detection but not in patient outcomes (Katon and Gonzales, 1994).

More recently, public health and professional groups have tried to develop improved classification systems for mental disorders to be used in primary care. Both the American Psychiatric Association, which publishes the "Diagnostic and Statistical Manual," fourth edition, and the World Health Organization's Division of Mental Health, have developed streamlined systems of classification for use by primary care clinicians. (APA, 1995; WHO, 1996) Whether these versions will improve detection and outcomes of treatment is not yet known.

Under mandate from the U.S. Congress, the Public Health Service supported development of treatment guidelines for common problems in primary care. The first set of guidelines included "Depression in Primary Care" (Agency for Health Care Policy and Research, 1992). A non-experimental study has found evidence to suggest that treatment following these guidelines did improve clinical outcomes for patients (Fortney et al., 2001). A formal trial of quality improvement programs in a collection of 46 managed primary care settings showed that quality of care, mental health outcomes, and employment improved over a one-year period, without increasing medical visits (Wells et al., 2000). This study employed a comprehensive set of educational initiatives, and even though participation in the QI programs was not mandatory, it is consistent with the suggestion that improved patient outcome may be related to the comprehensiveness of the intervention aimed at the primary care clinician (Anfinson and Bona, 2001).

Effectiveness Studies in Mental Health Settings

One of the most pressing issues in delivery of care is to find ways to help patients with severe mental disorders improve their lives in the community. One program that has shown tremendous promise is the Program for Assertive Community Treatment (PACT), which uses multidisciplinary teams, active outreach, and a variety of other measures such as job assistance. Initial studies its effectiveness have shown reduced hospitalization and improved stabilization in the community (Stein, 1992). An initial problem in having the program more widely adopted had been that replication studies had not taken place (Lalley et al., 1992).

In the past decade, that research gap has been filled, as multiple controlled trials of PACT have demonstrated its effectiveness in reducing hospital days, compared to standard case management. It also has been found to produce greater satisfaction for clients and their families (Bustillo et al, 2001; Marshall and Lockwood, 2000; Phillips et al. 2001; Ziguras and Stewart, 2000; Drake et al., 2000). In some circumstances, it may prove less expensive than standard care, but its greatest rationale in the age of evidence-based practice is in terms of effectiveness (Latimer, 1999).

Comparative studies of PACT with other, less intensive forms of case management have suggested that PACT can produce better outcomes for patients with substance use disorders as well, but the difference may appear only late in treatment, by the third year of follow-up (Clark, 1998). Subsequent analysis in this study suggested that closer adherence to the PACT model by individual programs provided superior outcomes compared to less faithful implementations of PACT (McHugo et al., 1999).

Another focus of controlled trials has been to test the effectiveness of outpatient commitment. Questions about the degree of coercion to use in requiring individuals with severe mental disorders to adhere to treatment have been debated from many perspectives, but a new one is from the viewpoint of effectiveness. Controlled studies have yielded mixed results, although even proponents acknowledge that a court order is only part of the necessary program, with intensive community treatment and other services also required (Applebaum, 2001; Allen and Smith, 2001; Torrey and Zdanowicz, 2001; Steadman et al., 2001b; Swartz et al., 2001).

CONCLUSION

At times, mental health services research has seemed close to fulfilling its promise of finding ways to improve the equity, efficiency, economy, and effectiveness of mental health services (Wing and Hailey, 1972; Taube et al., 1988a,b). At other times, it has seemed to fail (Leighton, 1982).

At the outset of the twenty-first century, the task of finding ways to deal with the problems that mental disorders cause for patients seems at least as acute as ever. With the base provided by new epidemiologic methods, with an emphasis by policy makers and funding agencies on the need for careful research on cost-effective care (Burke and Leshner, 1989; Sharfstein et al., 1993), and with the delineation of specific research agendas (NAMHC, 1991; Lalley et al., 1992), mental health services research now has its best opportunity to improve care for people with mental disorders. Even with better data, though, the treatment system must respond by implementing the approaches that can improve equity, efficiency, economy, and effectiveness. One way that clinical practice is being targeted to provide evidence-based interventions is through the use of guidelines, recommendations, and algorithms. (Torrey WC et al., 2001; Mellman et al., 2001) Whether these will change practice is uncertain. Beyond the clinical realm, as mental health services research becomes more fruitful, policy makers will also need to find ways to implement "evidence-based policies."

REFERENCES

Agency for Health Care Policy and Research (1992): "Depression in Primary Care:Clinical Practice Guidelines." Washington, DC: Government Printing Office.

Allen M, Smith VF (2001): Opening Pandora's box:the practical and legal dangers of involuntary outpatient commitment. Psychiatric Services 52:342–346.

American Psychiatric Association (1995): "Diagnostic and Statistical Manual of Mental Disorders," 4th ed, Primary Care Version. Washington, American Psychiatric Press.

Applebaum PS (2001): Thinking carefully about outpatient commitment. Psychiatric Services 52:347–350.

Anfinson TJ, Bona JR (2001): A health services perspective on delivery of psychiatric services in primary care including internal medicine. Med Clin North Am 85:597–616.

Baasher TA, Cooper JE, Davidian H, Jablensky A, Sartorius N, Stromgren E (eds) (1982): "Epidemiology and Mental Health Services: Principles and Applications in Developing Countries." Acta Psychiatrica Scand (Supp) 2961 65 1.

Borus JF (1986): Coverage, care, cost, and outcome. JAMA 256:1939.

Borus JF, Olendzki MC, Kessler L, Bums BJ, Brandt UC, Broverman CA, Henderson PR (1985): The "offset effect" of mental health treatment on ambulatory medical care utilization and charges. Arch Gen Psychiatry 42:573–580.

Brodey BB, Claypoole KH, Motto J, Arisas RG, Goss R (2000): Satisfaction of forensic psychiatric patients with remote telepsychiatric evaluation. Psychiatric Services 51:1305–1307.

Burke JD, Leshner Al (1989): New support for mental health services research. Focus Mental Health Services Res 3:1.

Burns BJ, Ryan Wagner H, Gaynes BN, Wells KB, Schulberg HC (2000): General medical and specialty mental health service use for major depression. Int J Psychiatry Med 30:127–143.

Buscema CA, Abbasi QA, Barry DJ, Lauve TH (2000): An algorithm for the treatment of schizophrenia in the correctional setting:the Forensic Algorithm Project. J Clin Psychiatry 61:767–783.

Bustillo J, Lauriello J, Horan W, Keith S (2001): The psychosocial treatment of schizophrenia:an update. Am J Psychiatry 158:163–175.

Center for Mental Health Services. (1996): In Manderscheid RW, Sonnenschein MA (eds): "Mental Health, United States, 1996." DHHS Pub. No. (SMA) 96–3098. Washington, DC Supt of Documents, U.S. Government Printing Office.

Clarke RE, Teague GB, Ricketts SK, Bush PW, Xie H, McGuire TG, Drake RE, McHugo GJ, Keller AM, Zubkoff M (1998): Cost-effectiveness of assertive community treatment versus standard case management for persons with co-occurring severe mental illness and substance use disorders. Health Serv Res 33:1285–1308.

Drake RE, Mueser KT, Torrey WC, Miller AL, Lehman AF, Bond GR, Goldman HH, Leff HS (2000): Evidence-based treatment of schizophrenia. Curr Psychiaty Rep 2:393–397.

Fortney J, Rost K, Zhang M, Pyne J (2001): The relationship between quality and outcomes in routine depression care. Psychiatric Services 52:56–62.

Frank RG, Goldman HH, McGuire TG (1992): A model mental health benefit in private insurance. Health Affairs 11:98–117.

Ginzberg E (ed) (1991): "Health Services Research:Key to Health Policy." Cambridge, MA:Harvard University Press.

Goldman HH, Adler DA, Beriant J, Docherty J, Dorwart R, Ellison JM, Pajer K, Slris S, Kapur S (1993): The case for a services-based approach to payment for mental illness under national health care reform. Hosp Commun Psychiatry 44:542–544.

Goldman HH, Morrissey JP, Ridgely MS, Frank RG, Newman SJ, Kennedy C (1992): Lessons from the program on chronic mental illness. Health Affairs 11:51–68.

Greenfield S, Nelson EC, Zubkoff M, Manning W, Rogers W, Kravitz RL, Keller A, Tarlov AR, Ware JE (1992): Variations in resource utilization among medical specialties and systems of care:Results from the medical outcomes study. JAMA 267:1624–1630.

Hankin JR, Oktay JS (1979): "Mental Disorders and Primary Medical Care:An Analytic Review of the Literature." Washington, DC: Government Printing Office.

Jones K, Vischi T (1979): Impact of alcohol, drug abuse, and mental health treatment on medical care utilization. A review of the research literature. Medical Care (Suppl) 17:ii–82.

Katon W, Schulberg H (1992): Epidemiology of depression in primary care. Gen Hosp Psychiatry 14:237–247.

Katon W, Gonzales J (1994): A review of randomized trials of psychiatric consultation-liaison studies in primary care. Psychosomatics 35:268–278.

Kessler RC, McGonagle KA, Zhao S, Nelson CF, Hughes M, Eshleman S, Wittchen HU, Kendler KS (1994). Lifetime and 12-month prevalence of DSM-III-R disorders in the United States; Results from the National Comorbidity Survey. Arch Gen Psychiatry 51:8–19.

Kessler LG, Cleary PD, Burke JD (1985): Psychiatric disorders in primary care. Arch Gen Psychiatry 42:583–587.

Kierman GL, Olfson M, Leon AC, Weissman MM (1992): Measuring the need for mental health care. Health Affairs 11:23–33.

Lalley TL, Hohmann AA, Windle CD, Norquist GS, Keith SJ, Burke JD (eds) (1992): A national plan to improve care for severe mental disorders. Schiz Bull 18:559–668.

Latimer EA (1999): Economic impacts of assertive community treatment:a review of the literature. Can J Psychiatry 44:443–454.

Leaf PJ, Bruce ML, Tischler GL, Freeman DH, Weissman MM, Myers JK (1988): Factors affecting the utilization of specialty and general medical mental health services. Med Care 26:9–26.

Leighton AH (1982): "Caring for Mentally III People:Psychological and Social Barriers in Historical Context." Cambridge, Cambridge University Press.

Manderscheid RW, Rae DS, Narrow WE, Locke BZ, Regier DA (1993): Congruence of Service Utilization Estimates from the Epidemiologic Catchment Area project and other sources. Arch Gen Psychiatry 50:108–114.

Manning WG, Wells KB (1992): The effects of psychological distress and psychological well-being on use of medical services. Med Care 30:541–553.

Manning WG, Wells KB, Duan N, Newhouse JP, Ware JE (1986): How cost sharing affects the use of ambulatory mental health services. JAMA 256:1930–1934.

Marshall M, Lockwood A (2000): Assertive community treatment for people with severe mental disorders. Cochrance Database Syst Rev 2:CD001089.

McHugo GJ, Drake RE, Teague GB, Xie H (1999): Fidelity to assertive community treatment and client outcomes in the New Hampshire dual disorders study. Psychiatric Services 50:818–824.

Mellman TA, Miller AL, Weissman EM, Crismon ML, Essock SM, Marder SR (2001): Evidence-based pharmacologic treatment for people with severe mental illness:a focus on guidelines and algorithms. Psychiatric Services 52:619–625.

Morris JN (1957): "Uses of Epidemiology." Edinburgh; Livingstone, 1957.

Mumford E, Schlesinger HJ (1987): Assessing consumer benefit:cost offset as an incidental effect of psychotherapy. Gen Hosp Psychiatry 9:360–363.

Mumford E, Schlesinger HJ, Glass GV, Patrick C, Cuerdon T (1984): A new look at evidence about reduced cost of medical utilization following mental health treatment. Am J Psychiatry 141:1145–1158.

Murray CJ, Lopez AD (eds) (1996): "The Global Burden of Disease: A Comprehensive Assessment of Mortality and Disability from Diseases, Injuries, and Risk Factors in 1990 and Projected to 2020." Cambridge, MA. Harvard University Press.

Myers JK, Weissman MM, Tischier GL, Holzer CE, Leaf PJ, Orvaschel H, Anthony IC, Boyd JH, Burke JD, Kramer M, Stoltzman R (1984): Six-month prevalence of psychiatric disorders in three communities: 1980–1982. Arch Gen Psychiatry 41:959–967.

Narrow WE, Regier DA, Rae DS, Manderscheid RS, Locke BZ (1993): Use of services by persons with mental and addictive disorders: Findings from the National Institute of Mental Health Epidemiologic Catchment Area Program. Arch Gen Psychiatry 50:95–107.

National Advisory Mental Health Council (1991): "Caring for People with Severe Mental Disorders: A National Plan of Research to Improve Services." Washington, DC :Government Printing Office.

National Advisory Mental Health Council (1993): Health care reform for Americans with severe mental illnesses. Am J Psychiatry 150:1447–1465.

Norquist GS, Wells KB (1991): How do HMOs reduce outpatient mental health care costs? Am J Psychiatry 148:96–10 1.

Novins DK, Beals J, Sack WH, Manson SM (2000): Unmet needs for substance abuse and mental health services among Northern Plains American Indian adolescents. Psychiatric Services 51:1045–1047.

Phillips SD, Burns BJ, Edgar ER, Mueser KT, Linkins KW, Rosenheck RA, Drake RE, McDonel Herr EC (2001): Moving assertive community treatment into standard practice. Psychiatric Services 52:771–779.

Regier DA, Boyd JH, Burke JD, Rae DS, Myers JK, Kramer M, Robins LN, George LK, Kamo M, Locke BZ (1988a): One-month prevalence of mental disorders in the United States:Based on five Epidemiologic Catchment Area sites. Arch Gen Psychiatry 45:977 –986.

Regier DA, Burke JD, Manderscheid RW, Bums BJ (1985): The chronically mentally ill in primary care. Psychol Med 15:265–273.

Regier DA, Goldberg ID, Taube CA (1978): The de facto US mental health services system: A public health perspective. Arch Gen Psychiatry 35:685–693.

Regier DA, Hirschfeld RMA, Goodwin FK, Burke JD, Lazar JB, Judd LL (1988b): The NIMH Depression Awareness, Recognition, and Treatment Program: Structure, aims, and scientific basis. Am J Psychiatry 145:1351–1357

Regier DA, Narrow WE, Rae DS, Manderscheid RW, Locke BZ, Goodwin FK (1993): The de facto U.S. Mental and Addictive Disorders Service System:Epidemiologic Catchment Area Prospective 1-year prevalence rates of disorders and services. Arch Gen Psychiatry 50:85–94.

Rice DP, Kelman S, Miller LS (1991): Estimates of economic costs of alcohol and drug abuse and mental illness, 1985, and 1988. Public Health Rep 106:280–292.

Robins LN, Heizer JE, Weissman MM, Orvaschel H, Gruenberg E, Burke JD, Regier DA (1984): Lifetime prevalence of specific psychiatric disorders in three sites. Arch Gen Psychiatry 41:949–958.

Rost K, Zhang M, Fortney J, Smith J, Coyne J, Smith GR (1998): Persistently poor outcomes of undetected major depression in primary care. Gen Hosp Psychiatry 20:12–20.

Sabin J (1991): Clinical skills for the 1990s: Six lessons from HMO Practice. Hosp Community Psychiatry 42:605–608.

Shapiro S, German PS, Skinner EA, VonKorff M, Turner RW, Klein LE, Teitelbaum ML, Kramer M, Burke JD, Burns BJ (1987): An experiment to change detection and management of mental morbidity in primary care. Med Care 25:327–339.

Shapiro S, Skinner EA, Kessler LG, VonKorff M, German PS, Tischler GL, Leaf PI, Benham L, Cottler L, Regier DA (1984): Utilization of health and mental health services:Three epiderniologic catchment area sites. Arch Gen Psychiatry 41:971–978.

Sharfstein SS, Stoline AM, Goldman HH (1993): Psychiatric care and health insurance reform. Am J Psychiatry 150:7–18.

Shepherd M, Cooper B, Brown AC, Kalton G, Clare A (1981): "Psychiatric Illness in General Practice," 2nd ed. Oxford; Oxford University Press.

Simon GE (1998): Can depression be managed appropriately in primary care? J Clin Psychiatry (suppl): 59 2:3–8.

Snowden LR, Cheung FK (1990): Use of inpatient mental health services by members of ethnic minority groups. Am Psychologist 45:347–355.

Snowden LR, Thomas K (2000). Medicaid and African-American outpatient mental health treatment. Ment Health Serv Res 2:115–120.

Steadman HJ, Deane MW, Morrissey JP, Westcott ML, Salasin S, Shapiro S (1999): A SAMHSA research initiative assessing the effectiveness of jail diversion programs for mentally ill persons. Psychiatric Services 50:1620–1623.

Steadman HJ, Stainbrook KA, Griffin P, Draine J, Dupont R, Horey C (2001a): A specialized crisis response site as a core element of police-based diversion programs. Psychiatric Services 52:219–222.

Steadman HJ, Gounis K, Dennis D, Hopper K, Roche B, Swartz M, Robbins PC (2001b): Assessing the New York City involuntary outpatient commitment pilot program. Psychiatric Services 52:330–336.

Stein LI (1992): On the abolishment of the case manager. Health Affairs 11:172–177.

Sturm R (2001): Economic grand rounds:the myth of medical cost offset. Psychiatric Services 52:738–740.

Surgeon General (1999): "Mental Health—A report of the Surgeon General. Rockville, MD, U.S. Department of Health and Human Services, Substance Abuse and Mental Health Services Administration, Center for Mental Health Services, National Institutes of Health, National Institute of Mental Health.

Swartz MS, Swanson JW, Hiday VA, Wagner HR, Burns BJ, Borum R (2001): A randomized controlled trial of outpatient commitment in North Carolina. Psychiatric Services 52:325–329.

Taube CA, Barrett SA (eds) (1985): "Mental Health, U.S. 1985." Washington, DC; U.S. Government Printing Office.

Taube CA, Goldman HH, Lee ES (1988a): Use of specialty psychiatric settings in constructing DRGS. Arch Gen Psychiatry 45:1037–1040.

Taube CA, Lave JR, Rupp A, Goldman HH, Frank RG (1988b): Psychiatry under prospective payment: Experience in the first year. Am J Psychiatry 145:210–213.

Teplin LA (1990): The prevalence of severe mental disorder among male urban jail detainees: Comparison with the Epidemiologic Catchment Area Program. Am J Public Health 1990:663–669.

Tiemens BG, Ormel J, Jenner JA, van der Meer K, Van Os TW, van den Brink RH, Smit A, van den Brink W (1999): Training primary-care physicians to recognize, diagnose and manage depression: Does it improve patient outcomes? Psychological Med 29:833–845.

Torrey EF, Erdman K, Wolfe SM, Flynn LM (1990): "Care of the Seriously Mentally Ill: A Rating of State Programs." Washington, DC: Public Citizen Health Research Group and National Alliance for the Mentally Ill.

Torrey EF, Zdanowicz M (2001): Outpatient commitment:what, why, and for whom. Psychiatric Services 52:337–341.

Torrey WC, Drake RE, Dixon L, Burns BJ, Flynn L, Rush AJ, Clark RE, Klatzker D (2001): Implementing evidence-based practices for persons with severe mental illnesses. Psychiatric Services 52:45–50.

Wells KB, Golding JM, Hough RL, Bumam A, Karno M (1988): Factors affecting the probability of use of general and medical health and social/community services for Mexican Americans and non-Hispanic whites. Med Care 26:441–452.

Wells KB, Hays RD, Burnam A, Rogers W, Greenfield S, Ware JE (1989): Detection of depressive disorder for patients receiving prepaid or fee-for-service care: Results from the Medical Outcomes Study. JAMA 262:3298–3302.

Wells KB, Sherbourne C, Schoenbaum M, Duan N, Meredith L, Unutzer J, Miranda J, Carney MF, Rubenstein LV (2000): Impact of disseminating quality improvement programs for depression in managed primary care: a randomized controlled trial. JAMA 283:212–220.

Wing JK, Hailey AM (1972): "Evaluating a Community Psychiatric Service:The Camberwell Regis 1964–1971." London: Oxford University Press.

World Health Organization (1996): "ICD-1O: Diagnostic and management guidelines for mental disorders in primary care." Seattle, WA and Gottingen, Germany. WHO/ Hogrefe and Huber.

Ziguras SJ, Stuart GW (2000): A meta-analysis of the effectiveness of mental health case management over 20 years. Psychiatric Services 51:1410–1421

CHAPTER 7

The Pharmacoepidemiology of Psychiatric Medications

PHILIP S. WANG, ALEXANDER M. WALKER, and JERRY AVORN

Division of Pharmacoepidemiology and Pharmacoeconomics, Brigham and Womens Hospital, Harvard Medical School, Boston, MA (P.S.W., J.A.); Department of Epidemiology, Harvard School of Public Health, Boston, MA (P.S.W., A.M.W.)

INTRODUCTION

Modern pharmacotherapy for psychiatric disorders began in the 1950s, with the development of chlorpromazine for psychotic disorders and its derivative, imipramine, for depressive disorders (Kuhn, 1958). Since then, numerous effective agents for mental disorders have been developed and have achieved widespread use. Psychopharmacologic drugs are now among the most widely consumed medications in general medical as well as psychiatric populations (Pincus et al., 1998).

Fairly soon after psychiatric medications were introduced, adverse effects were reported that were not anticipated, based on preapproval clinical trials. Such reports raised questions and hypotheses concerning the safety of psychiatric medications. Investigating possible unanticipated hazards from psychiatric drugs was the original impetus for the field of psychopharmacoepidemiology. Since then, the field has grown considerably to encompass a much wider array of studies, including: investigations of unanticipated benefits; descriptions of how psychiatric drugs are used in real-world populations; identification of unmet needs for psychopharmacologic treatment; examinations of the appropriateness and quality of psychotropic prescribing; studies of patient adherence to prescribed psychotropic regimens; pharmacoeconomic analyses; and studies of interventions to optimize psychiatric medication use. This chapter provides a brief overview of the field, potential data sources for investigators, examples of psychopharmacoepidemiologic studies, and some suggestions for future developments.

OVERVIEW OF PSYCHOPHARMACOEPIDEMIOLOGY

A Brief History

The history of psychopharmacoepidemiology generally parallels the history of the larger field of pharmacoepidemiology (Strom, 1994a). Both are relatively young

Textbook in Psychiatric Epidemiology, Second Edition, Edited by Ming T. Tsuang and Mauricio Tohen.
ISBN 0-471-40974-X

disciplines, born out of the thalidomide catastrophe in the 1960s. Thalidomide was originally marketed for its psychoactive properties of sedation and hypnosis. Soon after it was introduced, there were reports of deformed extremities among children who had been exposed to thalidomide *in utero* (McBride, 1961).

This public health disaster involving a psychotropic drug led to important policy changes and the establishment of systems for reporting unexpected hazards from marketed medications throughout the world (Wilholm et al., 1994). In the United States, The Kefauver–Harris Amendments were passed which established the federal Food and Drug Administrations (FDA) current regulatory requirements for all drug approvals (Baum et al., 1994). In an important step for the field of pharmacoepidemiology, these amendments also required the review of drugs that had already been approved and were being marketed at the time.

From these beginnings in the 1960s, pharmacoepidemiologic studies have grown in frequency, scope, and impact. Postmarketing pharmacoepidemiologic studies have occasionally been required by the FDA as a precondition at the time of approval (Mattison and Richard, 1987). In such studies, pharmacoepidemiologists have continued to uncover serious unanticipated adverse events from psychotropic medication use. For example, the antidepressant nomifensine was marketed in Europe during the 1980s and showed promise for treatment-resistant depression, but was found to cause fatal hemolytic anemia (Cole, 1988). The ultra short-acting benzodiazepine triazolam was frequently used as an hypnotic when it was found to be associated with anterograde amnesia (Morris and Estes, 1987). Results such as these have had a significant public health impact, leading to the withdrawal of hazardous agents as well as new recommendations and regulations to ensure the safe and effective use of psychotropic drugs that remain.

Pharmacoepidemiology has benefited from important methodologic advances in recent decades. Research groups have developed large automated databases with accurate drug exposure data for hundreds of thousands of patients. Such databases have in turn allowed psychopharmacoepidemiologists to study efficiently not only catastrophic adverse effects, but also more subtle adverse effects, effects occurring after longer lag periods, and adverse effects with higher background rates. New study designs have allowed investigators to study particular types of pharmacologic effects, such as the case cross-over and case-time-control designs to evaluate transient effects from intermittent drug exposures (Maclure, 1991; Suissa, 1995). Important advances have allowed investigators to deal more effectively with or at least quantify threats to the validity of pharmacoepidemiologic studies, such as the common problem of confounding by indication ("channeling bias") (Rosenbaum and Rubin, 1983a). These methodologic advances have also allowed psychopharmacoepidemiologists to focus not only on adverse effects but also turn their attention to many new types of study questions surrounding psychiatric medication use, as described in a following section, Psychopharmacoepidemiologic Studies for Specific Clinical Questions.

Advantages Offered by Psychopharmacoepidemiologic Studies

Psychopharmacoepidemiologic studies conducted after drug approval can add considerably to the knowledge gained in premarketing studies, and in fact are an indespensible complement to the clinical trials performed before drug approval.

Pharmacoepidemiologic studies may be the only type of study that can detect certain outcomes, such as those that are rare or occur only after long delays. Because of their larger sample sizes, pharmacoepidemiologic studies can allow investigators to estimate drugs effects with much greater precision. Psychopharmacoepidemiologists can examine how psychiatric drugs are used and their effects in populations that are often excluded from clinical trials, including patients with comorbid psychiatric and general medical disorders, the elderly, children, or pregnant patients. Psychopharmacoepidemiology makes it possible to evaluate psychiatric drug regimens that are typically used in the real world but may not be studied in clinical trials for practical or ethical reasons, including long-term exposures, cotreatment with other medications, no treatment, and even overdosages.

SOURCES OF DATA

The field of psychopharmacoepidemiology has depended critically upon the development of adequate data sources. Although hundreds of patients are often studied in clinical trials of psychiatric medications prior to drug approval, the number of subjects needed to answer psychopharmacoepidemiologic questions is often orders of magnitude greater. It has been crucial for the field to develop very large databases with accurate psychiatric drug exposure information. In addition, there is often great urgency to answering pharmacoepidemiologic questions, placing a premium on data that have already been collected. The often prohibitive costs of collecting data de novo have also made it necessary, where possible, to utilize secondary data collected for other purposes.

Clearly, some data sources will be more suitable for answering specific psychopharmacoepidemiologic questions than others. When choosing between the various data sources, investigators need to consider many factors (Strom, 1994b). First, are data on the drug exposure of interest available and is the exposure common enough to power the study adequately? How detailed and accurate are these exposure data? Are there adequate numbers of and accurate data on the outcomes of interest? Is there information that will allow the investigator to control for confounding and other biases? Are data available from the time periods of interest? How representative is the study population from which the data were drawn of other populations of interest? The following are brief descriptions of some types of data sources used in psychopharmacoepidemiologic studies, including some of their strengths and weaknesses.

Large Governmental Administrative Databases

An important source of data for psychopharmacoepidemiologists was created in the United States in the mid-1960s with the establishment of Medicaid entitlement programs for the indigent (Bright et al., 1989). Medicaid databases from specific states (e.g., New Jersey and Tennessee) as well as collections of states (e.g., the COMPASS consortium) have been employed as a relatively low cost source of data for pharmacoepidemiologic studies. Medicaid databases contain information on large numbers of psychiatric patients due to the poverty and disability experienced by many with mental illness, and make them ideal data sources for studies of specifically psychotropic medication use. The indigent status of recipients reduces out-of-pocket health care expenditures and contributes to the high level of completeness of Medicaid data for information on use of medications and other services (Lessler and Harris, 1984). Disadvantages of Medicaid data can include their lack of information on inpatient drug utilization, limited generalizability for certain investigations, and questions about the completeness and validity of recorded diagnoses (Roos et al., 1991). Other large governmental administrative databases collected for insurance purposes also exist, including data collected by the U.S. Veterans Administration and provincial governments in Canada (e.g., the Saskatchewan Health Database). These data sources may offer specific advantage in studies due to their inclusion of subjects with a wider range of socioeconomic and other characteristics. However, like all databases collected for administrative purposes, questions persist concerning the accuracy of their clinical information, especially on mental disorders.

Data from Health Maintenance Organizations

As increasing numbers of people in the United States receive their pharmacy benefits through health maintenance organizations (HMOs), use of HMO databases in psychopharmacoepidemiologic studies has become widespread. Automated databases from Group Health Cooperative of Puget Sound, the Kaiser Permanente Medical Care Program, United Health Care, Fallon Health Plan, and Harvard Pilgram Health Care have all been successfully used in psychopharmacoepidemiologic studies. As with other administrative data, these sources can be obtained at relatively low cost and reflect prescriptions actually filled by patients. One significant advantage of data from HMOs is that the clinical information collected for billing purposes can be supplemented with more complete or accurate information from review of patients primary medical records. HMO databases provide an ideal means to study psychotropic medication use in the increasingly important setting of primary care; however, because HMO membership often requires employment, HMO databases may not include use of psychiatric medications by those with serious mental illness. In addition, patient turnover is often high, hampering longitudinal studies.

Large-Scale Surveys

Data for psychopharmacoepidemiologic studies can also be obtained from large surveys of medication and other health services use. Surveys administered in multiple years in the United States include the annual National Ambulatory Medical Care Survey (NAMCS), which samples a nationally representative group of visits to physicians in office-based practices and records the prescriptions for medications given to patients. Advantages of data from such surveys include the ability to generate nationally representative estimates concerning psychiatric medication use. Disadvantages include the surveys' high costs, the possibility that patients may not have filled or consumed prescribed medications, the lack of longitudinal follow-up, and the lack of completeness and detail regarding clinical conditions. Psychiatric epidemiologic surveys such as the National Comorbidity Survey (NCS) and the Midlife Development in the U.S. survey (MIDUS) contain detailed information on mental disorders and also assess the use of psychotropic medications among respondents. Unfortunately, such surveys frequently lack detail concerning the medication regimens taken and require respondents to recall past medication use, raising the potential for information biases.

Practice-Based Networks

Another important source of information comes from practice-based networks, designed to study patterns and outcomes of health services use in typical practice settings. The General Practice Research Database (GPRD) contains computerized medical records of 683 general practices in the United Kingdom and has been extensively used in psychopharmacoepidemiologic analyses. Other practice research networks in the United States include the family practice Ambulatory Sentinel Practice Network (ASPN) and the Pediatric Research in Office Settings (PROS). Recently, the American Psychiatric Association established the Practice Research Network (PRN) to study a nationally representative sample of psychiatrists, their patients, and treatments used in routine psychiatric practice. Strengths of data from practice-based networks include their more accurate clinical information and the potential to develop nationally representative estimates; disadvantages include the high costs of maintaining networks and the uncertainty over whether patients actually consumed prescribed medications.

PSYCHOPHARMACOEPIDEMIOLOGIC STUDIES FOR SPECIFIC CLINICAL QUESTIONS

From its origins investigating adverse effects from psychotropic medications, the field of psychopharmacoepidemiology has broadened to now include a wider variety of study types. Mental health services researchers will notice that many of these clinical questions and types of studies bear resemblance to their own (Burke, 1995), in part because psychiatric medication use is but a specific form of mental health care.

Adverse Effects of Psychiatric Medications

Answering the question "Do psychiatric medications cause unanticipated adverse effects?" remains a mainstay for psychopharmacoepidemiologists. One area in which there has been considerable work has been the adverse effects of sedative-hypnotic use among older patients. Studies from the 1980s by Ray and colleagues (1989) identified that benzodiazepine users had significantly increased rates of hip fracture, a frequently disabling outcome in the elderly. However, the clinical implications of these findings have been complicated by the fact that benzodiazepines given for psychiatric indications may be quite beneficial in some patients. For this reason, it has been imperative to further identify particular agents, half-lives, dosages, and durations of use that may be especially dangerous and therefore avoided (Ray et al., 1989; Herings et al., 1995; Wang et al., 2001a). Because other classes of psychiatric medications can also be sedating and have adverse effects on cognition or balance, psychopharmacoepidemiologists have extended their investigations and identified risks for falls and fractures with use of antidepressants (Thappa et al., 1998) and newer, nonbenzodiazepine sedative-hypnotics (Wang et al., 2001d).

In addition to uncovering true hazards, an equally important question is "Has a psychiatric drug been wrongly accused of causing side effects?" Providing reassurance and accurate information concerning risks is vital, given the continuing stigma regarding psychiatric medication use and persistent underuse and delays in use by patients who would benefit. For example, case reports in the early 1990s reported the emergence of suicidality in patients taking selective serotonin reuptake(inhibitors (SSRIs) (Teicher et al., 1990). Subsequent psychopharmacoepidemiologic studies (Jick et al., 1995; Leon et al., 1999) as well as meta-analyses of randomized clinical trial data (Beasley et al., 1991) have been helpful in providing reassurance that these antidepressants do not cause this serious adverse effect. Other hypotheses concerning adverse effects from psychiatric medication use have come from animal studies, such as reports that SSRIs and tricyclic antidepressants act as tumor promoters in rodent models (Brandes et al., 1992). Psychopharmacoepidemiologic studies in humans have failed to corroborate these animal study results (Wang et al., 2001b), again providing needed reassurance regarding antidepressant use in the general and oncology populations.

Another related question that pharmacopidemiologists have begun answering with increasing frequency is, "Are there unanticipated benefits from psychiatric medication use?" In a recent example, Walker and colleagues (1997) found lower suicide rates among current versus prior clozapine users, raising the possibility of an underrecognized benefit for this very effective but often underutilized antipsychotic medication.

Patterns, Trends, and Predictors of Psychiatric Drug Use in Real-World Populations

Pharmaceutical companies have traditionally examined how their products are used and by whom, largely for marketing purposes. However, more recently a variety of other stakeholders, including insurers, health care policy makers, patients, and their advocates, have also begun to ask policy-relevant questions about psychiatric medication use, such as: "Has use of psychiatric medications in pediatric populations changed over time?" "Does use of psychiatric medications vary across racial groups?" and "What are potential barriers to receiving psychopharmacologic treatment?" Pharmacoepidemiologists have begun to address such questions through studies of patterns, time trends, and correlates of psychiatric medication use in real-world populations. Such studies have revealed important and, in some cases, actionable findings, including a dramatic recent rise in psychotropic medication use, much of it off-label, by preschool children in the United States (Zito et al., 2000) and the lower likelihood of racial minorities to receive newer expensive, but potentially more tolerable, psychotropic agents (Melfi et al., 2000; Wang et al., 2000a).

Assessing Unmet Needs for Psychopharmacologic Treatment

Another major agenda of mental health services research and psychopharmacoepidemiology is in the quantification of unmet needs for mental health care, identifying subpopulations in whom unmet needs are greatest and modifiable reasons for such undertreatment. Primary care patients with major depression have received considerable attention, in part because primary care settings are the most likely place for patients with this common and impairing condition to present. Earlier studies consistently found underuse of antidepressants and other treatments among such patients (Keller et al., 1982). Such findings have led to large-scale campaigns to increase awareness in the general public as well as educational programs to increase recognition of mental illnesses among primary care providers (Hirschfeld et al., 1997). However, recent data from the second half of the 1990s suggests that despite these efforts and the introduction of newer, more tolerable agents, psychiatric medications continue to be underused by patients with depression and other highly prevalent psychiatric disorders (Wang et al., 2000b). Another group in whom it has been critically important to assess unmet needs for psychopharmacologic treatment is the extremely vulnerable population with serious mental illness (SMI). Recent investigations of the SMI population in the United States have revealed disturbingly low rates of psychopharmacologic treatment and other mental health care (Kessler et al., 2001; Wang et al., 2002).

Growing constraints on health care resources, coupled with the rapid expansion in use of psychotropic medications by the general public, many without clear psychiatric indictions, will put increasing pressure on the need to shed light on the magnitude and determinants of overuse as well as underuse of psychiatric medications.

Quality and Appropriateness of Physician Prescribing of Psychotropics

A growing body of clinical trial data suggests that psychiatric medications should be prescribed in accordance with evidence-based guidelines regarding the type of drug, dosage, and duration of treatment, in order to be effective (AHCPR, 1993; APA, 1993; APA, 1994; APA, 1997; APA, 1998; Lehman and Steinwachs, 1998a). For this reason, a major new role for psychopharmacoepidemiology has been to monitor how well physicians follow such prescribing guidelines. Investigators have shown that prescribed antipsychotic (Lehman and Steinwachs, 1998b) and antidepressant regimens (Katon et al., 1992; Katz et al., 1998; Simon et al., 1993; Wells et al., 1994) frequently fall short of recommendations, exposing many patients with mental disorders to potentially ineffective and/or harmful treatments.

Patient Adherence with Psychiatric Medications

In addition to poor quality prescribing, patient nonadherence can also render drug treatment of mental illness ineffective. Patient compliance in clinical trials can be a poor estimate of adherence in the real world, due to the unique type of patients who volunteer for trials as well as investigators' efforts to ensure patient adherence. For these reasons, pharmacoepidemiologic studies of patient noncompliance with psychiatric medications are necessary. Such studies have shown that patient adherence to psychotropic regimens is frequently intermittent, and that this form of noncompliance can lead to increased risks of recurrence of mental disorders (Melfi et al., 1998). In related studies, investigators have examined the effects that psychopharmacotherapies can have on treatment dropout (Wang et al., 2000c), another highly prevalent form of noncompliance among patients with mental disorders. Pharmacoepidemiologists have also begun identifying the significant effects that various forms of psychopathology, such as depressive symptomatology, can have on medication compliance in general (Wang et al., to appear: a).

Pharmacoeconomic Analyses

As the cost of pharmaceuticals continues to increase rapidly, an increasingly important set of questions concerns the relative costs and benefits of psychiatric drugs: "Are they a good bargain?" "Would limited resources be better spent on these drugs or other health care interventions?" Answering such questions is increasingly a prerequisite before insurers and other stakeholders add new psychopharmacologic treatments to formularies. The antipsychotic medication clozapine has been extensively studied in this regard. Clozapine is more effective than conventional neuroleptics in patients with treatment-resistant schizophrenia, but also can cause potentially fatal agranulocytosis. As a result, its use requires ongoing monitoring of a patient's white blood count. Numerous pharmacoeconomic analyses have consistently shown clozapine to be more cost-effective than conventional neuroleptics, in spite of its higher costs and side effects (Meltzer et al., 1993; Rosenheck et al., 1997; Revicki et al., 1990; Davies et al., 1993). In addition to these head-to-head comparisons of clozapine versus other agents, the scope
of recent economic analyses of clozapine have expanded to include evaluations of the best monitoring strategy for agranulocytosis (Zhang et al., 1996) and the best sequence for trying clozapine in treatment-sensitive patients (Wang et al., submitted : a).

Interventions to Optimize Psychiatric Medication Use

In addition to identifying patterns, predictors, and outcomes of psychiatric medication use, psychopharmacoepidemiology has also increasingly used such information to develop, target, and then evaluate interventions to optimize the way psychiatric medications are used. Some interventions have focused on improving the psychotropic prescribing of clinicians, including one-on-one educational approaches such as "academic-detailing." In this approach, modeled on the promotional activities of drug companies, educational outreach workers such as pharmacists are deployed by a non-commercial organization, often a medical school, to visit physicians in order to teach them how to prescribe more appropriately. Field trials in nursing homes have shown these interventions to be highly effective in improving not only the quality of psychotropic prescribing but patient outcomes as well (Avorn et al., 1992). Recent interventions have also focused on patients, through patient education and care manager assistance with medication taking. Effectiveness trials among depressed patients in primary care settings have shown that these interventions can significantly improve the adequacy of antidepressant use, depressive symptomatology, and patient functioning as well (Katon et al., 1995; Wells et al., 2000).

Still other interventions have targeted health care systems or have focused on changing health care policies. For example, attempts to control unnecessary psychotropic drug use and costs have included requiring patients to share their psychotropic medication costs through copayments, and limiting the number of prescriptions patients can fill per month. However, evaluations of such policy experiments have been instructive in showing that interventions may not always have their intended effects. Investigators have shown that copayments deter use of needed psychotherapeutic drugs to a greater extent than comparable treatments for other general medical conditions (Reeder and Nelson, 1985). Soumerai and colleagues (1994) have shown that among patients with schizophrenia, prescription caps significantly reduced use of essential psychiatric drugs, increased use of mental health services, especially emergency care, and increased health care costs over drug cost savings by a factor of 17.

FUTURE DIRECTIONS

The growing field of psychopharmacoepidemiology already has a "full plate" of questions to investigate regarding currently marketed psychiatric drugs. Some have been raised only recently, such as whether some atypical antipsychotic medications can cause diabetes mellitus (Henderson et al., 2000; Wang et al., to appear: b). Others questions have persisted for decades, in spite of earlier attempts to answer them. For example, early animal studies raised the possibility that some anti-xxxpsychotic medications initiate or promote breast cancers through prolactin elevation, prompting the FDA to require product label warnings about a possible association for all conventional neuroleptics since the 1970s. Although psychopharmacoepidemiologic studies to date have been limited and produced inconsistent findings (Halbreich et al., 1996; Gulbinat et al., 1992; Kanhouwa et al., 1984; Mortensen, 1994), new impetus for answering this question (Wang et al., to appear: c) comes from the frequent use of antipsychotic medications in the general and oncology populations and the recent introduction of atypical agents which do not elevate prolactin levels. In addition to these existing questions, psychopharmacoepidemiologists should anticipate a steady stream of new hypotheses concerning unanticipated effects from both available and as yet to be introduced drugs. If use of psychiatric medications continues to expand as projected, results from rigorous and timely psychopharmacoepidemiologic investigations will become only more imperative.

To successfully answer these and other questions, methodologic advances will be required. New data sources need to be developed that contain detailed and accurate information on both medication use and clinical conditions. One option in this regard is to link the highly accurate information on drug utilization contained in existing administrative databases to more accurate and detailed clinical information from other sources (Wang et al., 2001c). Another option is to equip future psychiatric epidemiologic surveys, which do contain accurate clinical information, with improved assessments of medication use. Psychopharmacoepidemiology modules that collect comprehensive and detailed information on psychotropic use and also contain features that help minimize information bias have been added to upcoming surveys such as the National Comorbidity Survey Replication (NCS-R) and the WHO World Mental Health 2000 surveys.

To estimate validly the effects of psychotropic medications, it will be necessary to develop better means of dealing with important types of confounding and bias. Due to the nonrandom nature of drug exposures in observational studies, psychiatric drug use is often a marker of patients with peculiar risk profiles for outcomes of interest. To prevent"channeling bias" and other forms of confounding, psychopharmacoepidemiologists will need to develop better means of risk adjustment than those currently available (Wang et al., 2000d). Techniques such as propensity scores (Rosenbaum and Rubin, 1983b, 1984) and instrumental variable approaches (Newhouse and McClellan 1998; Greenland 2000) hold promise in this regard. Another example of a problem psychopharmacoepidemiologists must overcome in future studies is surveillance bias. Psychiatric medication use is recognized as a marker of patients who are less likely to be screened, diagnosed, and treated for a wide variety of medical disorders (Redelmeier et al., 1998; Adler and Griffith 1991; Druss et al., 2000). Effective methods are needed to deal with or at least quantify the magnitude and effect of this bias in future studies.

These and other needed methodologic advances will all help the field of psychopharmacoepidemiology contribute to the safe, effective, and optimal use of psychiatric medications.

REFERENCES

Adler LE, Griffith JM (1991): Concurrent medical illness in the schizophrenic patient. Epidemiology, diagnosis, and management. Schizophr Res 4:91–107.

Agency for Health Care Policy and Research (1993): "Depression in Primary Care," vol. 2. Treatment of Major Depression" Rockville, MD: U.S. Dept. of Health and Human Services.

American Psychiatric Association (1993): "Practice Guideline for Major Depressive Disorder in Adults." Washington, DC: American Psychiatric Association.

American Psychiatric Association (1994): "Practice Guideline for the Treatment of Patients with Bipolar Disorder." Washington, DC: American Psychiatric Association.

American Psychiatric Association (1997): "Practice Guideline for the Treatment of Patients with Schizophrenia." Washington, DC: American Psychiatric Association.

American Psychiatric Association (1998): "Practice Guideline for the Treatment of Patients with Panic Disorder." Washington, DC: American Psychiatric Association.

Avorn J, Soumerai SB, Everitt DE, Ross-Degnan DR, Beers MH, Sherman D, Salem-Schatz SR, Fields D (1992): A randomized trial of a program to reduce the use of psychoactive drugs in nursing homes. N Engl J Med 327:168–173.

Baum C, Kweder SL, Anello C (1994): The spontaneous reporting system in the United States. In: Strom BL (ed.) "Pharmacoepidemiology," 2nd ed. New York: Wiley, pp 125–137.

Beasley CM, Dornseif BE, Bosomworth JC, Sayler ME, Rampey AH, Heiligenstein JH, Thompson VL, Murphy DJ, Masica DN (1991): Fluoxetine and suicide: a meta-analysis of controlled trials of treatment for depression. Br Med J 303:685–692.

Brandes LJ, Arron RJ, Bogdanovic RP (1992): Stimulation of malignant growth in rodents by antidepressant drugs at clinically relevant doses. Cancer Res 52:3796–3800.

Bright RA, Avorn J, Everitt DE (1989): Medicaid data as a resource for epidemiologic studies: strengths and limitations. J Clin Epi 42:937–945.

Burke JD (1995): Mental health services research. In Tsuang MT, Tohen M, Zahner GEP (eds): "Textbook in Psychiatric Epidemiology." New York: Wiley, pp 199–207.

Cole JO (1988): Where are those new antidepressants we were promised? Arch Gen Psychiatry 45:193–197.

Davies LM, Drummond MF (1993): Assessment of costs and benefits of drug therapy for treatment-resistant schizophrenia in the United Kingdom. Br J Psychiatry 162:38–42.

Druss BG, Bradford DW, Rosenheck RA, Radford MJ, Krumholz HM (2000): Mental disorders and use of cardiovascular procedures after myocardial infarction. JAMA 283: 506–511.

Greenland S (2000): An introduction to instrumental variables for epidemiologists. Internat J Epidemiol 29:722–729.

Gulbinat W, Dupont A, Jablensky A, Jensen OM, Marsella A, Nakane Y, Sartorius N (1992): Cancer incidence of schizophrenic patients: results of record linkage studies in three countries. Br J Psychiatry (Suppl 18) 161:75–85.

Halbreich U, Shen J, Panaro V (1996): Are chronic psychiatric patients at increased risk for developing breast cancer? Am J Psychiatry 153:559–560.

Henderson DC, Cagliero E, Gray C, Nasrallah RA, Hayden DL, Schoenfeld DA, Goff DC (2000): Clozapine, diabetes mellitus, weight gain, and lipid abnormality: a five-year naturalistic study. Am J Psychiatry 157:975–981.

Herings RC, Stricker BH, de Boer A, Bakker A, Sturmans A (1995): Benzodiazepines and the risk of hip falling leading to femur fractures. Arch Intern Med 155:1801–1807.

Hirschfeld RMA, Keller MB, Panico S, Arons BS, Barlow D, Davidoff F, Endicott J, Froom J, Goldstein M, Gorman JM, Marek RG, Maurer TA, Meyer R, Phillips K, Ross J, Schwenk TL, Sharfstein SS, Thase ME, Wyatt RJ (1997): The National Depressive and Manic Depressive Association consensus statement on the undertreatment of depression. JAMA 277:333–340.

Jick SS, Dean AD, Jick H (1995): Antidepressants and suicide. Br Med J 310:215–218.

Kanhouwa S, Gowdy JM, Solomon JD (1984): Phenothiazines and breast cancer. J Natl Med Assoc 76:785–788.

Katon W, Von Korff M, Lin E, Bush T, Ormel J (1992): Adequacy and duration of antidepressant treatment in primary care. Med Care 30:67–76.

Katon W, Von Korff M, Lin E, Walker E, Simon GE, Bush T, Robinson P, Russo J (1995): Collaborative management to achieve treatment guidelines: impact on depression in primary care. JAMA 273:1026–1031.

Katz, SJ, Kessler RC, Lin E, Wells KB (1998): Medication management of depression in the United States and Ontario. J Gen Intern Med 13:77–85.

Keller MB, Klerman GL, Lavori PW, Fawcett JA, Coryell W, Endicott J (1982): Treatment received by depressed patients. JAMA 248:1848–1855.

Kessler RC, Berglund PA, Bruce ML, Koch JR, Laska EM, Leaf PJ, Manderscheid RW, Rosenheck RA, Walters EE, Wang PS (2001). The prevalence and correlates of untreated serious mental illness. Health Serv Res 36:987–1007.

Kuhn R (1958): The treatment of depressive states with G 22355 (imipramine hydrochloride). Am J Psychiatry 115:459–464.

Lehman AF, Steinwachs DM (1998a): Translating research into practice: the Schizophrenia Patient Outcomes Research Team (PORT) treatment recommendations. Schizophr Bull 24:1–10.

Lehman AF, Steinwachs DM (1998b): Patterns of usual care for schizophrenia: Initial results from the Schizophrenia Patient Outcomes Research Team (PORT) client survey. Schizophr Bull 24:11–20.

Leon AC, Keller MB, Warshaw MG, Mueller TI, Solomon DA, Coryell W, Endicott J (1999): Prospective study of fluoxetine treatment and suicidal behavior in affectively ill subjects. Am J Psychiatry 156(2):195–201.

Lessler JT, Harris BSH (1984): Medicaid data as a source for postmarketing surveillance information, final report. Research Triangle Park, NC: Research Triangle Institute.

Maclure M (1991): The case-crossover design: a method for studying transient effects of the risk of acute events. Am J Epidemiol 113:144–153.

Mattison N, Richard BW (1987): Postapproval research requested by the FDA at the time of NCE approval, 1970–1984. Drug Info J 21:309–329.

McBride WG (1961): Thalidomide and congenital abnormalities. Lancet ii:1358.

Melfi CA, Chawla AJ, Croghan TW, Hanna MP, Kennedy S, Sredl K (1998): The effects of adherence to antidepressant treatment guidelines on relapse and recurrence of depression. Arch Gen Psychiatry 55:1128–1132.

Melfi CA, Croghan TW, Hanna MP, Robinson RL (2000): Racial variation in antidepressant treatment in a Medicaid population. J Clin Psychiatry 61:16–21.

Meltzer HY, Cola P, Way L, Thompson PA, Bastani B, Davies MA, Snitz B (1993): Cost effectiveness of clozapine in neuroleptic-resistant schizophrenia. Am J Psychiatry 150:1630–1638.

Morris HH, Estes M (1987): Travelers amnesia: transient global amnesia secondary to triazolam. JAMA 258:945–946.

Mortensen PB (1994): The occurrence of cancer in first admitted schizophrenic patients. Schizophr Res 12:185–194.

Newhouse JP, McClellan M (1998): Econometrics in outcomes research: the use of instrumental variables. Ann Rev Public Health 19:17–34.

Pincus HA, Tanielian TL, Marcus SC, Olfson M, Zarin DA, Thompson J, Zito JM (1998): Prescribing trends in psychotropic medications: Primary care, psychiatry, and other medical specialties. JAMA 279:526–531.

Ray WA, Griffin MR, Downey W (1989): Benzodiazepines of long and short elimination half-life and the risk of hip fracture. JAMA 262:3303–3307.

Redelmeier DA, Tan SH, Booth GL (1998): The treatment of unrelated disorders in patients with chronic medical diseases. N Engl J Med 338:1516–1520.

Reeder CE, Nelson AA (1985): The differential impact of copayment on drug use in a Medicaid population. Inquiry 22:396–403.

Revicki DA, Luce BR, Weschler JM, Brown RE, Adler MA (1990): Cost-effectiveness of clozapine for treatment- resistant schizophrenic patients. Hospital Commun Psychiatry 41:850–854.

Rosenbaum PR, Rubin DB (1983a): Assessing sensitivity to an unobserved binary covariate in an observational study with binary outcome. J R Stat Soc B 45:212–218.

Rosenbaum PR, Rubin D (1983b): The central role of the propensity score in observational studies for causal effects. Biometrika 70:41–55.

Rosenbaum PR, Rubin DB (1984): Reducing bias in observational studies using subclassification on the propensity score. J Am Stat Assoc 79:516–524.

Rosenheck R, Cramer J, Xu W, Thomas J, Henderson W, Frisman L, et al. (1997): A comparison of clozapine and haloperidol in hospitalized patients with refractory schizophrenia. N Engl J Med 337:809–815.

Roos LL, Sharp SM, Cohen MM (1991): Comparing clinical information with claims data: some similarities and differences. J Clin Epidemiol 44:881–888.

Simon GE, Von Korff M, Wagner EH, Barlow W (1993): Patterns of antidepressant use in community practice. Gen Hospital Psychiatry 15:399–408.

Soumerai SB, McLaughlin TJ, Ross-Degnan D, Casteris CS, Bollini P (1994): Effects of limiting Medicaid drug-reimbursement benefits on the use of psychotropic agents and acute mental health services by patients with schizophrenia. N Engl J Med 331:650–655.

Strom BL (1994a): What is pharmacoepidemiology? In Strom BL (ed):" Pharmacoepidemiology," 2nd ed. New York Wiley, pp 3–13.

Strom BL (1994b): How should one perform pharmacoepidemiology studies?: choosing among the available alternatives. In Strom BL (ed) "Pharmacoepidemiology," 2nd ed. New York: Wiley, pp 337–350.

Suissa S (1995): The case-time-control design. Epidemiology 6:248–253.

Thapa PB, Gideon P, Cost TW, Milam AB, Ray WA (1998): Antidepressants and the risk of falls among nursing home residents. N Engl J Med 339:875–882.

Teicher MH, Glod C, Cole JO (1990): Emergence of intense suicidal preoccupation during fluoxetine treatment. Am J Psychiatry 147:207–210.

Walker AM, Lanza LL, Arellano F, Rothman KJ (1997): Mortality in current and former users of clozapine. Epidemiology 8:671–677.

Wang PS, West JC, Tanielian T, Pincus HA (2000a): Recent patterns and predictors of antipsychotic medication regimens used to treat schizophrenia and other psychotic disorders. Schizophr Bull 26: 451–457.

Wang PS, Berglund P, Kessler RC (2000b): Recent care of common mental disorders in the U.S. population: prevalence and conformance with evidence-based recommendations. J Gen Intern Med 15:284–292.

Wang PS, Gilman SE, Guardino M, Christiana JM, Morselli PL, Mickelson K, Kessler RC (2000c): Initiation and adherence to treatment for mental disorders: examination of patient advocate group members in eleven countries. Med Care 38:926–936.

Wang PS, Walker A, Tsuang M, Orav EJ, Levin R, Avorn J (2000d): Strategies for improving comorbidity measures based on Medicare and Medicaid claims data. J Clin Epidemiol 53:571–578.

Wang PS, Bohn RL, Glynn RJ, Mogun H, Avorn J (2001a): Hazardous benzodiazepine regimens in the elderly: effects of half-life, dosage, and duration on risk of hip fracture. Am J Psychiatry 158:892–898.

Wang PS, Walker AM, Tsuang MT, Orav EJ, Levin RL, Avorn J (2001b): Antidepressant use and the risk of breast cancer. J Clin Epidemiol 54: 728–734.

Wang PS, Walker A, Tsuang M, Orav EJ, Levin R, Avorn J (2001c): Finding incident breast cancer cases through U.S. claims data and a state cancer registry. Cancer Causes Control 12:257–265.

Wang PS, Bohn RL, Glynn RJ, Mogun H, Avorn J (2001d): Zolpidem use and hip fractures in the elderly. J Am Geriatr Soc 49:1685–1690.

Wang PS, Demler O, Kessler RC (2002): The adequacy of treatment for serious mental illness in the United States. Am J Pub Health 92:92–98.

Wang PS, Bohn RL, Knight E, Glynn RJ, Mogun H, Avorn J: Noncompliance with antihypertensive medications: the impact of depressive symptoms and psychosocial factors. J Gen Intern Med. To appear a.

Wang PS, Glynn RJ, Ganz DA, Schneeweiss S, Levin R, Avorn J: Clozapine use and the risk of diabetes mellitus. J Clin Psychopharmacol. To appear b.

Wang PS, Ganz DA, Benner JS, Glynn RJ, Avorn J: Should clozapine be a first-line therapy for schizophrenia?: a decision analytic model. Submitted a.

Wang PS, Walker AM, Tsuang MT, Orav EJ, Glynn RJ, Levin RL, Avorn J : Dopamine antagonists and the development of breast cancer. Arch Gen Psychiatry. To appear c..

Wells KB, Katon W, Rogers B, Camp P (1994): Use of minor tranquilizers and antidepressant medications by depressed outpatients: results from the medical outcomes study. Am J Psychiatry 151:694–700.

Wells KB, Sherbourne C, Schoenbaum M, Duan N, Meredith L, Unutzer J, Miranda J, Carney MF, Rubenstein L (2000): Impact of disseminating quality improvement programs for depression in managed primary care. JAMA 283:212–220.

Wilholm BE, Onsson S, Moore N, Wood S (1994): Spontaneous reporting system outside the United States. In Strom BL (ed). "Pharmacoepidemiology," 2nd ed. New York: Wiley, pp 139–155.

Zhang M, Owen RR, Pope SK, Smith GR (1996): Cost-effectiveness of clozapine monitoring after the first 6 months. Arch Gen Psychiatry 53:954–958.

Zito JM, Safer DM, dos Reis S, Gardner JM, Boles M, Lynch F (2000): Trends in the prescribing of psychotropic medication to preschoolers. JAMA 283:1025–1030.

CHAPTER 8

Peering into the Future of Psychiatric Epidemiology

EZRA SUSSER, MICHAELINE BRESNAHAN, and BRUCE LINK

Department of Epidemiology, Mailman School of Public Health, Columbia University, and New York State Psychiatric Institute

INTRODUCTION

Epidemiology has already contributed a great deal to psychiatric research. The discipline has been used extensively for studying the frequency of mental disorders in communities across the world. Increasingly, it is also being used to examine the causes of mental disorders, including biological and genetic causes, utilizing the major risk factor designs of case–control and cohort studies (Wyatt and Susser, 2000; Susser et al., to appear). Yet, even after risk factor methods are fully integrated into psychiatric research, we will have utilized only one small part of the potential contributions of epidemiology.

In this chapter, we explore some of the emerging trends in epidemiology and consider their implications for psychiatric research. The discipline is presently extending in a number of exciting directions that add intellectual depth and suggest new lines of questioning. As we venture into these realms, we are moving well beyond the established principles of contemporary risk factor epidemiology. Peering into the future, we anticipate that these new applications will be very important for psychiatric research in the coming decades.

The changes taking place are many but interrelated. Epidemiologists increasingly strive to integrate our understanding of disease and health across multiple levels of organization (Susser and Susser, 1996b; McMichael, 1999; Smith and Ebrahim, 2001). In a related transition, we are thinking about the development of disease over the life course, from conception to old age (Kuh and Ben-Shlomo, 1997; Kellam et al., 1998; Susser et al., 2000; Eaton, 2000). Related to both these themes, investigators are seeking to illuminate the relation of historical change to society's health (Stein and Karim, to appear; Marmot and Bobak, 2000; Bobak and Marmot, 1996).

Textbook in Psychiatric Epidemiology, Second Edition, Edited by Ming T. Tsuang and Mauricio Tohen.
ISBN 0-471-40974-X

To limit the scope of this chapter we will focus on the concept of levels of "causation." This concept enables us to specify causes at different levels of organization such as cellular, individual, or societal. We begin with a historical overview of thinking about levels of causation, showing how public health challenges led to what is now contemporary epidemiology and how new challenges are driving the emerging epidemiology. Then we describe thinking across multiple levels of causation and framing a research question in these terms. Finally, we provide examples from our own work, to demonstrate how our research on mental disorders could be enhanced by the multilevel perspective. In order to convey the main ideas, we concentrate on two levels of organization, the individual and the social context, but we indicate how the framework can be extended to biological studies and to more than two levels (for a more comprehensive treatment see Susser et al., to appear; Diez-Roux, 1998; Schwartz et al., 1999; Bryk and Radenbush, 1992).

LEVELS OF CAUSATION: A HISTORICAL OVERVIEW

The history of epidemiology has been marked by dramatic transitions in thinking, occurring in response to new public health challenges and/or scientific breakthroughs (Susser and Susser, 1996a, b; Susser and Bresnahan, 2001). These can be used to demarcate historical eras, characterized by prevailing causal paradigms. Below we trace the thinking about levels of causation over successive eras in epidemiology.

The crucible for the development of epidemiology was the Industrial Revolution in England in the early nineteenth century (Hamlin, 1998; Susser and Adelstein, 1975). In this early "Sanitary Era," epidemiologists adopted a very broad view of causation, with the focus mainly on societal factors. A dominant view was that the social transformation associated with industrialization had led to a concentration of human waste and other decaying organic matter in the new urban areas. At the societal level the thinking of the Sanitarians was valid enough; the societal transformation that they witnessed was indeed the underlying force behind the change in the health of England at that time. It motivated one of the most effective public health reforms ever enacted, the Public Health Act of 1848, an effort which culminated in the building of sewage and water systems throughout the newly industrialized towns and cities of England.

Despite its evident successes, sanitary epidemiology had fatal flaws. The Sanitarians lacked good explanations as to how societal factors led to disease in individuals. Most often, they relied upon the theory of "miasma," a kind of polluting vapor that emerged from the accumulation of decaying waste. [There were exceptions, for instance, the epidemiologist John Snow inferred the presence of microorganisms causing cholera as early as the 1840s (Snow, 1855)].

The epidemiology of the Sanitary Era was brought to a close by the development of a new science, microbiology, which did provide an explanation for disease at the individual level, and totally discredited the miasma theory (Winslow, 1943). Toward the end of the nineteenth century, Robert Koch and others made a series of stunning discoveries that demonstrated beyond any doubt that microbes played a crucial role in some of the most important diseases of the time. This ushered in the "Infectious Disease Era," in which epidemiology was actually redefined as the science of infectious diseases. In this period, epidemiologists primarily sought to identify microbial agents and their mode of transmission (Chapin, 1934). As infectious disease transmission is inherently a social process, the societal level of thinking remained important, but mainly within the narrow framework of the ways in which social factors influenced epidemic transmission (Ross, 1911). Some epidemiologists continued to focus on the implications of societal transformation for public health, but they no longer represented the mainstream of the discipline.

The next transition, to the Chronic Disease Era, was largely motivated by the changing health profile of developed countries in the mid-twentieth century (Susser, 1985; Morris, 1957; MacMahon et al., 1960). Infectious diseases were declining rapidly, whereas apparently noninfectious chronic diseases such as cardiovascular disease and cancer were increasing at an alarming rate. Infectious disease methods could not address the challenges presented by these frightening new causes of morbidity and mortality. Within a very short period after World War II, the discipline was again redefined, and its methodology transformed. The signal event was the demonstration that smoking was a "cause"—a "risk factor"—for lung cancer, using cohort and case–control designs developed for the purpose (Doll and Hill, 1950). Subsequently the notion of the risk factor became common parlance among epidemiologists, and these designs became standard methodology for investigating risk factors, especially individual exposures or lifestyles. What is most important for the present argument is that these designs brought the discipline to focus still further on the individual as opposed to the societal level influences on disease. As we shall explain below, the risk factor designs are individual level studies *par excellence*, and their very strength lies in isolating the individual level risk factor from all others.

Risk factor epidemiology is still dominant in textbooks and classrooms (e.g., Kelsey, 1996; Rothman and Greenland, 1998), but the field is rapidly changing once more. A perusal of the leading epidemiology journals or of funded grants will make it clear that investigators are taking up the challenge of thinking about multiple levels of causation (Susser and Susser, 1996b; McMichael, 1999; Smith and Ebrahim, 2001). Epidemiologists are not dispensing with risk factor investigations (nor should they), but rather, are subsuming them under a broader framework, and it is a framework that we believe to be especially well suited to psychiatric research (Susser et al., to appear). Thus, we now think systematically not only about risk factors, but also about the impact of family, community, society, and of gene, cell, tissue.

What is motivating the latest transition? Although the question is far beyond the scope of this chapter, it is worth noting that the AIDS pandemic has had more impact than any other single factor (Kuhn and Susser, 2001; Susser and Bresnahan, 2001; UNAIDS 2000). Today epidemiology and public health face the greatest challenge in their short history, a virtual holocaust as HIV sweeps through Africa and other developing regions. It is a challenge that simply cannot be met using risk factor methods alone. The war on AIDS requires research and intervention on every level: political leadership, deep social change, individual behavior change, and molecular genetics.

LEVELS OF CAUSATION

We now turn to introducing the concept of levels of causation which is coming to the fore in epidemiology. Before doing so, we should note that exceptional forward-thinking individuals have systematically considered causation at multiple levels throughout the history of epidemiology (Ross, 1911; Goldberger et al., 1918, 1920; Newsholme, 1927; Sydenstricker, 1933; Kermak et al., 1934 Susser, 1973). Historical eras are demarcated by prevailing paradigms but these are not the exclusive method in any given era. Nonetheless, it is only recently that this kind of thinking has received sustained attention from the field and been used as a foundation for training in epidemiology (Susser and Susser 1996a, b).

The idea of expanding the scope of psychiatric epidemiology "up" to social contexts and "down" to tissues and cells is immediately appealing for several reasons. It allows the possibility of integrating disparate orientations into an organic whole. A combined undertaking takes greater advantage of advances in understanding across levels of research and disciplines. In addition it releases us from prejudice that the "real causes" reside at any one level to conceive disease causation as occurring at many levels. Once we are able to specify the potential relevance of any particular level of analysis, the idea of excluding that level raises the specter of incompleteness, missed opportunity, model misspecification, and confounding.

Conceptualizing disease causation in this way does not mean that every study or even any study has to include many levels. Integrated understanding may be achieved through a series of studies with a much more limited purview. It does mean that every study has to begin by asking the question: what level or levels of organization are most relevant to the question at hand? Then the research is designed accordingly.

Individual Level

When trying to determine why some individuals are more likely to develop disease than others, we conduct "individual" level studies. An individual level observational study, whether it is cohort or case–control, is designed to see whether variation in the disorder among individuals within the population reflects variation in their exposure histories. It does not venture down to the level of the cell, where we might ask which cells are affected by the exposure and in what ways, nor up to the level of the society, where we might ask which societies are organized in such a way that their members are exposed.

Imagine that you posit a relation between exposure to sunlight and the risk of seasonal affective disorder. This model is appropriately conceptualized and investigated at the individual level. Individuals with more exposure to sunlight are hypothesized to be less vulnerable to this disorder, within the population of interest. To examine this hypothesis, it is sufficient to collect data on sunlight exposure and seasonal affective disorder for individuals within the population. The effects of sunlight exposure on cells, and the effects of social organization on sunlight exposure, are related topics but are not directly addressed by either the hypothesis or the study design.

Thus, the risk factor investigation is important, useful, and incomplete. We will mention three important limitations on what can be revealed about determinants of disease using individual level designs. This discussion will provide a segue to the next section on the contextual level, where we will see that these limitations can be partially overcome by research on other levels of causation.

First, not all risk factors of interest will vary between individuals within the study population. A factor which is universal in the study population, even if it participates in causing disease, cannot be readily examined in this framework. An interesting example of this limitation has emerged in studies of autism. One hypothesis that has been put forward and received much publicity is that childhood measles, mumps, and rubella (MMR) immunizations may play a role in some cases of autism (e.g., Wakefield et al., 1998). In developed countries, however, childhood MMR immunizations is government policy and nearly universal, so that there is little or no interindividual variation on this exposure. For a rare disease such as autism, it may be infeasible to collect a large enough cohort of individuals unexposed to MMR for comparison with a cohort of individuals exposed to MMR. In a case–control design, similarly, almost all cases and controls will be exposed to MMR, so it may not be feasible to collect a large enough number of cases and controls for meaningful results. Since the removal of ubiquitous risk factors may have an enormous impact on reducing risk, the inability to study them effectively is an important limitation.

A second limitation is that individual level risk factor designs are not well suited to discover the causes of an increase (or a decrease) in disease incidence in a population. A noticeable increase in the incidence of a disease is often what motivates an investigation. Generally the most parsimonious and useful explanation for a change in incidence is found at the societal level, albeit a societal change that brought about an increase (or decrease) in the population prevalence of an individual risk factor. An individual level study is ill equipped to identify the pivotal event, societal change. Consider our example of MMR immunization and autism. Some studies suggest that the prevalence of autism has increased markedly in developed societies over the last two decades (Gillberg et al., 1999). A purported explanation is the introduction of universal MMR vaccination as government policy. The MMR vaccination policy is clearly a societal factor, even though it is purported to affect disease risk by enforcing universal exposure to an alleged individual risk factor, MMR. There is little evidence to support this theory, but at the same time, it is extremely difficult to rule it out, using the methods of risk factor epidemiology. As noted earlier, a massive societal level effect of MMR may simply be undetectable by an individual risk factor study.

A third limitation is that the effect of an individual level determinant on the risk of disease is context dependent, even at the purely individual level of analysis. Under the paradigm of risk factor epidemiology, disease causation requires the participation of multiple risk factors, and individual cases may result from different constellations of risk factors, so that many different constellations may be "sufficient" to cause disease. The impact of each risk factor upon the disease risk will vary, depending upon the relative frequency of the other risk factors within the constellation, in the population being investigated. The more common risk factors of a sufficient constellation tend to appear less "influential" in disease causation than the rare risk factors of the same constellation (Schwartz and Carpenter, 1999). This occurs in spite of their joint contribution to disease occurrence in a given case.

Suppose that congenital neural tube defects (spina bifada, anencephaly) are caused by a combination of two risk factors: a genetic defect that increases the need for folate, and low folate in the maternal diet. (This causal model is not unrealistic though simplified for exposition; see van der Put et al., 1995). When the genetic defect is common and a low folate maternal diet is uncommon, in a crude analysis, the effect of the genetic defect on the risk of disease will appear to be much less than that of low folate diet. On the other hand, when the genetic defect is *uncommon* and a low folate maternal diet is common, the effect of the genetic defect will appear to be greater than that of low folate diet.

Yet, it may be precisely the common risk factors that carry the most implications for disease prevention. If we knew all the risk factors in the sufficient constellations, and had an extremely large number of individuals to study, we could reveal the full potential effects of all common risk factors, by examining their effects in the presence (and absence) of their necessary cofactors. In practice, however, we rarely have complete enough knowledge as well as large enough samples to do so.

A corollary result is that the magnitude of effect attached to a given risk factor can be expected to vary across populations due to variation in the prevalence of causal cofactors. Hence, we should not expect identical findings when we conduct the same study in two populations with a somewhat different constellation of risk factors. The findings may be similar in populations with similar risk factors, supporting the pursuit of replication of findings, but there *should* be some variation.

Contextual Level

We are naturally drawn to the level of social context and determinants when we seek to explain differences in rates of disease between populations. A social context may be any combination of individuals who are connected in some meaningful way, such as a family, a community, or a society. Thus, we move "up" from the individual level to higher levels, in order to gain access to causal determinants which may not be identifiable in individual level studies. As implied earlier, these include determinants that are invariant within a population and therefore obscured or even invisible at the individual level, as well as those determinants which are not defined in individuals but in the relationships and contexts that surround them.

The core idea in reasoning about contexts is that properties emerge as we move up from the individual to these higher levels of organization. For example, most of us are accustomed to thinking about the emergent properties of neighborhoods and intuitively understand their meaning. In New York City, "Harlem," "Greenwich Village," and "Chinatown" are examples of neighborhoods with particular attributes, although the individuals living in each of them are by no means homogeneous. Living in one or another of these neighborhoods will have a large influence on many dimensions of life, for example, the cost and quality of housing, the type of recreation available (e.g., parks, gymnasiums, cinemas, museums), the presence of noxious facilities (e.g., sewage treatment plants, power plants), the quality of schooling for children, and the amount and kind of police surveillance. Residents will also be affected by the perceptions of other people about these neighborhoods. In these and other ways, the emergent properties of the three neighborhoods will shape the experiences of people who live there. The same can be said of emergent properties of nations, regions of the country, cities, schools, work places, families, and dyadic relationships. The critical issue for epidemiologists is to identify the properties which are most central to health and then to measure those properties so as to test causal explanations that involve them.

The societal determinants of health may appear remote from the occurrence of a specific disease in an individual, and yet be of great consequence as a causal determinant. Consider the hypothetical example of sunlight and seasonal affective disorder, which we previously used to illustrate the individual level investigation. We could now elaborate our causal model by positing a relation between rates of seasonal affective disorder among women and societal determinants of women's work and leisure activities. Let us propose that societies which severely restrict women's access to outdoor occupations and recreations will have higher rates of seasonal affective disorder among women. This model is appropriately conceptualized at the societal level because the crucial determinant of health is societal constraints on women, and the outcome is the rate of disorder in the population. To examine the hypothesis, we might choose to compare several populations with different societal constraints on women, but similar geographic and climatic conditions, with respect to both pattern of sunlight exposure and rate of seasonal affective disorder among women. Note that while the risk factor investigation would provide the more "proximal" causal mechanism, the societal level investigation might be more likely to indicate an effective intervention. Unless the societal barriers can be reduced, individual women may find it difficult to change their work and leisure patterns.

When we turn attention from the individual to the contextual level we encounter great opportunities and enormous challenges. These opportunities exist in part because the conceptual and measurement work needed to capture variation in contexts like these has not been done. Current practice in collecting data for epidemiologic research has, perhaps, slowed their development. The standard approach is to sample and collect data on individuals; data is provided either through self reports or lab-based measures. As useful as this approach is, it does not give us direct access to information about contexts. We only learn about context indirectly through what people tell us about contexts, or what their biological measurements may reveal about contexts. Our attention is drawn towards individual level processes and away from the potential importance of processes at the contextual level. Consequently concepts and measurements at the contextual level do not come into the purview of the scientist on a regular basis when this approach is used.

Therein lies the challenge: to conceive of causal processes at the contextual level, and to successfully measure these processes. The best way to think about conceptual level causation is not yet entirely clear, and competing proposals have generated some excitement. Link and Phelan (1995) propose thinking of contexts as units that vary in the power they possess to secure health-enhancing living conditions—the capacity to secure good things for health and avoid bad things. The example of neighborhood suggests some possibilities along these lines in that well-heeled neighborhoods can resist noise, pollution, and crime in ways that neighborhoods that possess less social and political power cannot. Similarly, in a unionized workplace the union can negotiate for safe work conditions and better health care opportunities. These and other views have been supported by evidence, but the issues are far from resolved, and a vigorous debate is still underway (Wilkinson, 1992, 1996).

Combining Individual and Contextual Levels

Thinking about both individual and contextual levels at the same time frees us to ask different questions than we would in thinking at either level alone. Where before we were limited to two essential questions—Why do some individuals in a population develop disease and not others? and Why are the rates of disease higher/lower in some populations than others?—we can now ask about the interplay between determinants at different levels. Exemplary studies demonstrate the power of this approach for understanding disease causation and health phenomena (Goldberger et al., 1918, 1920; Diez-Roux et al., 1997; Sampson et al., 1997; Entwisle et al., 1986).

Studies of neighborhood social isolation and schizophrenia provide an example from contemporary mental health research. Following on early findings from the landmark ecologic studies of Faris and Dunham (1939), Hare (1956) demonstrated that in the city of Bristol, the incidence rate of schizophrenia was associated with neighborhood social isolation, measured by the proportion of people living alone. He proposed two explanations (not mutually exclusive): individuals might migrate to these neighborhoods, or, the social context of these neighborhood might foster the development of schizophrenia.

Recently, van Os and colleagues (2000) took up this line of enquiry in a study in the Netherlands, using a multilevel analysis that well reflects the emerging era of epidemiology. They too found an effect of neighborhood social isolation, measured by the proportion single and the proportion divorced, on the risk of schizophrenia. They also found an effect of marital status at the individual level. The neighborhood effects were not explained, however, by the individual effects of marital status, indicating that the measure of neighborhood social isolation tapped some emergent property of the neighborhood. Furthermore, neighborhood interacted with individual risk factors in the following manner: being single and living in a neighborhood with a lower proportion of single persons more than doubled the risk of schizophrenia over being single and living in a neighborhood with a higher proportion of single persons. That is, one is more at risk, perhaps one feels more alone, as a single person when living among couples.

Just as the association between marital status and risk of schizophrenia was modified by context, the association between a genotype and disease can be modified by context. Genetic susceptibility to alcohol dependence is associated with genes coding for enzymes involved in the metabolism of alcohol in the liver. In Asian populations, an allele coding for one of these enzymes, ALDH2*2, has repeatedly been shown to decrease alcohol consumption (Higuchi et al., 1996), and decrease the risk of alcohol dependence (Higuchi et al., 1994; Goedde et al., 1992).

The mechanism by which the allele reduces the risk of alcoholism involves an aversive reaction to alcohol consumption caused by a high concentration of acetaldeyde in the blood following consumption. The aversive symptoms can be very unpleasant, including intense flushing, palpitations and headache.

Individuals who are homozygous for the protective allele (ALDH2*2/*2) have such a strong aversive reaction that they drink very little if at all (Higuchi et al., 1996). This accounts for the fact that none were found in large samples of male alcoholics in Japan (Higuchi et al., 1994). Individuals who are heterozygous for this allele have a weaker and more variable aversive reaction. Consequently the biological effects of homozygous ALDH2*2 are so strong that they are little affected by cultural factors, whereas the effects of being heterozygous ALDH2*2 allow for an interaction of culture with the genotype. This is one possible explanation of observed changes in the proportion of ALDH2*2 heterozygotes in samples of male alcoholics in Japan (Higuchi et al., 1994). The protective effect of the heterozygous genotype may have become weaker as the strength of the social pressures for heavy drinking increased.

Examples

Rethinking existing epidemiologic research and outstanding questions in the field of psychiatry within a multilevel framework illustrates the relevance of this approach. Thinking about these issues in terms of levels of causation often adds intellectual interest and rigor and opens new perspectives on intervention. The examples which follow, drawn from our own research, show how multilevel reasoning evolved from a research question or finding and contributed to a new line of investigation.

Course and Outcome of Schizophrenia in Developing and Developed Countries. The course and outcome of schizophrenia have been found to be on average more benign in developing than developed countries (Jablensky et al., 1992). Thinking only in terms of individual level influences on course and outcome, these findings are counterintuitive. It has been shown that within populations, modern treatments (e.g., medication, family interventions) reduce the risk of relapse in patients with schizophrenia (Wyatt and Henter, 1998). And yet, in developed countries where individuals have greater access to those treatments, the mean outcome is comparatively worse.

To explain this difference in mean outcome across settings, researchers have had to consider societal level processes. Speculation has concentrated on three dimensions of context: family relationships, informal economies, and segregation of the mentally ill. First, in India and some other developing countries, families participate in care from the onset of illness through rehabilitation (Susser et al., 1996). This involvement helps maintain family relationships, and social integration of the mentally ill within the family settings. Other qualitative dimensions of the family context potentially related to recovery, such as expressed emotion, also may differ between developing and developed country settings (Leff et al., 1987; Wig et al., 1987). Second, in subsistence economies reintegration into work roles is common (Warner, 1985). Some evidence indicates that work can be beneficial for outcome of schizophrenia (Bell and Lysaker, 1997). Developing country economies may provide greater, more diverse opportunities for this to occur. Third, individuals with schizophrenia are far less likely to be segregated into hospitals and institutions in developing countries. At the societal level, segregation may encourage negative stereotypes and stigma, as well as promote social exclusion from family and work (von Zerssen et al., 1990).

Studies directed at these societal level factors will surely need to be conducted at the societal as well as the individual level. The findings will lead to a deeper understanding of the influences on course and outcome of schizophrenia. They also may open new possibilities for intervention. Perhaps we will learn that efficient delivery of modern treatments may not be the only appropriate goal or consideration in service systems addressing severe mental illness.

Nonaffective Acute Remitting Psychosis. Using the data of the WHO Ten Country Study, Susser and Wanderling (1994) found a dramatic tenfold higher incidence of nonaffective acute remitting psychosis (NARP) in developing than developed country settings. In seeking to explain the difference, they have suggested that the most meaningful explanation lies at the societal level, and formulated hypotheses about factors that are associated with many if not all developing societies (Collins et al., 1996).

One hypothesis was derived from the observation that developing countries have much higher rates of infectious diseases than developed countries, a difference that is attributable the overall socioeconomic milieu rather than to any one component of it. They posited that infectious disease may be a risk factor for NARP, perhaps due to fever and/or immune responses to infection, and that the high rate of infectious disease associated with developing country settings results in a high frequency of NARP. It was not yet established, however, that infectious disease was a risk factor for NARP.

In this instance, therefore, individual level studies were called for, as the most important next step, despite the fact that they were putting forward a societal explanation of the variation in incidence of NARP between populations. Using data from the Chandigarh, India sites of the WHO study, Collins et al. undertook such a study. They found that cases of NARP were more likely to have experienced fever in the 12 weeks preceding onset than controls (OR = 6.2) (Collins et al., 1999), supporting the view that infectious etiologies may be involved.

This example illustrates a point we have sought to emphasize throughout this chapter: considering multiple levels does not imply studying multiple levels at the same time. In any single study, what is most important is to make a reasoned and explicit choice to conduct research at one or more levels, and to appreciate the limitations that arise from having made that choice. Moreover, as in this instance, the primary question might reside at one level, whereas the most important next step requires a study at a different level.

Birth Weight and IQ. Recent evidence suggests that birth weight may be related to IQ, well into the normal birth-weight range (Breslau et al., 1996; Richards et al., 2001). Studies of the relationship between birth weight and IQ are shadowed, however, by the powerful and potentially confounding influence of family social environment. Removing the influence of family social environment is extremely difficult in individual level studies: controlling for parental attributes, and other measured family factors, does not fully capture the complex influence of family environment.

The aspects of family social environment that potentially confound these results are generally shared by siblings, and therefore, are better conceptualized as family level rather than individual level variables. So we are dealing with a family level variable (social environment) as a potential confounder of an individual level association (of birth weight and IQ). Once the cross-level nature of the confounding is recognized, it becomes possible to design studies so as to tightly control it. Sib-pair designs, examining individual level effects within families, offer a potential solution to this problem. Matte and colleagues used this strategy to examine the association of birth weight and IQ. Comparing individuals within same-sex sibships, they demonstrated that for boys, the increase in childhood IQ with birth weight extends well into the normal birth-weight range (Matte et al., 2001). Under this design, the birth-weight effect could not be confounded by family environment, as siblings within the same family share this environment. Although the effect is modest, the ramifications on a population level are important.

This example indicates still another way in which explicit thinking about multiple levels can be useful, that is, in the control of confounding. Causal determinants at one level can be confounders of findings at another level. Consequently, a clear conceptual framework that includes multiple levels of causation helps identify ways to control confounding, which is especially important for relatively small effects.

Violence and Mental Illness. There are many individual level risk factors for violent behaviors and severe mental illness is one of them (Stueve et al., 1997). At the same time, it is clear that the societal context exerts a powerful influence on violent behavior. This was demonstrated, for example, in an innovative study of Chicago neighborhoods, where collective efficacy (similar to social cohesion) of the neighborhood was inversely related to the rate of violent crime (Sampson et al., 1997). Consistent with this are findings from two studies by Link and colleagues, one in New York City and the other in Israel, using similar measures of violence (Link et al., 1992, 1999). They found modestly higher rates of violence among the mentally ill in both study populations; however, people with mental illness in Israel had rates of violence comparable to members of the public in New York City.

In light of these relationships, what do we do about higher rates of violence among people with schizophrenia and other severe mental illnesses? One answer is that we find out more about what predicts violence in samples of people who have been hospitalized for mental illnesses and we develop risk assessment tools to select out violent people for more thorough intervention and control. Individual risk factors do seem to play a role in the increased rates of violence that people with mental illness exhibit. Some investigators emphasize comorbid substance abuse (Steadman et al., 1998), while others emphasize the nature of psychotic symptoms (Link et al., 1999).

Such an approach is a reasonable and important one. But let us see how it can be enhanced by reasoning at a contextual level. Once we accept the possibility that context matters for violent behaviors we can begin to reason about the connection between mental illnesses and violent behaviors with a different frame of reference. Our vision is then shifted to thinking about the policies we implement and the structural arrangements these impose on people who develop serious mental illnesses.

Currently the most striking feature of policy toward individuals with schizophrenia in the United States is the scarcity of evidence-based treatments and the insufficient provision of even the most basic care such as shelter. Due in large part to the scarcity of supported housing, a very large number of mentally ill persons are presently residing in jails and prisons and municipal shelters. In these facilities, violent norms are well documented, and in such environments, mentally ill men and women are likely to adopt more violent behaviors. Moreover, those who can obtain supported housing generally are located in neighborhoods which have low social cohesion and high rates of violence; again these neighborhood characteristics can affect the behaviors of all residents including those who are mentally ill. To a large degree, these issues also pertain to individuals with other severe mental illnesses.

It may very well be, then, that policies shaped by irrational stigmatization and fear of people with schizophrenia and other severe mental illnesses have the ironic effect of contributing to high rates of violence in this group. The stigmatization of mental illness no doubt contributes a great deal to the policy of scarce services and supported housing, as it would be inconceivable for a developed society to impose the appalling conditions of prisons and shelters on individuals with less stigmatized illnesses (e.g., diabetes). In addition, the strong societal fear that people with mental illnesses will be dangerous, a fear that is entirely out of proportion to the real risk that people with these problems actually pose, breeds the Not In My Backyard (NIMBY) syndrome, ensuring that the available housing for people with mental illnesses will be mainly located in neighborhoods that do not have the clout to exclude this feared group from their midst.

Should these considerations change our viewpoint about policies to reduce violence among individuals with mental illness? Perhaps the most effective intervention of all would be at the societal level: make adequate care available including supported housing in safe neighborhoods. This policy would, at the same time, tend to reduce substance abuse and psychotic symptoms, which are among the important risk factors for violence that have been identified among mentally ill individuals. In addition, it might behoove us to address the antecedents of current policy, and advocate for change societal attitudes toward mental illness.

EXTENSION OF THE LOGIC

We have only considered moving "upward" to consider context as well as the individual. It is also very important to extend multilevel reasoning "downward" to include biological processes within the individual. In doing so, the reasoning recapitulates many of the same themes. In particular, it is useful to consider disease as an emergent property of individuals. An individual human being is not simply an aggregation of cells, but rather, a dynamic process. Health and disease are an emergent property of the ways in which the cells of the body interrelate. Placing biological determinants in the hierarchy of causation helps to remind us that individual and higher contextual level processes will influence biological phenomena. For example, animal studies suggest that an enriched social environment enhances dendritic branching and number of synapses in the developing brain (Rosenzweig and Bennett, 1996). While most of us are acutely aware that biological phenomena will influence higher level processes, we sometimes overlook the reciprocal relationship.

For clarity of exposition, we have explored multilevel reasoning within the simple framework of two levels, the individual and the social context. As noted earlier, the social context actually comprises many levels, and some studies may need to encompass more than one level of social context, for instance, the overall socioeconomic development of the country, the social cohesion of the neighborhood, and the relationships within the family. Similarly, biological determinants exist at many different levels of organization—molecule, cell, tissue, organ, system. The inclusion of many levels in a single investigation, however, greatly increases the complexity of design. As we argue below, carefully selecting the level of research is crucial to answering questions about causes.

FRAMING THE FUTURE

The possibilities for expansion both up and down are enormous, indeed endless. Take expansion up to contexts: there is the global context, the national context, the neighborhood context, the peer group context, the work context, the family context, even the context of a relationship with just one other person. Moreover, there is not just one facet to each of these contexts but rather a multitude of facets just as there are many, many characteristics of individuals. As a consequence, we are multiplying complexities.

This appealing expansion brings home two very critical points about epidemiological inquiry. First, we choose our focus. Because we cannot conceptualize, let alone accurately measure all influences, at all levels, we are forced to choose a focus whether we want to or not, whether we know it or not. Second, because we cannot include all variables at all levels, our statistical analyses are always misspecified by leaving out variables that would be included in a fully comprehensive model. This principle would apply even if we narrowed our focus to include only the individual level of analysis; it certainly applies when we expand our focus to include the cell and the society. Whatever choice we make, much will be left out, and the gap cannot be filled by any statistical analysis of the data collected.

The practical significance of the foregoing considerations is that to approach epidemiological questions wisely, we need to have causal explanations that involve multiple levels and the interconnections between those levels. This will require theory and conceptualization of what is salient for disease causation at the various levels. Thus, the era of multilevel inquiry will require the creative construction of rigorous causal explanations and the careful conceptualization and measurement of the variables implied by those explanations. We cannot hope to succeed by simply adding measures at other levels of analysis to the kinds of statistical manipulations used during the individually focused era of risk factor epidemiology. Furthermore, we cannot hope to succeed by simply adopting preexisting boundaries to define contexts: a census tract may or may not correspond to neighborhood. Significant effort must be invested in identifying the relevance and defining the actual boundaries of each level for a given research question.

Classical epidemiology before the primacy of multivariate methods is replete with examples of strategic inquiry focused on evaluating explanations for disease causation. Clever tests help us decide whether a causal explanation is consistent with observed facts or inconsistent with those facts. These examples from classical epidemiology tell us we need two things together: causal explanations and informative tests of those causal explanations. We need to bring this aspect of classical epidemiology to the new focus on multiple levels of inquiry.

REFERENCES

Bell MD, Lysaker PH (1997): Clinical benefits of paid work activity in schizophrenia: 1-year follow-up. Schizophr Bull 23:317–328.

Bobak M, Marmot M (1996): East-West mortality divide and its potential explanations: proposed research agenda. Br Med J 312(7028):421–425.

Bobak M, Pikhart H, Hertzman C, Rose R, Marmot M (1998): Socioeconomic factors, perceived control and self-reported health in Russia. A cross-sectional survey. Soc Sci Med 47:269–279.

Breslau N, Chilcoat H, DelDotto J, Andreski P, Brown G (1996): Low birth weight and neurocognitive status at six years of age. Biol Psychiatry 40:389–397.

Bryk AS, Raudenbush SW (1992): "Hierarchical Linear Models: Applications and Data Analysis Methods." Newbury Park, CA: Sage.

Chapin C (1934): "The Papers of Charles V. Chapin, M.D.: A Review of Public Health Realities." New York: The Commonwealth Fund, Oxford University Press.

Collins PY, Varma VK, Wig NN, Mojtabai R, Day R, Susser E (1999): Fever and acute brief psychosis in urban and rural settings in north India. Br J Psychiatry 173:520–524.

Collins PY, Wig NN, Day R, Varma VK, Malhotra S, Misra AK, Schanzer B, Susser E (1996): Psychosocial and biological aspects of acute brief psychoses in three developing country sites. Psychiatr Q 67:177–193.

Diez-Roux A, Nieto F, Muntaner C, Tyroler HA, Comstock GW, Shahar E, Cooper LS, Watson RL, Szklo M (1997): Neighborhood environments and coronary heart disease: a multilevel analysis. Am J Epidemiol 146:48–63.

Diez-Roux AV (1998): Bringing context back into epidemiology: variables and fallacies in multilevel analysis. Am J Public Health 88:216–222.

Doll R, Hill AB (1950).: Smoking and carcinoma of the lung. Preliminary report. Br Med J 2:739–148.

Eaton WW (2000): The 2000 Rema Lapouse Award: Continuities, contingencies, comorbidities, and latencies: evidence and logic for a national conception-to-death cohort study. 128th Annual Meeting of APHA (November 12–16, 2000).

Entwisle B, Mason WM, Hermali HI (1986): The multilevel dependence of contraceptive use on the socioeconomic development and family planning program strength. Demography 23:199–216.

Faris R, Dunham H (1939): "Mental Disorders in Urban Areas." Chicago: University of Chicago Press.

Gillberg C, Wing L (1999): Autism: Not an extremely rare disorder. Acta Psychiatr Scand 93:399–406.

Goedde HW, Agarwal DP, Fritze G, Meier-Tackmann D, Singh S, Beckmann G, Bhatia K, Chen LZ, Fang B, Lisker R, Paik YK, Rothhammer F, Saha N, Segal B, Srivastava LM,

Czeizel A (1992): Distribution of ADH2 and ALDH2 genotypes in different populations. Hum Genet 88:344–346.

Goldberger J, Wheeler GA, Sydenstrycker E (1920): A study of the relation of family income and other economic factors to pellagra incidence in seven cotton mill villages of South Carolina in 1916. Public Health Rep 35:2673–2714.

Goldberger J, Wheeler GA, Sydenstricker E (1918): A study of the diet of nonpellagrous and pellagrous households in textile mill communities in South Carolina in 1916. JAMA 71:944–949.

Hamlin, C (1998): "Public Health and Social Justice in the Age of Chadwick." Cambridge University Press. Cambridge, UK.

Hare EH (1956): Mental illness and social conditions in Bristol. J Mental Sci 102:349–357.

Higuchi S, Matsushita S, Imazeki H et al. (1994): Aldehyde dehydrogenase genotypes in Japanese alcoholics. Lancet 343:741–742.

Higuchi S, Matsushita S, Muramaysu T, Murayama M, Hayashida M (1996): Alcohol and aldehyde dehydrogenase genotypes and drinking behavior in Japanese. Alcohol Clin Exp Res 20:493–497.

Jablensky A, Sartorious N, Ernberg G, Anker M, Korten A, Cooper JE, Day R, Bertelsen A (1992): Schizophrenia: manifestations, incidence and course in different cultures. Psychological Medicine, Monograph Supplement 20. New York: Cambridge University Press.

Kellam SG, Ling X, Merisca R, Brown CH, Ialongo N (1998): The effect of the level of aggression in the first grade classroom on the course and malleability of aggressive behavior into middle school. Dev Psychopathol 10:165–185.

Kelsey J, Whittemore AS, Evans AS, Thompson WD (eds) (1996): "Methods in Observational Epidemiology," 2nd ed. New York: Oxford University Press.

Kermack WO, McKendrick AG, McKinley PL (1934): Death rates in Great Britain and Sweden: Expression of specific mortality rates as products of two factors, and some consequences thereof. J Hyg 3334:433–451.

Kuh E, Ben-Shlomo Y (1997): "A Live Course Approach to Chronic Disease Epidemiology." Oxford: Oxford University Press.

Kuhn L, Susser ES (2001): AIDS in Africa: the excruciating dilemma of breast feeding. P & S Medical Review 8(1):8–12.

Leff J, Wig NN, Gosh A, Bedi H, Menon DK, Kupiers L, Korten A, Ernberg G, Day R, Sartorius N, Jablensky A (1987): Influence of relatives expressed emotion on the course of schizophrenia in Chandigarh. Br J Psychiatry 151:166–273.

Link BG, Phelan J (1995): Social conditions as fundamental causes of disease. J Health Soc Behav (Extra Issue):80–94.

Link BG, Andrews H, Cullen FT (1992): The violent and illegal behavior of mental patients reconsidered. American Soc Rev 57:275–292.

Link BG, Monahan J, Stueve A, Cullen FT (1999): Real in their consequences: a sociological approach to understanding the association between psychotic symptoms and violence. American Soc Rev 64:316–332.

MacMahon B, Pugh TF, Ipsen J (1960): "Epidemiological Methods." Boston: Little Brown.

Marmot M, Bobak M (2000): International comparators and poverty and health in Europe. Br Med J 321:1124–1128.

Matte TD, Bresnahan M, Begg MD, Susser E (2001): Influence of variation in birth weight within normal range and within sibships on IQ at age 7 years: cohort study. Br Med J 323(7308):310–4.

McMichael AJ (1999): Prisoners of the proximate: Loosening the constraints on epidemiology in an age of change. Am J Epidemiol 149:887–897.

Morris JN (1957): "Uses of Epidemiology." London: Churchill Livingstone.

Newsholme A (1927): "Health Problems in Organized Society: Studies in the Social Aspects of Public Health." London: PS King and Son Ltd.

Richards M, Hardy R, Kuh D, Wadsworth MEJ (2001): Birth weight and cognitive function in the British 1946 birth cohort: Longitudinal population based study. Br Med J 322:199–203.

Rosenzweig MR, Bennett EL (1996): Psychobiology of plasticity: effects of training and experience on brain and behavior. Behav Brain Res 78:57–65.

Ross R (1911): "The Prevention of Malaria." London: Oxford University Press.

Rothman KJ, Greenland S (1998): "Modern Epidemiology" Philadelphia: Lippincott Williams and Wilkins.

Sampson RJ, Raudenbush SW, Earls F (1997): Neighborhood s and violent crime: A multilevel study of collective efficacy. Science 277:918–924.

Schwartz S, Carpenter K (1999): The right answer for the wrong question: consequences of type III error for public health research. Am J Public Health 89:1175–80.

Schwartz S, Susser E, Susser M (1999): A future for epidemiology? Ann Rev Public Health 20:1–19.

Smith GD, Ebrahim S (2001): Epidemiology—is it time to call it a day? Int J Epidemiol 30:1–11.

Snow J (1855): "On the Mode of Communication of Cholera," 2nd ed. London: Churchill. Reproduced in "Snow on Cholera." New York: New York. Commonwealth Fund, 1936.

Steadman HJ, Mulvey EP, Monahan J, Robbins PC, Appelbaum PS, Grisso T, Roth LH, Silver E (1998): Violence by people discharged from acute psychiatric inpatient facilities and by others in the same neighborhoods. Arch Gen Psychiatry 55:1–9.

Stein Z, Karim Q (2001): A decade of radical change: How HIV and liberation have affected the life course of women in South Africa. In Kuh D, Hardy R (eds): "A Life Course Approach to Womens Health." Oxford: Oxford Univeristy Press (to appear).

Stueve A, Link BG (1997): Violence and psychiatric disorders: Results from an epidemiological study of young adults in Israel. Psychiatr Q 68:327–342.

Susser E, Schwartz S, Bromet E, Morabia A, Gorman J (Eds.) (2001); "Concepts and Methods of Psychiatric Epidemiology." Oxford: Oxford University Press (to appear).

Susser E, Bresnahan M (2001): Origins of Epidemiology. In "Population Health and Aging: Strengthening the Dialogue Between Epidemiology and Demography." Annals of the NY Academy of Sciences, Volume 954. New York: New York Academy of Sciences.

Susser, E., Collins P, Schanzer B, Varma VK, Gittelman M (1996): Can we learn from the care of persons with mental illness in developing countries? Am J Public Health 86:926–928.

Susser E, Terry MB, Matte T (2000): The birth cohorts grow up: New opportunities for epidemiology. Pediatr Perinat Epidemiol 14:98–100.

Susser E, Wanderling J (1994): Epidemiology of nonaffective acute remitting psychosis vs schizophrenia. Arch Gen Psychiatry 51:294–301.

Susser, M (1973): "Causal Thinking in the Health Sciences: Concepts and Strategies of Epidemiology." New York: Oxford University Press.

Susser M (1985): Epidemiology in the United States after World War II: The evolution of technique. Epidemiol Rev 7:147–177.

Susser, M., Adelstein A (eds.) (1975): "Vital Statistics: A Memorial Volume of Sections from the Reports and Writings of William Farr." Metuchen, NJ: The Scarecrow Press.

Susser M, Susser E. (1996a): Choosing a future for epidemiology: I. Eras and paradigms. Am J Public Health 86:668–673.

Susser M, Susser E (1996b): Choosing a future for epidemiology: II. From black box to Chinese boxes in eco-epidemiology. Am J Public Health 86:674–677.

Sydenstricker E (1933): "Health and Environment." New York: McGraw-Hill.

UNAIDS (2000): "Report on the Global HIV/AIDS Epidemic June 2000."

van der Put NMJ, Steegers-Theunissen RPM, Frosst P, Trijbels FJ, Eskes TK, van den Heuvel LP, Mariman EC, den Heyer M, Rozen R, Blom HJ (1995): Mutated methlenetetrahydrofolate reductase as a risk factor for spina bifida. Lancet 346:1070–1071.

van Os J, Driessen G, Gunther N, Delespaul P (2000): Neighbourhood variation in incidence of schizophrenia. Evidence for person-environment interaction. Br J Psychiatry 176:243–248.

von Zerssen D, Leon CA, Moller HJ, Wittchen HU, Pfister H, Sartorius N (1990): Care strategies for schizophrenic patients in a transcultural comparison. Compr Psychiatry 31:398–408.

Wakefield AJ, Murch SH, Anthony A, Linnell J, Casson DM, Malik M, Berelowitz M, Dhillon AP, Thomson MA, Harvey P, Valentine A, Davies SE, Walker-Smith JA (1998): Illeal-lymphoid-nodular hyperplasia, non-specific colitis, and pervasive developmental disorder in children. Lancet 351:637–641.

Warner, R. (1985): "Recovery from Schizophrenia: Psychiatry and Political Economy." London: Routelage.

Wig NN, Menon DK, Bedi H, Leff J, Kupiers L, Ghosh A, Day R, Korten A, Ernberg G, Sartorius N, Jablensky A (1987): Distribution of expressed emotion component in relatives of schizophrenic patients in Aarhus and Chandigarh. Br J Psychiatry 151:160–165.

Wilkinson RG (1992): Income distribution and life expectancy. Br Med J 304:154–158.

Wilkinson RG (1996): "Unhealthy Societies. The Afflictions of Inequality." London: Routledge.

Winslow CEA (1943): "The Conquest of Epidemic Disease: A Chapter in the History of Ideas." Madison, WI: University of Wisconsin Press.

Wyatt RJ, Susser ES (2000): US birth cohort studies of schizophrenia: a sea change. Schizophr Bull 26:255–256.

Wyatt RJ, Henter ID (1998): The effects of early and sustained intervention on the long-term morbidity of schizophrenia. J Psychiatr Res 32:169–177.

PART II

ASSESSMENT

CHAPTER 9

Studying the Natural History of Psychopathology

WILLIAM W. EATON

Department of Mental Hygiene, Bloomberg School of Public Health, Johns Hopkins University, Baltimore, MD 21205

INTRODUCTION

The purpose of this chapter is to provide a conceptual framework for conducting studies of the natural history of psychopathology in the general population and to illustrate details of the framework with examples from research in the field of psychiatric epidemiology. The three major aspects of the natural history of psychopathology are *onset*, *course*, and *outcome*. Preventive actions directed at onset, course, and outcome are traditionally defined as *primary*, *secondary*, and *tertiary* prevention, respectively. This introductory section is followed by one section on each of the topics of onset, course, and outcome, followed by a section on methods, and a conclusion. The chapter has been revised from the 1995 version by reorganizing the methods into one section and adding new developments related to the conceptual framework for the natural history of psychopathology that have occurred since 1995.

This chapter is not intended as a review of studies on the natural history of psychopathology. A comprehensive review would be cumbersome and uninformative, because there is so much variation in methodologic quality of studies of natural course. If methodologic standards are set high for such a review (for example, by including only population-based studies with diagnostic information on an adequate number of subjects), there are very few studies that could be included. On the other hand, if methodologic standards are set low for such a review (for example, by including small studies of clinic samples and studies without diagnostic information), there would be a confusing morass of numerous studies with results so mixed and contradictory that the review would be of dubious value. This situation shows the state of the art in this area, indicating that we are still at the beginning stages of learning about the natural history of psychopathology.

Textbook in Psychiatric Epidemiology, Second Edition, Edited by Ming T. Tsuang and Mauricio Tohen. ISBN 0-471-40974-X

The *natural history of psychopathology* is a description, at the level of the population, of the ebbing and flowing of psychopathology from its earliest appearance to its final outcome. It includes signs and symptoms that occur before onset, the fluctuations in signs and symptoms that occur after onset, and consequences of the psychopathology, even those that may occur after remission. It does not include the study of risk factors except as they influence the course. Although there is not complete agreement on the issue, the stance is taken here that the natural history includes those treatments that are received by the general population in the natural setting. The definition leads to a focus in this chapter on descriptive population-based cohort studies. There is relatively little emphasis on cohort studies oriented toward specific risk factors, such as those comparing populations defined as exposed and not exposed to some risk factor. There is relatively little emphasis on cohort studies that include an intervention trial in an attempt to evaluate risk and protective factors, since the intervention trials are often not based in general populations and since the intervention itself may disrupt the natural history. The primary focus is on population-based studies, since many persons with mental disorder never seek treatment for it.

ONSET

Etiology and Pathology

In defining "onset," it helps to distinguish the *etiologic* process from the *pathologic* process. Pathology occurs when the sociobiologic dynamics have become abnormal and signifies a distinct change in the relationship among variables, the new influence of variables that were not important beforehand, or a new metabolism of some sort. The etiologic process is broader conceptually and includes the period of time when the probability of disorder is heightened, even though the process is still normal (Rothman, 1981). Causes may be present well before the pathologic process has begun. Onset occurs when the pathologic process begins.

The absence of firm data on the validity of the classification system enjoins us to be careful about operationally defining disease onset. It is particularly difficult to establish the validity of a threshold for the presence versus the absence of disorder, because signs and symptoms of psychiatric disorders are widespread in the population, not always reflecting the presence of a psychiatric disorder. From the clinical standpoint, subtle differences in approach to treatment may suggest quite varied thresholds; from the epidemiologic standpoint, subtle differences in threshold may produce widely varying prevalences. A simple definition is that onset occurs when the individual first enters treatment. A related definition is that onset occurs when the symptom is noticeable by a clinician. Another definition is the point when the symptom is first noticed by the individual. With the operational criteria of the *Diagnostic and Statistical Manual*, it is possible to conceive of onset as the time when full criteria are met for the first time in the life. This definition has been used in studies of incidence (e.g., Eaton et al., 1989a, b). But it omits that part of the pathologic process that takes place prior to meeting full criteria for disorder—the prodrome, as described below. Since the etiologic process may be extended in time, and the operation of etiologic factors distant from when full criteria for disorder are met, this may lead to missing important risk factors.

The definitions above are easy to operationalize but lack an explicit relationship to the pathologic process. Theoretically, onset is that point in time when the etiologic process becomes irretrievably pathologic, that is, the point when it is certain that the full criteria for disorder will eventually be met. This point of irreversibility is, unfortunately, very difficult to observe. Focus on population indicators for the force of morbidity leads to explicit consideration of the idea of a continuous line of development toward manifestation of disease with an as-yet-unknown point of irreversibility. At present we can only hypothesize where the disease begins, so that even the use of the word "symptom" is problematic in the strict medical sense, since we cannot ascribe the complaint or behavior to the disease with perfect accuracy. Studying the natural history of psychopathology may, in the end, lead to the conclusion that the disease concept is inappropriate or not useful, suggesting a shift to a more explicitly developmental framework (Baltes et al., 1981), with emphasis on normally distributed characteristics, and continuities in development, rather than rare dichotomies and discontinuities which the disease model entails.

There are at least two ways of thinking about the development toward disease. The first way is the increase in severity or intensity of symptoms. An individual could have all the symptoms required for diagnosis but none of them in sufficient intensity or severity as to meet the threshold for disease. The underlying logic of this conception is the relatively high frequency of the symptoms, at a mild level of intensity, in the general population, making it difficult to distinguish normal and subcriterial complaints from manifestations of disease. For many chronic diseases, including psychiatric disorders, it may be inappropriate to regard the symptom as ever having been absent (for example, deviant personality traits on axis II of the "Diagnostic and Statistical Manual"). This type of progression toward disorder is termed *intensification* and leads the researcher to consider whether a crucial level of intensity exists at which the rate of development toward disorder accelerates or becomes irreversible.

Figure 1 is an adaptation of a diagram used by Lilienfeld and Stolley (1994, Fig. 6.2) to visualize the concept of incidence as a time-oriented rate. Here the adaptation gives examples of the several distinct forms that onset can take when the disorder is defined by constellations of symptoms varying in intensity, as is the case with mental disorders. Compare cases No. 3 and No. 5, for example, which in the original diagram are situations of uncomplicated incidence. The bottom part of the figure shows how intensity, represented by the vertical width of the bars, might be different for these two new cases. It also shows how there might be intensifications occurring that are stronger in magnitude than that associated with incidence, which would not be recorded as new cases (bottom two "cases" in gray). Since the intensification of symptoms represents the force of morbidity in the population, use of a simple dichotomous measure of incidence will be misleading, unless the threshold of onset is placed precisely where the pathologic process begins.

A second conceptual approach toward the issue of disease development is the occurrence of new groups of symptoms where none existed. This involves the gradual *acquisition* of symptoms so that clusters are formed that increasingly approach the constellation required to meet specified definitions for diagnosis.

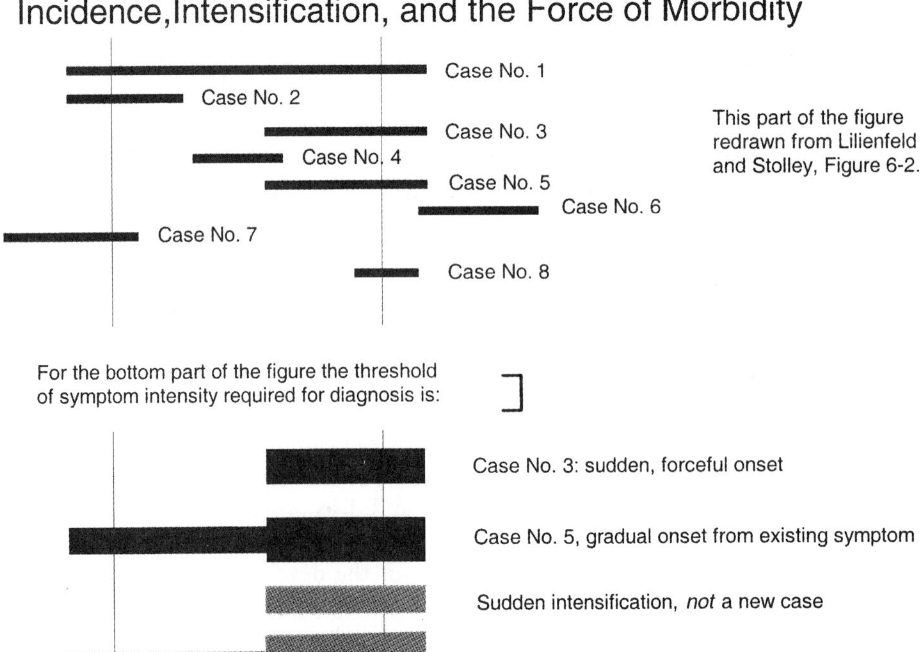

Figure 1. Onset of disorder through intensification of symptoms [adapted from Eaton et al., 1989b and Lilienfeld and Stolley, Figure 6.2 (top portion)].

"Present" can be defined as occurrence either at the nonsevere or at the severe level: thus, decisions made about the process of symptom intensification complicate this idea which focuses on symptom acquisition. This leads the researcher to consider the order in which symptoms occur over the natural history of the disease and, in particular, whether one symptom is more important than others in accelerating the process.

Conceptualizing the force of morbidity as time to a single dichotomous event (i.e., traditional concepts of incidence) is not flexible enough to deal with dimensional constructs, as shown in Figure 1. It is also not flexible enough to deal with changes through time in the covariation of indicators, which can be important aspect of the force of morbidity. *Emergence* is defined to be the development of new covariation of a group of symptoms to each other. Figure 2 shows a simplified view of this developmental phenomenon for the example of the depression syndrome. The vertical axis represents the intensity of mood disturbance, and the diagonal axis, slanting backwards from left to right, the intensity of somatic disturbance. Time is represented by the horizontal axis, passing from left to right. At some early stage of development, the correlation of mood to somatic disturbance is pictured as being 0.0 (round circle representing cross-sectional scatterplot with correlation equal to 0.0). Gradually the mood comes to be associated with the somatic disturbance, shown by the evolution of the circle into an ellipse. At this

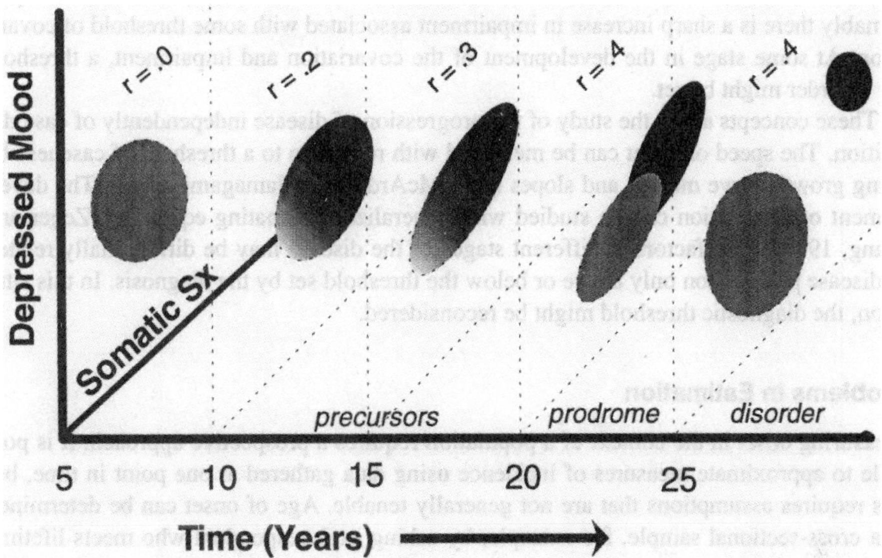

Figure 2. Onset of disorder through acquisition of symptoms. (Adapted from Eaton et al., 1989b.)

point, the normal and the abnormal have not split, and the disorder is not inevitable. At this stage both mood and somatic disturbance predict imperfectly to later onset of Major Depressive Disorder. Later, a group begins to emerge for whom mood and somatic disturbance are highly correlated. Finally, there emerges a group with very high covariation of mood and somatic disturbance, and a second normal group where little covariation remains. An increase in covariation can occur without an increase in mean levels of either mood or somatic disturbance. But presumably there is a sharp increase in impairment associated with some threshold of covariation. At some stage in the development of the covariation and impairment, a threshold for disorder might be set. These concepts allow the study of the progression of disease independently of case definition.

Prodromes and Precursors

The *prodrome* is the period prior to meeting full-blown criteria of disorder, when some signs or symptoms are nevertheless present. The prodome is defined only for those who eventually are diagnosed as cases, and can only be observed with complete certainty in a retrospective fashion. The *speed of onset* is the length of the prodromal period and can be measured in simple units of time (e.g., months or years). The presence of signs or symptoms below the criterion level may help to identify individuals at heightened risk for developing the full-blown disorder, who might be considered targets of prevention. Given the widespread prevalence of individual signs and symptoms of mental disorders in the general population, it is likely that many individuals with signs and symptoms of disorder will not go on to develop the full-blown criteria. In this situation the signs and symptoms are not quite prodromal, in the strict sense of the word, but it seems awkward to refer to them as risk factors. Signs and symptoms from a diagnostic cluster that precede

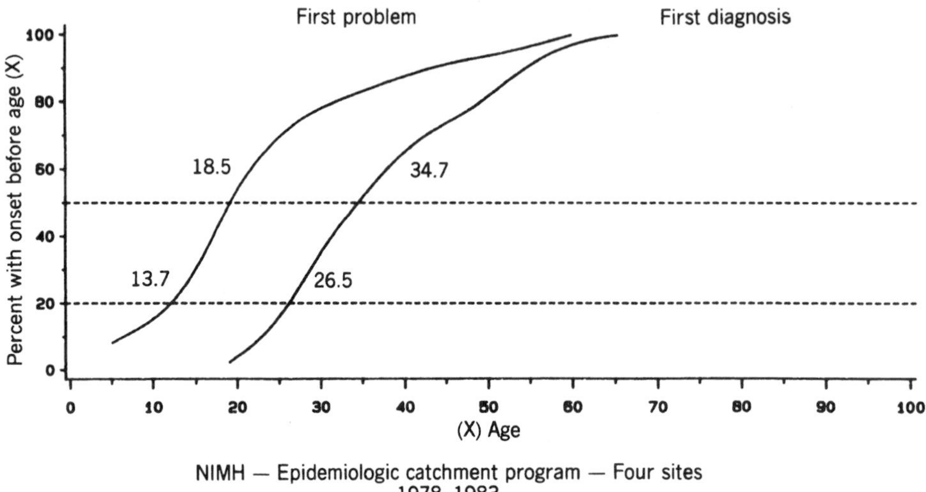

Figure 3. Prodromal period for panic disorder. The right curve is the cumulative age of onset for the disorder; the left curve is the cumulative age of onset for the first problem associated with the disorder; the area between the curves is the prodromal period. (Adapted from Eaton et al., 1995.)

disorder, but do not predict the onset of disorder with certainty, are referred to here as *precursor signs and symptoms*. At the present state of our knowledge of the onset of mental disorders, there are few or no signs and symptoms that predict onset with certainty, but precursor signs and symptoms may be helpful in identifying groups at higher risk for onset than the general population. Converting what is known about precursors into true prodromes is an important topic of research for epidemiologists interested in longitudinal research and in prevention.

An illustration of these issues is presented in Figure 3 and Table 1. Figure 3 shows two cumulative distributions for panic disorder. The distribution on the right focuses on the age at which the individual first meets full criteria for DSM-III Panic Disorder. For this distribution, onset must occur during the one-year follow-up period of the ECA Program, that is, a true prospective design. The population at risk includes those who had never met criteria for the diagnosis at the beginning of the follow-up period. Thus, the at-risk group includes those with no symptoms, as well as those with some symptoms of disorder, but not meeting full DSM-III criteria. The distribution on the left focuses on the age at which panic first occurred, as reported by the new cases. The dotted line marks the 20th and 50th percentiles, and age values for these are recorded. The area between the two curves gives a rough outline of the prodromal period.

Panic disorder has onset in young adulthood (Fig. 3). Twenty percent of cases meet criteria for diagnosis for the first time before the age of 27 years and 50% before they are 35. Twenty percent have their first panic attack before the age of

TABLE 1. Relative and Attributable Risk for Panic Disorder Due to Precursors: Epidemiologic Catchment Area Program

Precursor	Precursor Relative Risk	Precursor Prevalence (%)	Precursor Attributable Risk (%)
Nervous person	8.2	24.3	64
Panic attack	24.9	3.8	48
Attack with breathing difficulty	32.9	1.2	28
Attack with heart pounding	30.9	2.7	45
Attack with dizziness	25.1	1.0	19
Attack with fingers tingling	23.4	0.7	14
Attack with pain in chest	24.0	1.0	19
Attack with choking sensation	28.5	0.9	19
Attack with fainting sensation	25.7	1.0	20
Attack with sweating	24.6	2.0	32
Attack with shaking	23.4	2.2	33
Attack with derealization	27.7	1.4	27
Attack with fear of dying	30.4	1.6	32
Attack with hot/cold flashes	27.7	1.8	32

Source: Adapted from Eaton et al., 1995.

14 and 50% before the age of 19. The prodromal period is about 13 years long for those with early onset and about 16 years for those with later onset.

Symptoms associated with onset of panic disorder, defined above as precursors, are associated with accelerated onset of the disorder. Table 1 shows the prevalence of the precursor, its relative risk in predicting onset of panic disorder during the one year of follow-up in the ECA Program, and the attributable risk that can be estimated with the prevalence and the relative risk. The standard formula for attributable risk can be applied here (e.g., Kleinbaum et al., 1982) and is useful because it might prioritize precursors for screening or other prevention programs, but this use of the term is conceptually different from other uses because of the limited duration of the follow-up. Therefore, the duration of the follow-up is used to qualify the attributable risk. A panic attach with breathing difficulty displays the highest relative risk (32.9), but, due to rarity in the population (prevalence of 1.2% in the population), the one-year attributable risk is only 28%. The occurrence of a simple panic attack is a strong precursor of panic disorder because the relative risk is high (24.9) and the prevalence is not too low (3.8%). A positive response to the question "Are you a nervous person?" is also a strong precursor of panic disorder. This strategy of searching for precursors is applicable for most disorders. It has been applied to depression previously (Dryman and Eaton, 1991; Horvath et al., 1992).

Many mental disorders have long prodromal periods, as shown in Figure 3 for panic disorder. The symptomatic picture of the prodromal period is efficiently summarized with a horizontal bar chart, as shown in Figure 4, in this case for depression (Eaton et al., 1997). As required for prodromes, only new cases, from the Baltimore ECA Follow-up, are included. The bars show the durations of time that symptoms in the DSM-IV symptom groups have endured prior to onset. The

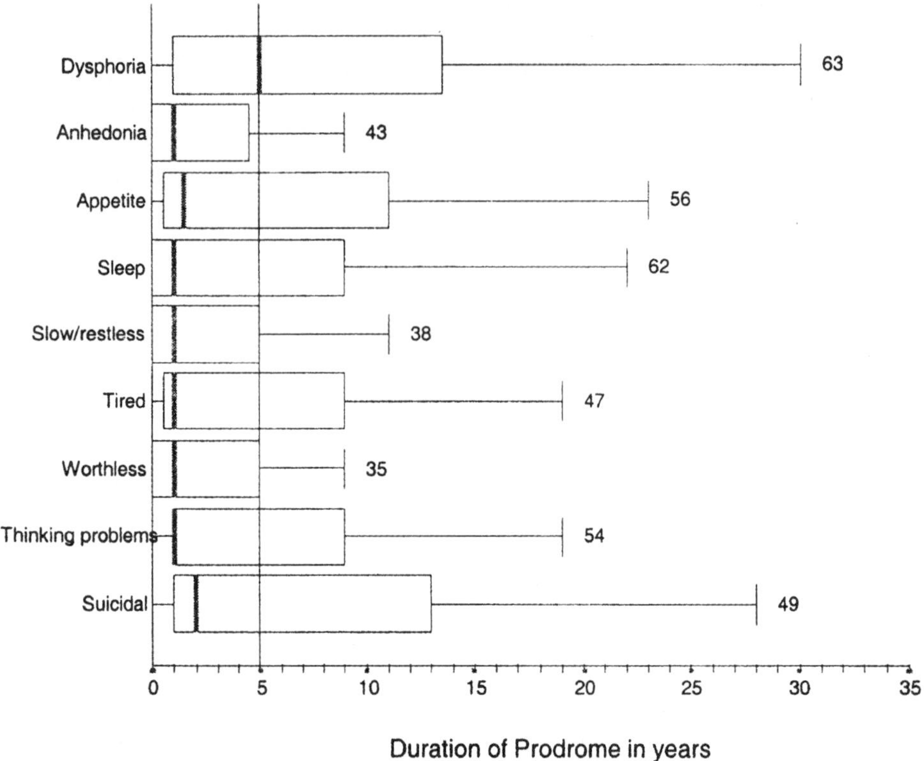

Figure 4. Prodromal period for depression in 71 new cases from the Baltimore Epidemiologic Catchment Area Follow-up. The open horizontal bars enclose 50% of the cases, and the vertical bar is the median. (Adapted from Eaton et al., 1997.)

median time is designated by the vertical line inside the bar, and the quartiles are designated by the ends of the bars. Most symptom groups have prodromes lasting one or two years, but for dysphoria and suicidal ideation, there is much heterogeneity, with over half the prodromes being more than five years long.

Population Measures of Onset

Incidence is the rate at which new cases develop in the population. It is essential to distinguish *first incidence* from *total incidence*. The distinction itself is commonly assumed by epidemiologists, but there does not appear to be consensus on the terminology. Most definitions of the incidence numerator include a concept such as new cases (Lilienfeld and Lilienfeld, 1980), illness commencing (Expert Committee, 1959), cases that come into being (MacMahon et al., 1960), or persons who develop a disease (Mausner and Kramer, 1985) or have onset (National Center for Health Statistics, 1977). Sartwell and Last (1980) imply total incidence when they state the necessity of allowing for an individual being counted more than once, if the condition is one for which this is possible (e.g., accidents, colds). Lilienfeld and

Lilienfeld (1980) also occasionally equate incidence with attack rate. Kleinbaum et al. (1982) hint at the distinction between first and total incidence, but are not explicit on the issue. Morris (1975) defines incidence as equivalent to our first incidence and attack rate as equivalent to our total incidence. Except for the latter text, in none of these definitions is it explicit whether or not an individual who is healthy now, but has had episodes of the disorder over the life course, qualifies for a new onset. First incidence corresponds to the most common use of the term "incidence," but since the usage is by no means universal, the prefix is recommended.

The numerator for first incidence is composed of those individuals who have had an occurrence of the disorder for the first time in their lives during a specified time period; the denominator excludes all persons who start the period with any prior history of the disorder. The numerator for total incidence includes all individuals who have a new occurrence of the disorder during the time period under investigation whether or not it is the initial episode of their lives or a recurrent episode. The denominator for total incidence excludes only persons who are active cases at the beginning of the follow-up period.

The preference for first or total incidence in etiologic studies depends on hypotheses and assumptions about the way causes and outcomes important to the disease ebb and flow. If the disease is recurrent and the causal factors vary in strength over time, then it might be important to study risk factors not only for first but for subsequent episodes (total incidence). For example, one might consider the effects of changing levels of stress on the occurrence of episodes of neurotic illness (Tyrer, 1985) or of schizophrenia (Brown and Birley, 1968). For a disease with a presumed fixed progression from some fixed starting point, such as dementia, the first occurrence might be the most important episode to focus on, and first incidence is the appropriate rate. In the field of psychiatric epidemiology, there are a range of disorders with both types of causal structures operating, which leads to discussion of the two distinct types of incidence.

The two types of incidence are functionally related to different measures of prevalence. Kramer et al. (1981) have shown that lifetime prevalence (i.e., the proportion of the population who have ever had an occurrence of a disorder) is a function of first incidence and mortality in affected and unaffected populations. Point prevalence (i.e., the proportion of persons in a defined population at a given time who manifest the disorder) is linked to total incidence by the queuing formula $P = I * D$ (Kramer, 1957; Kleinbaum et al., 1982): that is, point prevalence is equal to the total incidence multiplied by the average duration of episodes.

Incidence data on specific psychiatric disorders are expensive to gather. A minority of individuals, not necessarily representative of those with disorder, receive treatment, and therefore a field survey is required. Many of the disorders are rare and many well individuals have to be evaluated, at two distinct points in time to estimate the incidence rate. The number of prospective studies with sufficiently large samples to estimate rates of incidence is small. If 5,000 person-years of observation is set as the minimum requirement, there are only a handful of studies that cover a range of disorders. These include the ECA study in the United States (Eaton et al., 1989a, b), the Stirling County study in Canada (Murphy et al., 1987), the Traunstein study in Germany (Fichter et al., 1987), the Lundby Study in Sweden (Hanell et al., 1990), the Baltimore ECA Follow-up

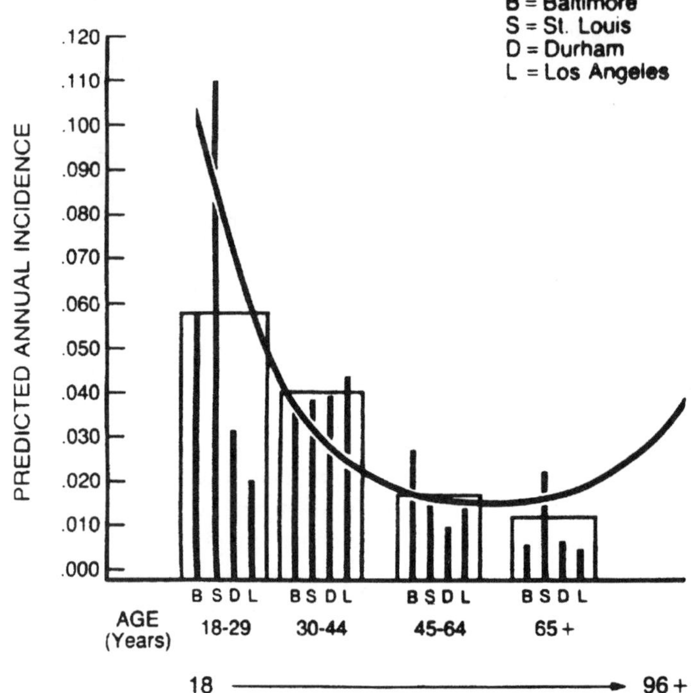

Figure 5(*a*). Age of onset for alcohol abuse or dependence among males. Prospective data from four sites of the Epidemiologic Catchment Area Program. (Adapted from Eaton et al., 1989.)

(Eaton et al., 1997), and, soon, the Follow-up of the National Comorbidity Survey (Kessler et al., 1995).

Comparison of results between these studies is important because the numerators are so small that the findings from any one study are statistically volatile. Analysis of the onset of alcohol abuse or dependence in the ECA cohort (Figure 5) shows sharply declining incidence after young adulthood and a slight rise at the beginning of the seventh decade. The rise is caused by only five individuals who had onset in that age range. A similar curve from the Lundby study has the same shape (Ôjescho et al., 1982), with the rise after age 60 based on only three individuals who had incidence in that age range. These results suggest etiologic clues and have implications for prevention efforts. The results of each study might not be convincing, but the replication of the identical pattern is credible.

COURSE

Remission

Careful definition of terms is essential for studying the course of psychopathology (Frank et al., 1991). Conceptualizing and measuring the ebb and flow of psychopathology after onset necessitates focus on duration, measured by units of time,

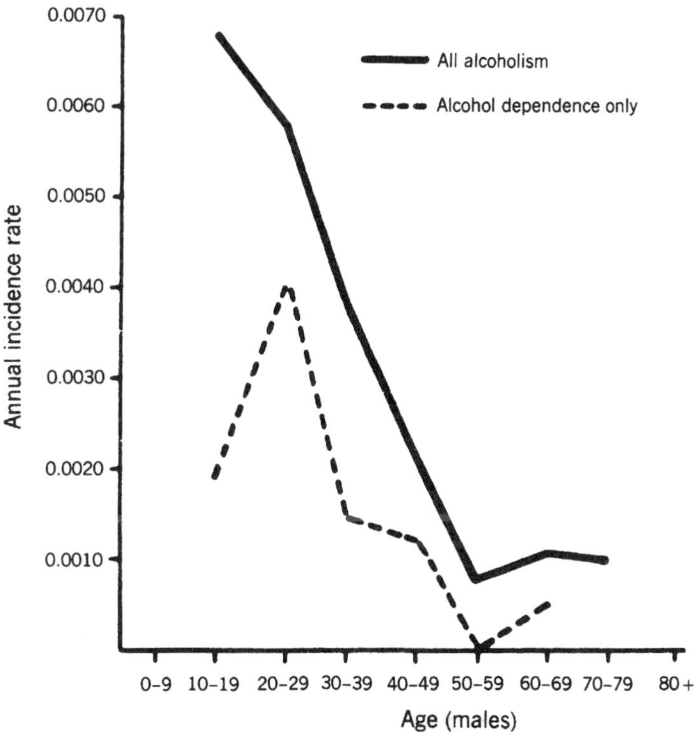

Figure 5(*b*). Age of onset of alcoholism among males. Prospective data from the Lundby study. (Adapted from Ojesjo et al., 1982. Reprinted with permission from *Journal of Studies on Alcohol*, vol. 43, pp 1190–98, 1943. (© Alcohol Research Documentation, Inc., Rutgers Center of Alcohol Studies, Piscataway, NJ 08855.)

and on recurrence, which is measured in the manner similar to incidence. *Remission* is a point in time after onset when signs and symptoms diminish sharply. After the first onset has occurred, it is useful to have a measure of level of symptomatology that defines remission unambiguously. Only after setting a threshold for remission can the duration of the episode be studied (Philipp and Fickinger, 1993). The definition of remission has all the complexities of the definition of onset. But as well as a threshold for the presence and absence of signs and symptoms, defined by both intensity and breadth, the definition of remission requires that a threshold of a minimum time period be set, below which a remission does not occur. For example, a remission may be defined as a continuous period of three months or more during which the individual is not meeting full criteria for disorder; or, a stricter definition might be three months during which the individual has no symptoms of the disorder at all.

The measure of remission will be most useful if it uses the diagnostic criteria as a comparison or standard value, because that will facilitate meaningful comparison of qualities of remission between disorders. As an example, an operational measure of completeness of remission is proposed to describe that point between episodes that is most free of signs and symptoms. It requires that thresholds be established for the intensity of signs and symptoms, as in, for example, the SCAN (rating scale one value of 1 versus 2 or 3; Wing et al., 1990). The measure of completeness of remission can be used even if the threshold levels are set differently in different research studies. The measure below takes advantage of the SCAN definitions to set thresholds of symptom intensity and sets three months as the minimum time period during which the individual must fail to meet complete diagnostic criteria in order for a remission to be defined and measurable. The proposed levels of completeness of remission are the following:

Level 1: No signs and symptoms present.

Level 2: At least one sign or symptom present, but none above the threshold of intensity.

Level 3: One and only one sign or symptom present above the threshold of intensity; other signs and symptoms may or may not be present below the threshold of intensity.

Level 4: More than one sign or symptom present above the threshold.

Level 5: Full criteria for disorder are present continuously (i.e., remission does not occur) ("continuously" is defined as having no gaps greater than three months).

The *speed of remission* is defined similarly to the speed of onset and the prodromal period. It is the time from the point at which the disorder is at its symptom peak to the beginning of the remission. The symptom peak is best defined similarly to the concept of acquisition, discussed above: the point in time where the highest number of signs and symptoms are above the threshold of intensity. The speed of remission can be measured in standard units of time (e.g., weeks and months).

Recurrence

A *relapse* occurs if the individual meets criteria for disorder after a remission. Relapse requires careful work on terminology and operational definition, as with remission (Falloon et al., 1983). The speed of relapse is the time required to move from the state of remission to the symptom peak. As with other duration measures, the metric for speed of relapse is standard units of time. *Recurrence* is the risk for relapse and is analogous to the incidence in expressing a dynamic or time-oriented risk for onset, as discussed above regarding attack rate. The rate of recurrence can be estimated similarly to incidence, with the risk set for recurrence being comprised of all those not currently meeting criteria for disorder.

The natural course is advantageously displayed in quasi-continuous fashion, as in Figure 6. Here the horizontal dimension is time, measured in yearly increments, and the vertical dimension is an ordinal measure of the frequency of panic attacks during the year. The graph shows every bit of data obtained on the course for the 33 new cases in the Baltimore ECA Follow-up (Eaton et al., 1998). The points in the graph are randomly jittered so that the course for each individual can be observed. The graph displays the great heterogeneity of the natural history, without reducing information, as would occur with the calculation of remission or recurrence rates. Individuals representing certain typical types of natural course

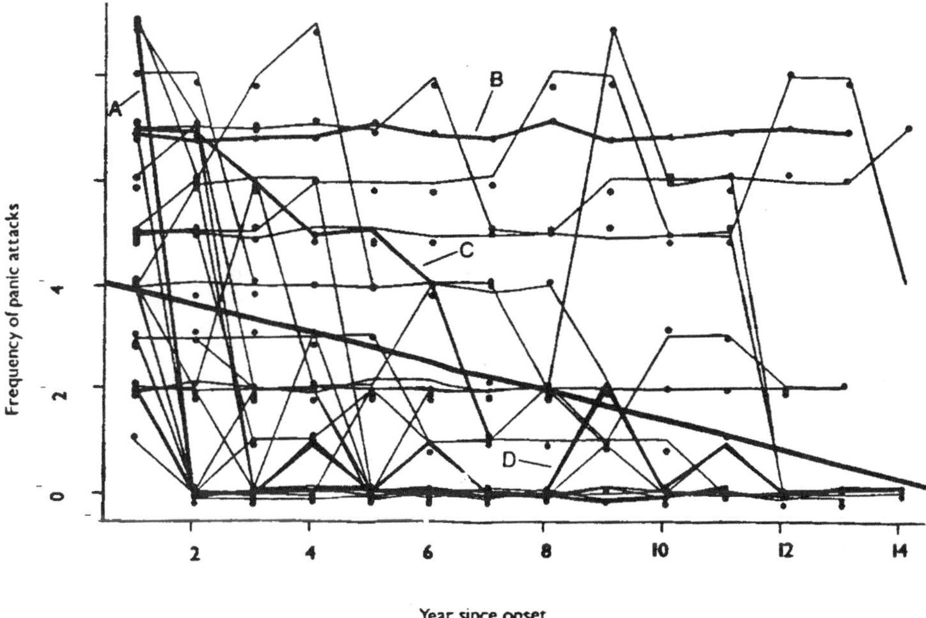

Figure 6. Natural course of panic following onset in 33 new cases in the Baltimore ECA Follow-up: abscissa is years following onset; ordinate is frequency of panic attacks (0 = no attacks that year; 1 = once that year; 2 = several times that year; 3 = once a month; 4 = 2–3 times a month; 5 = once a week; 6 = 2–3 times a week; 7 = 4–6 times a week; 8 = every day; 9 = more than once per day). Cases A, B, C, D, represent prototypical courses; heavy descending line represents least-squares fit line.

can be identified (as for the quick and enduring recovery for case A; the stable chronic case B; the gradual recovery in case C; and case D, who crosses the threshold of panic attacks back and forth repeatedly). These data can serve as the basis for random effects models, which estimate a slope for each individual (average slope portrayed in Figure 6, declining from ordinal frequency Level 4 to level zero over the 14 years of follow-up.

Many of the concepts discussed above present a simplistic point of view by not taking the long-term course into account. For example, incidence, remission, and relapse are all dichotomous outcomes that can be measured with only two waves of observations. One wave defines the sample at risk, which comprises the denominator, and the second wave estimates the numerator. These approaches involve severe reductions in the complexity of data, such as that displayed in Figure 6. Attempts have been made to categorize or quantify the entire course of psychopathology for a given disorder—what might be termed the *career of psychopathology*. For example, Ciompi (1980) has proposed eight categories for the course of schizophrenia that combine the three dichotomies of onset (acute vs. insidious), course (stable vs. episodic), and outcome (good vs. bad). A visual description of these categories, adapted from Ciompi, is shown in Figure 7. These figures stimulate questions as to the nature of the course. For example, what is the ultimate outcome? Is the course steadily, progressively deteriorative or progres-

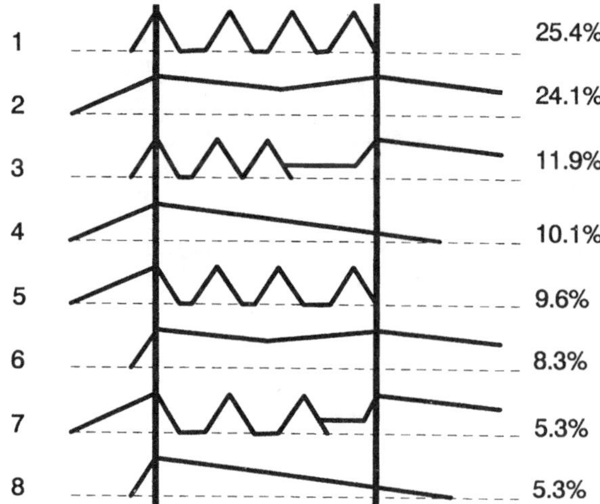

Figure 7. Typologies of course of schizophrenia, according to dichotomous criteria for onset, course, and outcome. (Redrawn from Ciompi, 1980.)

sively ameliorative (Eaton et al., 1992b)? Is the rate of remission related to the speed of onset? Is the risk for recurrence related to the duration of the episode or to the speed of onset? Answers to these questions would be important for clinical treatment, but not much is known because of the difficulties of conducting research on the natural history of psychopathology.

Risk factors may have differential effects on incidence, duration, and recurrence, and it is informative to combine the study of all three indicators for any given risk factor. For example, prevalence studies uniformly show that female gender is associated with higher prevalence of major depressive disorder. Analysis from the Baltimore ECA cohort showed that the gender difference existed only for incidence, not for duration of episodes, nor for the risk for recurrence (Eaton et al., 1997).

OUTCOME

Outcome refers to the consequences of the psychopathology. These consequences can be immediate, such as impairment and disability resulting from the disorder. The focus here is on important and pernicious consequences of disorder that occur afterward and that are not included in the defining phenomena of the disorder, that is, future psychopathology of other types and physical illness (comorbidity), overall functioning, and death.

Comorbidity

Comorbidity is the occurrence of two or more disorders in one individual. There has been increasing interest in narrowly defined disorders since the introduction of the DSM-III. Since psychopathology does not always fit into the DSM categories and is highly overlapping, the increased splitting of disorders has led to increasing interest in psychiatric comorbidity: the occurrence of two or more disorders in the same individual. The disorders can occur simultaneously in the same individual, or they can occur at different points in time: so-called *lifetime comorbidity*. Comorbidity over the lifetime presumably expresses a genetic diathesis, an early and enduring risk factor, or a long-standing environmental cause. Patterns of differential comorbidity will contribute, eventually, to improved nosology. Cross-sectional study of comorbidity focuses on the increase in lifetime prevalence for one disorder, given the presence of another (Merikangas et al., 1996). Studies of natural history focus on risk, either through retrospective recall of the timing of one disorder versus the other, or through a true prospective design. For example, in the ECA data, the risk for onset of DSM-III major depressive disorder is 3.4 times higher if the individual has had a panic attack than if the person has not suffered a panic attack (Andrade et al., 1996).

Many mental disorders have their peak periods of onset in adolescence and young adulthood (e.g., depressive disorder, panic disorder, alcohol disorder, substance use disorder, and schizophrenia), while many important chronic physical conditions have peak onset in middle age or later (e.g., heart diseases, cancers, type 2 diabetes, and strokes). Therefore, physical illness is another type of comorbidity and a possible consequence of psychopathology. In follow-ups based on psychiatric case registers, the systems of registration are usually based on the structure of the treatment systems, which tend to separate psychiatry from other areas of medicine. Thus, only highly specialized registration systems, such as the Oxford Record Linkage Study (Acheson, 1967), or the use of two or more illness-based registers, such as the Danish Psychiatric and Cancer registration systems (Mortensen and Juel, 1993), is effective. In population-based follow-ups, such as the Baltimore ECA Follow-up, a difficulty has been anticipating the range of potential consequences. Table 2 shows the range of consequences of depression for selected physical conditions and symptoms. Each relative risk in the table was the result of a separate analysis that compared depressive disorder to other forms of psychopathology, and which adjusted for other known risk factors for the physical condition. For most conditions, depressive disorder was the only nontrivial

TABLE 2. Depression as Predictor of Onset of Physical Conditions: Baltimore ECA Follow-up

Condition	First Author	Relative Odds[a]	Journal
Type II diabetes	Eaton	2.2	*Diabetes Care*
Heart attack	Pratt	4.0	*Circulation*
Breast cancer	Gallo	3.9	*Cancer Causes and Control*
Stroke	Larson	3.6	*Stroke*
Migraine	Swartz	1.0	*Archives of General Psychiatry*

[a]Relative odds are adjusted for age, sex, and other major risk factors. See references for full citations.

predictor from the range of psychopathology. Consistent with the developmental approach taken above, the effects of psychopathology below the threshold of diagnosis were also important for some physical conditions (not shown). The sizes of the relative risks are large enough to place depressive disorder on a par with other risk factors such as high cholesterol for heart attack, family history for breast cancer, hypertension for stroke, and obesity for type 2 diabetes. Since depressive disorder is mostly not treated, in spite of the availability of effective treatments, and since it is relatively easy to screen for it, these data have implications for the practice of preventive medicine in the primary care setting.

Functioning

Functioning is the ability to deal with the normal demands of everyday life. Persons with psychopathology are sometime less able to function effectively than the general population. The term as used here includes the WHO definition of disability (WHO, 1980). Impairment and disability resulting from a given disorder such as schizophrenia is widely variable (Jablenski et al., 1980; Eaton, 1991), and most of the costs associated with psychiatric problems come from the reduced functioning, not from the signs and symptoms themselves. The conversion of psychopathology to impairment and disability is thus an important area of study. A growing number of longitudinal studies show that psychopathology has strong consequences for disability, comparable to, or greater than, consequences of chronic physical conditions (Hays et al., 1995; Kouzis and Eaton, 1995, 1997; Armenian et al., 1998).

Mortality

Mortality, or the rate of death in the population, is usually higher in individuals with psychopathology than in the general population. Increased mortality is associated with schizophrenia (e.g., Babigian and Odoroff, 1969), mood disorders (e.g., Murphy at al., 1987; Black et al., 1985; Harris and Barraclough, 1998; Wulsin et al., 1999), anxiety disorders (Weissman et al., 1989), cognitive impairment (Badawi et al., 1999) and substance use disorders (Kouzis et al., 1995; Neumark et al., 2000). For some disorders the increased mortality is associated with the signs and symptoms of the disorder itself, as is the situation for suicide with depression. But the risk for suicide is also high for disorders where the connection is less obvious, as in the controversy over panic and suicide (Weissman et al., 1989; Anthony and Petronis, 1991) and suicide in schizophrenia (Herrman et al., 1987). The rate of accidental death is also sometimes higher among persons with psychopathology. Other causes of death related to psychopathology are more subtle still. For example, it may be the case that individuals with psychopathology are less likely to engage in illness prevention and health promotion behaviors, such as curtailment of smoking or lowering of cholesterol intake, due to preoccupation with psychopathology or less effective functioning generally. Finally, the mortality rate is raised due to the association with physical conditions which raise risk for death, as discussed above and in Table 2.

METHODOLOGIC CONCEPTS FOR STUDYING THE NATURAL HISTORY OF PSYCHOPATHOLOGY

Measuring onset, course, and outcome in the context of population benefits from a prospective approach. The traditional design for natural history is the cohort study in which a population of individuals are observed prospectively over years, decades, or even a lifetime (Breslow and Day, 1987; Samet and Munoz, 1998). The minimum design requirement is two waves of data collection. For example, to estimate incidence, the lifetime history of pyschopathology is determined at the first wave in order to exclude individuals who have already met the criteria for caseness. At the second wave, those who have become new cases form the numerator of the incidence rate, and those who were never cases at wave 1 form the risk set, or denominator.

Attrition

Major sources of error in cohort studies are due to attrition, censoring, and recall. *Attrition* is the loss of subjects in longitudinal research usually due to one of three causes: individual mobility outside the study area or to an unknown residence, death, and refusal to participate after some threshold of response burden is reached. In field surveys such as the ECA, attrition after even so short a period as one year can be large enough to threaten the credibility of results. The ECA attrition in one year of follow-up was mostly due to refusal (about 15%) and partly to failure to locate individuals (about 5%). Since the time period was short, there was relatively little attrition due to mortality (less than 1%). In the Baltimore ECA Follow-up, in which the follow-up interview was thirteen years after the baseline, the proportions shifted: nearly 25% had died, 12% could not be located, and 8% refused (Badawi et al., 1999).

Attrition can bias results. In the one year follow-up of the ECA, older white women and younger black males had about twice the rate of attrition than other respondents, and these differences in attrition were larger than baseline differences related to psychopathology (Eaton et al., 1992a). In the Baltimore ECA Follow-up of thirteen years, older persons were more likely to die, but there were also biases connected to psychopathology, such as the tendency for those with cognitive impairment to die, and for those with antisocial characteristics not to be located (Badawi et al., 1999). Attrition forestalls studying the effect of psychopathology during the interval between baseline and follow-up: For example, there may be a tendency for those with new episodes of disorder to move to another location (e.g., a young person might move to another city to live with parents during recovery). Since both the episode of psychopathology and the attrition occur between waves of interviews, attrition eliminates the possibility of studying this tendency.

In population-based psychiatric case registers, attrition is likely to have different causes and a different structure. In a survey study, persons with psychosis may be more likely to refuse to be interviewed, and more likely to change address and be lost to follow-up after the passage of time. For a psychiatric case register, refusal is less likely to be important if the level of psychopathology is such as to need or even require treatment, such as might be argued is the case for psychosis. For disorders such as depression, where treatment is often not sought, register data will be severely biased by attrition. For registers of limited geographic spread, mobility will be important; for case registers that cover an entire country, such as in Denmark or Israel, mobility will be much less important. The upshot of these comparisons is that population-based psychiatric case registers are a useful source of information on the natural history of severe mental disorders such as psychosis.

Censoring

Censoring is the bias that results from the fact that the period of observation is limited in time. The extreme version of censoring is the cross-sectional study. It is possible to approximate measures of incidence, remission, and recurrence using data gathered at one point in time, but this requires assumptions that are not generally tenable. Age of onset can be determined in a cross-sectional sample, for example, by asking each respondent who meets lifetime criteria for disorder when the symptoms began. Even if the recall is accurate (discussed below), episodes of individuals who have onsets after the data collection is complete will be omitted, and this will lead to a downward bias in the estimate of age of onset. The problems of censoring are less severe with a cohort study, but exist nevertheless in any study which begins after birth and ends before all members of the cohort have died. In estimating the duration of an episode of psychopathology, for example, there will always be a small portion of the cohort who are in an episode at the time the data

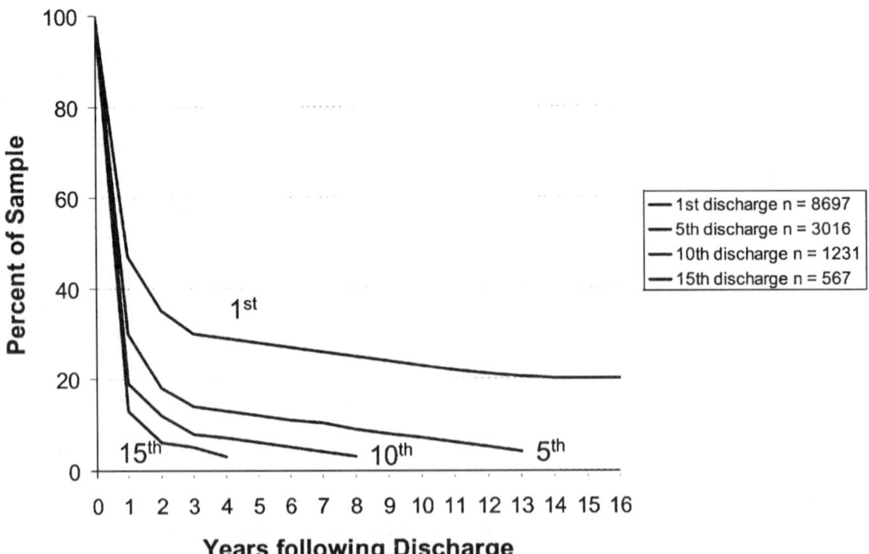

Figure 8. Probability of remaining in the community for schizophrenics after discharge from hospital in first, fifth, tenth, and fifteenth episodes. (Adapted from Mortensen and Eaton, 1994.)

collection concludes, making it impossible to estimate the average duration of the episode in the cohort. Since the mean is highly influenced by observations on the tail of the distribution, the bias in the mean can be strong.

The problems of attrition and censoring are illustrated in Figure 8 with data from the Danish Psychiatric Case Register on hospital admissions during the period 1973 to 1988. In contrast to the display of course in Figure 6, this method requires a dichotomous indicator for presence or absence of disorder. The cohort begins with the first episode in the individual's lifetime wherein the diagnosis of schizophrenia was given. The figure shows survival curves for the first, fifth, tenth, and fifteenth episodes. Each curve shows the percentage of individuals who remain outside the hospital (vertical axis) according to time since discharge (horizontal axis). Relapse from the first episode tends to occur in the first few years after discharge; by the fifth year, over three-fourths of the cohort have had a second episode of hospitalization. The manner of presentation is immune from the censoring bias, since it correctly portrays the lack of information for the individuals who have not suffered a relapse by the end of the follow-up in 1988. Later curves reveal the effects of attrition, however, since they are only computed for individuals suffering 4 or more, 9 or more, and 14 or more relapses, respectively. Survival in the community is less likely for these cohorts because they represent an increasingly severe subsample of the first admission cohort. These data show, in contrast to ECA data discussed previously, that attrition can bias toward portraying more severe psychopathology.

Recall

Recall bias is the error in measurement due to inaccuracies in the respondent's memory of events. The cross-sectional approach is compromised because it relies on the respondents autobiographical memory to recall the time of the onset, which may be quite distant from the time of the data collection. It is likely that those with more recent onsets are less likely to forget the occurrence of the disorder, which biases the onset distribution toward later onset. But it is also likely that those with severe cases of disorder are less likely to forget the occurrence of disorder; if severity is associated with earlier onset, this bias would be toward earlier onset. The study of risk factors will be further complicated because individuals may not remember the order of occurrence of the risk factor and the onset. Thus, retrospective data from a cross- sectional approach include a mixture of biases that are sometimes undecipherable. The same mistakes in recall can occur in the cross-sectional or prospective design. But in the prospective design, the mistakes made by an individual are likely to be smaller than in the cross-sectional design, because the time of data collection is closer to the present for the individual, especially at the second or later waves where new onsets are determined.

The effects of error are complex in the prospective design, because the biases can concatenate in so many different ways. For example, in the East Baltimore ECA panel cohort, there were 2,622 individuals who had never in their lifetimes met criteria for diagnosis of panic disorder by the time of the interview at Wave 1; 20 of these met criteria at Wave 2, giving a cumulative annual incidence rate of about 7 per 1,000 per year (Eaton et al., 1989b). There were 40 individuals at Wave 1 who met criteria for past or present diagnosis; of these, 20 reported never having experienced a panic attack at Wave 2. These 20 might be labeled "reverse incidence." They represent half (20/40) of those meeting criteria for diagnosis at Wave 1; they match exactly the number (20) of incident cases. This phenomenon is not unique to the ECA surveys. The existence of reverse incidence is due to forgetting and, while disquieting, does not negate the existence of the 20 cases in the numerator of the incidence rate. It does suggest that forgetting of episodes occurs, a tendency that would bias prevalence rates downward and incidence rates upward. The upward bias in incidence would occur because cases that belong in the numerator of the attack rate would be mixed in with the numerator of the first incidence rate.

Lack of blind measurement is an important problem in estimation as regards outcome. The dependence of outcome on initial state is a central focus of research on natural history, but it may be difficult to measure outcome independently of initial state. If the respondent or the interviewer remembers the initial measurement session, the results of that session are likely to bias measurement of outcome. For example, an interviewer may probe more persistently for the occurrence of panic attacks if it is known that they have occurred in the recent, or even distant, past. Impairment and disability are likely to be rated downward if it is known that the individual once met the criteria for diagnosis of schizophrenia, even if no signs and symptoms are present at the time of the follow-up. Thus, bias due to lack of blindness is likely to overestimate the relationship of early indicators of psychopathology to later outcomes.

Random error has counterintuitive pernicious effects in prospective research on the natural history of disorder. Indeed, in the context of estimating incidence in field surveys, the concept of random error is not very useful. If by random error is meant an equiprobable response, then it is straightforward to show that, for a sample, the bias resulting is moderately upward for prevalence and strongly upward for incidence. The rates of false-positive and false-negative answers to a given question will depend on the question and will not be equiprobable, in general; but many other types of errors in the survey process—mistakes in data entry, for example—will have an equiprobable character to them. Thus, the tendency is for seemingly random errors to bias the incidence and recurrence rates upward.

There has been an explosion of statistical techniques over the last several decades which address many of the problems of prospective studies. A body of statistics called survival analysis has grown up around the problems of censoring (e.g., Lawless, 1982). The development of covariation over time can be studied with generalized estimating equations (Zeger and Liang, 1986). Risk factors at different stages of the disease may be differentially related to disease progression only above or below the threshold set by the diagnosis. In this situation, the diagnostic threshold might be reconsidered. Statistical techniques to locate a threshold are being developed (Scharfstein et al., 2001). Statistical techniques suitable for four or more waves of analysis are being developed and will be very useful in future studies (Diggle, Liang, and Zeger, 1994; Bollen, 1989; McArdle and Hamagami, 1992).

CONCLUSION

Studying the natural history of psychopathology in the general population requires large resources of effort and expense because of the combination of population-based sampling, long-term commitment, and intensity of measurement. Perhaps for these reasons the field is in its infancy. Most data on natural history are based on clinical samples, which are not representative of the population of persons with mental disorders. There are few benchmark estimates for the incidence of most major mental disorders that have been replicated and for which there is a consensus among investigators. The estimates for parameters of long-term course of disorders are widely varying. Thus, there is plenty of progress to be made!

ACKNOWLEDGMENTS

This work was supported by NIMH grants MH47447 and MH53188.

REFERENCES

Acheson ED (1967): "Medical Record Linkage." London: Oxford University Press.

Allison P (1984): "Event History Analysis: Regression for Longitudinal Data." Beverly Hills: Sage.

Andrade L, Eaton WW, Chilcoat H (1996): Lifetime comorbidity of panic attacks and major depression in population-based study: Age of onset. Psychol Med 26:991–996.

Andrade L, Eaton WW, Chilcoat H (1994): Lifetime comorbidity of panic attacks and major depression in a population based study: Symptom profiles. Br J Psychiatry 165:363–369.

Anthony JC, Petronis KR (1991): Panic attacks and suicide attempts. Arch Gen Psychiatry 48:11–14.

Armenian HK, Pratt LA, Gallo JJ, Eaton WW (1998): Psychopathology as a predictor of disability: a population-based follow-up study in Baltimore, Maryland. Am J Epidemiol 148:269–275.

Babigian HM, Odoroff CL (1969): The mortality experience of a population with psychiatric illness. Am J Psychiatry 126:470–480.

Badawi MA, Eaton WW, Myllyluoma J, Weimer L, Gallo JJ (1999): Psychopathology and attrition in the Baltimore ECA follow-up 1981–1996. Soc Psychiatry Psychiatric Epidemiol 34:91–98.

Baltes PB, Reese HW, Lipsitt LP, (1980): Life-span developmental psychology. Ann Rev Psychol 31:35–110.

Berkson J (1946): Limitations of the application of fourfold table analysis to hospital data. Biom Bull 2:47–53.

Birley JLT, Brown GW: Crises and life changes preceding the onset of relapse of acute schizophrenia: Clinical aspects. Br J Psychiatry 116:327–333.

Black DW, Warrack G, Winokur G (1985): The Iowa record linkage study. I. Studies and accidental deaths among psychiatric patients. Arch Gen Psychiatry 42:71–75.

Bohrnstedt GW (1983): Measurement. In Rossi PH, Wright JD, Anderson AB (eds): "Handbook of Survey Research." Orlando: Academic Press, pp 69–121.

Bollen KA (1989): "Structural Equations with latent variables." New York: Wiley.

Breslow, NE, Day NE (1987): Statistical methods in cancer research. II. The design and analysis of cohort studies. Lyon: International Agency for Research on Cancer.

Brown GW, Birley JLT (1968): Crises and life changes and the onset of schizophrenia. J Health Social Behav 9:203–214.

Ciompi L (1980): Catamnestic long-term study on the course of life and aging of schizophrenics. Schiz Bull 6:606–618.

Diggle PJ, Liang K-Y, Zeger SL (1994): In Atkinson AC, Copas JB, Pierce DA, Schervish MJ, Titterington DM (eds) "Analysis of longitudinal data. Oxford Statistical Science Series." New York: Oxford University Press.

Dryman A, Eaton WW (1991): Affective symptoms associated with the onset of major depression in the community: Findings from the U.S. NIMH Epidemiologic Catchment Area Program. Acta Psychiatr Scand 84:15.

Eaton WW (1991): Update on the epidemiology of schizophrenia. Epidemiol Rev 13:320–328.

Eaton WW, Anthony JC, Tepper S, Dryman A (1992a): Psychopathology and attrition in the epidemiologic Catchment Area Surveys. Am J Epidemiol 134:1041–1059.

Eaton WW, Anthony JC, Gallo J, Cai G, Tien A, Romanoski A, Lyketsos C, Chen L-S (1997): Natural history of DIS/DSM major depression: The Baltimore Epidemiologic Catchment Area follow-up. Arch Gen Psychiat 54:993–999.

Eaton WW, Anthony J, Romanoski A, Tien A, Gallo J, Cai G, Neufeld K, Schlaepfer T, Laugharne J, Chen L-S (1998): Onset and recovery from panic disorder in the Baltimore Epidemiologic Catchment Area follow-up. Brit J Psychiat 173:501–507.

Eaton WW, Armenian, HK, Gallo JJ, Pratt L, Ford D (1996): Depression and risk for onset of type II diabetes: A prospective, population-based study. Diabetes Care 19(10):1097–1102.

Eaton WW, Badawi M, Melton B (1995): Prodromes and precursors. Epidemiologic data for primary prevention of disorders with slow onset. Am J Psychiatry 152(7):967–972.

Eaton WW, Bilker W, Haro JM, Herrman H, Mortensen PB, Freeman H, Burgess P (1992b): The long-term course of hospitalization for schizophrenia: Change in rate of hospitalization with passage of time. Schiz Bull 18:185–207.

Eaton WW, Kramer M, Anthony JC, Dryman A, Shapiro S, Locke BZ (1989a): The incidence of specific DIS/DSM-III mental disorders: Data from the NIMH Epidemiologic Catchment Area Program. Acta Psychiatr Scand 79:163–178.

Eaton WW, Kramer M, Anthony JC, Chee EML, Shapiro S (1989b): Conceptual and methodological problems in estimation of the incidence of mental disorders from field survey data. In Cooper B, Helgason T (eds): "Epidemiology and the Prevention of Mental Disorders." London: Routledge, pp 108–127.

Eaton WW, Whitmore GA (1977): Length of stay as a stochastic process: A general approach and application to hospitalization for schizophrenia. J Math Sociol 5:273–292.

Expert Committee on Health Statistics (1959): Sixth Report. Geneva: World Health Organization.

Falloon RH, Grant N, Marshall JLB et al. (1983): Relapse in schizophrenia: A review of the concept and its definitions (editorial). Psycholo Med 13:469–477.

Fichter MM, Koch HJ, Rehm J, Weyerer S (1987): Adversity and the risk of mental illness: preliminary results of the Upper Bavarian Restudy. In Angermeyer MC (ed): "From Social Class to Social Stress." Berlin: Springer.

Frank E, Prien RF, Jarrett RB et al. (1991): Conceptualization and Rationale for consensus definitions of terms in major depressive disorder. Arch Gen Psychiatry 48:851–855.

Gallo JJ, Armenian HK, Ford DE, Eaton WW, Khachaturian AS (2000): Major depression and cancer: the 13-year followup of the Baltimore Epidemiologic Catchment Area sample. Cancer Causes and Control 11:751–758.

Hagnell O, Essen-Moller E, Lanke J et al. (1990): The Incidence of Mental Illness Over a Quarter of a Century. Stockholm: Almqvist and Wiksell International.

Harris EC, Barraclough B (1998): Excess mortality of mental disorder. Br J Psychiatry 173:11–53.

Hays RD, Wells KB, Sherbourn CD, Rogers W, Spritzer K (1995): Functioning and well-being outcomes of patients with depression compared with chronic general medical illnesses. Arch Gen Psychiatry 52:11–19.

Herrman HE (1987): Re-evaluation of the evidence on the prognostic importance of schizophrenic and affective symptons. Aust NZ J Psychiatry 21:424–427.

Horvath E, Johnson J, Klerman GL, Weissman MM (1992): Depressive symptoms as relative and attributable risk for first-onset major depression. Arch Gen Psychiatry 49:817–823.

Jablenski A, Schwartz R, Tomov T (1980): WHO collaborative study on impairments and disabilities associated with shizophrenic disorders. Acta Psychiatr Scand (Suppl 285) 62:152–163.

Kessler RC (1995): Epidemiology of psychiatric comorbidity. In Tsuang MT, Tohen M, Zahner GEP (eds) "Textbook in Psychiatric Epidemiology." New York: Wiley pp 179–197.

Kleinbaum DG, Kupper LL, Morgenstern H (1982): "Epidemiologic Research: Principles and Quantitative Methods." Belmost, CA: Lifetime Learning.

Kouzis AC, Eaton WW, Leaf P (1999): Psychopathology and mortality in the general population. Social Psychiatry and Psychiatric Epidemiology 30:165–170.

Kouzis AC, Eaton WW (1999): Psychopathology and the development of disability. Social Psychiatry and Psychiatric Epidemiology 32:379–386.

Kouzis AC, Eaton WW (1995): Disability Days and Psychopathology. Am J Public Health 84:1304–1307.

Kramer M (1957): Discussion of the concepts of prevalence and incidence as related to epidemiologic studies of mental disorders. Am J Public Health 47:826–840.

Kramer M, Von Korff M, Kessler L (1981): The lifetime prevalence of mental disorders: Estimation, uses and limitations. Psychol Med 10:429–436.

Larson SL, Owens PL, Ford DE, Eaton WW (2001): Depressive disorders, dysthymia risk of stroke: a thirteen year follow-up from the Baltimore ECA. Stroke 32:1979–1983.

Lawless JF (1982): "Statistical Models and Methods for Lifetime Data." New York: Wiley.

Liang KY, Zeger SL (1989): A class of logistic regression models for multiple binary time series. J Am Stat Assoc 84:447–451.

Lilienfeld AM, Lilienfeld DE (1980): "Foundations of Epidemiology." 2nd ed New York: Oxford University Press.

Lilienfeld DE, Stolley PD (1994): "Foundations of Epidemiology." New York: Oxford University Press.

Lyketsos CG, Mestadt G, Cwi J, Heithoff K, Eaton WW (1994): The Life Chart Interview: A standardized method to describe the course of psychopathology. Int J Methods Psychiatr Res 4:143–155.

MacMahon B, Pugh TF, Ipsen J (1960): "Epidemiologic Methods." Boston, MA: Little, Brown.

Mausner JS, Kramer S (1985): Epidemiology: An Introductory Text. Eastbourne, England: WB Saunders.

McArdle JJ, Hamagami F (1992): Modeling incomplete longitudinal and cross-sectional data using latent growth structural models. Exp Aging Res 18:145–166.

Merikangas KR, Angst J, Eaton W, Canino G, Rubio-Stipec M, Wacker H, Wittchen H-U, Andrade L, Essau C, Whitaker A, Kraemer H, Robins LN, Kupfer DJ (1996): Comorbidity and boundaries of affective disorders with anxiety disorders and substance misuse: results of an international task force. Br Psychiatry (Supp) 30 168:58–67.

Morris JN (1975): "Uses of Epidemiology." 3rd ed Edinburg: Churchill Livingstone.

Mortensen PB, Eaton WW (1994): Predictors for readmission risk in schizophrenia. Psychol Med 24:223–232.

Mortensen PB, Juel K (1993): Mortality and causes of death in first-admitted schizophrenic patients. Br J Psychiatry 163:183–189.

Murphy J, Monson RR, Olivier DC, Sobol AM, Leighton AH (1987): Affective disorders and mortality: A general population study. Arch Gen Psychiatry 44:473–480.

National Center for Health Statistics (1977): Health Interview Survey Procedures (1957–1974): Vital and Health Statistics, Ser 1, No. 11. Washington, DC: U.S. Government Printing Office.

Neumark YD, Van Etten ML, Anthony JD (2000): Drug dependence and death: survival analysis of the Baltimore ECA sample from 1981 to 1995. Substance Use and Misuse 35:49–63.

Ojesjo L, Hagnell O, Lanke J (1982): Incidence of alcoholism among men in the Lundby Community Cohort. Sweden 1957–1972. J Stud Alcohol 43:1190–1198.

Pratt LA, Ford DE, Crum RM, Armenian, HK, Gallo JJ, Eaton WW (1996): Depression, psychotropic medication and risk of heart attack: prospective data from the Baltimore ECA Follow-up. Circulation 94:3123–3129.

Philipp M, Fickinger MP (1993): The definition of remission and its impact on the length of a depressive episode. Arch Gen Psychiatry 50:407–408.

Rothman KJ (1981): Induction and latent periods. Am J Epidemiol 114:253–259.

Samet JM, Munoz A, and editors, editors (1998): Epidemiologic Reviews: Cohort Studies. Baltimore, Maryland: The Johns Hpkins University School of Hygiene and Public Health.

Sartwell PE, Last JM (1980): Epidemiology. In Last JM (ed): "Maxcy-Rosenau Public Health and Preventive Medicine." 11th ed New York: Appleton-Century-Crofts, p 985.

Schorfstein (2001).

Swartz KL, Pratt LA, Armenian HK, Lee LC, Eaton WW: Antecedent affective disorders do not predict incident migraine headaches in the Baltimore ECA Followup study. Archives of General Psychiatry (in press).

Tyrer P (1985): Neurosis divisible? Lancet 8430:685–688.

Weissman MM, Klerman GL, Markowitz JS, Ouelette R, Phil M (1989): Suicidal ideation and suicide attempts in panic disorder and attacks. N Engl J Med 321:1209–1214.

World Health Organization (1980): International Classification of Impairments, Disabilities, and Handicaps. Geneva: World Health Organization.

Wing JK, Babor T, Brugha T, Burke J, Cooper JE, Giel R, Jablenski A, Regier D, Sartorius N (1990): SCAN: Schedules for clinical assessment in neuropsychiatry. Arch Gen Psychiatry 47:589–593.

Wulsin LR, Vaillant GE, Wells V (1999): A systematic review of the mortality of depression. Psychosomatic Medicine 61:6–17.

Zeger SL, Liang K-Y (1986): Longitudinal data analysis using generalized linear models. Biometrics 7313–7322.

CHAPTER 10

The Developmental Epidemiology of Psychiatric Disorders

MARY CANNON, MATTI HUTTUNEN, and ROBIN MURRAY

Division of Psychological Medicine, Institute of Psychiatry. London, UK (M.C., R.M.); Department of Mental Health and Alcohol Research, National Public Health Institute, Helsinki, Finland (M.H.).

> To view lives in cross-section is like trying to understand traffic by standing in the middle of Times Square. The confusion is bewildering and external events seem critical. The time of day, the traffic lights, rain, and adventitious accidents seem all-important. But if each car is viewed in the perspective of time, suddenly each one acquires a defined, if not fully predictable trajectory, and seen from afar, this trajectory is governed far more by the driver of the vehicle than by the complex outer social forces that affect Times Square.
>
> —George E. Vaillant, *Adaptation to Life*

DEVELOPMENTAL EPIDEMIOLOGY

Developmental or life-course epidemiology is concerned with early life risk factors for adult diseases and the accumulation of risks for disease over the life span (Kuh and Ben-Schlomo, 1997). This far-reaching longitudinal approach is transforming our understanding of a number of physical disorders, such as coronary heart disease and diabetes (Barker, 1992; Kuh and Ben-Schlomo, 1997), and is already doing the same for psychiatric illness (Susser et al., 2000). The life-course model incorporates such elements as cumulative insults over the life span, critical periods of susceptibility throughout life, and the interaction between early and late risk factors. Biological and social risk factors at each life stage may be linked to form pathways between early life experiences and adult disease.

The term "developmental epidemiology" was first coined in the 1970s (Kellam et al., 1983) and was originally confined to the study of the distribution and risks of childhood disorders (Scott et al., 1994; Costello and Angold, 1995). However, the term has now extended to include the study of early antecedents and risk factors for adult-onset and chronic diseases as well as childhood conditions (Buka and Lipsitt, 1994).

Textbook in Psychiatric Epidemiology, Second Edition, Edited by Ming T. Tsuang and Mauricio Tohen. ISBN 0-471-40974-X

DEVELOPMENTAL PSYCHOPATHOLOGY

Where the study of psychiatric illness is concerned there is a great deal of overlap between developmental epidemiology and the field of developmental psychopathology (Cicchetti, 1984; Rutter, 1988). Developmental psychopathology has been defined as "the study of the origins and course of individual patterns of behavioral maladaptation" (Sroufe and Rutter, 1984). The key elements of developmental psychopathology are that the study of normal development informs the study of psychopathological conditions (and *vice versa*). Thus, rather than development being predetermined or "canalized," individuals are viewed as developing along flexible trajectories which can be influenced at any point in the lifespan to either increase or reduce the risk of disorder (Hollis and Taylor, 1997). According to this perspective, psychological disorders do not emerge from the inevitable unfolding of a disease process but arise out of a dynamic, transactional relationship between the development of the individual and the changing demands of the environment. The path between risk and outcome is not inevitable. The same risk factor may have multiple possible outcomes; this principle is known as multifinality. Equally, multiple pathways can lead to the same outcome; this principle is known as equifinality (Cicchetti, 1990).

The common features of developmental epidemiology and developmental psychopathology include an interest in the process of disorder causation in the context of development, causal chain mechanisms and person–environment interaction. A developmental perspective posits a continuum between normality and abnormality, unlike the traditional "disease model" of illness. The main difference is that the research issues in developmental psychopathology are often formulated in ways that depart in some respects from traditional epidemiologic methods (Rutter, 1988). Although major advances have been made in both disciplines, much work remains to be done to create measurement techniques and classification systems that are developmentally sensitive, and generate analytic and design methods that assess the impact of multiple causes and/or multiple outcomes. The relatively new discipline of developmental epidemiology will therefore lead to an enrichment of study design and analytic techniques (Buka and Lipsitt, 1994).

STUDY DESIGN STRATEGIES IN DEVELOPMENTAL EPIDEMIOLOGY

Two main analytic study designs are currently used in developmental epidemiology: cohort studies, which proceed from cause to effect, and case–control studies, which look from effect to cause.

Cohort Studies

Cohort studies can be either prospective or retrospective. A *prospective cohort study* is one in which researchers define an exposure that may be associated with a given outcome and then select exposed and unexposed subjects before the outcome of interest has occurred. The subjects are observed for a defined period of time during which all newly occurring cases of the outcome are identified. The prospective cohort study design is a powerful tool. It permits direct measurement of the incidence of a given condition within a population. The time sequence is clear and strengthens the inference than the specific risk factor may be a cause of the outcome. A further advantage is that multiple outcomes of interest can be examined within a single study.

However, in relating this study design to the study of childhood risk factors for adult illness, two main problems emerge. First, if the outcome of interest does not occur frequently in the population (e.g., schizophrenia), the cohort study must include very large numbers of subjects in order to accrue a meaningful number of cases. The second important disadvantage relates to the fact that prospective cohort study designs often require a great deal of time for follow-up and data collection. If there is a long latency period between exposure and outcome, the study will require sufficient resources for a follow-up period lasting many years, even decades.

Two strategies have been used to circumvent these problems and allow the use of the prospective cohort design for investigating the developmental epidemiology of adult psychiatric disorders. One strategy is to use enriched cohorts such as genetic high risk cohorts where the yield of cases will be considerably higher. The second strategy is to use existing birth cohorts that have already "matured" or at least "semimatured." Considerably less time and expense are involved as the long latency period has already occurred. The design therefore becomes a type of *retrospective cohort study* as both the exposure and the outcome have occurred before the study has begun, and investigators "scavenge" the cohort for childhood risk factors that may be of interest from a developmental viewpoint. It shares the advantages of a prospective cohort study in that there are clear temporal associations between exposure and outcome and an ability to measure incidence and relative risk. However, because of the reliance on existing historical information, researchers have minimal control over the quality and nature of the data collected. Data may have been measured and recorded in ways that are not optimal for answering the current research questions or certain information may not have been recorded at all.

Case–Control Studies

Case–control studies choose subjects based on outcome status and look retrospectively from effect to cause. Study subjects are identified and grouped on the outcome of interest (cases and controls) and retrospective exposure and demographic data are used to identify possible risk factors. Cases and controls are compared with respect to the ratios of those having a history of an exposure or risk factor. A major strength of the case–control study design is its efficiency in terms of cost and length of the study compared to the cohort design. Case–control studies can effectively examine outcomes of interest with a very long latency period of expression. A second major strength of the case–control design is that it is efficient compared to other designs in the examination of rare or low prevalence outcomes. A final strength is that such a design allows for the examination of multiple potential risk factors.

The case–control methodology is not without weaknesses: The temporal link is not as clearly established as in a cohort design and only one outcome can be evaluated. However, the biggest drawback to the case–control design, and a genuine threat to its validity, is the increased potential for bias. Bias in epidemiological studies is a systematic error in the design, conduct, or analysis that results in a distortion or masks the true association between risk factors and outcomes. While bias can occur in any study design, traditional case–control studies are particularly vulnerable to selection and information biases.

There are several steps that an investigator can take to prevent the occurrence of bias or minimise its effect within a case–control design. First, selection bias can be prevented or reduced by using cases and control groups sampled directly from the defined populations of "all cases" and "all controls." This design is known as a "nested" case–control study or a population-based case-control study, (Rothman and Greenland, 1998; Langholtz and Thomas, 1990). These population-based case-control studies are relatively free of selection bias and have higher statistical power than traditional cohort designs. A nested case–control study design was used by Cannon et al (1999) to investigate the relationship between school performance and later schizophrenia in Helsinki, Finland. In this study, all cases of schizophrenia born in Helsinki over a ten-year period (1951–1960) were identified from national health care registers and one control per case was randomly chosen from the same population base. In this way a sample of over 400 cases of schizophrenia, diagnosed according to accepted diagnostic criteria, was available for study with high statistical power. In contrast, conventional birth cohort studies yield much smaller numbers of cases, usually less than one tenth that amount.

One type of information bias that is of particular concern for developmental epidemiology is recall bias—a situation in which the cases are more likely to report exposures that have occurred to overestimate their exposure levels relative to the self-report of the control subject. The effect of such differential reporting would be to overestimate the association between the exposure and the outcome. Information bias can be reduced or prevented by the use of extant sources of information collected before the outcome of interest, such as archived school or child health records.

Record linkage is a means of joining two independent data sets, recorded at different times or places, with information about the same individuals or families. This methodology has a number of advantages when applied to developmental epidemiology. It is useful in studying diseases or outcomes that have a long latency period and for studying low-prevalence conditions, and researchers can select an adequate sample size available from an extant database while incurring minimal time and financial burden. Despite its advantages, it is important to note some limitations of record linkage methodology. The use of extant databases limits the information available and the accuracy and completeness of the data entered are out of the control of the researcher. In addition, when linking two or more databases from different agencies, the data format may be discrepant and poses a challenge in assuring correct linkages, data analysis and interpretation.

ANALYTIC METHODS IN DEVELOPMENTAL EPIDEMIOLOGY

Major advances have been made in the study of large, complex datasets that include categorical variables, repeated waves of data collection, nested variables (i.e., children within families or schools), and missing data, all of which are likely to occur in developmental epidemiology. The data analytic methods used in developmental epidemiology draw on a variety of approaches recently described for the analysis of longitudinal observational data (Diggle et al., 1994).

Repeated Observations

The distinguishing feature of a longitudinal study is that the response variable of interest and a set of covariates are measured repeatedly over time. Because repeated observations are made on the same individual, the repeated measurements on the response variable will usually be (positively) correlated. This within-subject correlation or autocorrelation must be accounted for in order to make correct inferences. Therefore, a model for longitudinal data has two components: a regression model for the dependence of the response variable on time and the covariates of interest; and a model for the autocorrelation among the repeated observations for an individual. In most cases the parameters of the regression model are of prime interest but estimates of these and their standard errors, and consequently inferences about them, will be affected by the model chosen to describe the autocorrelation (Everitt, 1998). Fortunately it is now relatively simple to build models for longitudinal data that allow consideration of a richer variety of correlational structures for the autocorrelation than older techniques such as ANOVA or MANOVA (Diggle et al., 1994; Everitt, 1998). The generalized estimating equation method (Liang and Zeger, 1986) has been introduced for the analysis of longitudinal, nonnormal data where data consist of clusters of intercorrelated observations (for an example, see Cannon et al., 2002). In this approach, any required covariance structure and any link structure may be assumed, robust estimates of standard errors are provided and quasi-likelihood is generalized to take account of covariances of responses within clusters.

Growth Curve Models

Sometimes the amount of variability within individuals is the main focus of the analysis, for instance in the analysis of cognitive development. Mixed and multilevel models including growth curve models can be used for such analyses (Goldstein, 1995; Taylor et al., 1998). Methods for the analysis of growth have become more easily accessible with the development of software for multilevel models such as MLwiN (Goldstein et al., 1998), and other programs for random effects modelling such as STATA (StatCorp, 1999; Rabe-Hesketh and Everitt, 2000). These programs require neither the number of observations nor the intervals of time between observations to be the same for all subjects, making them applicable to a much wider range of clinical and epidemiological studies than their less flexible predecessors (Taylor et al., 1998).

Data Hierarchies

Many kinds of data have a nested or clustered structure; for example, children are nested within families and will therefore tend to be more alike than children from different families for a variety of reasons both genetic and environmental. Students are nested within classes or schools, or individuals and families are nested within neighborhoods (Goldstein, 1995). Repeated measures data can also be viewed as data clustered within one individual. A hierarchy consists of units grouped at different levels. Thus school grades over time may be clustered within students which are the level 2 units, clustered within schools which are the level 3 units (see Cannon et al., 1999). Multilevel analysis will allow the optimal examination of this type of data (Goldstein, 1995). Software packages such as MLwiN (Goldstein et al., 1998) have been developed for use with such hierarchial data.

Missing Values

A considerable problem with the analysis of longitudinal data is the opportunity for missing values. The "older" approach of complete case analysis uses only the subset of subjects with no missing values. The procedure is valid only when the values are missing completely at random (which is rarely the case) and even then is highly inefficient if a large proportion of subjects have to be discarded. If the values are not missing completely at random, then the results of the analysis will be seriously biased. An alternative is to replace the missing values with imputed values such as cross-sectional means or "last observation carried forward," neither of which are particularly satisfactory (Everitt, 1998). Fortunately, the more recently developed techniques for analyzing longitudinal data (Diggle et al., 1994) are specifically formulated so that they can accommodate noninformative missing values in the models used. Consequently, such missing values raise no problems in the estimation of parameters or their standard errors.

THE APPLICATION OF DEVELOPMENTAL EPIDEMIOLOGY TO PSYCHIATRIC DISORDERS

In this section we propose to give examples of how developmental epidemiological techniques have enriched our understanding of some psychiatric disorders.

Schizophrenia

From its earliest descriptions, schizophrenic psychosis had a longitudinal dimension (Clouston, 1892; Southard, 1915). Both Kraepelin (1896) and Bleuler (1911) noted that people who developed the psychotic syndrome were often different from their peers before psychosis began. The so-called "neurodevelopmental hypothesis" of schizophrenia came to prominence in the late 1980s and has proved highly influential in revitalizing developmental epidemiological approaches to psychosis. It proposes a subtle deviance in early brain development whose full adverse consequences are not manifest until adolescence or early adulthood (Murray and Lewis, 1987; Weinberger, 1987). Central to the neurodevelopmental hypothesis is the existence of neurological or behavioral abnormalities during childhood or adolescence before the overt symptoms of the illness appear (Marenco and Weinberger, 2000). In fact, as Jones (1999) points out, the neurodevelopmental hypothesis is "not really a hypothesis at all, rather an aetiological model that directs research towards early life in terms of causation."

Several different research strategies have been used to examine the developmental precursors of adult schizophrenia, including the genetic high-risk cohort design, the use of archived information, and follow-up studies of existing birth cohorts (Cannon and Jones, 1996). Each of these strategies has uncovered evidence of childhood motor, language, cognitive, and behavioral precursors to schizophrenia (Fish et al., 1992, Marcus et al., 1993; Jones et al., 1994; Done et al., 1994; Walker et al., 1994; Hollis, 1995; Crow et al., 1995; Olin and Mednick, 1996; Kremen et al., 1998; Malmberg et al., 1998; Hans et al., 1999; Amminger et al., 1999; Cannon et al., 1999, 2000a; Erlenmeyer-Kimling et al., 2000; Rosso et al., 2000a; Bearden et al., 2000; Isohanni et al., 2001). Childhood developmental impairments most likely reflect the expression of schizophrenia susceptibility genes (Jones and Murray , 1991), echoing the earlier theoretical concept of "schizotaxia," a "neural integrative defect" that is the neurobiological consequence of the genetic origins of schizophrenia, (Meehl, 1962, 1989; Tsuang et al., 2000). Early neuromotor, language, and cognitive developmental impairment appear to show some specificity to schizophreniform disorder, whereas childhood emotional and interpersonal difficulties are associated with a range of psychiatric disorders in adulthood (Cannon et al., 2002). Self-reported psychotic symptoms at age 11 strongly predict later schizophreniform disorder, reinforcing the view that schizophrenia is an illness with a longitudinal phenotype (Poulton et al., 2000).

Prenatal and perinatal risk factors for schizophrenia have been extensively studied (for review see Jones and Cannon, 1998; Jones, 1999). Obstetric complications involving hypoxia and fetal growth retardation are significantly related to the risk of later developing schizophrenia (Dalman, 1999; Jones et al., 1997; Cannon et al., 2000b; Rosso et al., 2000b, Zornberg et al., 2000). Prenatal exposure to influenza increases the risk of later schizophrenia by approximately two-fold (for review see McGrath et al., 1995; Jones, 1999), and this effect may extend to schizotypal personality disorder also (Machon et al., 2002). Severe stress during pregnancy (as indexed by loss of a spouse) has been associated in one study with a six-fold increase in risk of schizophrenia among the offspring (Huttunen and Niskanen, 1978). However, these intriguing prenatal, perinatal and childhood developmental risk factors have yet to be integrated into a coherent etiological mechanism.

Affective Disorder

The classification of depression into mutually exclusive "reactive" and "endogenous" types was common until very recently. However depression is now being recognized as a multifactorial illness caused by multiple, and possibly interacting, environmental, genetic, and developmental risk factors (O'Keane, 2000). Although adverse life experiences undoubtedly play a role in the genesis of depressive disorder, there is good evidence that genetic factors influence the experience of and reaction to those life events (Kendler and Karowshi-Shuman, 1997; Thapar et al., 1998). A developmental perspective is provided by case–control and longitudinal birth cohort studies which demonstrate early childhood risk factors for both childhood-onset and adult-onset affective illness (Rodgers, 1990; Cannon et al., 1997, 2001; van Os et al., 1997).

It has long been known that overdrive of the hypothalamic-pituitary-adrenal (HPA) system is associated with depression (Gold et al., 1988). Recent evidence from animal studies shows that stress during critical periods of brain development, such as fetal life or early childhood, can lead to abnormal functioning of the HPA axis and thus may be linked to an increased sensitivity to stress in adulthood and possibly depression (for review see Sapolsky, 1996; Graham et al., 1999). This effect could be mediated through persistent changes in glucocorticoid receptor density in the hippocampus (Owens and Nemeroff, 1991). Glucocorticoids can exert an adverse effect on growth and neuronal myelination (Sapolsky, 1996, 2000), and high circulating levels of glucocorticoids have been reported to accelerate death of hippocampal neurons. (Sapolsky and Meaney, 1986). Rats prenatally exposed to stress demonstrate a reduction in hippocampal pyramidal neurons (Uno et al., 1989), abnormal turnover of catecholamines (Huttunen, 1971), persistent hyperactivity of their HPA axis, and a vulnerability towards later sensitivity to stressful stimuli (Fride et al., 1986).

Much of the literature on the effects of early stress is derived from animal studies but some findings are emerging from human studies to support this model (Graham et al., 1999). Women who were sexually and physically abused in childhood have been shown to exhibit increased pituitary adrenal and autonomic responses to stress (Heim et al., 2000). Even mode of delivery appears to alter HPA axis responses—salivary cortisol responses to the stress of inoculation at eight weeks postdelivery were increased in neonates who had assisted deliveries compared to those delivered by elective caesarian section (Taylor et al., 2000). Maternal depression has important effects on the development of the offspring (Field, 1998). This new and exciting model of depression and other stress-related psychopathology will require innovative studies spanning the disciplines of neuroendocrinology, epidemiology and psychology (Rutter et al., 1997; O'Keane, 2000).

Post-Traumatic Stress Disorder

The original definition of post-traumatic stress disorder (PTSD) awarded causal pre-eminence to the traumatic event: The definition of a traumatic stressor was one "that would evoke significant symptoms of distress in almost everyone" (American Psychiatric Association, 1980). However, it has subsequently emerged that only about 25% of individuals who experience a traumatic event such as a traffic accident (Koren et al., 1999; Ursano et al., 1999), a mass shooting (North et al., 1997), or an earthquake (Wang et al., 2000) subsequently meet criteria for PTSD. What are the risk factors for development of PTSD among survivors of trauma? What places some individuals at risk for PTSD while others appear to be protected?

In recent years research has begun to focus on vulnerability factors for PTSD (McNally, 2001). It is becoming evident that events from early childhood or even prenatal life may "sensitize" individuals to develop PTSD in response to later trauma in adulthood (Bramsen et al., 2000). A history of childhood abuse has been shown to increase the risk for PTSD by about four-fold among Vietnam veterans (Bremner et al., 1993; Zaidi and Foy, 1993). A community survey (based on retrospective data) has shown that history of previous exposure to traumatic events before age 15 years was associated with a two-fold increase in risk of developing PTSD from the index trauma (Breslau et al., 1999). Reduced hippocampal volumes have been noted in combat veterans with PTSD (Bremner et al., 1995; Gurvits et al., 1996) indicating either that stress has directly damaged the brain, causing reduced brain volume, or alternatively that individuals who had smaller hippocampi as a result of earlier trauma or disruption to intrauterine growth (as discussed above) may be more vulnerable to developing PTSD in adulthood. As with affective disorder, research with a developmental perspective has transformed our conceptualization of the etiology of PTSD.

Violence and antisocial behaviour

Violent behavior has also begun to be viewed from a developmental neurobiological perspective (Buka and Earls, 1993, Volavka, 1995, 1999; Farrington et al., 1996). A promising line of enquiry involves the relationship between early environmental events and later criminal behavior (Brennan and Mednick, 1997). Moffitt (1993) recognized that age at onset is a key differentiating feature in antisocial behavior and drew a distinction between life-course persistent antisocial behavior and adolescence-limited antisocial behavior. The life-course persistent variety is much more common in males and characterized by markedly disruptive behavior in the preschool years, an association with hyperactivity-inattention, poor peer relations and mild cognitive impairment. This type of antisocial behavior is associated with a poor outcome. By contrast the adolescence-limited type is characterized mainly by poor parental supervision and being part of an antisocial peer group, the sex ratio is nearer parity and the outcome usually good. Recognition of this distinction between life-course persistent antisocial behavior and adolescence-limited antisocial behavior was possible by longitudinal study of a representative birth cohort of 1037 children from Dunedin, New Zealand (Moffitt, 1993).

Raine and colleagues have published a series of papers demonstrating that biological factors predispose individuals to violent behavior specifically in adverse early environments, (Raine et al., 1994, 1996, 1997a), and have outlined a "biosocial interaction" theory of crime causation, (Raine et al., 1997b). The first finding from this series was that birth complications in combination with early maternal rejection predisposed to violent crime among males (odds ratio. 2.3) in a Danish general population birth cohort, (Raine et al., 1994). A subsequent follow-up examination on 10% of the original cohort, found that males who had both early neuromotor deficits and unstable family environments showed high rates of violence and academic and behavioral problems in adulthood, and accounted for 70.2% of all crimes committed in the entire cohort (Raine et al., 1996). This "biosocial interaction" effect held for a follow-up period through age 34, and predicted violent but not nonviolent offending among males, (Raine et al., 1997a). Brennan et al. (1997) showed that males in the same Danish cohort with both delivery complications and early institutionalization had higher rates of persistent criminal and violent offending. Investigators have to a greater or lesser extent replicated these findings in other samples (Piquero and Tibbetts, 1999; Tibbetts and Piquero, 1999; Arseneault et al., 2000, 2002). As a body of evidence, these studies suggest that early developmental factors are involved in the predisposition to later violence and criminal offending.

Temperament, Adaptation and Resilience

Longitudinal developmental research has shown that behavioral and temperamental characteristics among children as young as three years of age can predict adult psychiatric disorders. Children with undercontrolled temperament at age 3 were more likely at 21 years to meet diagnostic criteria for antisocial behavior whereas inhibited 3 year olds were more likely to meet diagnostic criteria for depression (Caspi et al., 1996). The roots of temperament and psychiatric disorder can be traced back even further, to prenatal life. Maternal distress in pregnancy was associated with ratings of negative emotionality at age 5 years in the Helsinki Longitudinal Temperament Project (Martin et al., 1999).

Study of protective factors and resilience is very relevant to a developmental epidemiological approach but has been relatively neglected in comparison to the study of risk factors and disorder (Cicchetti, 2000). Resilience has been conceptualized as three dolls made respectively of glass, plastic, and steel that were exposed to the same standard blow from a hammer (Anthony, 1968). Under impact the glass doll shattered, the plastic one showed a dent and the steel one remained unscarred. We should be just as interested in the steel dolls as those made of glass or plastic. Knowledge about how children appear to have overcome or been protected from negative consequences of early childhood adversities has important implications for the development of prevention and treatment programs. Why do some of us cope so well with the portion life offers us, while others, who have had similar advantages (or disadvantages) cope badly or not at all?

Between 1939 and 1942, one of America's leading universities recruited 268 of its healthiest and most promising undergraduates to participate in a longitudinal study. The originators of the program, which came to be known as the Grant Study, felt that medical research was too heavily weighted in the direction of disease, and their intent was to chart the ways in which a group of promising individuals coped with their lives over the course of many years. Nearly 40 years later, George E. Vaillant, director of the study, reviewed the Grant Study men in the classic text, *Adaptation to Life* (Vaillant, 1977). He concluded that mental health exists as a continuum, like intelligence, not just as the absence of psychiatric symptoms, and that adaptation to life means continued growth. In fact, isolated traumatic events rarely seem to mould individual lives. What truly impinges upon health is the continued interaction between ones choice of adaptive mechanisms and ones sustained relationships with other people. Much of what is termed "mental illness" is merely outward evidence of inward struggles to adapt to life. The use of mature adaptive mechanisms such as sublimation, humor, altruism, suppression and anticipation are crucial for a good outcome (Vaillant, 1976).

CONCLUSION

The application of developmental epidemiological techniques to the study of mental illness psychiatry has shown that even disorders thought to have a purely "environmental" origin , such as PTSD, have significant developmental components. Development is not a straightforward process. While they set the program, genes do not by any means determine the outcome (Rutter et al, 1997). Each individual develops at his or her own rate within certain broad parameters and we need to study causal processes, or what has been termed a "self-perpetuating cascade of abnormal development" (Jones et al., 1994), rather than individual risk factors. There are usually many mediating factors to be considered, not least the impressive plasticity of the brain during development. We need to understand how certain events at critical periods can alter the course of development. We need to find out more about protective factors and resilience. The good news is that our biology is not our destiny and vulnerabilities, if identified and understood, need not turn into psychiatric disorders

REFERENCES

American Psychiatric Association (1980): "Diagnostic and Statistical Manual of Mental Disorders," 3rd ed. Washington, DC: American Psychiatric Association.

Amminger GP, Pape S, Rock D, Roberts SA, Ott SL, Squires-Wheeler E, Kestenbaum C, Erlenmeyer-Kimling L (1999): Relationship between childhood behavioral disturbance and later schizophrenia in the New York High Risk Project. Am J Psychiatry 156:525–530.

Anthony EJ (1968): The developmental precursors of adult schizophrenia. In: Rosenthal D, Kety SS (eds): "The Transmission of Schizophrenia." London: Pergamon Press, p 293.

Arseneault L, Tremblay RE, Boulerice B, Seguin JR, Saucier J-F (2000): Minor physical anomalies and family adversity as risk factors for violent delinquency in adolescence. Am J Psychiatry 157:917–923.

Arseneault L, Tremblay RE, Boulerice B, Saucier J-F (2002): Obstetric complications and adolescent violent behaviors: testing two developmental pathways. Child Development 73:496–508.

Barker DJP (1992): "Fetal and Infant Origins of Adult Disease." London: BMJ Publishing Group.

Bearden CE, Rosso IM, Hollister JM, Sanchez LE, Hadley T, Cannon TD (2000): A prospective cohort study of childhood behavioral deviance and language abnormalities as predictors of adult schizophrenia. Schizophr Bull 26:395–410.

Bleuler E (1911): "Dementia Praecox or the Group of Schizophrenias." Leipzig: F Deutsche. Transl. Zenkin J, New York International University Press, 1950.

Bramsen I, Dirkzwager AJE, Van der Ploeg HM (2000): Predeployment personality traits and exposure to trauma as predictors of posttraumatic stress symptoms: A prospective study of former peacekeepers. Am J Psychiatry 157:1115–1119.

Bremner JD, Southwick SM, Johnson DR, Yehuda R, Charney DS (1993): Childhood physical abuse and combat-related posttraumatic stress disorder in Vietnam veterans. Am J Psychiatry 150:235–239.

Bremner J, Randall P, Scott T, Bronen R, Seibyl J, Southwick S, Delaney R, McCarthy G, Charney D, Innis R (1995): Magnetic resonance imaging based measurement of hippocampal volume in patients with combat-related posttraumatic stress disorder. Am J Psychiatry 152:973–981.

Brennan P, Mednick SA (1997): Medical histories of antisocial individuals. In Stoff D, Breiling J, Maser J (eds): "Handbook of Antisocial behavior." New York: Wiley, pp 269–279.

Brennan P, Mednick S, Raine A (1997): Biosocial interactions and violence: a focus on perinatal factors. In Raine A, Brennan P, Farringdon D, Mednick S (eds): "Biosocial Bases of Violence." New York: Plenum Press, pp 163–174.

Breslau N, Chilcoat HD, Kessler RC, Davis GC (1999): Previous exposure to trauma and PTSD effects of subsequent trauma: results from the Detroit Area Survey of Trauma. Am J Psychiatry 156:902–907.

Buka S, Earls F (1993): Early determinants of delinquency and violence. Health Affairs, Winter, 47–64.

Buka Sl, Lipsitt AP (1994): Towards a developmental epidemiology. In Friedman SL, Haywood HC (eds). "Developmental, Follow-up Concepts, Domains and Methods" New York: Academic Press, pp 331–350.

Cannon M, Jones P (1996): Schizophrenia. J Neurology, Neuropsychiatry and Neurosurgery 61:604–613.

Cannon M, Jones P, Gilvarry C, Rifkin L, McKenzie K, Foerster A, Murray RM (1997): Premorbid social functioning in schizophrenia and bipolar disorder: similarities and differences. Am J Psychiatry 154:1544–1550.

Cannon M, Jones PB, Huttunen MO, Tanskanen A, Huttunen T, Rabe-Hesketh S, Murray RM (1999): School performance in Finnish children and the later development of schizophrenia. Arch Gen Psychiatry 56:457–463.

Cannon M, Caspi A, Moffitt TE, Harrington HL, Taylor A, Murray RW, Poulton R (2002): Evidence for early, specific, pan-developmental impairment in schizophreniform disorder: results from a longitudinal birth cohort. In press. Arch Gen Psychiatry May 2002.

Cannon TD, Bearden CE, Hollister JM, Rosso IM, Sanchez LE, Hadley T (2000a): Childhood cognitive functioning in schizophrenia patients and their unaffected siblings: A prospective cohort study. Schizophr Bull 26:379–393.

Cannon TD, Rosso IM, Hollister JM, Bearden CE, Sanchez, Hadley T (2000b): A prospective cohort study of genetic and perinatal influences in the etiology of schizophrenia. Schizophr Bull 26:249–256.

Caspi A, Moffitt TE, Newman D, Silva PA, (1996): behavioral observations at age 3 years predict adult psychiatric disorders. Arch Gen Psychiatry 53:1033–1039.

Cicchetti D (1984): The emergence of developmental psychopathology. Child Development, 55:1–7.

Cicchetti D (1990): An historical perspective on the discipline of developmental psychopathology. In Rolf, A, Masten D, Cicchetti D, Neuchterlein K, Weintraub S (eds): Risk and Protective Factors in the Development of Psychopathology. New York: Cambridge University Press, pp 2–28.

Cicchetti D, Sroufe LA (2000): The past as prologue to the future: 'The times, they've been a changin.' Dev Psychopathology 12:255–264.

Clouston TS (1892): "Clinical Lectures on Mental Diseases.," 3rd Ed. London, Churchill.

Costello EJ, Angold A (1995): Developmental epidemiology. In Cicchetti D, Cohen DJ (eds): "Developmental Psychopathology" Vol 1. New York: Wiley, pp 23–56.

Crow TJ, Done DJ, Sacker A (1995): Childhood precursors of psychosis as clues to its evolutionary origins. Eur Arch Psychiatry Clin Neurosci 245:61–69.

Dalman C, Allebeck P, Culberg J, Grunewald C, Kster M (1999): Obstetric complications and the risk of schizophrenia: A longitudinal study of a national birth cohort. Arch Gen Psychiatry 56:234–240.

Diggle PJ, Liang KY, Zeger SL (1994): "Analysis of Longitudinal Data." Oxford: Oxford University Press.

Done DJ, Crow TJ, Johnstone EC, Sacker A (1994): Childhood antecedents of schizophrenia and affective illness: Social adjustment at ages 7 and 11. Br Med J 309:699–703.

Erlenmeyer-Kimling L, Rock D, Roberts SA, Janal M, Kestenbaum C, Cornblatt B, Adamo UH, Gottesman II (2000): Attention, memory and motor skills as childhood predictors of schizophrenia-related psychoses: The New York High Risk Project. Am J Psychiatry 157:1416–1422.

Everitt BS (1998): Analysis of longitudinal data. Beyond MANOVA. Br J Psychiatry 172:7–10.

Farrington DP, Loeber R, Van Kammen WB (1996): Long term criminal outcomes of hyperactivity-impulsivity-attention deficit and conduct disorder in childhood. In Robins L, Rutter M (eds): "Straight and Devious Pathways from Childhood to Adulthood," Cambridge: Cambridge University Press, pp 62–81.

Field T (1998): Maternal depression effects on infants and early interventions. Preventive Med 27:200–203.

Fish B, Marcus J, Hans SL, Auerbach JG, Perdue S (1992): Infants at risk for schizophrenia: sequelae of a genetic neurointegrative defect. A review and replication analysis of pandysmaturation in the Jerusalem Infant Development Study. Arch Gen Psychiatry 49:221–235.

Fride E, Dan Y, Feldon J, Halevy G, Weinstock M (1986): Effects of prenatal stress on vulnerability to stress in prepubertal and adult rats. Physiology and behavior, 37:681–687.

Gold PP, Goodwin F, Chrousos G (1988): Clinical and biochemical manifestations of depression. New Eng J Med 319:414–420.

Goldstein H (1995): "Multilevel Statistical Models." 2nd ed. London: Arnold.

Goldstein H, Rasbash J, Plewis I , Draper D, Browne W, Yang M, Woodhouse G, Healy M (1998): A users guide to MLwiN (Version 1.0). London: Institute of Education

Graham YP, Heim C, Goodman SH, Miller AH, Nemeroff CB (1999): The effects of neonatal stress on brain development: implications for psychopathology, Dev and Psychopathology 11:545–565.

Gurvits T, Shenton M, Hokama H, Ohta H (1996): Magnetic resonance imaging study of hippocampal volume in chronic combat-related posttraumatic stress disorder. Biological Psychiatry 40:193–199.

Hans SL, Marcus J, Nuechterlain KH, Asarnow RF, Styr B, Auerbach JG (1999): Neurobehavioral deficits at adolescence in children at risk for schizophrenia: The Jerusalem Infant Development Study. Arch Gen Psychiatry 56:741–748.

Heim C, Newport DJ, Heit S, Graham YP, Wilcox M, Bonsall R, Miller AH, Nemeroff CB (2000): Pituitary-adrenal and autonomic responses to stress in women after sexual and physical abuse in childhood. JAMA 284:592–597.

Hollis C (1995): Child and adolescent (juvenile onset) schizophrenia. A case control study of premorbid developmental impairments. Br J Psychiatry 166:489–495.

Hollis C, Taylor E (1997): Schizophrenia: a critique from the developmental psychopathology perspective. In Keshavan MS, Murray RM (eds): Neurodevelopment and adult psychopathology. Cambridge: Cambridge University Press, pp 213–234.

Huttunen MO (1971): Persistent alteration of turnover of brain noradrenaline in the offspring of rats subjected to stress during pregnancy. Nature 230–233.

Huttunen MO, Niskanen P (1978): Prenatal loss of father and psychiatric disorders. Arch Gen Psychiatry 35:429–431.

Isohanni M, Jones PB, Moilanen K, Rantakallio P, Veijola J (2001): Early developmental milestones in adult schizophrenia and other psychoses. A 31-year follow-up of the North Finland 1966 Birth Cohort. Schizophrenia Research 52:1–19.

Jones P, Murray R (1991): The genetics of schizophrenia is the genetics of neurodevelopment, Br J Psychiatry, 158:615–623.

Jones P, Rodgers B, Murray R, Marmot M (1994): Child developmental risk factors for adult schizophrenia in the British 1946 birth cohort. Lancet 344:1398–402.

Jones PB, Cannon M (1998): The new epidemiology of schizophrenia. Psychiatr Clin N Am 21:1–27.

Jones PB, Rantakallio P, Hartikainen A-L, Isohanni M, Sipila P (1998) Schizophrenia as a long-term outcome of pregnancy, delivery and perinatal complications: a 28-year follow-up of the 1966 North Finland General Population birth cohort. Am J Psychiatry 155:355–364.

Jones PB (1999): Longitudinal approaches to the search for the causes of schizophrenia: past, present and future. In Gattaz WF, Häfner H (eds.): "Search for the Causes of Schizophrenia." Vol. IV. "Balance of the Century," Steinkopf: Darmstadt; Springer: Berlin. pp. 91–119.

Kellam SG, Brown CH, Rubin BR and Ensminger ME (1983): Paths leading to teenage psychiatric symptoms and substance use: Developmental Epidemiological studies in Woodlawn. In Guze SB, Earls FJ, Barrett JE (eds): "Childhood Psychopathology and Development." New York: Raven Press, pp 17–51.

Kendler KS, Karkowski-Shuman L (1997): Stressful life events and genetic liability to major depression: Genetic control of exposure to the environment? Psychol Med 27:539–547.

Koren D, Arnon A, Klein E (1999): Acute stress response and posttraumatic stress disorder in traffic accident victims: a one-year prospective, follow-up study. Am J Psychiatry 156:367–373.

Kraepelin E (1896): Dementia praecox. "Psychiatrie" 5th ed. pp 426–441. Barth: Leipzig. Transl Cutting J, Shepherd M (1987): "The Clinical Roots of the Schizophrenia Concept." pp 13–24. Cambridge: Cambridge University Press.

Kremen WS, Buka SL, Seidman LJ, Goldstein JM, Koren D, Tsuang MT (1998): IQ decline during childhood and adult psychotic symptoms in a community sample: A 19-year longitudinal study. Am J Psychiatry 155:672–677.

Kuh D, Ben-Schlomo Y (1997): A Life Course Approach to Chronic Disease Epidemiology. Oxford: Oxford University Press.

Langholz R, Thomas S (1990): Nested case-control and case-cohort methods of sampling from a cohort: a critical comparison. Am J Epidemiol 31:169–176.

Liang KY, Zeger SL (1986): Longitudinal data analysis using generalised linear models. Biometrika 73:13–22.

Machón R, Huttunen MO, Mednick SA, Sinivuo J, Tanskanen A, Bunn Watson J, Henriksson M, Pyhälä R (2002): Adult schizotypal personality characteristics and prenatal influence in a Finnish birth cohort. Schizophrenia Research 54:7–16.

Malmberg A, Lewis G, David A, Allebeck P (1998): Premorbid adjustment and personality in people with schizophrenia. Br J Psychiatry, 172:308–313.

Marcus J, Hans SL, Auerbach JG, Auerbach AG (1993): Children at risk for schizophrenia: the Jerusalem Infant Development Study II: neurobehavioral deficits at school age. Arch Gen Psychiatry 50:797–809.

Marenco S, Weinberger DR (2000): The neurodevelopmental hypothesis of schizophrenia: Following a trail of evidence from cradle to grave. Development and Psychopathology 12:501–527.

Martin RP, Noyes J, Wisenbaker J, Huttunen MO (1999): Prediction of early childhood negative emotionality and inhibition from maternal distress during pregnancy. Merrill-Palmer Quarterly 45:370–391.

McGrath JJ, Castle D, Murray RM (1995): How can we judge whether or not prenatal exposure to influenza causes schizophrenia. In Mednick SA, Hollister JM (eds): "Neural Development and Schizophrenia. Theory and Research." Plenum Press: New York. pp. 203–246.

McNally RJ (2001): Vulnerability to anxiety disorders in adulthood. In Vulnerability to Psychopathology. Risk across the Lifespan. Ingram RE, Price JM (eds): Guilford: New York. pp. 304–321.

Meehl PE (1962): Schizotaxia, schizotypy, schizophrenia. Am Psychologist 17:827–838.

Meehl PE (1989): Schizotaxia revisited. Arch Gen Psychiatry 46:935–944.

Moffitt TE (1993): Adolescence-limited and life-course persistent antisocial behavior: A developmental taxonomy. Psychol Rev 100:674–701.

Murray RM, Lewis SW (1987): Is schizophrenia a neurodevelopmental disorder? Br Med J 295:681–682.

North CS, Smith EM, Spitznagel EL (1997): One-year follow-up of survivors of a mass shooting. Am J Psychiatry 154:1696–1702.

O'Keane V (2000): Evolving models of depression as an expression of multiple interacting risk factors. Br J Psychiatry 177:482–483.

Olin SS, Mednick SA (1996): Risk factors of psychosis: identifying vulnerable populations premorbidly. Schizophrenia Bulletin 22:223–240.

Owens M, Nemeroff C (1991): Physiology and pharmacology of corticotrophin-releasing factor. Pharmacol Rev 43:425–473.

Piquero A, Tibbetts S (1999): The impact of pre/perinatal disturbances and disadvantaged familial environment in predicting criminal offending. Studies on Crime and Crime Prevention 8:52–70.

Poulton R, Caspi A, Moffitt TE, Cannon M, Murray RM, Harrington H-L (2000): Childrens self-reported psychotic symptoms and adult schizophreniform disorder: A 15-year longitudinal study. Arch Gen Psychiatry 57:1053–1058.

Rabe-Hesketh S, Everitt BS (2000): "A Handbook of Statistical Analyses using Stata." Chapman and Hall/CRC Press: Boca Raton, FL.

Raine A, Brennan P, Mednick SA (1994): Birth complications combined with early maternal rejection at age 1 year predispose to violent crime at age 18 years. Arch Gen Psychiatry 51:984–988.

Raine A, Brennan P, Mednick B, Mednick SA (1996): High rates of violence, crime, academic problems and behavioral problems in males with both early neuromotor deficits and unstable family environments. Arch Gen Psychiatry, 53:544–549.

Raine A, Brennan P, Mednick SA (1997a): Interactions between birth complications and early maternal rejection in predisposing individuals to adult violence: specificity to serious, early-onset violence. Am J Psychiatry. 154:1265–1271.

Raine A, Brennan P, Mednick B, Mednick SA (1997b): Biosocial bases of violence: conceptual and theoretical issues. In. Raine A, Brennan P, Farrington D, Mednick SA (eds). Biosocial Bases of Violence, New York, Plenum, pp 1–20.

Raine A, Reynolds C, Venables P, Mednick SA, Farrington DP (1998): Fearlessness, stimulation-seeking and large body size at age 3 years as early predispositions to childhood aggression at age 11 years. Arch Gen Psychiatry 55:745–751.

Rodgers B (1990): Adult affective disorder and early environment. Br J Psychiatry 157:539–550.

Rosso IM, Bearden CE, Hollister JM, Gasperoni TL. Sanchez LE, Hadley T, Cannon TD (2000a): Childhood neuromotor dysfunction in schizophrenia patients and their unaffected siblings: a prospective cohort study. Schizophr Bull 26:367–378.

Rosso IM, Cannon TD, Huttunen T, Huttunen MO, Lnnqvist J, Gasperoni TL (2000b): Obstetric risk factors for early-onset schizophrenia in a Finnish birth cohort. Am J Psychiatry 157:801–807.

Rothman K. Greenland S (1998): Case-control studies. In: Rothman K, Greenland S (eds): "Modern Epidemiology," 2nd. Philadelphia: Lippincott-Raven, pp 93–114.

Rutter M (1988): Epidemiological approaches to developmental psychopathology. Arch Gen Psychiatry 45:486–495.

Rutter M, Dunn J, Plomin R, Simonoff E, Pickles A, Maughan B, Ormel J, Meyer J, Eaves L (1997): Integrating nature and nurture: Implications of person-environment correlations and interactions for developmental psychopathology. Development and Psychopathology 9:335–364.

Sapolsky R, Meaney M (1986): Maturation of the adrenocortical stress response: neuroendocrine control mechanisms and the stress hyporesponsive period. Brain Res Rev 11:65–76.

Sapolsky R (1996): Why stress is bad for your brain. Science 273:749–750.

Sapolsky RM (2000): Glucocorticoids and hippocampal atrophy in neuropsychiatric disorders. Arch Gen Psychiatry 57:925–935.

Scott KG, Shaw KH, Urbano JC (1994): Developmental epidemiology. In Friedman SL, Haywood HC (eds): Developmental follow-up concepts, domains and methods. New York: Academic Press, pp 351–374.

Southard EE (1915): On the topographic distribution of cortex lesions and anomalies in dementia praecox with some account of their functional significance. Am J Insanity 71:603–671.

Sroufe LA, Rutter MR (1984): The domain of developmental psychopathology. Child Dev 55:17–29.

StataCorp (1999): Intercooled Stata 6.0 for Windows 98/95/NT. Stata Corporation: College Station TX.

Susser E, Brown A, Matte T (2000): Prenatal antecedents of neuropsychiatric disorder over the life course: Collaborative studies of United States birth cohorts. In Rapoport J (ed): "Childhood Onset of Adult Psychopathology," Washington, DC, American Psychiatric Press.

Taylor A, Pickering K, Lord C, Pickles A (1998): Mixed and multilevel models for longitudinal data: Growth curve models of language development. In Everitt BS, Dunn G (eds) "Statistical Analysis of Medical Data." London, Arnold, pp 127–145.

Taylor A, Fisk NM, Glover V (2000): Mode of delivery and subsequent stress response (research letter). Lancet 355:120.

Thapar A, Harold G, McGuffin P (1998): Life events and depressive symptoms in childhood: Shared genes or shared adversity? J Child Psychol Psychiatry 39:1153–1158.

Tibbetts S, Piquero A (1999): The influence of gender, low birth weight and disadvantaged environment in predicting early onset of offending: A test of Moffitts interactional hypothesis. Criminology 37:843–877.

Tsuang MT, Stone WS, Faraone SV (2000): Towards the prevention of schizophrenia. Biological Psychiatry 48, 349–356.

Uno H, Tarara R, Else J, Suleman M, Sapolsky R (1989): Hippocampal damage associated with prolonged and fetal stress in primates. J Neurosci 9:1705–1711.

Ursano RJ, Fullerton CS, Epstein RS, Crowley R, Kao T-C, Vance K, Craig KJ, Dougall AL, Baum A (1999): Acute and chronic posttraumatic stress disorder in motor vehicle accident victims. Am J Psychiatry 156:589–595.

Vaillant GE (1976): Natural history of male psychological health. V. Relation of choice of ego mechanisms of defense to adult adjustment. Arch Gen Psychiatry 33:535–545.

Vaillant GE (1977): "Adaptation to Life: How the Best and Brightest Came of Age." Boston: Little, Brown. (Reprinted 1995, Harvard University Press).

van Os J, Jones P, Lewis G, Wadsworth M, Murray R (1997): Developmental precursors of affective illness in a general population birth cohort. Arch Gen Psychiatry 54:625–631.

Volavka J (1995): "Neurobiology of Violence." Washington, DC, American Psychiatric Press.

Volavka J (1999): The neurobiology of violence, an update. J Neuropsychiatr Clin Neurosci 11:307–314.

Walker E, Savoie T, Davis D (1994): Neuromotor precursors of schizophrenia. Schizophr Bull 20:441–451.

Wang X, Gao L, Shinfuku N, Zhang H, Zhao C, Shen Y (2000): Longitudinal study of earthquake-related PTSD in a randomly selected community sample in North China. Am J Psychiatry 157:1260–1266.

Weinberger DR (1987): Implications of normal brain development for the pathogenesis of schizophrenia. Arch Gen Psychiatry 44:660–669.

Zaidi LY, Foy DW (1993): Childhood abuse experiences and combat-related PTSD. J Traum Stress 7:33–42.

Zornberg GL, Buka SL, Tsuang MT (2000): Hypoxic-ischaemia-related fetal/neonatal complications and risk of schizophrenia and other nonaffective psychoses: A 19-year longitudinal study. Am J Psychiatry 157:196–202.

CHAPTER 11

Birth and Development of Psychiatric Interviews

LEE N. ROBINS

Department of Psychiatry, Washington University School of Medicine, St. Louis, MO 63110

INTRODUCTION

Psychiatric epidemiology had a long history before potential cases in and out of treatment were interviewed to estimate the number of affected persons in the population. And it was even longer before these interviews allowed assigning cases to specific disorders. Such personal interviews with members of the general population are now the standard method for assessing the frequency of specific disorders in the population. Let us look at their history.

BEFORE PERSONAL INTERVIEWS

Hospital Records

At first, ascertaining the size of the population with any psychiatric disorder was based on choosing a short period, sometimes only one day, and counting the patients in public pyschiatric hospitals. Cases that remitted slowly or were held longer because they were violent or suicidal were overrepresented as compared with those quickly discharged, because they had a better chance of being in the hospital during the time period selected. The prevalence of specific disorders was ascertained by looking at diagnoses in the hospital records. Prevalence rates were calculated for the whole population, for men and women, natives and immigrants, blacks and whites, by dividing these counts of hospital patients by the populations in the area from which the hospital patients came. Similar calculations were carried out to see whether specific diagnoses were more common in one gender, in one ethnic group, or in immigrants versus natives. Those who could afford private hospitals were missed. So were the less severe cases, who were hospitalized on medical floors or treated as outpatients. Because the responsible physician's

Textbook in Psychiatric Epidemiology, Second Edition, Edited by Ming T. Tsuang and Mauricio Tohen.
ISBN 0-471-40974-X

prejudices and preconceptions could play a part in the assignment of the diagnoses found in the records, conclusions about the distribution of specific disorders in the population were suspect.

All Patients Currently in Care

When researchers became dissatisfied with reliance on public hospital records, they began to broaden the source of treated subjects to include all patients, whether inpatients or outpatients. They did this by interviewing all local doctors who treated psychiatric cases, to learn about the symptoms of each patient known to those doctors. The New Haven study by Hollingshead and Redlich (1958) was done in this way. It relied on hospital records and doctors' notes to decide on diagnoses. The coverage of doctors known to specialize in psychiatric patients was complete, but of course, patients diagnosed by nonspecialists were missed.

Another such study was done by Thomas Helgason in Iceland (1964) while he was a resident in psychiatry in Denmark. He quite easily collected names of all the psychiatric patients in Iceland because his father was the only psychiatrist in that country! Data about each patient were submitted to the psychiatrists with whom Helgason had trained, who then reached a consensus on the proper diagnosis. Diagnoses in these studies were more objective than in studies that accepted hospital diagnoses. These two studies were elegantly carried out, but such studies are feasible only in small geographical areas. They also omit untreated and unrecognized cases of mental disorder.

A Single Household Informant

The National Health Survey in its earlier days had a few questions to cover mental illness, but there was no personal interview. One informant per household was asked about medical illnesses, including mental disorders, for the whole household. The questions were not organized into diagnostic categories.

Questionnaires

Self-administered questionnaires provided standardized items that research subjects judged as typical or not typical of themselves. An important example is the Minnesota Multiphasic Personality Inventory (MMPI) (Oltmanns and Emery, 2001, pp. 132–136). The MMPI was composed of items grouped into 26 categories describing the respondent's personality. Nine of the categories resembled the symptoms of clinical syndromes. For each of these syndromes, a scale provided information about how far above or below the median score for a sample of Minnesota residents were the respondent's answers. However, there were no cutoffs to specify when diagnostic criteria had been met. When the respondent was high on multiple clinical scales, there were no rules for deciding the chief diagnosis.

PERSONAL INTERVIEWS TO ASSESS PREVALENCE OF MENTAL DISORDERS

The NSA

Interest in standardized personal interviews was engendered in World War II by the very different rates of rejection for psychiatric disorder in men evaluated by different draft boards. Starr (1950) thought it highly unlikely that there was so large a difference in the prevalence of psychiatric disorder by geographic area. In 1945 she used items from the MMPI as the basis for designing an interview, the Neuropsychiatric Screening Adjunct (NSA), to be used by doctors at every draft board to standardize the psychiatric examination of prospective soldiers. Specific diagnoses were not made, perhaps because they were irrelevant to the goal of deciding suitability to serve in the military. The NSA was never actually used for the purpose intended because the war had ended by the time it was completed. Nonetheless, several studies later used questions from the NSA, or similar questions based on the original MMPI to ascertain the rate of mental illness in a defined population.

The HIS

These descendants of the NSA, like the NSA itself, did not cover all psychiatric diagnoses. The best known of these interviews is the Home Inventory Schedule (HIS) written about 1953 for the Midtown Manhattan Study (Srole et al., 1962). In the Midtown Manhattan study, psychologists and graduate students acted as interviewers and psychiatrists reviewed their results to grade the severity and certainty of the presence of some mental disorder. Toward the end of the study, a computer program was substituted for the psychiatrists. In all, 80% of this New York City sample were found to have a mental disorder. At the severest and most certain end of the scale, a more probable 20% were positive. The HIS, like the NSA, asked about *current* symptoms. Presumably if symptom *history* had been asked, the rate of positives might have reached virtually 100%.

The Midtown Manhattan study illustrates problems that arise even in studies that make use of well-standardized questions. In those days it was assumed that persons with psychiatric problems would try to hide them from interviewers and minimize those they reported, because the interviewer was a stranger. This assumption encouraged interviewers to elicit as many symptoms as they could. Since the interview provided no criteria for deciding whether a symptom had clinical significance, trivial and transient life problems may have been recorded as psychiatric symptoms. These beliefs about how subjects would behave and the failure to exclude trivial and transient symptoms may explain the extraordinary number of positive cases detected.

The lack of interest in diagnosis in the Midtown Manhattan study probably reflected the prevailing Freudian views in American departments of psychiatry in the 1950s and 1960s. Freudians believed that reaction to infantile and childhood trauma could be expressed in a variety of adult psychiatric symptoms (Kolb, 1973). They also believed that psychoanalysis was the treatment of choice for all patients motivated to change who were not psychotic or of low IQ. Since careful descriptions of psychiatric syndromes was thought irrelevant to both understanding the etiology of psychiatric disorders and selecting an appropriate treatment, making psychiatric diagnoses had low priority.

STANDARDIZED AND SEMISTANDARDIZED DIAGNOSTIC INTERVIEWS

The HOS

The Stirling County study in Nova Scotia devised its Health Opinion Survey (HOS) (Murphy, 1986) hoping to make diagnoses. But the authors discovered that writing an interview based on the description of disorders in the then current *Diagnostic and Statistical Manual* (American Psychiatric Association, 1952) presented insurmountable problems. Many of the disorders were very incompletely described; most diagnoses included a statement about etiology of the disorder, that could not be reliably ascertained by interview; although only a single "primary" diagnosis was allowed, there was no guidance as to how to decide which disorder was "primary" in persons who qualified for more than one disorder. Given these difficulties, the Stirling County study substituted the phrase "symptom pattern" for "diagnosis." The symptom pattern was based on interviews plus hospital records and information from general practitioners.

The PSE

A lack of interest in diagnosis was not characteristic of studies conducted in Europe. Although the mental disorders chapter of ICD-8 was almost as abbreviated and vague as DSM-I, John Wing and his group in London constructed a complex diagnostic interview, the Present State Examination (PSE) (Wing and Sturt, 1978). It consisted of specific questions to be asked by psychiatrists, and followed up as they saw fit, to decide whether each specific symptom was present. A computer program then examined the pattern of positive symptoms to assign the case to its most probable diagnosis.

The CIS/GHQ

David Goldberg was responsible for two interviews (Goldberg et al., 1976). The long interview was the Clinical Interview Schedule (CIS), a general purpose psychiatric interview later used in a large general population assessment. The short version of the CIS, the General Health Questionnaire (GHQ), was designed to be filled in by patients while in the waiting room before a doctor's appointment. Its purpose was to alert the general practitioner to likely psychiatric problems in this patient. Both interviews focused mainly on depression and anxiety.

The Lundby Interview

A number of Scandinavian studies interviewed subjects to assess the psychiatric disorders found in a defined geographic area. An example is the Lundby study

(Hagnell, 1966; Hagnell et al., 1990), which consisted of two resurveys of the entire population, including children, living in two Swedish counties. In the first follow-up, one psychiatrist did all the interviewing. He carried a card on which were listed all the symptoms and personality characteristics he intended to assess. He phrased questions as he chose to ascertain the presence or absence of these symptoms. There were no formal algorithms for combining symptoms into diagnoses. Diagnoses were made by the psychiatrist interviewer, who used answers to questions, information from informants, hospital records, and observations of the respondent's behavior as his data.

Epidemiological Diagnostic Instruments in the United States

One event that changed the attitude of American researchers toward the utility of diagnosis was the discovery of drugs that controlled hallucinations and delusions. To use the drugs appropriately, a doctor had to be able to separate schizophrenia and other psychoses from the remainder of mental disorders. To estimate how many persons would require such treatment, epidemiologists needed to distinguish psychoses from other disorders. Similarly, the later discovery of drugs for treating depression, for treating and preventing manic attacks, and for treating anxiety interested clinicians and epidemiologists in accurate diagnosis.

The CESD

The National Institute of Mental Health (NIMH) sponsored the Center for Epidemiological Studies—Depression (CESD) questionnaire (Radloff, 1977). It asked questions about depressive symptoms experienced within the last two weeks. Like earlier structured instruments, it did not ask about course, change from the usual state, or the duration of symptoms, three topics necessary for the diagnosis of depression. Nonetheless, it has been used extensively because it is quick to administer, and it provides an indication that positive responses should be investigated further.

The "Department Interview"

Another important player in the development of standardized diagnostic interviews was the outlier American psychiatric department at Washington University in St. Louis. This department's view was that psychiatric disorders should be treated like medical disorders, that is, be diagnosed and given disorder-specific treatment. This view was rare in the United States but common in Scandinavian, German, and British departments of psychiatry.

The Washington University Department of Psychiatry devised a diagnostic interview to be used for both clinical and epidemological research, as well as in clinical practice (Feighner et al., 1972). The clinical studies followed up patients and expatients and compared them with control subjects without a known psychiatric history, a group much like respondents in epidemiological studies in the general population. The Department Interview looked much like the Lundby interview—a list of topics to be covered by the interviewing psychiatrist. However, every symptom was assigned to one of 14 disorders. Its occurrence over the whole lifetime was explored, as well as its current presence. Interviewers learned a standard method for deciding whether a positive symptom was clinically significant and for exploring whether it might be explained by physical illness or injury or by ingestion of any substance. These interviews lasted about four times as long as the Lundby interviews had (2 hours vs. 30 minutes).

The scoring of the diagnosis was not left up to the clinical judgment of the psychiatrist interviewer, as it had been in the Lundby study. Instead, the Department had reached a consensus on how many symptoms, for how long a duration, were required for each specific disorder. These criteria were applied in each psychiatrist's diagnostic evaluation. At that time, psychiatrists gave only a single diagnosis per patient. Therefore, rules were set to choose a diagnosis for cases who met criteria for two or more disorders. The criteria included the seriousness of the disorder (schizophrenia had the highest priority, mild depression the lowest) and the order in which the symptoms of multiple disorders had first appeared. The disorder with the earlier appearance was considered "primary," later appearing disorders "secondary."

SADS-L

Eli Robins, the principal author of the Department Interview, was part of a large NIMH collaborative study on the course of depression. He worked with Drs. Robert Spitzer and Jean Endicott of Columbia University on the diagnostic criteria for depression. Together they created the Research Diagnostic Criteria (RDC) (Spitzer et al., 1978), which spelled out and amplified the Department's diagnostic criteria. Dr. Spitzer's group at Columbia University then constructed an interview, the SADS-L (1977), to operationalize the RDC. The SADS-L was to be given by clinically trained personnel. It suggested questions, but the clinical interviewer could ask any desired follow-up questions. Also, the interviewer was not bound to accept the respondents' answers in scoring disorders, and was allowed to take into account treatment records and informants' observations.

When Dr. Spitzer was named to head the construction of the American Psychiatric Association's *Diagnostic and Statistical Manual*, Third Edition (DSM-III) (1980), he used the RDC as a model for specifying the requirements for each disorder.

The DIS

DSM-III was the first edition of the DSM with a fully spelled out set of symptoms for each disorder, and criteria for how many symptoms had to be present for how long. It set priorities specifying how to choose among disorders when criteria were met for more than one.

Publication of DSM-III radically changed the opportunities for the construction of an epidemiological diagnostic interview. For the first time it was possible to consider face validity; that is, does each question adequately serve the criterion in DSM-III for which it was intended?, and does the diagnostic scoring of each disorder follow the algorithms in the Manual?

The Epidemiologic Catchment Area (ECA) (Robins and Regier, 1991) was a very large collaborative epidemiological study supported by NIMH. It was designed to assess the rate of specific disorders in the general population according to

DSM-III criteria. At the time that an interview was to be selected for that project, a group at Washington University had recently devised a new interview, the Renard Diagnostic Interview (RDI) (Helzer et al., 1977), to provide specific questions to cover each symptom item in the Department Interview. The group had also formalized the questions to be asked to decide whether each symptom was clinically significant and whether it might have a physical explanation. Symptoms were dated in terms of their first occurrence and last appearance. A test–retest of the RDI had just been completed (Helzer et al., 1981). Each respondent had received three interviews, either by two lay interviewers and one psychiatrist, or by one lay interviewer and two psychiatrists. This design allowed measuring agreement between lay interviewers, between pyschiatrists, and between lay interviewers and psychiatrists. Agreement between diagnoses based on two lay interviewers' interviews was high, and agreements between a lay interviewer and a psychiatrist were as high as agreements between two psychiatrists. Thus the interview appeared to be both reliable and valid when administered by lay interviewers. This finding was important in selecting an interview for the ECA, which called for a sample size much too large to consider using psychiatrists as data collectors. The Washington University group was asked to modify the RDI to make it appropriate for assessing disorders in DSM-III, which was still under construction at that time.

Since the Department Interview had been the father of the RDC, which in turn was the father of DSM-III, many of the RDI's questions were appropriate to criteria in the DSM-III. Some questions were added to cover disorders that were not among Washington University's traditional 14. Like Starr's NSA, the RDI was never used further under its own name. The RDI became the Diagnostic Interview Schedule (DIS-II) (Robins et al., 1979).

Questions were again modified once a final version of DSM-III became available. After these revisions to match DSM-III criteria, DIS-II became DIS-III, and was the official interview for the ECA. Scoring programs were also modified to match the DSM-III algorithms.

The DIS has been published in three additional versions: DIS-III-A (Robins and Helzer, 1985), which added the diagnoses of generalized anxiety and post-traumatic stress disorder (PTSD); DIS-III-R (Robins et al., 1989) to make it compatible with DSM-III-R (American Psychiatric Association, 1987); and DIS-IV (Robins et al., 1995) to make it compatible with DSM-IV (American Psychiatric Association, 1994).

The CIDI

Inspired by the ECA, the World Health Organization decided to produce a similar entirely structured interview that would serve the International Classification of Diseases (ICD) as well as DSM-III. I was asked to collaborate with John Wing in England to create an interview that assessed ICD disorders, as well as DSM-III disorders. Its basis was to be a combination of questions from the PSE and DIS-III. We were joined by clinicians from many countries to assure that our interview would be applicable in different cultures. The resulting interview was named the World Health Organization's Composite International Diagnostic Interview (CIDI) (Robins et al., 1983).

At that time, the ICD-10 Classification of Mental and Behavioural Disorders (World Health Organization, 1992) was being developed. As criteria for ICD-10 were finalized, we had to make changes in the CIDI. The result was CIDI 1.0 (WHO, 1990). Because the ICD-10's Mental Disorders chapter had been greatly influenced by DSM-III, it was necessary to add relatively few symptom questions to cover items where the two systems diverged. However, DSM-III was then revised, making it necessary to modify the questions and scoring programs for the CIDI. The modified version was CIDI 1.1 (WHO, 1993). CIDI 1.1 became the basis for three related interviews, the University of Michigan CIDI, the Fresno CIDI, and the Munich CIDI, each of which made significant changes in its procedures. The CIDI has been modified once more to make it compatible with DSM-IV. Its current DSM-IV version is CIDI 2.1 (WHO, 1997).

STABILITY AND INNOVATION IN THE CURRENT VERSIONS

The revisions necessitated by the publication of DSM-IV were applied to both the CIDI and DIS. Many of the characteristics of earlier versions have been preserved in these new versions. As before, they can be given by lay interviewers trained for one week, they are fully structured, and they do not require medical records or informants. Both still discourage interviewers' improvisation of symptom questions and follow-up questions about symptoms' clinical significance and physical explanations, in order to maintain consistency across interviewers. Both have data entry computer programs and both are scored by computer. Both are available in a computerized as well as a paper and pencil version. The new CIDI computer version is called CIDI-Auto (WHO, 1999); the new DIS computer version is called the C-DIS (Robins et al., 1999). Both computer versions allow the interview to be self-administered or given by an interviewer. The structure of both interviews remains a separate module for each disorder, so that disorders of no interest to a study can be dropped. Both typically take one to two hours to complete.

Both CIDI 2.1 and DIS-IV now determine whether a specific disorder was present in the last 12 months, the CIDI through a special 12-month version, the DIS as a standard part of the full interview. Both interviews have an abbreviated form, the CIDI Short-Form and the DIS Screener. The DIS Screener is integrated into the computer version so that some disorders can be abbreviated while others are given in full. The methods of abbreviation differ. The CIDI Short-Form reduces the symptom set to those symptoms that were most highly correlated with the diagnosis in its full version. The DIS includes all symptom questions, but discontinues questioning for each diagnosis as soon as it can be shown that if all subsequent answers were positive the diagnosis still would not be positive, and discontinues questioning for each criterion as soon as it can be shown that it is positive. It skips all subsequent questions for a disorder once any criterion is known to be negative. This method has been shown to produce no misdiagnosis when about 1000 computer-generated "interviews" were scored in full and screener versions.

A number of features have also been added to DIS-IV that were not available for DIS-III-R and are not available in CIDI 2.1.

1. *Additional Diagnoses.* Added are four childhood disorders: attention deficit/hyperactivity, oppositional disorder, conduct disorder, and separation anxiety. Subtyping of positive disorders has been added where suggested in DSM-IV.

2. *Dated Risk Factors.* DIS-IV asks about additional risk factors: broken homes, offspring, sibships, parents' educational level, marital history, chronic physical illness, past maximum use of each substance of abuse. These and previously available risk factors are dated so that it is possible to tell whether or not they predated the onset of any specific disorder.

3. *Additional Information about Course.* DIS-IV asks about periods of remission lasting a year or longer. This allows ascertaining whether people with more than one disorder experienced the symptoms of both during the same time interval. And it makes it possible to describe multiple disorders as concurrent or sequential. The periods of remission are subtracted from the time between the first and last symptom of a disorder to estimate its lifetime duration. At the end of the interview, the respondent reviews all positive disorders beginning about the same time to clarify their order of appearance.

4. *Use of Medical Services.* While consulting a doctor about a disorder has from the beginning been used in both the DIS and CIDI as one indicator of its clinical significance, responses to that specific question had not previously been coded. DIS-IV now codes medical contacts for each disorder so that disorders can be compared with respect to the probability that they will lead to care-seeking. For each disorder, recent unmet need for care is ascertained by asking whether symptoms for which medical care was desired but not received were experienced in the last 12 months.

5. *Impairment.* The respondent is asked about each disorder's significant contribution to disability at work or with family and friends ever and in the current year.

6. *Subsyndromal and Borderline Cases.* These cases are identified through a modification of the scoring program. The report created after an interview is completed now shows which criteria were met by persons who did not receive a positive diagnosis (subsyndromal cases). Borderline cases are identified by a count of positive symptoms, so that "almost positives" can be identified and "barely positive" cases distinguished from prototypic cases.

Fully structured epidemiological psychiatric interviews have improved over the 56 years since Starr first constructed one. This review of DIS-IV's unique features suggests that it has moved further than other interviews along the route of solving problems and improvising ways of meeting needs revealed in past studies. That is not unexpected since it is more recent than CIDI 2.1. However, the drafting of epidemiological interviews is still ongoing. A new version of the CIDI, now under construction, promises to include many of these innovations, while preserving the advantage of making ICD-10 diagnoses as well as DSM-IV diagnoses.

PSYCHOMETRIC PROPERTIES

Interviews are judged not only by what they can do, but also by how reliable and valid they are. We want the interview to measure what it purports to measure (be valid), and to do so in a variety of settings and regardless of individual characteristics of interviewers (be reliable). Only if it is reliable can results be adequately compared across studies. Only if it is valid is communication of results to others meaningful. Yet measuring these qualities has been problematic. I will argue that our methods of assessing the reliability and validity of our interviews have not shown the progress that we achieved in meeting other criteria for a satisfactory interview.

Reliability

Reliability is measured by the replicability of an interview's results, usually when administered at a later date by an interviewer who is blind to answers to the initial interview. If the initial results are not confirmed in the second interview, we assume that the initial interview was not answered fully or correctly. If the agreement between the two interviews is high, the initial interview is judged to have been little influenced by the personality of the interviewer, the place and time of interview, and therefore to be reliable, that is, immune to variation idiosyncratic to its use in a particular study or in a particular setting. By this criterion of agreement between an initial and a retest interview, fully structured interviews like the CIDI and DIS are found to have much higher levels of agreement than do less structured interviews. But is this satisfactory evidence for their reliability?

Suppose that test–retest agreement is high. The agreement level could be high because the respondent remembers what he said in the previous interview and is trying to be consistent, whether or not the previous answers were correct. This tells us little about whether our goal of showing that an interview is immune to situation or interviewer effects has been met. Suppose test–retest agreement is low. If the second interview reveals symptoms not mentioned previously, the first interview may have prompted the respondent to continue to think about the questions and remember events not previously reported. Or the second interview may omit symptoms reported in the first interview, a common finding. The recall of symptoms not reported initially suggests that the interview was not completely *valid*, because it did not prompt complete reporting of the symptom history. The omission of symptoms previously reported has been attributed to the respondents' finding the reinterview boring and trying to shorten it by denying previously reported symptoms that led to a series of follow-up probe questions. But there are a number of other possibilities: The respondent may not understand that the reliability of the first interview is being tested, but instead may assume that the second interviewer is looking for new information, and so feels free to omit information already provided. Another possibility is that the respondent believes that he or she has learned which responses were of interest to the first interviewer, and so tries to screen out positive responses that the second interviewer can be expected to find irrelevant or not severe enough to be of interest. If any of these explanations are correct, note that it accounts for errors in the *reinterview*, not in the initial interview. It has not shown that the *initial* interview was reliable.

Validity

The usual way in which the validity of epidemiological instruments is evaluated is by comparing the diagnoses it produces in a sample of respondents with the diagnoses produced by clinicians evaluating the same respondents later. The problem with this method is that it does not identify the source of disagreements, nor whether the fault lies with the epidemiological instrument or with the clinician's reinterview.

Note that the validity of the diagnoses produced by an epidemiological instrument is the product of the validity of decisions made at a series of steps. A satisfactory measure of validity provides evaluation at each of these steps so that authors are guided to make necessary improvements.

Steps at Which to Assess the Validity of a Diagnostic Interview

1. Do the interview's questions accurately and exhaustively map onto the symptoms and other criteria in the Diagnostic Manual?
2. Are the skip rules correct, so that respondents are not asked questions to which only one answer is logically possible?
3. Do respondents understand the questions as intended?
4. Do the respondents have the information necessary to answer the questions?
5. Are the questions acceptable to respondents?
6. Was the interviewing situation conducive to frank and complete answers?
7. Have the respondent's responses been correctly entered into the data base?
8. Does the computer diagnostic program accurately map onto the diagnostic algorithms in the Manual?
9. Does the computer program distinguish cases where a disorder's absence is equivocal from cases known to be negative?

Validity should be assessed at each of these steps through a method appropriate to that particular step. Such methods have not yet been fully specified, but some useful suggestions can be made.

For Step 1, a panel of experts can evaluate interview questions against the Manual's description of each symptom and criterion to see whether the questions are precisely on target and the target is fully covered. When the experts are not satisfied, the questions need to be rewritten and reevaluated.

Errors at Step 2 can be detected by considering whether an instruction to skip a subsequent question has been inserted wherever a past response signifies that the respondent cannot meaningfully answer that question or that the answer would only repeat information already obtained. Obversely, there must be no skip instruction before a question to which an answer can be informative. Careful editing can discover skip errors.

Step 3. Judging whether questions are understood as the authors intended can be determined by asking a small group of members of the population to be sampled to rephrase the questions in their own words. Experts must judge whether the rephrasing means the same thing as the original question. If it does not, they can pursue the source of the misinterpretation, rewrite the question, and retest it in the same way. Lack of shared meanings is particularly likely when an interview is given to respondents who have different educational levels or come from regions with their own idioms. To overcome these differences in understanding, interviews should be written in simple language and should not contain idiomatic expressions.

Evaluating the validity of questions written in a different language is particularly challenging. Currently, the most popular method of testing correctness of translation is back-translation, that is, having a bilingual speaker who is unfamiliar with the interview in its original language translate the translation into the original language. Discrepancies are taken to mean that the translation is incorrect. That conclusion is probably justified. What is not justified is assuming that agreements with the original interview show that the translation is adequate. This is because it may be easier for a bilingual back-translator to guess the form of the question in the original language when the translation is particularly poor, that is, when it uses the grammatical structure and idioms of the original language and uses cognates that have a different meaning in the two languages. Several solutions have been suggested, for example, translating both the original and the translation into the same third language, or having the translation done independently by several bilingual persons who then meet to reach consensus for each question on which translation best matches the meaning of the original.

Step 4. An abundance of "I don't know" responses to any question indicates that respondents do not have the information necessary to answer the question. Examples of questions likely to have this problem concern the etiology of symptoms and their dating and frequency. A solution is to ask the question in a form that minimizes demands for precision. Instead of "What caused (SYMPTOM)?" ask "Did any of your lab tests have positive results?" Instead of "How often did that happen?" ask "Did it happen more than 10 times?" Instead of "How old were you the first time it happened?" ask "Did it happen for the first time before you were 30?"

Step 5. Unacceptability of a question can be judged by frequent refusals of respondents to answer or breaking off the interview after it was asked, or not answering it honestly. Honesty can be judged by comparing answers with data from other sources such as vital statistics and criminal justice records, and by inconsistent responses.

Step 6. Invalidity due to a poor interviewing situation can be reduced by requiring that the interviewer find a time and place to be alone with the respondent. Privacy has been found in a number of studies to be a major factor in honesty.

Step 7. Being sure that the data entered into a data set are complete and accurate requires an editor who reviews each interview for omissions and legibility. It also requires a data entry and cleaning program that prevents violation of the skip rules and prevents illogical entries, such as the end of a symptom's predating its onset. Typing errors can be minimized by double entry of interview responses into the computer.

Step 8. The validity of diagnostic programs is enhanced by their transparency. Transparent programs allow persons other than experienced computer programmers to compare the program to the Manual's algorithms and check to be sure that the correct variables are used to evaluate each criterion. Techniques that improve transparency include using question numbers as names of variables and the Manual's names for the criteria as the computer's names for these criteria. Transparency is also enhanced by avoiding difficult-to-understand computer languages, even when they may be more efficient.

There has been little development of formal methods for assessing the accuracy of scoring programs, a serious lack (Marcus and Robins, 1998). One solution suggested requires two independently constructed scoring programs which are then applied to the same data set. Discrepancies in their results require making corrections in one program or the other.

Step 9. Scoring programs must give a distinctive code to cases with too much missing information to justify a negative diagnosis. This code will make it possible to drop these cases from the denominator when calculating prevalence rates.

If no problem is found with any of these nine steps, a study using this interview will produce valid results; that is, it will accomplish what the interview's authors intended. However, there is no guarantee that the diagnoses it produces will be correct. That will depend on whether the Manual's criteria are correct and correspond to real disorders. This distinction between an interview's validity, that is, its ability to assess the Manual's criteria correctly, and the Manual's validity is seldom made.

The usual test for validity of a standardized interview, rather than validating each step of its application as recommended above, is to compare its results with those obtained by an interview given by a mental health clinician. Disagreement of the epidemiological instrument's results with a clinician's diagnosis is not necessarily evidence for invalidity because clinicians do not always apply criteria as specified in the manuals. They often ignore some of the disorders covered by the interview, and may make diagnoses based on presenting complaints, ignoring disorders now in remission. However, there are now structured clinical interviews —the WHO SCAN for ICD010 and DSM-IV and the SCID for DSM-IV (Spitzer et al., 1988)—that guarantee that the clinicians administering them consider all the relevant diagnoses. They have been shown to have reasonably good agreement between clinicians trained to use them (Williams, 1992). These clinical instruments are certainly better "gold standards" than ordinary clinical interviews for evaluating the validity of lay-interviewer or self-administered interviews. But they are not immune to problems.

Clinicians using these interviews are free to ignore any positive response they feel is irrelevant to the "real" diagnosis. They may also press the respondent further if they doubt that the denial of a symptom was correct. These, of course, are the strengths of a clinical interview, the very reason that they may serve as a test of a standardized interview. But it is impossible to tell whether a clinician's disagreement with the lay interview is due to the invalidity of the lay interview or to the clinician's idiosyncratic interpretation of the Manual. Fully standardized interviews like the CIDI and DIS are committed to following the Manual precisely as written, with no room for interpretation. Clinicians' inclination to vary in their interpretations of the Manual, even when using a semistructured interview, was shown in validity studies of DIS-III as used in the Epidemiological Catchment Area project (Robins, 1985). In St. Louis and Baltimore, the DIS produced almost identical prevalences of specific disorders. Yet psychiatrists in the two cities, who reinterviewed subjects using different semistructured interviews both intended to make DSM-III diagnoses, produced very different patterns and rates of disorder, depending on where they had been trained. It was obvious that they applied the DSM-III rules very differently. Thus, disagreements between clinicians' results and results from the DIS and CIDI might reflect psychiatrists' dissatisfaction with some of the criteria in the Manual, rather than the invalidity of the epidemiological interview.

The validity criteria offered by Robins and Guze (1970); elevated rates of the disorder in family members, stability of the diagnosis over time, forecasting known outcomes, consistent laboratory findings; are frequently cited as excellent ways of assessing validity. Unfortunately for our purposes, these criteria were designed to validate the descriptions of disorders that one might find in a Diagnostic Manual, not the validity of interviews that try to represent these descriptions. They are not helpful in assessing how well a diagnostic interview achieves the goal of validly operationalizing the Manual.

THE FUTURE

CIDI 2.1 and DIS-IV are now being used in both paper-and-pencil and computerized versions in many epidemiological studies in North America, elsewhere, and in multinational studies. Of course, some day there will be DSM-V and ICD-11. Their publication will immediately create a market for interviews based on the criteria in the new manuals for both epidemiological research and for computerized versions that can be self-administered in a doctor's waiting room. For those who assume the burden of converting the existing instruments to serve the new manuals, there will at least be a great deal of experience to draw on concerning ways of presenting and scoring questions. There will also be many experienced users to offer suggestions to the new authors.

REFERENCES

American Psychiatric Association (1952): "Diagnostic and Statistical Manual."

Feighner JP, Robins E, Guze SB, Woodruff RA, Wijinokur G, Munoz R (1972): Diagnostic criteria for use in psychiatric research. Arch Gen Psychiatry 26:57–63.

Goldberg D, Kay C, Thompson L (1976): Psychiatric morbidity in general practice and the community. Psychol Med 6:565–569.

Hagnell O (1966): "A Prospective Study of the Incidence of Mental Disorder." Norstedts, Sweden: Svenska Bokforlaget.

Hagnell O, Essen-Moller E, Lanke J, Ojesjo L, Rorsman B (1990): "The Incidence of Mental Illness over a Quarter of a Century." Stockholm: Alqvist and Wiksell.

Helgason T (1964): Epidemiology of mental disorders in Iceland. Acta Psychiatrica Scandinavica (Suppl. 173) 40:11–257.

Helzer JE, Robins LN, Croughan J, Welner A (1981): Renard Diagnostic Interview: Its reliability and procedural validity with physicians and lay interviewers. Arch Gen Psychiatry 38:393–398.

Helzer JE, Robins LN, Croughan JL (1977): "Renard Diagnostic Interview" (with general description and instructions). St. Louis: Washington University.

Hollingshead AB, Redlich FC (1958): "Social Class and Mental Illness: A Community Study." New York: Wiley.

Kolb LC (1973): "Modern Clinical Psychiatry," 8th ed. Philadelphia: W.B. Saunders, pp. 590f.

Marcus S, Robins LN (1998): Detecting errors in a scoring program: A method of double diagnosis using a computer-generated sample. Social Psychiatry and Psychiatric Epidemiol 33:258–262.

Murphy JM (1986): The Stirling County Study. In Weissman MM, Myers JK, Ross CE (eds.): "Community Surveys of Psychiatric Disorders." New Brunswick: Rutgers University Press.

Radloff LS (1977): The CES-D scale: A self-report depression scale for research in the general population. Applied Psychol Measurement, 1:385–401.

Robins E, Guze SB (1970): Establishment of diagnostic validity in psychiatric illness: Its application to schizoprenia. Am J Psychiatry, 126:107–111.

Robins LN (1985): Epidemiology: Reflections on testing the validity of psychiatric interviews. Arch Gen Psychiatry 42:918–924.

Robins LN, Helzer JE (1985): "The Diagnostic Interview Schedule," Version III-A. St. Louis.

Robins LN, Helzer JE, Cottler L, Goldring E (1989): "The Diagnostic Interview Schedule," Version III-R. St. Louis.

Robins LN, Regier DA (eds) (1991): "Psychiatric Disorders in America." New York: The Free Press.

Robins LN, Wittchen H-U, Cottler L et al. (1990): "Composite International Diagnostic Interview," Version 1.0. Geneva: World Health Organization.

Robins LN, Helzer J, Croughan J, Williams J, Spitzer RL (1979): "The NIMH Diagnostic Interview Schedule," Version II. ADM-42-12-79, with History and Introduction (1980), Instructions (1979), and Computer Programs (1980).

Robins LN, Wing J, Helzer J (1983): "The Composite International Diagnostic Interview (CIDI)." Geneva: World Health Organization. Revised 1985.

Robins LN, Cottler L, Bucholz K, Compton W (1995): "The Diagnostic Interview Schedule," Version IV. St. Louis.

Robins LN, Slobodyan S, Marcus S et al. (1999): "The C-DIS-IV (Computerized full and screening DISIV)". St. Louis.

Spitzer RL, Endicott J (1977): "Schedule for Affective Disorders and Schizophrenia (SADS-L)." New York: New York State Psychiatric Institute.

Spitzer RL, Endicott J, Robins E (1978): "Research Diagnostic Criteria (RDC) for a Selected Group of Functional Disorders." New York: New York State Psychiatric Institute.

Spitzer RL, Williams JBW, Gibbon M, First MB (1988): "Structured Clinical Interview for DSM-III-R." New York: New York State Psychiatric Institute.

Srole L, Langner TS, Michael ST, Opler MK, Rennie TAC (1962): "Mental Health in the Metropolis." New York: McGraw-Hill.

Starr SA (1950): The screening of psychneurotics: Comparison of psychiatric diagnoses and test scores at all induction stations. In Stouffer SA, Guttman L, Suchman EA, Lazarsfeld PF, Starr SA, Clausen JA (eds): "Measurement and Prediction." New York: Wiley.

WHO Editorial Committee (1993): "CIDI-AUTO," Version 1.1. Sydney, Australia: WHO Research and Training Center.

WHO Editorial Committee (1993): "Composite International Diagnostic Interview," Version 1.1. Washington, DC: American Psychiatric Press.

Williams JBW (1992): The Structured Clinical Interview for DSM-III-R (SCID). II Multisite test-retest reliability. Arch Gen Psychiatry, 49:630–636.

Wing JK, Sturt E (1978): "The PSE-ID-CATEGO System Supplementary Manual." London: MRC Social Psychiatry Unit.

CHAPTER 12

Symptom Scales and Diagnostic Schedules in Adult Psychiatry

JANE M. MURPHY

Department of Psychiatry, Massachusetts General Hospital, Harvard Medical School, and Department of Epidemiology, Harvard School of Public Health, Boston, MA 02115

INTRODUCTION

This chapter concerns assessment of the psychiatric status of adults by means of systematic questions. A set of such questions along with preestablished categories for the subject's response—or for the interviewer's evaluation of the response—is called an *instrument* or *test*. An individual question in an instrument is referred to as an *item*. Such instruments are of two types. One type focuses on a dimension of psychopathology and is called a *scale* while the other type deals with diagnostic categories and is called a *schedule*.

The chapter begins with general information about scales and schedules. This is followed by a review of the field that focuses on the evolution of such methods over the past 50 years in different geographic locations and different research and treatment settings. The historical period as a whole is described in terms of landmarks and trends that are important for understanding the instruments.

A central feature of the chapter is Figure 1. This figure shows a selection of instruments according to time and place of design. It serves as a guide to descriptions of the characteristics of the instruments, the studies in which they have been used, their evolution over time, and the role they play in the history as a whole. Both clinical and epidemiologic instruments are covered. In keeping with the goal of providing a textbook for psychiatric epidemiology, somewhat greater emphasis is placed on instruments used in epidemiologic investigations.

An overview of reliability and validity follows the description of instruments. Then controversial issues are discussed. A final section points to unanswered questions and directions for future work.

Textbook in Psychiatric Epidemiology, Second Edition, Edited by Ming T. Tsuang and Mauricio Tohen.
ISBN 0-471-40974-X

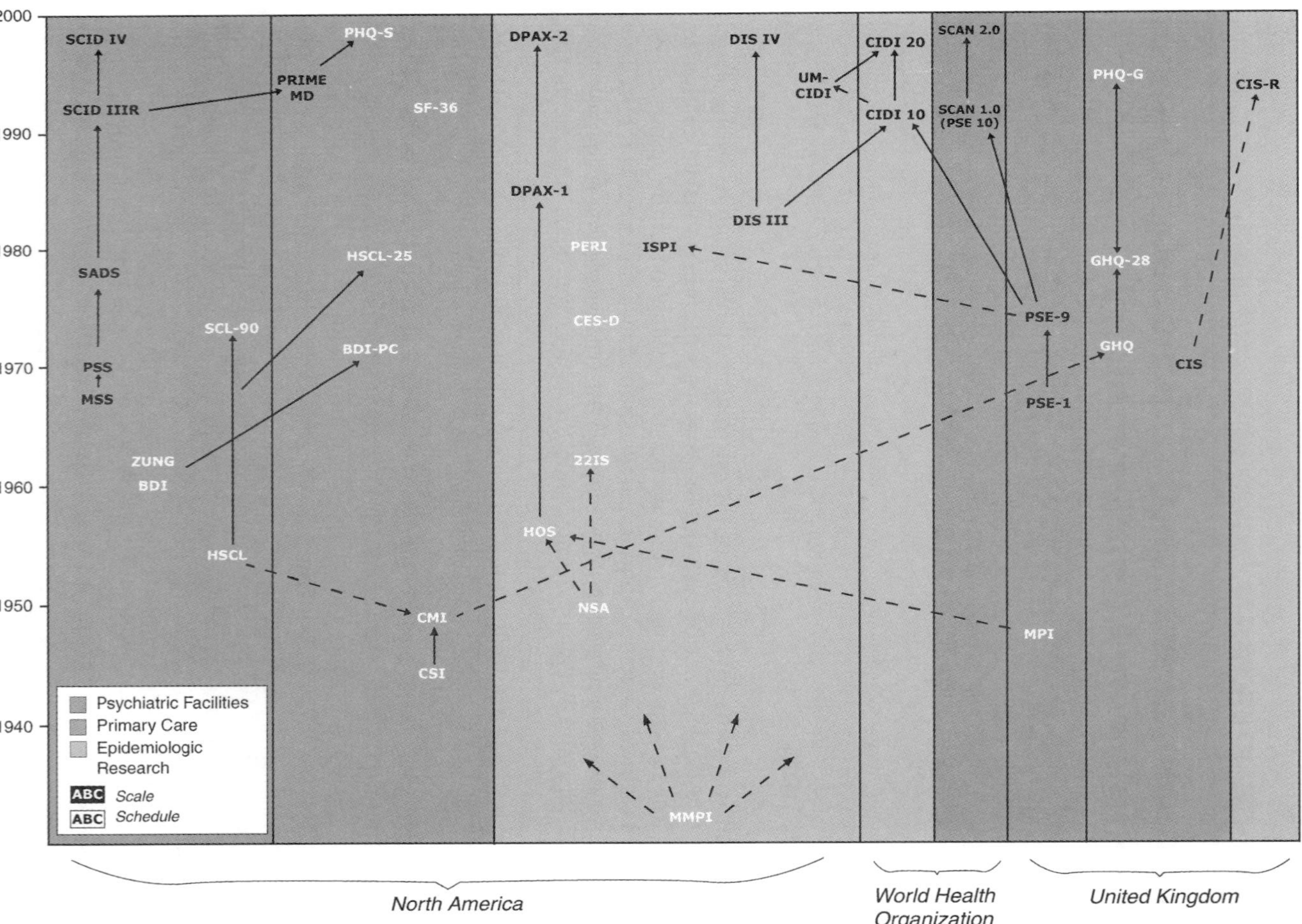

Figure 1. Time, place, and purpose of instruments developed for adult psychiatry.

DIMENSIONS AND SYNDROMES

The difference between a dimension and a syndrome is critical to understanding scales and schedules. A scale involves a series of questions about symptoms from one or more dimensions of psychopathology. A dimension, sometimes called a domain, is a collection of interrelated symptoms about a given aspect of psychopathology that constitutes a continuum from a few to many symptoms. Thus a dimension involves a quantitative gradient based on symptoms representing a qualitative theme. Many scales reflect influence from psychometric theory and survey methodology, and psychologists and sociologists have been more prominent as their designers than psychiatrists.

The concept of a syndrome is fundamental to diagnostic classification as illustrated in the recent *Diagnostic and Statistical Manuals* (DSM-III, DSM-III-R, DSM-IV (American Psychiatric Association, 1980, 1987, 1994). The clinical tradition of psychiatry indicates that a disorder is usually identified by a pattern of symptoms that is made of some central symptoms that define the syndrome and other symptoms that frequently accompany the defining features. The central symptoms are called *essential features* and the symptoms that accompany the *essential features* are called *associated symptoms*.

Anxious and depressive symptomatology has been assessed in virtually all scales and schedules and will frequently be used for illustration. The type of anxiety involved at the beginning of this history was called *free-floating* but would now be called *generalized* anxiety. The type of depression would now be called *unipolar*.

Where anxiety is concerned, frightened and nervous apprehension is at the heart of the syndrome and constitutes its essential feature. The associated symptoms involve autonomic hyperactivity such as palpitations and cold sweats, motor tension such as trembling and muscle-twitching, and vigilance such as being "keyed-up" or easily startled. Where depression is concerned, the essential features involve dysphoria and anhedonia (the former referring to pervasive sadness and the latter to loss of interest and pleasure) and the associated symptoms involve disturbances of sleep, appetite, energy, and concentration as well as lack of self-esteem and thoughts about death and suicide.

The syndrome concept also takes the *duration* of symptomatology into account. In DSM-IV, *disability* or *distress* was added as a requirement for many diagnostic categories. The full complement of components for syndrome recognition and diagnosis includes *essential features*, *associated symptoms*, *duration*, *distress* and *disability*. Depending on the completeness of the pattern, the syndrome is considered to be present or absent thereby reflecting dichotomous measurement. Schedules are oriented to syndrome recognition for different diagnostic categories, and psychiatrists have played active roles in their construction.

Scales

Psychiatric scales are simpler than schedules, and historically they emerged earlier. Sometimes a scale is referred to as a *screening instrument*, a *symptom inventory*, or a *questionnaire*, although the latter is usually reserved for a paper and pencil test of the type which a patient might fill out while waiting to see a doctor. The scales used in epidemiologic research have mainly been administered verbally, face-to-face, by a trained interviewer.

While scales concern dimensions of psychopathology, most of them include questions about both the essential features and associated symptoms of a syndrome. A scale for anxiety, for example, may include items for nervousness and fearfulness as well as for autonomic and tension indicators. A few scales include items for impairment in everyday functioning, and several of them ask about the degree to which the symptom is bothersome. Thus they include information about disability and distress. Further, most scales establish duration by asking the subject to report about symptoms experienced over a given period of time such as a week or month. Thus a scale includes information that is used in a diagnostic category, but the way the information is processed is quite different from the procedures for syndrome recognition.

Each question in a scale is asked of each subject, and specific categories of response are spelled out in advance. Sometimes the response categories refer simply to the presence or absence of a symptom. In others, the presence or absence of the symptom is expanded to cover the frequency of its occurrence or the degree to which it is distressing.

Responses are given numerical values that are added together to form a *score* or linear combination. Sometimes each symptom that is positively endorsed is given the value of 1 while the symptoms not so endorsed are given the value of 0. Other times the value is weighted for frequency or distress. A symptom that is "very distressing" will be given a higher value than one that is only a "little bit distressing." Each scale has a score range, and sometimes scores for selected subjects are presented in terms of the mean value for the group. In psychiatric epidemiology it is more customary for the score range to be described as having a *threshold score* or *cutting-point* that allows cases to be separated from noncases. The scoring of symptoms represents a continuum, but the application of a cutting-point means that the final product is often dichotomous.

A major difference between the way a scale functions and the manner in which syndrome recognition occurs is that each symptom is treated equally in a scale. A symptom like palpitations is scored in exactly the same way as the symptom of fearful apprehension. Scales do not, in other words, require the essential feature of a syndrome to be present. When a cutting-point is applied it divides cases from noncases in terms of an indiscriminate set of symptoms. A case can be identified based only on associated symptoms or only essential features.

Two types of procedures have been used in order to select symptoms for scales. One is based on consulting the clinical literature or on borrowing from earlier instruments. The other method involves a second step that has come to be called *calibration* (Goldberg, 1972). A large number of questions are asked of a *known ill* group and a *presumed well* group. The questions are then tested to see which ones discriminate between these groups at an adequate level of statistical significance. If the known ill group is homogeneous in regard to psychiatric diagnosis, the symptoms selected are interpreted as being useful for identifying people who suffer from that disorder.

Because of their foundation in psychometrics, many scales use strategies to control response styles or response biases. *Response styles* refer to personal characteristics that interfere with the subject's ability to understand the question adequately, consider it thoughtfully, interpret it meaningfully, and answer it truthfully.

For many years, response styles were of concern to designers of psychiatric scales. The styles that received attention were, for example, *acquiescence*, *social desirability*, *lying*, and the *error of central tendency* (Nunnally and Bernstein, 1994). For example, it has been thought that some subjects may not pay attention to the questions and merely answer in a rote fashion as "Yes, yes, yes" or "No, no, no." One method thought useful for overcoming such inattention was called *balancing* and involved reversing the wording of selected questions so that the pathological response was sometimes "yes" and sometimes "no."

It was also thought that a simple"yes" versus "no" response pattern was more likely to foster "acquiescence" than a set of categories requiring more discrimination on the part of the subject. For instance, four categories of response are often used so that the subject will differentiate between the symptom being "not at all distressing," "a little bit distressing," "quite a bit distressing," or "extremely distressing."

Further, a trichotomous response pattern was thought to promote the "error of central tendency" in that subjects would automatically and without thinking about it choose the middle category rather than either extreme (Guilford, 1936). It can be appreciated that if a widespread tendency exists for people to respond on the basis of middle-category preference, the distribution of scores for a three-category scale would form a bell-shaped curve. There is no evidence, however, that such is the case. Drawing on a large body of data from one of the studies that used a scale with three categories, the common profile of responses was that 7% of the subjects said they "often" experienced a psychiatric symptom, 23% said "sometimes," and 70% said never (Murphy, 1993).

Where "evidence" about score distribution has been published or can be calculated, marked skewness appears. This means that the majority of people report that they do not have any psychiatric symptoms, or have only a few, and a minority of people report that they suffer from quite a few to many symptoms. This pertains across instruments that have used different numbers of response categories and other forms of reducing the influence of response styles.

It is a solid fact of history that the shape of the score distributions for psychiatric scales is the pattern one would expect from an indicator of abnormal pathological processes. Psychiatric symptoms are not normally distributed as are height, weight, IQ, and some social attitudes. It is not a matter of most people having an average amount of psychiatric symptomatology, with some people having more, and some less.

A voluminous literature exists on response styles from the early 1930s through the 1960s (Rorer, 1965). Thereafter, psychometric interest in the topic dwindled. This was due to the fact that response styles were found to account for very little variance (Nunnally and Bernstein, 1994). Also, it seemed clear that procedures for reducing the effects of such styles introduced unnecessary complexity into scale measurement. Modern psychometricians have turned attention to more subtle evidence about what generates certain patterns of response and deal with such issues through an approach called Item Response Theory (IRT) (Hambleton and

Swaminathan, 1985). As yet, there is not much evidence that IRT is being used to assess psychiatric scales. This is partly because schedules have become more commonly applied, especially in epidemiologic research, than are scales.

Schedules

Diagnostic schedules are more comprehensive in psychiatric coverage than scales in that all of them deal with psychotic disorders as well as depression and anxiety disorders. Increasingly they have come to include substance abuse and personality disorders.

Sometimes an interview guided by a diagnostic interview is called an *examination* because it is similar to a clinical examination. The history of such schedules began with the requirement that a clinician conduct the interview and evaluate the responses. At the present time, most schedules have been formatted so that they can be used in large-scale epidemiologic studies when administered by a lay interviewer. A *lay interviewer* is one who has not received formal clinical training but who has been trained in the administration of the schedule. While scales owe much of their heritage to psychometric theory and survey methodology, the schedules owe most of their early development to the clinical experiences of psychiatrists.

A schedule is not only more comprehensive it is also more complex than a scale. This pertains to the way the questions are formulated, the manner in which they are administered, and in the analysis of responses. In all these regards, a schedule follows a diagnostic algorithm that requires the presence of essential features and determines the syndrome's completeness by a threshold for the associated symptoms. The duration requirements are often built into the question about essential features. The questions and algorithm also take into account the degree to which the symptoms impose distress or disability. Criteria for each component of the algorithm establish the boundaries of what is considered to be a diagnosable disorder and what is not.

The schedules differ in terms of whether they focus on the clinical status at the time of the interview or on the subject's history of psychiatric disorders. The schedules used in epidemiologic studies tend to utilize the lifetime approach in response to the need for population norms in family genetic studies where the lifetime experience of disorders among family members is compared to the lifetime disorders of index cases.

It is helpful in understanding the lifetime schedules to consider the concept of an *episode* that typically involves a *florescence of symptoms* that can be described as having a particular time of occurrence and a duration. DSM-III makes use of this concept for many diagnostic categories through requirements for a minimum duration of symptomatology. Major depression, for example, is considered to be an episodic disorder for which two weeks is a minimum duration.

The schedules designed for epidemiologic research are highly structured so that clinical judgment need not be applied during the course of the interview. Most of them have *modules* for the separate diagnoses thereby allowing the researcher to select certain diagnoses for study. In some schedules, the module opens with one or two *stem* questions about the essential features of that diagnosis. In other schedules, a series of stem questions appear at the beginning of the interview as a whole and deal with the essential features of many diagnoses.

If the subject responds negatively to the stem questions, the module for that diagnosis can be skipped. The schedules contain careful instructions to the interviewers about *skip-outs*. Even if a given module is started, skip-outs occur as it becomes clear that the subject will not meet the criteria for a given diagnosis. If the interview continues, additional questions are asked about the number of associated symptoms, their clustering together in an episode, the number of episodes, the age of onset at the first and most recent episodes and various characteristics of the worst episode.

A diagnostic schedule usually contains special routines called *probes*. The probes are intended to insure that reported symptoms are serious enough to contribute to a diagnosis and that they are psychiatric in their nature. For example, questions about lack of self-esteem, feeling guilty, or having thoughts about death and suicide do not require probes because they are inherently of psychiatric significance. On the other hand, questions about appetite, fatigue, sleep, and so on, require probing. The subject is usually asked if a doctor was told about the symptom and if so what the doctor's diagnosis was. If the symptom was, in the doctor's view or by default in the subject's view, always caused by taking drugs or alcohol or by a physical illness or injury, the response does not count toward reaching the criterion threshold.

It can be appreciated that a diagnostic schedule guides an interview that is quite different from one based on a scale. Where a scale is concerned, all subjects are asked all questions but with a schedule only a few subjects are asked all questions about all diagnoses, and even for the many who may respond positively to several stem questions, the modular skip-outs will reduce the number of questions they are asked. However, for those with evidence of psychopathology, the schedule interview is much more demanding to the subject since it may require keeping one's whole life in mind and continually reviewing it for discrete time periods of given durations when symptoms were present in specified clusters.

SELECTION OF INSTRUMENTS

Most instruments are known by an acronym standing for the full name of the instrument, and sometimes by the name of the designer. Table 1 gives a list of acronyms and names of the instruments discussed in this chapter along with a reference for each that describes construction and basic attributes.

The selection is intended to provide a historical overview since many of the schedules and scales in use today are outgrowths or revisions of earlier instruments. The selection is not, however, exhaustive. Rather, it provides examples for several key points about the evolution of this type of methodology (Murphy, 1981, 1986, 1990, 1993).

Specifically excluded are rating scales for use by observers rather than for asking direct questions. The Hamilton Rating Scale for Depression (Hamilton, 1960) and the Brief Psychiatric Rating Scale (Overall and Gorham, 1962) are examples of well-known instruments excluded on this basis.

TABLE 1. Scales and Schedules Discussed in This Chapter

BDI	Beck Depression Inventory (Beck et al., 1961)
BDI-PC	Beck Depression Inventory for Primary Care (Beck and Beck, 1972)
CES-D	Center for Epidemiologic Studies Depression Scale (Radloff, 1977)
CIDI 1.0	Composite International Diagnostic Interview, Version 1.0 (Robins et al., 1988)
CIDI 2.1	Composite International Diagnostic Interview, Version 2.1 (World Health Organization, 1997)
CIS	Clinical Interview Schedule (Goldberg et al., 1970)
CIS-R	Clinical Interview Schedule Revised (Lewis et al., 1992)
CMI	Cornell Medical Index (Brodman et al., 1949)
CSI	Cornell Selectee Index (Weider et al., 1944)
DIS-III	Diagnostic Interview Schedule for DSM-III (Robins et al., 1981)[a]
DIS-IV	Diagnostic Interview Schedule for DSM-IV (Washington University in St. Louis Website, Diagnostic Interview Schedule Homepage, 2002)
DPAX-1	Depression and Anxiety Schedule, Version 1 (Murphy et al., 1985)
DPAX-2	Depression and Anxiety Schedule, Version 2 (Murphy et al., 1998)
GHQ	General Health Questionnaire (Goldberg, 1972)
GHQ-28	General Health Questionnaire 28-Item Scaled Version (Goldberg and Hillier, 1979)
HOS	Health Opinion Survey (Macmillan, 1957)
HSCL	Hopkins Symptom Checklist (Parloff et al., 1954; Derogatis et al., 1974)
HSCL-25	Hopkins Symptom Checklist: 25 Items (Hesbacher et al., 1980)
ISPI	Iowa Structured Psychiatric Interview (Tsuang et al., 1980)
MPI	Maudsley Personality Inventory (Eysenk, 1947)
MMPI	Minnesota Multiphasic Personality Inventory (Meehl and Hathaway, 1946; Dahlstrom et al., 1972)
MSS	Mental Status Schedule (Spitzer et al., 1967)
NSA	Neuropsychiatric Screening Adjunct of the U.S. Army (Star, 1950)
PERI	Psychiatric Epidemiological Research Instrument (Dohrenwend et al., 1980a, 1986)
PHQ-G	Personal Health Questionnaire (Goldberg and Simpson, 1995; as published in Rizzo et al., 2000)[b]
PHQ-S	Patient Health Questionnaire (Spitzer, et al., 1999)[b]
PRIME-MD	Primary Care Evaluation of Mental Disorders (Spitzer, et al., 1994)
PSE-1	Present State Examination, Version 1 (Wing et al., 1967)
PSE-9	Present State Examination, Version 9 (Wing et al., 1974)
PSS	Psychiatric Status Schedule (Spitzer et al., 1970)
SADS	Schedule for Affective Disorders and Schizophrenia (Endicott and Spitzer, 1978)
SCAN 1.0	Schedules for Clinical Assessment in Neuropsychiatry, Version 1.0 (Wing et al., 1990)
SCAN 2.0	Schedules for Clinical Assessment in Neuropsychiatry, Version 2.0 (includes PSE-10) (Wing et al., 1998)
SCID-IIIR	Structured Clinical Interview for DSM-III-R (Spitzer et al., 1992)
SCID-IV	Structured Clinical Interview for DSM-IV (First et al., 1997)
SCL-90	Symptom Checklist: 90 Items (Derogatis et al., 1973)
SF-36	Short-Form Health Survey - 36 items (Ware and Sherbourne, 1992)
UM-CIDI	University of Michigan Version of the Composite International Diagnostic Interview (Kessler et al., 1994a, 1998a)
Zung	Zung Depression Scale (Zung, 1963)
22IS	Twenty-Two Item Scale, (Langner, 1962)

[a] DSM stands for *Diagnostic and Statistical Manual.*

[b] The instruments developed by Goldberg and Simpson and by Spitzer et al. have different names but the same acronym. For purposes here, the former is called PHQ-G and the latter PHQ-S.

For full appreciation of the number, variety, and history of the types of instruments discussed here, the Buros *Mental Measurements Yearbook* should be consulted (Plake, 2001). In addition, there are several books or articles that cover instruments not included here (Thompson, 1989; McDowell and Newell, 1996; Salek, 1998). Others describe a portion of the history in greater detail (Üstün and Tien, 1995; Wing et al., 1998; Cooper and Oates, 2000).

TECHNICAL DEVELOPMENTS

At the beginning of the this 50-year history, most of the symptom scales were developed as paper and pencil questionnaires since they were intended to be used in clinical settings or in the armed forces. For epidemiologic research, the face-to-face interview has been the typical mode of data-gathering for both scales and schedules. Increasingly in recent years, data-gathering has been carried out by means of telephone interviews or by computer-assisted methods. Considerable experimentation is going on regarding the use of interactive computer methods where the subject reads the questions from a screen and enters a response (Blouin et al., 1987). Another type of computer method is for the interviewer to conduct a verbal interview that is guided by a computerized version of the schedule that automatically carries the interview through complex skip-outs and probes.

In addition, there have been technical changes in the way information is shared. In the early part of the 50 years, several of the instruments were described in hardcover books with little or no effort to expand this to the readership of professional journals. Shortly, however, the most common mode of dissemination was through journal articles. More recently, the Internet has played a prominent role. As will be seen, some of the references for this chapter are shown as Website addresses.

Medline is another technological development. For example, a search using the acronym DIS identifies 1556 articles. The number of citations generated from acronyms varies considerably and should not, however, be taken as showing full coverage. Limitation in the number of citations may relate to the fact that Medline goes backward in time only to 1966. It can also mean that the search needs more descriptive information than simply an acronym. With the availability of Medline coupled with the fact that some of the instruments have been used or discussed in a very large number of articles, the references for this chapter are far from being exhaustive. They have been selected as background for specific points.

GUIDE TO FIGURE 1

Figure 1 gives a general overview of the field and introduces the individual instruments in the context of their development. Time is shown horizontally and is marked by dates to the left of the figure. As indicated at the bottom, the figure is divided into three main parts. Two of these are the geographic areas of the United States and the United Kingdom. The third, the World Health Organization (WHO), represents an international perspective. Each of these parts is subdivided into the types of settings where an instrument was developed: population-based epidemiologic research, psychiatric facilities, and primary care settings.

The instruments are shown by their acronyms. The scales are shown in white letters and the schedules in black letters. Solid lines that end in an arrow show the evolution of an instrument or series of instruments carried out by a given group of researchers with one or two leaders remaining a constant contributor. Dotted lines that end in an arrow reflect that an instrument developed by one group of researchers influenced a subsequent instrument designed by a different group of researchers.

The Figure is organized so that, to the extent possible, the lines representing the influence of one group of researchers working together or in close collaboration with another group are in adjacent columns. The dates used to position the instruments are those for a first published report that describes the process of construction and gives evidence about reliability and validity. Many of the instruments were being designed over a considerable period of time before being presented in such published articles and some of them were even used in major studies prior to publication.

The figure shows that the earliest instruments were scales and that more of them were developed in the United States than the United Kingdom. However, in both the United Kingdom and the United States, the first of the diagnostic schedules appeared at about the same time, the late 1960s. In the last decade, WHO has taken a prominent role in instrument development and sponsorship of research.

Almost without exception, instruments designed for one setting have been used in one or another of the other settings. Further, each new instrument has been influenced to some degree by prior instruments, and there are several lines of influence that flow across the boundaries for the United States, the United Kingdom and WHO. Sometimes the influence has been a matter of borrowing items. Other times it has been a matter of starting a new approach as a reaction to perceived faults in an earlier instrument.

The instruments have been used in a number of case–control studies within both psychiatric and medical settings. Where population-based studies are concerned, it is important to distinguish three types of epidemiologic investigations in which an instrument has been employed. One is the use of a population register, such as National Health Insurance in the United Kingdom, where both diagnoses by physicians and ratings by an instrument can be used to give prevalence estimates. The other types are single- and two-stage investigations. Single-stage studies involve the administration of an instrument to each individual selected for a population sample. A two-stage design involves the use of a short instrument at the first stage in which each member of a sample is contacted followed by the administration of a more complete psychiatric work-up for a subset of subjects. The subset contains an oversampling of those subjects who reported positively at the first stage and is biassed toward psychopathology. In order to project backward to the whole sample, the subset also contains a known portion of those who reported negatively.

A two-stage design typically involves the use of a scale for the first step and a schedule for the second. Such a design has the attractiveness of economy while at the same time providing a more thorough examination of those who are probably afflicted with a psychiatric disorder. Such a design suffers, however, by providing two points at which subject attrition can occur. Nevertheless, the use of a two-stage design means that sizeable numbers of subjects have been assessed by both a scale and a schedule in the same investigation. Because this review is intended to be international in scope, it is of interest that no major epidemiologic study in North America has used a two-stage design while such a design is common elsewhere. There are, however, a number of North American studies where a clinical instrument has been used for a subset of subjects in order to assess the validity of the epidemiologic findings.

LANDMARKS AND TRENDS

Over the 50 years of this review, three important landmarks influenced the field. The Second World War was the first in that it revealed the magnitude of the number suffering from a psychiatric disorder that had never been diagnosed or treated. Initial efforts in both the United States and the United Kingdom were carried out to create scales appropriate for assessing recruits into the armed forces. In the postwar era, similar scales were designed for general population studies.

The next landmark took place over a period of a few years in the United States but had wide repercussions elsewhere. It was initiated by President Carter's Commission on Mental Health (1978) and was brought to fruition in the publication of DSM-III (1980). The Commission drew attention to the need for improved epidemiologic research and paved the way for appropriation of funds. In the year when the report of the Commission was published, an issue of the *Archives of General Psychiatry* highlighted the significance of the report. The editor, Daniel Freedman (1978), wrote that the Commission demonstrated an "earnest public quest for sound information" of the type that could only be generated in carefully planned psychiatric epidemiologic studies.

That same issue of *Archives* included two important articles that set the stage for a change from symptom scales to diagnostic schedules (Weissman and Klerman, 1978; Robins, 1978) as well as a report on the evolution of diagnostic criteria that culminated in DSM-III (Spitzer et al., 1978). Unlike its predecessors and its international partner, the *International Classification of Diseases* (ICD-9) (World Health Organization, 1977), DSM-III provided explicit criteria that represented considerable consensus on the part of nosologists and practicing psychiatrists. Prior to DSM-III, the term *diagnosis* stood for a theoretical formulation based on assumed etiology but in the new manual *diagnosis* stood for the application of descriptive criteria. Such criteria revolutionized the task of instrument development by giving a standard, nationally-accepted nomenclature. Questions, formulated to implement the criteria, could be brought together in what was now appropriately called a *diagnostic schedule*. The combined influences of the Commission and DSM-III led to the largest of the US epidemiologic investigations, the Epidemiologic Catchment Area Program (ECA) (Regier et al., 1984).

The third landmark took its initiation from the publication, on behalf of WHO, of *The Global Burden of Disease* (Murray and Lopez, 1996). Where hitherto the health of nations had been gauged largely by death rates, this new approach added disability and focussed as much attention on the quality of life as on its duration. The inclusion of disability had the immediate effect of highlighting the *burden* imposed by psychiatric disorders. In worldwide perspective, it was estimated that by 2020 unipolar depression would become second only to ischemic heart disease in terms of the level of *burden* involved.

The importance of disability had also been emphasized a few years earlier in the U.S. Medical Outcomes Study (MOS) where depression was found to be associated with more everyday impairment than any of the chronic medical conditions other than advanced coronary heart disease (Tarlov et al., 1989; Wells et al., 1989). However, the global estimates called for empirical investigation, and this need launched a vastly larger psychiatric epidemiologic program than heretofore envisaged. Named World Mental Health 2000 (WMH2000), this project is currently underway and will probably involve the participation of many nations and a very large number of subjects (World Health Organization, 2000).

Other events influenced the course of instrument development but their effects appeared more slowly and they can best be thought of as trends. One was the gradual acceptance of *symptoms* as important for diagnosis in contrast to *intrapsychic dynamics*. Psychoanalytic psychiatry, that in the United States was in ascendancy during and after World War II, emphasized the unconscious and intrapsychic dynamics. The symptoms on which the early scales concentrated by virtue of the fact that the subject was *aware* of them were thought to be superficial and non-informative in regard to "real" issues.

A member of one of the early studies observed that symptomatic information of the type elicited in psychiatric scales "offered no firm perceptual footing to discern intrapsychic dynamics that are the *sine qua non* of operable data for diagnosis within psychiatry's rapidly evolving nosological framework" (Srole et al., 1962, p. 134). As the dominance of psychoanalytic psychiatry receded, however, psychiatrists began to pay increased attention to overt symptoms and how they combined into clinical syndromes.

A related trend was a gradual shift of attention away from anxiety to depression. Anxiety played a pervasive role in psychodynamic psychiatry as the "alpha and omega" of psychopathology (Lewis, 1970). It was considered to be the hallmark of a neurotic disorder as presented in the psychoanalytically influenced DSM-I (American Psychiatric Association, 1952). Anxiety was very visible in the early scales, and the phrase *anxious neurotic* was used to characterize the kind of patient who measured positively on them (Lipman et al., 1969).

As psychoanalytic thinking became less influential, anxiety lost much of its prominence. More than that, however, it was not until the mid-1960s that milder forms of depression began to appear in psychiatric outpatient services (Muncie, 1963; Rosenthal, 1966; Paykel, 1971; Klerman,1978). Prior to this, the term *depression* tended to be reserved for more serious illnesses, especially those affective disorders with psychotic features. In DSM-I, nonpsychotic depression received little attention and was described briefly as a psychoneurotic depressive reaction in which the anxiety involved in the reaction was allayed by self-depreciation. DSM-III contributed to the changing view of anxiety in that *neurosis*, with its link to underlying anxiety, was no longer shown as a category, and the anxiety and affective disorders were separated and specified. A shift from focus on generalized anxiety to depression will be seen in the history of instrumentation. It should be noted, however, that specific anxiety disorders are beginning to receive more attention and several scales and schedules have been constructed that focus on the panic–agoraphobic spectrum or obsessive–compulsive symptoms, and so on, (Goodman et al., 1989; Cassano et al., 1999).

Another change in conceptualization that has impinged on the design of instruments concerns depression itself, over and above the changing focus away from anxiety. DSM-III gave two main categories of depression: major depressive disorder and dysthymia. Major depressive disorder was presented as an episodic disorder and dysthymia as a chronic one. Major depression received by far the greater amount of attention, and many psychiatrists viewed depression as mainly an acute illness. In the decades since DSM-III, this view changed as evidence came forward indicating that chronicity was common. Much of contemporary instrumentation presents depression as episodic, and it remains a question as to how best to deal with the chronic versus acute issue.

Another influential trend was the emergence of psychotropic medication. Barbiturates were the only available psychopharmacological products when this history began. The methods of psychiatry were therefore focussed on psychotherapy and hospitalization. General physicians were limited mainly to making referrals or offering reassurance. In the mid-1950s, new psychotropic medications began to be discovered (Healy, 1997). By 1970, the anxiolytics and antidepressants were being used by many general physicians and had become widely known to the public at large. Some of the psychiatric scales were used to help monitor the effectiveness of such medication in clinical trials.

There have also been marked historical changes in the role of substance abuse in psychiatry. Alcoholism was shown as a sociopathic personality disturbance in DSM-I but its description was meager compared to those for the psychoses and neuroses. Also there were few treatments for substance abuse that had become part of standard psychiatric practice. Since then, alcohol and drug abuse have become major health problems, and the field responded by creating instruments to assess such disorders (Teitelbaum and Mullen, 2000). Further, the frequent comorbidity between substance abuse and other psychiatric disorders influenced the planning of mental health services and fostered the next large U.S. epidemiologic study after the ECA—the National Comorbidity Survey (NCS) (Kessler et al., 1994a).

Throughout its history, clinical psychiatry has understandably given major attention to psychotic disorders, especially schizophrenia. For the most part the early instruments used in epidemiologic research did not attempt to gather information about psychoses. This led to some misinterpretation. Because schizophrenia is the mental illness *par excellence* in the public mind, many of the scales that focussed on anxiety and depression were criticized for not measuring mental illness (Dohrenwend and Dohrenwend, 1965; Tousignant et al., 1974). The psychotic disorders were, however, central in the evolution of the diagnostic schedules. Two important studies, the U.S./U.K. Diagnostic Project (Cooper et al., 1972) and the *International Pilot Study of Schizophrenia* (World Health Organization, 1973) emphasized the need for systematic schedules to assess such disorders. Thereafter, the diagnostic schedules developed for epidemiologic research have included such disorders as well as personality disorders. Thus, progressively over time, the full spectrum of psychiatric disorders has been incorporated into the field of instrument development.

As a final trend to be noted, it is useful to perceive that there have been changes in the sponsorship of instrument development. While the designers have regularly been affiliated with academic departments, there has been an increase in sponsorship by government and other types of institutions such as WHO. This has introduced a level of coordination that did not exist in the early years and that has improved possibilities for meaningful comparative research.

In the next sections of this chapter, the instruments will be described from the earliest to the most recent as shown in the columns of Figure 1. In order to deal with important lines of influence, the following order will be used for these descriptions:

The Second World War
Epidemiologic Instruments: United States and Canada
Clinical Instruments: United Kingdom and WHO
Epidemiologic Instruments: WHO
Clinical Instruments for Primary Care Settings: United States and United Kingdom
Clinical Instruments: United States
Epidemiologic Instruments: United Kingdom

The Second World War

The question and answer mode of inquiry regarding psychopathology dates back to the 1930s when the Minnesota Multiphasic Personality Inventory (MMPI) was constructed by a group of psychometricians at the University of Minnesota (Meehl and Hathaway, 1946; Dahlstrom et al., 1972). Although the MMPI was concerned with measuring personality rather than psychopathology *per se*, it is often thought of as the grandfather of psychiatric instrumentation, and numerous later efforts borrowed items from it. In this chapter, however, attention will mainly be given to the proliferation of instruments that has taken place since the Second World War.

The needs and experiences of the Second World War led to the development of three scales that had profound influence on subsequent work. In the United States, these were the Cornell Selectee Index (CSI) (Weider et al., 1944) and the Army's Neuropsychiatric Screening Adjunct (NSA) (Star, 1950). In the United Kingdom, Eysenck (1947) developed the Maudsley Personality Inventory (MPI). As a field, personality measurement has distinctive features that will not be traced here except as they relate to the identification of psychiatric disorders. Nevertheless, the earliest version of the MPI had more in common with the other wartime scales than did subsequent revisions.

The CSI and NSA were designed to screen for evidence of psychopathology among recruits to the Armed Forces. They set the style of question formulation that characterized virtually every scale that was later developed in that each question focussed on a given symptom. Typical questions were: "Are you bothered by your heart racing?" or "Are you bothered by nervousness?" The CSI used a "yes" and "no" response pattern while the NSA asked about frequency of occurrence in terms of whether the symptom was experienced "often," "sometimes," or "never."

The construction and testing of the NSA was described in detail in the volume on *Measurement and Prediction* of the series on *The American Soldier* (Stouffer et al., 1950). Even now, this volume serves well as a textbook by illustrating issues that need to be faced in developing a psychiatric scale. Items for the NSA were selected by the calibration method. The large number of initial questions used in this procedure included several items based on psychodynamic concepts about early life experiences and potential unconscious conflicts. The calibration procedure used soldiers who were hospitalized with a diagnosis of "psychoneurosis" as the known ill group and a sample of active-duty soldiers as a presumed well group.

The 15 items that did the best job of discriminating between these groups were those in a subscale named "Psychosomatic Complaints." These questions constituted the core of the NSA. Looking back at the scale, aided by language that has now become standard, it is clear that the scale measures generalized anxiety of the type that might turn into panic. It asks about nervousness and registers all the physiologic signals that accompany intense fear in a panic disorder: racing heart, choking, dizziness, and in the earliest version, uncontrollable incontinence.

There is probably no psychiatric syndrome more likely to interfere with a soldier's ability to function in combat than panic. If the scale had been named specifically for its focus on generalized anxiety and panic, its course in the postwar era might have been quite different. Because the scale had the broad name of *neuropsychiatric screening* and the subscale from which it was mainly drawn was named *psychosomatic complaints*, the NSA was later criticized as lacking face validity. It was dominated by symptoms of autonomic hyperactivity and motor tension items, and as a consequence it was also thought to be biased toward identifying physical disorder. These criticisms tended to override evidence that the NSA carried credentials of reliability and validity that were as good or better than many produced later.

Turning to the CSI, it contained a larger number of questions than the NSA, and the items were selected solely from the clinical literature rather than by the further step of actuarial testing by calibration. Although the CSI included questions about autonomic anxiety, it also contained items about depression. Its construction and characteristics were not, however, described in the same amount of detail as pertained for the NSA.

An interesting feature of history that has not always been appreciated is that neither the CSI nor the NSA was actually used to screen recruits during the war. The war was over by the time the instruments were ready. All U.S. recruits were examined by psychiatrists rather than some of them not being examined because they screened negative. Thus a test of the ability of these scales to identify recruits who would or would not perform adequately in the army was never actually made, and decisions about rejection and acceptance remained in the hands of clinical psychiatrists.

At one induction center, however, a study was carried out in which the CSI and NSA were administered to the same recruits (Leavitt, 1946). The correlation between the two instruments was very high, and recommendations were made for the development of a new psychiatric instrument that would incorporate what appeared to be the best features of each. Unfortunately such an instrument was never developed. Like the absence of reference to generalized anxiety and panic for the NSA, the absence of later work to combine the best of the CSI and NSA can, in retrospect, be seen as having retarded the growth of the field.

Each of the wartime instruments had a distinctive postwar history. The CSI became the Cornell Medical Index (CMI) for use in general medical settings (Brodman, et al., 1949). The British MPI continued to evolve as one of the major instruments for assessment of personality and came to be known as the Eysenck Personality Questionnaire (Eysenck and Eysenck, 1975). The NSA was never changed or updated but it had extraordinarily strong influence on the evolution of instruments for population-based epidemiology in North America.

Epidemiologic Instruments: United States and Canada

The first two instruments published after the war were scales for screening large populations. One was the Health Opinion Survey (HOS) (Macmillan, 1957) and the other was the Twenty-Two Item Scale (22IS) (Langner, 1962). Each was designed as part of the first psychiatric epidemiologic investigations to utilize structured interviews administered by lay interviewers: the Stirling County Study (Leighton, 1959) and the Midtown Manhattan Study (Srole et al., 1962).

There were several similarities in the construction and content of these two screening instruments. Both were designed under the sponsorship of Cornell University which was active in the field during this early period with the Cornell Selectee Index (CSI) already given as an example. However, each instrument was designed by a separate group of researchers.

An important similarity between the HOS and the 22IS is that items were selected by the calibration method described in *The American Soldier*. Because the intent was to create instruments appropriate for community research, the known ill and presumed well groups were comprised of both men and women and exhibited a broad age range. While the Army's Neuropsychiatric Screening Adjunct (NSA) had been developed for young men, its 15 items were included in the pools of questions. The 75-item pool from which the HOS was derived contained questions not only from the NSA but also from a psychiatric behavior checklist and from the Maudsley Personality Inventory (MPI). The contribution of the MPI to the HOS constituted the first of the transatlantic influences shown in Figure 1. The 120-item instrument for the 22IS contained questions from the NSA and several other instruments.

Indicative of the importance of the NSA items on generalized anxiety for distinguishing between the ill and well in the era after World War II is the fact that the NSA items were 16 times more likely than the other items to be selected for the HOS and they were 7 times more likely to be selected for the 22IS (Murphy, 1981). The known ill group for the HOS calibration consisted of psychiatric patients with all types of diagnoses but it was not until the group was limited to those diagnosed as psychoneurotic that discrimination was possible. The known ill group for the 22IS consisted of patients described as "neurotics and remitted psychotics." The content of both instruments was congruent with a primary focus on neurotic disorders, as was characteristic of that period.

In noting that the NSA concerned anxiety and that its items worked well in distinguishing neurotic patients from normals in community research, it would be misleading to suggest that depression was completely absent. Included were the "vegetative" or "vital" signs of depression such as disturbances of sleep, appetite, and energy. On the other hand, dysphoria, lack of self-esteem, and suicide ideation were not nearly as well represented as in later instruments. The dearth of items about lowered mood and dysphoria needs to be seen in light of what was said earlier about depression more often being seen in severely ill psychotic patients.

For example, items about depression were included in the MMPI but it was considered to be a clinical instrument for assessment of psychotic patients. The designers of the HOS were advised against using the MMPI as a source of questions for community research because of the MMPI's affiliation with severe mental illness. Further, there were no items on dysphoria *per se* in the early version of the British MPI. The closest approximation was an MPI item about "mood swings." Although the mood swings item was used in the calibration of questions for the HOS, it was not selected as a statistically significant discriminator.

During the 1960s and 1970s, the HOS with some questions from the 22IS was adapted for studying a U.S. national sample as reported in *Americans View Their Mental Health* (Gurin et al.,1960) and subsequently another national sample presented in *The Inner American* (Veroff et al.,1981a) and in *Mental Health in America* (Veroff et al.,1981b). These investigations were carried out by the University of Michigan's Institute for Social Research, an organization that has a long history of national sample studies and of continuing improvement of survey methods. Neither the early nor the more recent of these studies was strictly an epidemiologic study, however, since prevalence was not estimated. The population profiles were mainly presented as the proportions of the sample who answered individual questions in particular ways.

There were, however, a number of investigations that used the HOS for prevalence estimates by the application of a cutting-point on the score range (Myers et al., 1971; Schwab et al., 1979). However, the 22IS was used more than any other scale in North American epidemiologic studies during this period (Manis et al., 1964; Phillips, 1966; Prince et al., 1967; Shader et al., 1971; Dohrenwend and Crandell, 1970) Also, both the 22IS and the HOS were analyzed in several methodologic studies (Seiler, 1973; Tousignant et al., 1974; Gove et al., 1976; Roberts et al., 1976). Questions were raised about what the instruments "really" measure. As mentioned earlier, many users mistakenly assumed that the instruments were intended to identify the full range of psychopathology. Under such an assumption, both instruments were ill-fated. A contributing factor to this fate was that neither scale was named in such a way as to indicate the type of phenomena that it did, in fact, identify well.

The HOS is mainly affiliated with the Stirling County Study and 22IS with the Midtown Manhattan Study. The findings in both of these studies were, however, based on a considerably larger body of data than the screening instruments. For case-identification, each study used a procedure described as a psychiatric evaluation whereby the survey results were read and assessed by psychiatrists for the purpose of presenting epidemiologic findings. A major difference between the two studies is that Stirling gave attention to diagnostic categories based on differences among syndromes while Midtown produced general mental health ratings. Despite these differences, the overall rates of psychiatric disorders were similar, being 20% for Stirling County (Leighton et al., 1963a, 1963b) and 23% for Midtown (Srole et al., 1962). These rates were much higher than expected and this aspect of the early work, like discussion of what the scales measure, led to considerable critical assessment (Lapouse, 1967). Various efforts within the studies themselves as well as by others were carried out to test the degree to which such rates could be considered reasonable.

Both of these early investigations were able to conduct longitudinal research. Midtown carried out a cohort follow-up giving a 20-year perspective from 1954 to 1974 (Srole and Fischer, 1980a). For this, the longer interview schedule was readministered and the analysis was conducted by statistical procedures that essentially treated the items as a scale through multiple regression (Singer et al., 1976). The product was thus consistent over time in being a rating of general mental health.

The Stirling Study has been able to continue with both repeated cross-sectional surveys and cohort follow-up investigations so that now it provides a 40-year perspective from 1952 to 1992 (Murphy et al., 1984, 1988, 2000a, 2000b). The interview schedule for the 1952 survey includes most of the items that were later published as the HOS as well as several others. The absence of an item about lowered mood in the HOS was viewed by the investigators as a serious weakness. As a consequence they added a question about being in poor spirits to the existing questions about the vital signs of depression. With this addition, it was hoped that both the depression and the anxiety syndromes would be sufficiently covered. The interview schedule, as a whole, includes questions for a general health history with onset and termination information provided for medical conditions as well as periods of impairment in everyday functioning. The complete interview for the Stirling County Study was thus an early version of a schedule, while the HOS that it contains was a scale.

For the longitudinal research, a computerized algorithm was prepared for the interview schedule. The algorithm replicates the products of the psychiatric evaluation and has steps for essential features, associated symptoms, duration, and impairment. In order to specify that the schedule focuses on depression and anxiety the name was changed to DPAX with the DP standing for depression and the AX for anxiety (Murphy et al., 1985).

The first version (DPAX-1) was used for the research carried out between 1952 and 1970. A second version (DPAX-2) was designed to make use of changes introduced in 1970 (Murphy et al., 1998). In the course of this, the original schedule was maintained intact, but several questions were added that use different words for describing depressed and anxious mood. The schedule now includes a supplement that expands the questions about duration, distress, and disability. The supplement is used only for those who report positively about the essential features. Thus the schedule now has a skip-out feature.

The second version (DPAX-2) was used for research carried out between 1970 and 1992. Products of the two versions were comparable in the 1970 period and showed good agreement. The agreement and comparability were reduced in the 1992 period due to decline in familiarity with the idiom of "being in poor spirits" as a way to represent depressed mood. A reasonable 40-year perspective on the epidemiology of depression and anxiety has been made possible by using both versions (DPAX-1 for 1952 and DPAX-2 for 1970 and 1992). The line of instrument development that started with the HOS, as shown in Figure 1, is the only one to date in which a scale constituted part of a schedule for which analytic procedures were designed to produce diagnoses that bear a reasonable degree of comparability to DSM-III and DSM-IV.

In regard to the screening instruments—the HOS and the 22IS—it was mentioned that absence of clarity on the part of many users as to what was being measured and the attendant lack of face validity were problematic. These factors contributed to the fact that the next epidemiologic instrument to appear on the US scene was presented as explicitly concerned with depression.

The Center for Epidemiologic Studies Depression Scale (CES-D) differed from its predecessors on several accounts over and above its specific focus on depression (Radloff, 1977). Among these is the fact that it was designed at the National Institute of Mental Health (NIMH) and had government rather than university sponsorship. Also it was not designed by the actuarial methods characteristic of the NSA, HOS, and 22IS but rather by drawing on the clinical literature and by borrowing items from one of the instruments that had become well known in psychiatric facilities, the Beck Depression Inventory (BDI) (Beck et al., 1961). The CES-D, possibly because of how it originated, was better accepted by clinical psychiatry than the earlier scales. It is affiliated with a period when psychiatrists began to take a more central role in the construction of instruments based partly on the profession's increasing appreciation of the importance of overt symptoms.

The CES-D was first used in a comparative psychiatric epidemiologic study of Kansas City, MO and Washington County, MD (Markush and Favero, 1974; Comstock and Helsing, 1976). It has continued to be used in many studies, both clinical and epidemiological, where assessment of the current level of depressed mood is needed. It has taken the place of the 22IS as the most commonly used short instrument in U.S. studies (Weissman et al., 1977; Berkman et al., 1986; Lyketsos et al., 1996; Li et al., 2001).

The most recent scaled instrument for use in psychiatric epidemiology is the Psychiatric Epidemiologic Research Instrument (PERI) (Dohrenwend et al., 1980a, 1986). The PERI is much broader in scope than the earlier instruments in that it consists of 17 scales that cover, for example, false beliefs and perceptions, manic characteristics, suicide ideation, distrust, rigidity, sex problems, problems due to drinking, as well as depression and anxiety. Its focus is on the dimensions of psychopathology and its heritage is in the psychometric tradition. Many of its items were, however, suggested by the psychiatric clinicians who collaborated in its design. The main goal of the PERI is to produce empirically distinct scales of adequate internal reliability in community subjects who represent different ethnic and racial groups.

The PERI contains most of the items that had earlier appeared in the NSA, HOS, and 22IS. The Dohrenwend group suggests that these scales measure "nonspecific psychological distress" (Dohrenwend et al., 1980a, b). They propose that such distress be named demoralization (Link and Dohrenwend, 1980). The term *demoralization* was suggested in a formulation offered by Jerome Frank (1974) who indicated that diagnosis *per se* is rarely useful in selecting a particular type of psychotherapy and that, in contrast, the phenomena that many different types of psychotherapies treat is demoralization. The Dohrenwend group distinguishes between demoralization and diagnosable psychiatric disorder even though the syndromes of depression and anxiety form the crux of the demoralization idea.

The PERI was presented as an instrument composed of *screening scales* that would be especially useful in two-stage designs of psychiatric epidemiologic research (Dohrenwend and Dohrenwend, 1982). While the PERI has not been used in a two-stage study in North America, one of the main studies in which it figures is the Israeli Study of Psychiatric Disorder and Social Status, a large two-stage investigation of the relationships between the prevalence of most types of psychiatric disorders and socioeconomic status in Israel (Dohrenwend et al., 1992).

At about the same time that the PERI appeared in a published report, another broad-range psychiatric instrument was described that had already been used in the Iowa 500 Study (Tsuang and Winokur, 1975; Tsuang et al., 1980). This instrument is named the Iowa Structured Psychiatric Interview (ISPI) and it was the first of the diagnostic instruments developed in the United States that was intended for use in the general population. It reflected another instance of transatlantic influence, as shown in Figure 1, in that it drew heavily on the model provided by the Present State Examination (PSE) that had been developed in the United Kingdom (Wing et al., 1974).

The ISPI is built around a core of 20 screening questions for depression, mania, schizophrenia, and neurosis. Today these 20 items would probably be called stem questions. In the body of the interview, attention is given to the duration and history of each symptom. The ISPI was designed so that it would be acceptable to subjects who did not suffer from psychiatric disorder. The main study with which it is affiliated, however, is the Iowa 500 follow-up and family history investigation of patients selected from mental hospital records with diagnoses of schizophrenia and affective psychosis as well as normal controls selected from surgical services.

The next phase of instrument development per se demonstrated the shift from symptom scales to diagnostic schedules and was linked to the second landmark. Based on the recommendations of the President's Commission on Mental Health, the NIMH Epidemiologic Catchment Area (ECA) Program was initiated as an investigation of unprecedented scale. Most of the earlier studies had drawn samples of 1000 to 1500 subjects, but the ECA's sample consisted of more than 20,000 subjects from 5 mental health catchment areas in different parts of the United States: New Haven, CT; Baltimore, MD; the Piedmont area of North Carolina; St. Louis, MO; and Los Angeles, CA (Regier et al, 1984; Eaton et al., 1984).

The Diagnostic Interview Schedule (DIS) was designed for the ECA (Robins et al, 1981). Its construction was sponsored by the government but it also reflected university influence in that it was developed by a group of researchers led by Lee Robins at Washington University in St. Louis. Its most direct progenitor was the Renard Diagnostic Interview (Helzer et al.,1981) which had been developed and used in the Department of Psychiatry there. Under the headship of Eli Robins, this department had taken the lead in developing explicit criteria for different diagnostic categories that came to be known as the Feighner criteria (Feighner et al., 1972). Subsequently the Washington University group collaborated with a group at Columbia University headed by Robert Spitzer to produce an improved set of criteria known as the Research Diagnostic Criteria (RDC) (Spitzer et al., 1978). The development of DSM-III under the chairmanship of Spitzer drew on both the Feighner criteria and the RDC. While there was considerable overlap between these sets of criteria, the DIS was designed so that the diagnostic products could implement each of these sets through the computerized algorithms.

Considerable encouragement about the prospects of using a diagnostic schedule in a general population study came from a group of researchers at Yale University who had recently used lay interviewers to administer a clinical instrument (Weissman et al., 1978). The instrument chosen for this experimental effort was one designed by the Columbia group, the Schedule for Affective Disorders and

Schizophrenia (SADS) (Endicott and Spitzer, 1978). The demonstration that a complex instrument such as the SADS could be used successfully in a community study was the beginning of what is now nearly a quarter of a century of sustained work in using diagnostic schedules.

The demonstration was not, however, welcomed by all of the participants in the psychiatric epidemiology community. A lively exchange of letters to the editor of the *Archives of General Psychiatry* ensued between Weissman and Klerman on the side of diagnostic specification and Srole and Fischer representing the Midtown Manhattan Study's continued use of general mental health ratings (Weissman and Klerman, 1980a, b; Srole and Fischer, 1980b, c). It was clear, however, that the tenor of the times favored diagnostic schedules and analysis by means of DSM criteria. In so far as the defense of psychiatric scales has been maintained, it has appeared in arguments such as those of the Dohrenwends for two-stage epidemiologic studies in which dimensional scales would be used at the first stage and instruments for categorical diagnoses at the second (Dohrenwend and Dohrenwend, 1982).

The DIS was ready for use when the ECA studies got started. It has gone through several revisions, mainly revisions that adjusted for changes in diagnostic criteria shown between DSM-III and the subsequent versions, DSM-IIIR and DSM-IV. The original DIS dealt with 40 diagnoses that covered a wide range from schizophrenia, mania, depression, panic, phobias, obsessive–compulsive, somatization, alcohol and drug abuse as well as antisocial personality. It was the first of the U.S. epidemiologic instruments to include assessment of a personality disorder. Because each version has been concerned with multiple diagnostic categories, its format has continued to be one of having discrete modules.

Using the module for depression as illustration, the first question concerns both the essential features and duration for major depression: "Over your lifetime, have you ever had two weeks or more when you felt sad, blue, or depressed or when you lost all interest and pleasure in things you usually enjoyed?" The second question is similar but involves a two-year duration for dysthymia. These are followed by questions regarding the eight groups of associated symptoms that deal with disturbances of appetite, sleep, energy, psychomotor activity, loss of interest in sex, disturbances of concentration and of self-worth, as well as preoccupation with death.

For each of the associated symptoms a two-week duration is employed and a probing system is used to rule out instances in which the symptom might have been caused by physical illness or injury or due to taking drugs or alcohol. The module is terminated at this point if the subject did not report at least three associated symptoms. If three such symptoms were reported, however, the remainder of the module deals with whether the symptoms clustered together in time and whether the episode occasioned seeing a doctor, taking medication, or being impaired. Information about the timing of the first and most recent episodes is also gathered.

Because the DIS is more complex than the earlier instruments, special training of interviewers was needed. A central training center was created at Washington University. As use of the DIS has increased, this center has served as a clearinghouse for information about the instrument through the publication of a regular newsletter that offers continual updates. The number of reports published on the ECA data is very extensive. A general overview of findings is provided in the book,

Psychiatric Disorders in America, where a useful bibliography is provided (Robins and Regier, 1991).

Both the original versions and the updated versions of the DIS have also been used in different countries around the world (Helzer and Canino, 1992; Weissman et al., 1996). One of the largest of these was carried out in Canada, the Edmonton Psychiatric Epidemiology Study (Bland et al., 1988). Due to comparability in design, size, and methods, this study can be thought of as adding another site to the ECA and making it possible to compare recent work carried out in the United States and Canada. While there were differences in findings among these sites, the overwhelming impact was of general similarity. For example, the six-month prevalence rates across the six sites varied only from 17% to 23% (Bland et al., 1988) and were quite comparable to the 20% and 23% reported for the Stirling and Midtown Studies. Overall rates that had seemed very high in the early 1950s were corroborated in the 1980s.

If the overall and diagnostic-specific rates from these studies had been widely different, the variation would have been viewed as probably due to methodologic artifacts indicating that the same phenomena were *not* being measured from study to study. Because the overall rates were roughly comparable, correlations between risk factors and prevalence could be taken more seriously. All of these North American studies show an association between low socioeconomic status (SES) and high prevalence of several different types of psychiatric disorders.

Of all the findings of psychiatric epidemiologic studies, the SES association is the most robust over time and across sites (Dohrenwend and Dohrenwend, 1969; Dohrenwend et al., 1980b, 1992; Holzer et al., 1986; Bruce et al., 1991; Murphy et al., 1991). The inverse relationship between SES and prevalence is now commonly acknowledged as an important contribution to knowledge about the distribution of psychiatric disorders in the general population of North America and of several other populations as well. Suggestive evidence has been presented to the effect that the association is due in part to the handicaps imposed by suffering certain diagnoses (the "social drift" or "social selection" hypothesis) and in part to the social stresses affiliated with low SES (the social causation hypothesis), but confirmation of the causal processes is still needed.

While the SES association is well accepted, other associations are more problematic. Studies using the DIS have consistently indicated an association between increasing age and low prevalence. The reliance of the DIS on long-term recall has raised questions about whether the low prevalence among older people is due to reporting inaccuracy (Rogler et al., 1992; Fennig and Bromet, 1992; Giuffra and Risch, 1994; Simon et al., 1995). The use of retrospective reconstruction remains an active methodological issue.

The next step in epidemiologic instrument development reflects international collaboration, as will be described more fully below in discussing the contributions of WHO. This collaboration produced the Composite International Diagnostic Interview (CIDI) (Robins et al., 1988). This section on epidemiologic instruments used in America would be incomplete, however, if it did not include a description of a modified version of the CIDI, the University of Michigan CIDI (UM-CIDI) (Kessler et al., 1998a).

The UM-CIDI was used in the National Comorbidity Survey (NCS) which is the first nation-wide sample of the United States to be investigated with a diagnostic schedule (Kessler et al., 1994a). The UM-CIDI was also used in the first province-wide sample in Canada, the Ontario Mental Health Survey (Offord et al., 1996).

Like the ECA, the NCS was sponsored by NIMH but the work was carried out through the Michigan University Institute of Social Research. It was mentioned earlier that the 1956 and 1976 national studies that used a version of the HOS were carried out by the Michigan Institute as part of its long history of involvement in surveys and survey methodology. The modifications introduced into the UM-CIDI grew out of this tradition and reflected a return to input from sociology and psychometrics, but in this case relevant to an instrument designed within the tradition of clinical psychiatry.

The modifications focussed on strategies for increasing comprehension of the questions and for motivating accurate reporting, especially through careful retrieval of autobiographical memories about illness episodes (Kessler et al., 1998a). One example concerns the question about the essential features of depression. The DIS question combined the feature of dysphoria (feeling sad, blue, or depressed) with the feature of anhedonia (losing interest and pleasure in things one usually enjoyed). In the UM-CIDI, these two features were presented in separate questions. This follows the standard principle of survey methodology to avoid complex, two-pronged questions to which a person can answer affirmatively to one part and negatively to the other.

Another modification was that all the stem questions were brought to the opening section of the interview rather than being positioned at the beginning of each pertinent module. This change was based on the view that the DIS format made it possible for subjects to learn that if they responded positively to a stem question they would be asked many more questions that followed from that response, but if they responded negatively they would not need to answer so many questions. By bringing all the stem questions to the front of the interview, subjects would be inclined to answer more truthfully because they could not perceive that a negative response would lead to a shorter and possibly more comfortable interview.

Still another modification was a technique called a *commitment question* for motivating accurate retrieval of autobiographical memory. Early in the interview, interviewers are instructed to read slowly the following statement and question: "This interview asks about your physical and emotional well-being and about stress in your life that could affect your physical and emotional well-being. It is important for us to get accurate information. In order to do this, you will need to think carefully before answering the following questions. Are you willing to do this?" Interviewers were instructed to close their interview booklets and leave if a subject answered negatively, but it appears that such termination rarely, if ever, happened.

A key aim of the NCS was to investigate further the evidence produced by the ECA that there is much more comorbidity among psychiatric disorders than expected. The frequent combination of substance-abuse disorders with other psychiatric disorders was of special interest because of its relevance for mental health service planning. Also building on the ECA findings about low prevalence among older subjects, the NCS limited its focus to those between the ages of 15 and 54.

The rates produced by the NCS were higher than those from the ECA. This applied across most diagnoses and for lifetime as well as current prevalence. For example, the 1-year overall rate from the NCS was 29% while for the ECA it was 20%. This led to further analysis of the ECA and NCS data (Regier et al., 1998). The magnitude of difference was reduced by controlling for various factors and by combining results from the initial and one-year follow-up of the ECA but questions remain about whether the higher NCS rates reflect the influence of the various strategies used to motivate subjects.

Shortly after the NCS data-gathering was concluded, the UM-CIDI was used in the Ontario Mental Health Survey. In order to lay the foundation for comparison, staff from the Michigan Institute provided interviewer training for the Ontario group. While the Ontario sample was not identical to the NCS, it was similar in excluding older subjects by limiting the age range from 15 to 64. The rates from Ontario were, however, much more like those from the ECA and Edmonton than the NCS. For example the overall annual rate was 19% in contrast to NCS's 29%. This finding has raised further methodologic questions focussed on trying to understand why the NCS rates were higher than any of the other North American studies. Nevertheless, the NCS and Ontario data bases have been used for numerous reports, including some that involve direct comparison (Kessler et al., 1994b, 1995, 1997; Goering et al., 1996).

To conclude this section on psychiatric epidemiologic instruments used in the United States and Canada, the need for continued attention to methodologic precision remains active. Nevertheless, several general patterns can be discerned. The change from scales to schedules appears to be complete as is also the change from focus on anxiety and depression to a much expanded purview that includes not only alcohol abuse but also many of the rarer disorders. While two-stage designs have not been used in any of the well-known North American studies, the size of samples has become larger so that the rarer disorders have a greater likelihood of being represented. At the same time, the importance of high completion rates has been emphasized by evidence that subjects who refuse or are repeatedly unavailable are not a representative subset but rather that they are more likely to have a psychiatric disorder than the more willing members of the sample (Kessler et al., 1994a; Horton et al., 2001).

Clinical Instruments: The United Kingdom and WHO

The Present State Examination (PSE) was mentioned as having been an influence on the Iowa Structured Psychiatric Interview (ISPI) and as a partner with the Diagnostic Interview Schedule (DIS) in contributing to the World Health Organization's Composite International Diagnostic Interview (WHO-CIDI).

The PSE was developed over a period of years by Wing and his coworkers at the British Medical Research Council. The first publication appeared in 1967 and indicated that its purpose was to provide a guide for a psychiatrist wishing to "cross-examine" a patient for evidence of schizophrenia (Wing et al., 1967). It expresses the European psychiatric tradition, especially in its indebtedness to Jaspers and Schneider, and it has been affiliated with the 9th and 10th versions of the *International Classification of Diseases* (ICD) (Wing et al., 1974; 1998).

The PSE is named for the fact that the recent month is the focus of inquiry. Prior experimentation suggested that recall of subjective experiences over a longer period of time was often faulty. Unlike most of the instruments described thus far, the results of the PSE reflect the decisions of the interviewer rather than the report given by the subject. The schedule consists of preformulated questions, but the responses of the subject are not used in analysis. Rather diagnosis is based on the interviewer's evaluation of the subject's responses as guided by a glossary of differential definitions. The interviewer decides if the symptoms are sufficiently severe to warrant contributing evidence to a syndrome and is free to vary the order of the questions or to ask about past experiences if pertinent.

In the early phases of its history, the PSE was used mainly by psychiatrists concerned with psychotic disorders. Gradually the coverage was expanded to include neuroses, and ultimately it was found that adequate levels of interrater reliability could be achieved when the schedule was administered by other types of professionals who had received training in the clinical tradition on which the PSE rests.

Like many other instruments, the PSE went through several versions. It was used in two prominent international studies conducted in the late 1960s. The seventh version was used in the U.S./U.K. Diagnostic Project (Cooper et al., 1972) which demonstrated that many of the differences in diagnosis comparing the United States and the United Kingdom disappeared when structured interviews were employed. The eighth version was used in the *International Pilot Study of Schizophrenia* (World Health Organization, 1973), which contributed evidence that schizophrenia seems to be found in most parts of the world. Shortly thereafter, the ninth revision was published along with a description of a computer program named CATEGO that had been developed for standardized analysis (Wing et al., 1974). Then, in order to use the PSE in population-based epidemiology, an Index of Definition was constructed to differentiate between cases and noncases (Wing et al., 1978).

PSE-9 was translated into more than 40 languages, and it has been used extensively in clinical research and in several one- and two-stage epidemiologic studies (Brown and Harris, 1978; Henderson et al., 1979; Bebbington et al., 1981; Rogers and Mann, 1986). Throughout this phase, it continued to focus on psychoses and neuroses and to exclude substance abuse and personality disorders.

Not long after the U.S. President's Commission on Mental Illness, the WHO Division of Mental Health and the U.S. Alcohol, Drug Abuse, and Mental Health Administration (ADMAHA) joined forces in order to carry out a worldwide review of diagnoses and classification of psychiatric disorders. In 1982 a WHO-ADMAHA Task Force was formed to develop diagnostic interviews that would implement the definitions embodied in the 10th revision of the ICD that was in preparation at the time (World Health Organization, 1992) as well as the criteria employed in DSM-III and the principles used in the PSE-CATEGO system. One goal was to develop a schedule for studying clinical samples. The product of this endeavor consisted of a series of schedules and the overall name is Schedules for Clinical Assessment in Neuropsychiatry (SCAN) (Wing et al., 1990).

SCAN provides a comprehensive procedure for clinical examination appropriate for use throughout the world. It incorporates the 10th version of the PSE along with other schedules. PSE-10 retains its character as a semi-structured guide for the interviewer to make decisions about the presence and severity of symptoms. Other components of the package include, for example, a schedule for rating the possible pathologies and causes involved in an episode (PATHEP), a schedule of extra items to be asked specifically for the ICD (SF), and one for extra items related to DSM-III-R (SD). Further, it is suggested that still other schedules be employed as needed. These include the International Personality Disorder Examination (IPDE) (Loranger et al., 1994) and the Disability Assessment Schedule (DAS) (Jablensky, et al., 1980).

The SCAN has been assessed in field trials in a large number of international centers. Translation into other languages continues to be aided by a systematic set of procedures. Training manuals are available and several training centers have been instituted. The most current version of the package is SCAN 2.1 (Wing et al., 1998).

Epidemiologic Instrument: WHO

In addition to developing the Schedules for Clinical Assessment in Neuropsychiatry (SCAN), the WHO-ADMAHA Task Force was charged with the preparation of an instrument that could be administered by lay interviewers and used in large-scale epidemiologic studies. The Composite International Diagnostic Interview (CIDI) is the product of this work (Robins et al., 1988).

The CIDI was intended to bring together the best features of both the Diagnostic Interview Schedule (DIS) and the Present State Examination (PSE). Like the DIS, the CIDI does not allow variation in order or changes in the way the questions are asked but it contains 35 PSE items that could be transformed into the type of close-ended questions employed by the DIS. Because the CIDI is highly structured and does not allow interviewers to interpret responses it is much more similar to the DIS than the PSE. In fact, some PSE items, especially those dealing with delusion, were not incorporated because they required clinical judgment based on the glossary definitions.

Like the SCAN, the CIDI went through numerous field trials and a variety of special topics were investigated. These included, for example, analysis of comparability with the PSE (Farmer et al., 1987); issues of recall and dating symptoms (Wittchen et al., 1989); appropriateness and feasibility for cross-cultural investigations (Cottler, et al., 1991; Wittchen et al., 1991; Rubio-Stipec et al., 1993), as well as reliability and validity (Wittchen, 1994; Andrews and Peters, 1998; Breslau et al., 1998).

At the same time, the CIDI began to be used in epidemiologic studies. Mention was made of the two North American studies that used the UM-CIDI: the National Comorbidity Survey and the Ontario Mental Health Survey. In addition, the CIDI was used in a national survey of Australia (Andrews et al., 2001), a two-stage investigation in Norway (Sandanger et al., 1999a), and in a large WHO-sponsored study conducted in primary care settings located in 15 different sites (Sartorius et al., 1993).

The CIDI is modular in format and covers 50 diagnoses. There are, however, several other types of versions. A computerized version called CIDI-AUTO was created and tested (Peters and Andrews, 1995). A short form named CIDI-SF was also designed and evaluated (Kessler et al., 1998b). A screening version named CID-S has also been presented and assessed (Wittchen et al., 1999). In addition to the UM-CIDI developed in the United States, a version known as the M-CIDI has been designed by a group of researchers in Munich (Reed et al., 1998).

At the present time, CIDI version 2.1 is being employed in the World Mental Health 2000 (WMH2000) Project (World Health Organization, 2000). This investigation is much larger than any undertaken before. Because the work is ongoing, the final features are not altogether known, but there may be as many as 20 participating nations and it is expected that approximately 100,000 subjects will have been interviewed using the CIDI. The WMH2000 research is coordinated by a representative Advisory Committee chaired by Ronald Kessler of the United States and Bedirhan Üstün of WHO.

WMH2000 is the outgrowth of the third landmark. The *Global Burden of Disease* provided a new, worldwide perspective on psychiatric disorders by defining *burden* as a combination of reduced quality of life (disability) and reduced quantity of life (death). At the same time, the Global Burden consists in estimates that are based on limited data. Thus a goal of WMH2000 is to provide empirical evidence about the prevalence of psychiatric disorders found throughout the world. It is unlikely that a project of this magnitude could have been planned and undertaken without the availability of an instrument like the CIDI that is sponsored by WHO and that has benefitted from numerous collaborative modifications and improvements.

Clinical Instruments for Primary Care Settings

Returning to the first landmark, it is now possible to trace the development of instruments for use in primary care settings. The link between the Second World War and primary care came about because the Cornell Selectee Index was modified for use in general medicine and renamed the Cornell Medical Index (CMI) (Brodman et al., 1949).

The developers of the CSI, Harold Wolff and colleagues, had a strong commitment to the whole person orientation and to studying the relationships between emotional problems and medical conditions. Influenced by this approach, the CSI was expanded into the 101-item CMI. The first parts of the revised instrument included questions about a wide range of medical conditions and physical symptoms while the last sections were concerned with psychological symptoms, mainly those involving depression and anxiety.

The CMI was widely used throughout the early part of this history and dominated the primary care scene for many years. In addition, however, it was used in several epidemiologic investigations (Brodman et al., 1952; Arthur et al., 1966; Eastwood and Trevelyan, 1972; Levav et al., 1977). It is one of the few instruments where prediction of outcome was tested. In this regard, the CMI performed well in forecasting subsequent psychiatric and psychosomatic problems (Brodman et al., 1954). From the vantage point of this review, the most prominent investigation to use the CMI was a study in the United Kingdom concerned with the identification of psychiatric illness in a sample of 40 general practices in London (Shepherd et al., 1966).

The London General Practice Study was carried out by the General Practice Research Unit of the Institute of Psychiatry at the Maudsley Hospital, a unit that has played a significant role in the history of psychiatric instrumentation. Because National Health Insurance was instituted in the United Kingdom after the Second World War and involved nearly complete population registration, general practices provided opportunity for making epidemiologic estimates. The London study made use of the psychiatric diagnoses given by general practitioners but it also drew on information from the CMI.

In Figure 1, the only line of transatlantic influence that tracks from the United States to the United Kingdom is the link between the CMI and the General Health Questionnaire (GHQ). The GHQ was developed by David Goldberg (1972), a member of the General Practice Research Unit, who designed the GHQ mainly to overcome perceived flaws in the CMI. It was noted in the London study that the CMI had a very high test–retest coefficient over a one-year period (0.87). This suggested that the CMI measured stable personality traits rather than the types of psychiatric episodes thought to be of primary concern in general medical settings. The CMI tended to ask if a person was "usually" bothered by such and such a symptom, a feature that fostered a high test–retest value and probably did, in fact, incline this instrument toward identifying chronic illness if not personality traits as suggested in its predictive capability. To overcome the perceived problem of focussing on stable features, the GHQ asks if the person has the symptom "more than usual." The intent is to identify a change from the patient's normal state and to register the kinds of episodes that might be influential in bringing the patient to the general physician.

The construction of the GHQ was described in the book, *Detection of Psychiatric Illness by Questionnaire* (Goldberg, 1972). In many regards this book is a text for psychiatric scale development, being on a par with the sections of *The American Soldier* that deal with the construction of the U.S. Army's Neuropsychiatric Screening Adjunct (NSA). No other psychiatric scales have been so extensively and usefully described as the NSA and GHQ.

The validation study for the NSA involved comparison of test results with assessments provided by clinical psychiatrists using their own typical interviewing procedures. Where the GHQ is concerned, test results were compared with the results of a clinician-administered structured interview named the Clinical Interview Schedule (CIS) that was also produced in the General Practice Research Unit (Goldberg et al., 1970). Although of a rather similar vintage as the Present State Examination (PSE), the focus of the CIS was on the disorders commonly found in primary care in contrast to the PSE's initial focus on schizophrenia. The CIS did not become as prominent as the PSE but has recently experienced a revival in population-based epidemiology, as will be described later.

Item selection for both the NSA and the GHQ was based on calibration. It will be recalled that the NSA calibration produced a scale focussed on the autonomic indicators of generalized anxiety, items that were later found to be preferentially selected for the Health Opinion Survey (HOS) and the Twenty-Two Item Scale (22IS). The GHQ is singularly devoid of those types of symptoms, possibly because patients diagnosed as depressed were heavily represented among the known ill group. It may also reflect the secular trend mentioned earlier whereby milder forms of depression came to be seen more frequently in psychiatric clinics during the 1960s.

In the original publication, it was emphasized that the GHQ measures general psychopathology of a non-psychotic type such as might underlie diverse syndromes. In light of growing interest in diagnosis, however, Goldberg and Hillier (1979) developed a 28-item scaled version of the GHQ that was intended to be useful in distinguishing between depression and anxiety. The scaled version was created by factor analysis and yielded four domains: anxiety and insomnia; severe depression; social dysfunction; and general illness.

The anxiety and insomnia factor highlights the fact that the kind of anxiety described in the GHQ is much more cognitive than in the other anxiety scales. It focuses on symptoms like "being under strain" and "everything getting on top of me." The associated symptoms for GHQ anxiety are limited to sleep difficulties rather than including symptoms like "heart pounding" and "cold sweats." In the full GHQ, sleep receives a larger number of items than in any other of the scales. The severe depression scale reveals that thinking about death and suicide ideation are more extensively and explicitly covered than in most of the GHQ's earlier counterparts. Another distinctiveness shown in the scaled version is that the GHQ represents impairment in everyday functioning better than any other scale of its era.

At the present time, the GHQ has been used in more primary care studies than any other instrument, and its use around the world in both epidemiologic and clinical studies far exceeds what was achieved by its predecessor, the CMI. Using "GHQ" for a Medline search identified 841 references, among which the following illustrate the sustained used of the GHQ (Prince and Miranda, 1977; Mari and Williams, 1984; Von Korff et al., 1987; Piccinelli et al., 1993, Schmitz et al, 1999; Furukawa et al., 2001). The GHQ was also used in the first stage of the WHO Primary Care Study mentioned earlier as having also used the CIDI (Sartorius et al., 1993). Recently, Goldberg and Simpson (1995) developed the Personal Health Questionnaire (PHQ), a 10-item instrument designed to elicit information specifically about depression according to ICD-10 (Rizzo et al., 2000).

It should be noted that a group of U.S. researchers have also designed a primary care instrument with a rather similar name. It is called the Patient Health Questionnaire (Spitzer et al., 1999). Because the acronyms for these two instruments are the same, they are distinguished in Figure 1 by a letter standing for the main developer: G for Goldberg (PHQ-G) and S for Spitzer (PHQ-S). Figure 1 also indicates that many of the U.S. instruments used in primary care are adaptations of instruments developed to assess psychiatric patients. These will be described in conjunction with their parent instruments.

Recently, however, an instrument designed independently and with somewhat different goals has been created. It is an outgrowth of the instrument used in the U.S. Medical Outcomes Study (MOS) (Tarlov et al., 1989) and is therefore linked to the third landmark. It is named the MOS 36-Item Short-Form Health Survey (SF-36) (Stewart et al., 1988; Ware and Sherbourne, 1992; McHorney et al., 1993). Like the CMI, the SF-36 is intended to be useful in assessing both physical and emotional health but its special focus is disability.

The SF-36 was created mainly by factor analytic techniques. It is a multi-item scale that is concerned with eight health concepts. These include limitations in physical activities due to health problems, limitations in social activities because of physical or emotional problems, limitations in usual role activities due to physical health problems, bodily pain, psychological distress and well-being, limitations in usual role activities due to emotional problems, vitality, and general health perception. Limitations in physical activities are identified through questions about walking, carrying or lifting objects, bending, bathing or dressing self. The questions about role activities focus on "cutting down" or "accomplishing less."

The questions about distress and well-being illustrate the psychometric technique of *balancing* in that a positive answer is sometimes the pathological indicator and sometimes a negative response is. The questions to which a positive response is indicative of illness concern "nervousness," "being in the dumps," "feeling downhearted and blue," "feeling worn out," "feeling tired." The questions to which a negative response points in the direction of illness are "feeling full of pep," "feeling calm and peaceful," "feeling full of energy," "being a happy person."

The questions about "being in the dumps" and "feeling down-hearted" are typical of those shown in many of the reviewed scales for the essential features of depression but the SF-36 associated symptoms are limited to energy disturbance. Anxiety is less completely represented, being limited to the references to nervousness and calmness, and there are no questions about autonomic and tension features of anxiety. By using the words "distress" and "well-being" to indicate what these items measure, the SF-36 is more affiliated with the concept of a demoralization scale than with the diagnostic approach. While it gives indicators of depression, it would not be as good a candidate for a study with a special interest in depression as the Center for Epidemiologic Studies Depression Scale (CES-D).

At the same time, the fact that the special focus of the SF-36 is disability makes the presentation of this instrument very timely. This stems from the general increase in attention to the burden of disease in disability terms and to the fact that DSM-IV requires evidence of disability for many diagnoses. Thus, there is evidence of fast-growing use of the SF-36 in a variety of types of studies (Johnson et al., 1995; Arocho and McMillan, 1998; Simon et al., 2001).

Clinical Instruments: The United States

The main pre-World War II instrument used in psychiatric clinics was the MMPI. Like the other scales described here, it consisted of questions to be answered by the patients themselves. After the war, Lorr et al. (1952) developed a Multidimensional Scale for Rating Psychiatric Patients that, like the Brief Psychiatric Rating Scale that came later (Overall and Gorham, 1962), was a guide for clinicians to assess patients rather than a series of direct questions. The first post-war instrument for use in psychiatric clinics that is of the genre described here was one developed by a group of researchers in the Department of Psychiatry at the Johns Hopkins Medical School.

Borrowing items from the CMI and the Lorr scale, the Hopkins researchers designed a scale to monitor the effectiveness of psychotherapy (Parloff et al., 1954). Several psychometric improvements were introduced, such as specifying the time frame and changing the response pattern from "Yes/No" to four categories concerned with the degree to which the symptom bothered the patient. Originally this instrument was called simply the "Discomfort Scale" because of its focus on bothersome symptoms. It was also the intent of this group to develop instruments for measuring disability and insight but only the symptom-oriented scale reached fruition. It came to be called the Hopkins Symptom Checklist (HSCL) and was the subject of what Derogatis et al. (1974) called a "programmatic sequence" of instrument improvements based largely on factor analytic studies.

Many of the early HSCL reports concerned patients described as "anxious neurotics." The subscale for somatization consisted mainly of the autonomic equivalents of anxiety. The psychometric properties of this scale were among the best achieved in terms of internal consistency, test–retest reliability, and correspondence with psychiatrists' assessments (Derogatis et al., 1971, 1972, 1974). In many ways, the somatization scale of the HSCL was similar to the Army's Neuropsychiatric Screening Adjunct (NSA), and its credentials seem to fit with what has been said about patients being highly aware of these symptoms and able to report accurately about them. However, the HSCL was not limited to somatization but included factors for anxiety, depression, obsessive–compulsive symptoms, and interpersonal sensitivity.

Indicative of the prominent role the HSCL has played is the fact that it was often used in the early drug trials that characterized the period when psychotropic medications were first being developed in the late 1950s and 1960s (Lipman et al., 1965; Rickels et al., 1971a; Covi et al., 1973). During this time, it was one of the most frequently used instruments in clinical research.

An important study regarding the evolution of instruments was a comparison of the HSCL with the General Health Questionnaire (GHQ) (Goldberg et al., 1976). There are several differences between these two instruments that might have led to their being poorly correlated. The language of the HSCL is much simpler than that of the GHQ; the HSCL does not have the focus on "change from usual state" that characterizes the GHQ; the HSCL covers the autonomic and vegetative signs more adequately than the GHQ; and the GHQ deals with social dysfunction more adequately than the HSCL. Despite the differences, the two instruments were quite highly correlated (0.78). This was another historical instance when two scales were administered to the same individuals and were found to be sufficiently correlated to suggest that a new instrument might be designed by taking the best features of each. This did not happen, however, and each kept to its separate track, with the HSCL never becoming as well-known internationally as the GHQ.

The evolution of the HSCL led to a 25-item version for use in Primary Care (Hesbacher et al., 1980). HSCL-25 consists of a factor for anxiety and one for depression. Somewhat longer versions were used in epidemiologic studies (Uhlenhuth et al., 1974; Mellinger et al., 1978). Data from a national study was used for one of the first demonstrations of applying a diagnostic algorithm based on DSM-III guidelines to a psychiatric scale (Uhlenhuth et al., 1983). This application resembled the work that led to the DPAX procedures for the Stirling County Study in that the algorithm required the presence of essential features, a minimum number of associated symptoms, and a minimum duration. Algorithmic assessment did not, however, become the standard procedure, and most HSCL studies continue to use a simple score and a cutting-point. Because of the simplicity of the HSCL language, it has been a good candidate for translation into other languages (Mollica et al., 1987), and recently the HSCL-25 was used for the first stage of the two-stage Norwegian investigation that employed the CIDI in its second stage (Sandanger et al., 1999b).

There have been a number of studies in which one of the short scales was compared to the Diagnostic Interview Schedule (DIS). One of these studies compared three scales that were among the most promising to screen for depression and anxiety disorders as identified by the DIS. The three chosen were the HSCL, the GHQ, and the Center for Epidemiologic Studies Depression Scale (CES-D). The results of this investigation indicated that the three scales were indistinguishable one from the other in terms of relationship to the DIS (Hough et al., 1990). Each performed similarly, and none perfectly.

The ultimate version of the Hopkins instrument is known now as the Symptom Checklist 90-items (SCL-90) (Derogatis et al., 1973). The SCL-90 covers a wider range of psychopathology than earlier versions. The additional factors concern hostility, phobic anxiety, paranoid ideation, and psychoticism. Many of the improvements embodied in the SCL-90 derive from further use of factor analysis to clarify the dimensional properties of psychopathology.

Some years after the launching of the HSCL, the Beck Depression Inventory (BDI) (Beck et al., 1961) and the Zung Depression Scale (Zung, 1963) were constructed in psychiatric settings. In each case, the focus was exclusively on depression and they reflect the growing attention on this disorder as antidepressant medications were developed and marketed. A version of the BDI has been prepared for use in primary care (Beck and Beck, 1972). The original BDI continues to be used extensively in studies carried out in psychiatric settings and, along with the Hamilton Rating Scale, is probably the best known to psychiatric residents of any of the psychiatric scales. In recent years, the program of national screening for depression in the United States has drawn heavily on both the BDI and the Zung (Baer et al., 2000).

The evolution of structured clinical interviews in the United States began at the same time as the advent of the Present State Examination (PSE) in the United Kingdom. In the United States, this line of development has been carried out by a group of psychiatric researchers at the New York Psychiatric Institute of Columbia University under the direction of Spitzer. Their first version was named the Mental Status Schedule (MSS) (Spitzer et al., 1967). Unlike the HSCL, the BDI, and the Zung, the intent of the MSS was to provide a schedule for systematic assessment by clinicians.

The next version was named the Psychiatric Status Schedule (PSS) (Spitzer et al., 1970). For its analysis, Spitzer and Endicott (1968, 1969) created a system of differential diagnosis to be carried out by a computerized set of algorithms. The computer programs were named DIAGNO. The PSS was used in the U.S./U.K. Diagnostic Project along with the PSE and helped produce the evidence that many of the diagnostic differences between the two countries disappeared when clinicians used a structured schedule (Cooper et al., 1972).

The U.S./U.K. Project offered several opportunities for clarification of nosological issues. One of these was the long-standing question about whether anxiety and depression can be differentiated. The PSE definition of anxiety involves a syndrome in which the autonomic hyperactivity and motor tension items are well represented while the PPS definition was more cognitive with a focus on anxious mood, worry, and feeling under strain. Zubin and Fleiss (1971) found that depression and anxiety were better discriminated by the PSE than by the PPS. This suggests that the autonomic indicators may contribute to distinguishing between the two syndromes despite the fact that the two syndromes are often comorbid. This point harkens back to what was said about the GHQ where anxiety is also represented mainly by cognitive expressions. It is possible, in other words, that the absence of autonomic features in the GHQ may underlie the fact that it was originally described as focusing on the general features of nonpsychotic disorders rather than their specific differentiation into the anxiety and depression components of nonpsychotic disorder.

Next the Columbia group produced the Schedule for Affective Disorders and Schizophrenia (SADS) (Endicott and Spitzer, 1978). Coupled with the Research Diagnostic Criteria (RDC) (Spitzer et al., 1978), this schedule played a special role in the developments that led to DSM-III and is therefore a fundamental part of the second landmark. As Chair of the American Psychiatric Association Task Force that produced DSM-III, Spitzer was in many regards the key architect of the new Manual. His experience in instrument development as well as in designing criteria for diagnosis contributed significantly to the work of the Task Force.

It has been mentioned that the use of the SADS in a community study contributed to the view that diagnostic schedules could be used for population-based epidemiology such as the ECA (Weissman et al., 1978; Regier et al., 1984). The most important study in which the SADS has been used, however, is the Psychobiology of Depression Study (Katz and Klerman, 1979; Keller et al., 1982; Coryell et al., 1984; Hirschfeld et al., 1986; Mueller et al., 1994; Solomon et al., 2000). This investigation continues to contribute useful information about the course and outcome of treated cases of depression.

Most of the diagnostic schedules, including the SADS, inquire about depression in the framework of its being an episodic illness. The Psychobiology of Depression study has emphasized, however, that empirical follow-up suggests that depression is often chronic and that the episodic features frequently emerge out of and return to a chronic base, as in double depression (Keller and Shapiro, 1982). The findings of this study contributed much of the evidence that led a former director of NIMH to comment that the most recent and important paradigm shift is the acceptance of unipolar MDD—Major Depressive Episode—as primarily a chronic rather than an acute illness (Judd, 1997).

After publication of DSM-III-R, Spitzer and colleagues produced the Structured Clinical Interview for DSM-III-R (SCID) (Spitzer et al., 1992). SCID has been assessed through a number of field trials (Williams et al., 1992), and versions for use among patients as well as nonpatients were created. Later, a version was designed to be congruent with DSM-IV (First et al., 1997). SCID has become the most commonly used schedule in US clinical studies (Swinson et al., 1992; Kendler and Roy, 1995; Zimmerman et al., 2000). SCID was designed more recently than the GHQ but rivals it in the number of citations shown in a Medline search.

Spitzer and colleagues have also prepared an instrument named Primary Care Evaluation of Mental Disorder (PRIME-MD) (Spitzer et al., 1994). Geared to DSM-III-R, PRIME-MD is a guide for general physicians to evaluate disorders frequently encountered in primary care settings: depression, anxiety, somatoform, alcohol and eating disorders. The recommended procedure is for the patient to respond to a one-page paper and pencil test that serves as a screen and determines which modules of the PRIME-MD the physician should administer. Subsequently, this group presented a revision that was entirely self-administered (Spitzer et al.,

1999). The self-report version was named the Patient Health Questionnaire (PHQ-S). In line with the growing attention to disability, both the PRIME-MD and the PHQ-S studies used the Short-Form 36-Items (SF-36) as a measure of functional status.

Epidemiologic Instruments: The United Kingdom

Studying large samples of the population by means of a structured instrument does not have as long a tradition in the United Kingdom as in the United States. Until recently only a few household surveys were carried out and they tended to focus on segments of the population such as women (Brown and Harris, 1978; Surtees et al., 1983) or residents of special housing areas (Taylor and Chave, 1964; Hare and Shaw, 1965). In the 1990s, however, a very large investigation was conducted and named the National Psychiatric Morbidity Surveys of Great Britain (Lewis et al., 1992; Meltzer et al., 1995; Jenkins et al., 1997a, b).

Like the national sample studies in the United States and Australia (Kessler et al., 1994a; Andrews et al., 2001), the Great Britain study involved a large carefully drawn sample and the use of lay interviewers to administer a structured interview. Like the ECA, it included a sample of institutions but, in addition, it included a sample of homeless persons. The British study differs from the national sample studies in the United States and Australia, however, by not using the CIDI. The decision to reject the CIDI was motivated primarily due to its length and reliance on complex questions that attempt to elicit information about psychopathology across the subject's whole life. Instead, the British group chose to revise the Clinical Interview Schedule (CIS) that, as mentioned earlier, had been prepared by the General Practice Research Unit (Goldberg et al., 1970).

The original CIS was intended to be used by psychiatrists for identifying the common disorders that are found in primary care and community settings (Lewis and Williams, 1989). The schedule consists of two halves. The first is based on self-report and is directed toward establishing the frequency, duration, and intensity of 10 groups of symptoms: somatic symptoms, fatigue, sleep disturbance, irritability, lack of concentration, depression, anxiety and worry, phobias, obsessions and compulsions, and depersonalization. The second half concerns manifest abnormalities and provides opportunity for the psychiatrist to record clinical observations about features such as agitation, defensiveness, and impaired intellectual functioning. When used as a validating standard in the assessment of the GHQ, the CIS did not give a diagnosis but rather a rating of severity along with a cutting-point to separate cases from noncases. The CIS approach was thus congruent with the GHQ focus on identifying general nonpsychotic disorder. In several other CIS studies, however, diagnostic information was provided by psychiatrists.

For the new study, the CIS was revised so that it could be administered by lay interviewers, and it was given the name Clinical Interview Schedule, Revised (CIS-R) (Lewis et al., 1992). The emphasis on general neurosis was retained, and in this regard it differs from both the DIS and the CIDI. As with its parent, the CIS-R uses a cutting-point to identify those who suffer from general neurotic psychopathology. Additional analytic routines allow, however, the application of diagnostic designations for generalized anxiety disorder, depressive episode, phobias, obsessive-compulsive disorders, panic disorder, and nonspecific neurotic disorder. The algorithms for identifying these diagnoses are based on ICD-10.

To avoid long-term recall, the time frame is the previous week, but subjects are asked to give the date of onset of key symptoms. The CIS-R is described as a bottom-up schedule that gathers information about the basic phenomena to which classification algorithms can be subsequently applied. This contrasts to instruments that build the classification rules into the questions as illustrated by the presence of the criteria for a minimum duration of two weeks in questions about the essential features of depression in the DIS and CIDI. The rationale for the CIS-R approach relates to the objective of conducting subsequent surveys for comparison over time when the specific criteria may be modified. The CIS-R is similar in this regard to the DPAX schedule used in the Stirling County Study where comparison over time has been a primary consideration.

In addition to using the CIS-R, a screening instrument for psychosis was developed for the survey, and those who scored positively were subsequently interviewed with the SCAN. Like most of the instruments designed before 1980, the CIS-R itself does not include a section on substance abuse. A separate schedule was therefore developed in order to give estimates of the prevalence of such disorders and their comorbidity with psychotic and neurotic disorders.

It is unknown at the present time whether or not researchers in other countries will elect to use the CIS-R. Nevertheless, a number of substantive reports have already been produced from the extensive database generated by this U.K. investigation (Lewis et al., 1998, Paykel et al., 2000; Weich et al., 2001).

RELIABILITY AND VALIDITY

Estimates of reliability and validity have been reported for all of the instruments. While there is voluminous information on these issues, none of it allows an unequivocable statement that, in its class, a given instrument is the best. The choice of an instrument depends, however, on the purpose of the investigation in which it will be used. For any epidemiologic study where the goal is to be able to draw comparisons about prevalence with other areas, the CIDI would obviously be the best choice because of the large amount of comparative data that will be available through the WMH2000 Project.

Other goals would dictate other choices but they should be made knowing that some issues about reliability and validity still remain unresolved. But at a level of abstraction that looks at the field as a whole over time, it is possible to offer some general conclusions about reliability and validity.

Symptom Scales

The reliability of scales is tested both for internal and test–retest consistency. Everything else being equal, internal consistency is higher when the scale contains a larger number of items. For scales that include 20 to 30 items, it has often been found that internal consistency measures at about 0.85 by Cronbach's *alpha* (1951). For longer scales, the values can easily go above 0.90. As far as can be determined, none of the scales has failed a test of this kind of consistency. The reason for such good performance is that most of the scales concentrate on depression and/or anxiety. There is some evidence that the two syndromes can be distinguished, but the presence of both depressive and anxious symptomatology in a scale does not appear to reduce internal consistency probably because the two syndromes are often affiliated with each other.

The picture of test–retest consistency is different because of variability in the amount of time between test and retest and in whether the scale seeks usual or unusual symptoms. In the initial assessment of the GHQ, which is the only scale that specifically calls for a change from the subject's normal condition through asking that symptoms be "more than usual" effort was made to insure that the person was in the same clinical condition at both the first and second test. Under those circumstances, the test–retest performance of the GHQ was excellent. However, in a less structured situation stemming from a primary care study, the one week test–retest coefficient was 0.44 and as such was one of the lowest reported for the scales (Duncan-Jones and Henderson, 1978). This suggests that if the instrument identifies a change from normality it will probably not take very long for the subject to return to normality. Bearing in mind that the GHQ was specifically designed so as to avoid identifying chronic disorders, its low retest coefficient might be considered desirable. On the other hand, it can be argued that the identification of time-limited episodes is not an appropriate target because such episodes, by their nature, disappear and probably do not require clinical intervention.

Where the other scales are concerned, the test–retest results tend to be well over 0.80 if the duration between tests is a month or less. Even for longer durations, the retest consistency is probably higher than most researchers would expect. In keeping with its goal of monitoring the course of illness during therapy, the HSCL asks about symptoms experienced over the recent week. Yet at 6 months, the HSCL was found to have a retest coefficient of 0.72 suggesting that the types of symptoms registered tend to be chronic (Rickels et al., 1971b). On the whole, then, test–retest consistency for the scales tends to be in line with the trend of recognizing depression as a chronic rather than a necessarily episodic disorder.

In regard to validity, most of the scales have been tested using some form of concurrent validity in contrast to predictive validity. Numerous examples exist of two or more scales being administered to the same subjects in order to test discriminant and convergent validity (Campbell and Fiske, 1959; Dinning and Evans, 1977; Radloff, 1977; Link and Dohrenwend, 1980). More weight has been attached, however, to validity tests that employ a clinical standard.

In the early part of this history, it was not uncommon to consider that a scale was validated if the responses of patients differed from presumed normals. This was followed by using as the criterion a clinical psychiatrist's judgment based on an unstructured interview. More recently validation studies have employed clinical judgment guided by a structured interview such as the SADS or the CIS.

On the whole, the greater the number of validation studies performed for a given scale, the greater the range of validity values. This indicates that a scale can be shown to perform both well and poorly if tested enough times under enough different circumstances. Also in general, the validity results have been better when the criterion standard is close to the intent of the scale. In so far as one scale can be separated out as having shown good validity credentials over several trials, it is the GHQ. Several of these trials employed the CIS as the standard. Because the CIS and GHQ embody similar orientations, the results illustrate the point that a scale performs better when the validating standard is in line with the scale's intent.

Lay-Administered Diagnostic Schedules

A diagnostic schedule does not lend itself to a test of internal consistency in the same manner as pertains when Cronbach's *alpha* is applied to a scale. This stems from the fact that the schedules focus on multiple, discrete diagnoses involving skip-outs. Because many subjects do not answer all the questions, it is not possible to calculate internal consistency in the conventional way. Grade of Membership (GOM) analysis has, however, been employed for a somewhat similar purpose. Among those who answered positively to a minimum number of DIS somatization questions, for example, GOM was used to see if the symptoms cluster empirically to support the clinical syndromes they were intended to measure, and encouraging results were reported (Swartz et al., 1986).

Because the DIS and CIDI deal with lifetime experience of illness, it is commonly expected that retest reliability should be very high. If the report of lifetime symptoms is accurate, symptoms reported in a first interview should not disappear by the time of the second interview, although new symptoms can be acquired. Problems about the reliability of lifetime recall were brought to attention when the SADS was used as a lay-administered schedule in a study that required a follow-up profile to be compared with a baseline profile (Bromet et al., 1986). Also where the DIS is concerned, the one-year follow-up of the ECA sample indicated that fewer lifetime symptoms were reported in the second compared to the initial administration (Robins, 1985). Now numerous reports have been presented giving evidence both for and against the accuracy of the lifetime approach.

Many of these tests of the reliability of lifetime reports focus on the ability of the subject to identify the same episode of illness in both interviews. This constitutes a very rigorous test because the subject needs to be reliable not only about the date of onset but also about all of the components of diagnosis: essential features, associated symptoms, duration, and disability. It can be appreciated that this type of test places a much greater burden on subject reliability than does test–retest reliability of a scale where consistency is based on similarity in the number and ordering of symptoms reported. It would be desirable if a test–retest examination could be designed for the diagnostic schedules that would focus exclusively on the stem questions that are asked of all subjects. This would give a middle ground reading on reliability that might help resolve the issues about reliability of lifetime recall. As far as can be determined, this type of test has not been carried out, and the reliability of lifetime recall constitutes one of the major methodologic issues with regard to diagnostic schedules.

Where the validity of diagnostic schedules is concerned, the typical strategy has been to compare the results of a lay-administered schedule with the results of a clinician-administered schedule. It has been suggested that such a strategy be referred to as *procedural validity* (Spitzer and Williams, 1980). Procedural validity refers to the congruence in results from two procedures designed to implement the same diagnostic criteria. It is not concerned with the validity of the criteria themselves. Reports on the procedural validity of lay-administered schedules have raised more questions than they have answered. This is partly because agreement has not been consistently good and has varied considerably by diagnosis as illustrated in the validity studies carried out for the ECA in Baltimore and in St. Louis for the DIS (Anthony et al., 1985; Helzer et al., 1985).

More than that, however, the results have called into question the value of clinical judgment as the "gold standard." In reviewing such validity information about the DIS, Robins (1985) pointed out that there was more variability in the clinical results across the two sites than there was according to the lay interviews. A similar test was made regarding the CIS in which the first half is devoted to self-reported symptoms and the second half to using clinical judgment about manifest abnormalities. It was found that there was more variability and less reliability where clinical judgment was used compared to self-report (Lewis and Williams, 1989).

From the first use of lay-administered schedules in epidemiological studies, questions have been raised about their validity because the resultant prevalence rates were perceived as unrealistically high. This perception was strengthened when the National Comorbidity Survey reported higher overall and diagnostic-specific rates than the other North American studies (Regier et al., 1998). In view of the high rates, it has been suggested that epidemiologic surveys might be identifying normal and transient reactions to stressful life events rather than clinical disorders. If clinicians were to examine the subjects, it was thought that they would be able to differentiate between normal and pathological reactions and would identify smaller numbers of subjects and therefore produce lower prevalence rates.

Two recent studies indicated, however, that prevalence rates based on clinician assessments about lifetime depression would be considerably higher than those based on lay-administered schedules. Both studies involved a design whereby community subjects were selected for a clinical interview based on the results of a lay-administered schedule. One of the studies was part of the longitudinal follow-up of the Baltimore ECA project where the DIS was compared to the SCAN (Eaton et al., 2000). The other was part of the Stirling County Study where the DPAX schedule as well as the DIS were compared to the SCID (Murphy et al., 2000c). In each, the clinicians identified a much larger number of cases than did the lay-interview methods. In each study, specificity was high but sensitivity was low. In other words, the clinicians rarely negated a case identified in the lay interviews but they identified many additional cases.

A different result appeared in a study that compared the lay-administered CIDI with the clinician-administered SCAN in the United Kingdom (Brugha et al., 2001). This investigation focused on the current clinical state in regard to both depression and anxiety. Unlike the North American investigations, estimated prevalence rates were somewhat lower when based on the SCAN than on the CIDI. It is possible that the emphasis on current in contrast to lifetime diagnosis contributed to the findings. It was noted, however, that many of the symptoms rejected as lacking sufficient severity by the clinician had been reported in the CIDI. This suggests that the application of clinical judgment in this study contributed to the lower prevalence rate.

These contradictory findings raise new questions. It will be important to gain further understanding of how clinical judgment functions in a structured interview and ultimately to determine if results from such an interview have greater prognostic value than one in which the focus is on providing an accurate record of what the subject says about symptoms in response to highly structured interviews.

Clinician-Administered Structured Interviews

The credentials of schedules like SCAN and SCID have mainly been limited to tests of inter rater reliability. This follows from the fact that most of the impetus for developing structured interviews grew out of evidence that psychiatrists frequently did not agree about what diagnosis characterized a given case. On the whole, inter-rater reliability for SCID and SCAN has been found to achieve acceptable levels.

Having largely solved the problem of the reliability of psychiatric diagnoses in the two decades since DSM-III was published, attention has been increasingly turning to issues of validity. The clinician-administered schedules have rarely been subjected to criterion validation because they are themselves often thought of as providing the "gold standard." In view of the continuingly unresolved questions about the validity of psychiatric diagnoses, the concept of a lead standard has been proposed (Spitzer, 1983). The "lead standard" draws upon Longitudinal evidence evaluated by a panel of Experts who have access to All available Data. The concept of a "lead standard" moves the focus away from concurrent validity to predictive validity through its emphasis on longitudinal information. It suggests that the validity of a diagnosis depends on the clinical outcome that follows from a given diagnosis rather than on the cross-sectional profile of clinical syndromes. Ultimately, diagnosis will need to be confirmed through knowledge about its etiology (what has come before the cross-sectional expression of symptoms) but until such knowledge becomes available, a useful way to confirm a diagnosis will be through knowledge about outcome (what comes after the cross-sectional expression of symptoms). In the final section of this chapter, the lead standard will be discussed in the context of future directions.

A CONTROVERSIAL ISSUE

In addition to concern about the reliability and validity of instruments, another issue that remains unresolved concerns the relative merits of dimensional versus categorical measurement. Those who favor dimensional approaches argue that most psychiatric disorders involve more than one dimension and that research can be more fruitfully conducted if the focus is on individual dimensions or traits rather than on their complex integration in a category. Those who support the use of dimensional measurement are often opposed to the dichotomies inherent in separating cases from noncases and distinguishing one diagnosis from another. They suggest that a "more or less" approach is truer to nature.

Diagnostic measurement implements a categorical approach in which effort is made to discover which syndromal pattern best describes the subject's disorder. Much of the criticism of the categorical approach relates to the fact that under the influence of hierarchical classification, effort was made to use one and only one diagnostic category. Inherent in the hierarchical approach was the goal of using the most informative of all the possible categories which pertain. For example, if a patient exhibited four syndromal patterns (schizophrenia, alcohol abuse, depression and anxiety), it was customary to use only schizophrenia. A major achievement of the ECA was demonstrating the pervasiveness of multiple categories (Boyd et al.,1984). This has led to recognizing the value of relaxing exclusionary criteria in situations where hiding such comorbidity should be avoided.

With the publication of DSM-III, diagnostic measurement largely replaced the dimensional approach in psychiatric epidemiology. Now researchers are beginning to question whether research needs, especially those of genetic studies, are being adequately served by commitment to categorical assessment. Such questions formed the theme of the Annual Meeting of the American Psychopathological Association in 2000. In explaining the selection of this theme, the Association's President wrote "We have made great strides in creating categorical definitions of psychopathology that can be applied reliably. Paradoxically, genetics and other contemporary research made possible by reliable diagnoses calls into question the adequacy of a strictly categorical system" (Helzer, 2000). Several of the presentations at this meeting dealt with the limitations of the diagnostic model and the need to explore new approaches or to revive old approaches.

It is important to be aware, however, that continuous versus categorical may be a false dichotomy. Psychiatric scales involve continuous measurement, but they are routinely converted to categorical statements by the application of a cutting-point. Also categorical assessment, insofar as it involves algorithmic steps, almost always involves some dimensional features. Creative use of combinations of the two approaches may offer some resolution of these controversies.

A comparison and evaluation of the two approaches can be illustrated through an experiment involving Receiver Operating Characteristic (ROC) Analysis (Swets et al., 1979; Hanley and McNeil, 1983). The illustration draws on materials from the Stirling County Study where the DPAX schedule incorporates the HOS scale. Figure 2 shows an ROC analysis of the two bodies of data (Murphy et al.,1987). The standard for assessment in this illustration consists of agreed-upon decisions provided by teams of two psychiatrists who read the results of the research protocol in order to determine who should be counted as a case of depression and/or anxiety and who not.

ROC analysis produces a curve based on the calculation of all possible sensitivity and specificity values as the threshold is moved across the score range. The value named Area Under the Curve (AUC) is a statistical assessment of the congruence between the test and the standard. If the sensitivity and specificity values track across the line of no information, it means that the test is unable to discriminate the ill from the well as identified by the standard. The more the curve arches toward the upper left corner, the better the test.

The continuous scoring of the HOS gave a curve that arches well above the line of no information, indicating that the test provided information that was useful to the psychiatrists. With a low score of only two symptoms, everyone who was judged to be a case was identified and sensitivity was perfect. As the threshold was moved from low to high scores, sensitivity deteriorated while specificity became perfect. When the threshold was set at the highest possible score, everybody judged not to be a case was excluded. While the AUC value for this curve was significantly different from the line of no information, it needs to be emphasized that, in this curve and in all such curves based on continuous scoring, a constant relationship

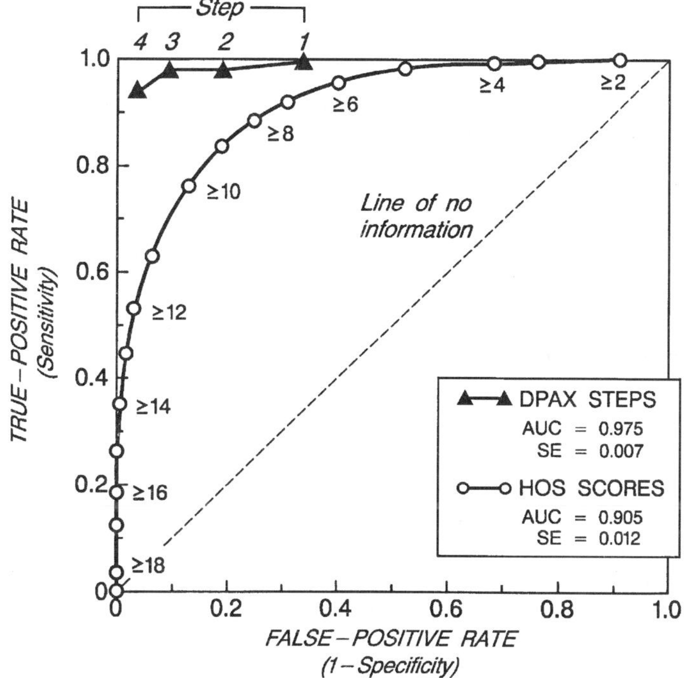

Figure 2. Receiver Operating Cuvce (ROC) analysis for continuous and categorical scoring. DPAX (DP standing for depression and AX for anxiety) is a schedule that uses a computer program consisting of four steps that implement a categorical algorithm for diagnosis (Murphy et al., 1985). HOS (Health Opinion Survey) is a continuously scored sychiatric scale (Macmillan, 1957). These instruments were developed as part of the Stirling County Study, a longitudinal investigation of psychiatric epidemiology. The ROC analysis of these scoring procedures was first reported by Murphy et al. (1987).

between sensitivity and specificity pertains. If the threshold is raised to improve specificity, there is an automatic loss in sensitivity.

The ROC curve for the DPAX program involved four steps. The first step was the application of discriminant function coefficients which were tested in split-half designs and by application to samples other than the test sample. The discriminant function results were based on using all HOS items but with heavy weighting of the items for the essential features of depression and/or anxiety. This first step captured everyone who exhibited the essential features and who had an appreciable amount of associated symptomatology. The second step established that the essential features were present; the third applied criteria for impairment and duration; and the fourth established that the symptoms were sufficiently intense and frequent to warrant clinical recognition.

The curve indicated that the first step cast a wide net identifying virtually everyone who could possibly be a case, and then with each successive step, the mesh was tightened by the application of more criteria. Accordingly, the algorithm began with high sensitivity and then improved specificity without serious loss of sensitivity. By the fourth step, the program had 92% sensitivity and 98% specificity based on the standard utilized. These values did not, in and of themselves, imply validity because the standard was not independent of the test material. They did, however, give an image of the thought processes involved in reaching a categorical decision. In implementing the thought process by computer algorithms, cutting-points on continuous dimensions were employed. For example, the items for essential features constituted a dimension as did the items for associated symptoms. Duration is inherently a dimension, and the concept of a minimum duration illustrates the application of a cutting-point on a continuum.

Earlier it was mentioned that the CIS-R and DPAX schedules are similar in that a series of structured questions are asked of all subjects and, depending on the responses, other questions are asked for the purpose of applying diagnostic criteria. It is possible that application of ROC analysis to the two parts of the CIS-R would generate curves similar to the continuous and categorical ones shown in Figure 2 for DPAX.

On the other hand, if the results of the DIS and CIDI were to provide a curve for their categorical approach that would give comparable evidence of maintaining sensitivity without loss of specificity, it is clear that the stem questions would need to provide almost perfect sensitivity. This follows from the fact that the response to a stem question serves either to initiate the rest of the module or to skip-out and the skip-out means that the subject cannot be given that particular diagnosis.

To achieve nearly perfect sensitivity for a stem, it is probable that several questions would need to be asked on the stem's theme. It can be appreciated that if the essential features of a syndrome need to be registered in a response to only one question, the burden of sensitivity for that question is very heavy. A series of questions would yield greater potential for achieving the necessary level of sensitivity. At the same time, the availability of several questions would provide an array of idioms about the theme so that subjects would have several options for revealing that they had experienced the central feature of a syndrome and should therefore be asked the rest of the questions about that syndrome. The symptom scales provide models for what is meant by an array in that they ask questions about dysphoria using such diverse idioms as "down in the dumps," "downhearted." "blue," "in poor spirits," "depressed and sad," and the like. Such a series would constitute the basis for a continuous score on which a cutting-point could be applied for the first categorical step of a diagnostic algorithm. Where depression is concerned, the evolution of the CIDI has moved away from having only one question for the essential features to having one question for dysphoria and another question for anhedonia. It is possible that an even larger array would be beneficial.

SUMMARY AND CONCLUSIONS

Considerable progress was made over the past 50 years in psychiatric measurement but improvement is still needed. In the following points, major achievements are outlined and suggestions are offered regarding ways in which progress might be carried even further.

Interdisciplinary Collaboration

The history of instrumentation began with psychologists and sociologists taking the more formative role. For the first half of the period, most psychiatrists stood aside and viewed these developments with skepticism. The reasons for their distance were multiple and complex. They included the influence of psychodynamic psychiatry, doubt that asking questions was enough, and belief that nonpsychiatrists were unable to interpret answers accurately or to perceive the nuances of facial expression and body movement that are necessary for an adequate psychiatric work-up.

There is no doubt that visual information about appearance and comportment contributes to a psychiatric assessment. The time may come when the process of observation will achieve sufficient standardization by both lay and clinical interviewers to be useful in epidemiologic research. But that approach is not yet on the horizon. Similarly with biological markers. The time may also come when they will have been identified and proven sufficiently accurate and efficient to be used in large-scale studies. But that approach is also not yet on the horizon. The face-to-face interview or some other form of question and answer interaction (by paper and pencil, telephone, or computer) remains the most useful mode of gathering data.

Measurement Strategies and Reliability

Major advances in the question and answer approach were achieved when clinical criteria, such as now exist in the DSM and the ICD, became foremost as guides for the formulation of questions. There were, however, some losses. Psychometric principles tended to be ignored as did also the principles of survey methodology. These principles are beginning to re-emerge as additional guides for helping the subject give as accurate a report as possible about psychiatric experiences.

The concept of a psychiatric syndrome is at the heart of the classification systems of DSM and ICD. By nature categorical, the syndrome is either present or absent, or more accurately it is complete enough to say that it is present or sufficiently incomplete to warrant saying it is not. There are numerous aspects of syndrome recognition, however, that draw on dimensional models. It is possible that dimensions will play a stronger role in measurement strategies of the future than they do now, especially if they can be seen to heighten the value of certain kinds of research.

A question raised in this chapter is whether there is any future role for scales *per se*. It seems exceedingly unlikely that scales will be entirely eclipsed by schedules. Instruments such as the CES-D and the GHQ continue to be used in numerous studies where assessment of the current clinical state is needed. Where assessment of disability is desirable, scales will also prevail. Disability is not like a syndrome; it does not have an essential feature but rather is a multifaceted continuum. As more attention is paid to disability, the scales that have done a good job of measuring it, such as the social dysfunction factor in the scaled GHQ and the impairment parts of the SF-36, are likely to be increasingly called upon in and of themselves and as models for further scale development.

If two-stage designs become more common, a scale will be a natural candidate for the first stage. In referring to two-stage designs, however, a word of caution is in order. As more is learned about the psychiatric profiles of subjects who refuse an interview, it becomes increasingly compelling to avoid subject attrition. Incompleteness of data is one of the serious problems faced by psychiatric epidemiology at the present time, and two-stage designs are more subject to its perils than are single-stage investigations.

A feature of the diagnostic schedules that needs further thought concerns the use of lifetime recall. There is evidence of international tension on this point. The schedules developed in the United Kingdom (PSE and CIS-R) focus on the current clinical state. The U.S. and WHO schedules (DIS and CIDI) elicit information about lifetime experiences. The lifetime approach in psychiatric epidemiology appeared about the same time as an upsurge in genetic research in which lifetime population norms were needed for family studies. With the changing face of genetic research, as it moves away from family studies toward molecular studies, the need and rationale for lifetime rates may recede. Thus it deserves thought as to whether psychiatric instrumentation would be able to take important steps forward in reliability if assessment of the current clinical state became the first order of inquiry.

Reliability is fostered when the subject comprehends the interview situation and is well motivated to give accurate answers. Both psychometric theory and survey experience suggest that the best ways to reduce misunderstanding on the part of the subject and to decrease error and variability on the part of interviewers is to provide clear instructions and use simple language (Choi and Comstock, 1975; Nunnally and Bernstein, 1994). The diagnostic schedules may need to give increased attention to these principles and to carry out procedures for the reduction of complexity.

Validity

The major challenges that lie ahead for both lay and clinician interviews have to do with validity. New questions have been raised by the fact that the use of well-recognized clinical interviews (SCID and SCAN) in epidemiologic studies gave considerably higher rates of depression than did lay interviews. The clinical approach did not invalidate the lay results, as was expected, but rather the clinicians indicated that the lay-administered schedules missed numerous cases.

Many of the questions asked by clinicians were the same as those asked by lay interviewers. This raises the problem of whether use of a question-oriented "gold standard" provides an adequate test of validity. Campbell and Fiske (1959, p 83) emphasize that validity depends upon using independent and different information: "Reliability is the agreement between two efforts to measure the same trait through maximally similar methods. Validity is represented in the agreement between two attempts to measure the same trait by maximally different methods."

Given the fact that the interviews involved similar questions, the differences must result from features other than the questions asked. What is maximally different about them? Do clinicians ask the same questions in a different manner from lay interviewers? Do subjects answer the same question with a different response when interviewed by a clinician? Do clinicians interpret the same response to the same question in ways that are distinctively different from the record of the response left by a lay interviewer. It would be useful if research could be carried out in which clinicians studied their own interviews side-by-side with the accompanying lay interviews in order to suggest reasons for the difference, especially as it may involve interpretation. Such research could be useful in sharpening the questions and format of a lay interview or it might point to inferences on the part of clinicians that are unwarranted.

Evidence suggests that schedules like SCID and SCAN have achieved the objective of reliability when applied in clinical settings. In such settings, it is a matter of determining what kind of diagnosis is pertinent rather than whether the person is a case or not. In community settings, the situation may be sufficiently different that a different kind of approach will be needed. Over and above investigation of interpretative differences when the same questions are asked, efforts at validation need to seek materials that are genuinely dissimilar from the question and answer format.

Such material may reside in the "lead standard" mentioned earlier as involving longitudinal assessment by a panel of clinical experts who have access to all available data (Spitzer, 1983). The lead standard has been employed to assess certain CIDI diagnoses in a clinic-based study. A group of psychiatrists (the "panel of experts") who had known the patients over considerable time provided consensus diagnoses that agreed well with the CIDI results (Peters and Andrews, 1995). Given the fact that many people in the community who suffer a psychiatric disorder do not seek treatment for it, another type of application of the "lead standard" may be needed. For example, it may be possible to use prospective evidence about the course and outcome of illness identified by structured lay interviews to confirm or reject the diagnosis.

There are, as yet, only a few longitudinal population studies that have employed a diagnostic schedule that can be put to such a test. Some evidence has, however, been given by the Stirling County Study through the DPAX schedule (Murphy, 1995). At the time of the first survey in 1952, the prevalence of acute and chronic depression according to the DPAX schedule was 5% of the adult population using a sample of 1003 subjects. At that time, there was very little difference in the rates for men and women, with women having only a slightly higher rate. Over the first sixteen years of the longitudinal study, the prognosis for these depressed subjects was poor. Depressed men, none of whom had comorbid alcohol abuse, were found to have experienced twice the expected number of deaths. Depressed women did not have a significantly elevated mortality rate but one of them had committed suicide. Among those who survived, three-fourths had a poor clinical outcome. The majority of the men remained chronically depressed while it was more typical of the women to remain ill but with anxiety becoming the prominent diagnostic feature. For both men and women, there was evidence of continuing and increasing impairment in everyday functioning.

These results have not yet been replicated in similar longitudinal studies, and the second half of the Stirling County Study has not yet been analyzed in this regard. Nevertheless, the findings do *not* support the view that transient and normal reactions are being identified as illness in epidemiologic surveys. Rather these findings appear to offer support for the view that asking questions about symptoms and disability in the community has considerable validity as a method for identifying disorders that have the same characteristics of morbidity and mortality that are seen in clinically identified cases of serious disorder.

Three Landmarks

Each of three landmarks influenced the course of instrument development and, in turn, the use of these instruments has thrown light on the issues raised. The first landmark indicated that the prevalence of psychiatric disorders among those recruited to serve in the armed forces was higher than expected, but it was unknown whether this magnitude should be estimated as 1 in 40, or 1 in 20, or what. The answer provided, where such instruments have been used in epidemiologic studies of general populations in North America and Europe, has an impressive amount of consistently across time and place. It puts overall prevalence at approximately 1 in 5.

The second landmark joined clinical and epidemiologic psychiatry together around the diagnostic standards of DSM-III. Using these standards, the diagnostic schedules opened the door to better understanding of the different types of disorders that make up the yearly overall rate of 1 in 5. For example, numerous studies suggest that about a quarter of the overall rate is composed of people suffering either from a major episode of depression or from a chronic dysthymia. The mandate embodied in the President's Commission ushered in a period when the questions about psychiatric symptoms were asked of larger and larger samples, thus giving a firmer basis for generalization. While these aspects of the second landmark took place mainly in the United States, it was becoming increasingly apparent that psychiatric disorders were found in all parts of the world where studies had been carried out. Collaborative work with WHO soon laid the foundation for extending the use of instruments across diverse cultures.

The third landmark drew attention to the fact that the burden of disability carried by many types of psychiatric disorders is exceedingly heavy. The work of the third landmark is going on now, and one of its clearest messages is that the application of question and answer techniques can no longer be limited to North America and Europe. The perspective must be global and the techniques need to be adapted for studies in all parts of the world.

The impact of the three landmarks led to research in which the scales and schedules described here have shown that psychiatric disorders are common, diverse in character, widely distributed, and heavily burdensome.

ACKNOWLEDGMENT

This chapter is based on a course taught at the Harvard School of Public Health. From 1987 through 1999, the course was titled "Psychiatric Screening and Diagnostic Tests" after which the title was changed to "Psychiatric Diagnosis in Clinic and Community Populations." The chapter also draws on a report prepared for the National Institute of Mental Health under contract 80M014280101D titled "Psychiatric Instrument Development for Primary Care Research: Patient Self-Report Questionnaire," 1981. In addition, the chapter draws on materials from the Stirling County Study through NIMH Grant R01 MH39576.

REFERENCES

American Psychiatric Association (1952): "Diagnostic and Statistical Manual," 1st ed. Washington, DC: American Psychiatric Association.

American Psychiatric Association (1980): "Diagnostic and Statistical Manual of Mental Disorders," 3rd ed. Washington, DC: American Psychiatric Association.

American Psychiatric Association (1987): "Diagnostic and Statistical Manual of Mental Disorders," 3rd ed. Revised. Washington, DC: American Psychiatric Association.

American Psychiatric Association (1994): "Diagnostic and Statistical Manual of Mental Disorders," 4th ed. Washington, DC: American Psychiatric Association.

Andrews G, Henderson S, Hall W (2001): Prevalence, comorbidity, disability and service utilisation: Overview of the Australian National Mental Health Survey. Br J Psychiatry 178:145–153.

Andrews G, Peters L (1998): The psychometric properties of the Composite International Diagnostic Interview. Soc Psychiatry Psychiatr Epidemiol 33:80–88.

Anthony JC, Folstein M, Romanoski AJ, Von Korff MR, Nestadt GR, Chahal R, Merchant A, Brown CH, Shapiro S, Kramer M, Gruenberg EM (1985): Comparison of the lay Diagnostic Interview Schedule and a standardized psychiatric diagnosis: Experience in eastern Baltimore. Arch Gen Psychiatry 42:667–675.

Arocho R, McMillan CA (1998): Discriminant and criterion validation of the US-Spanish version of the SF-36 Health Survey in a Cuban-American population with benign prostatic hyperplasia. Med Care 36:766–772.

Arthur RJ, Gunderson EKE, Richardson JW (1966): The Cornell Medical Index as a mental health survey instrument in the naval population. Milit Med 131:605–610.

Baer L, Jacobs DG, Meszler-Reizes J, Blais M, Fava M, Kessler R, Magruder K, Murphy J, Kopans B, Cukor P, Leahy L, O'Laughlen J (2000): Development of a brief screening instrument: The HANDS. Psychother Psychosom 69:35–41.

Bebbington P, Hurry J, Tennent C, Sturt E, Wing JK (1981): Epidemiology of mental disorders Camberwell Psychol Med 11:561–579.

Beck AT, Beck RW (1972): Screening depressed patients in family practice: A rapid technique. Postgrad Med 52:81–85.

Beck AT, Ward CH, Mendelsohn M, Mock J, Erbaugh J (1961): An inventory for measuring depression. Arch Gen Psychiatry 4:561–571.

Berkman LF, Berkman CS, Kasl S, Freeman DH, Leo L, Ostfeld AM, Cornoni-Huntley J, Brody JA (1986): Depressive symptoms in relation to physical health and functioning in the elderly. Am J Epidemiol; 124:372–388.

Bland RC, Newman SC, Orn H (eds) (1988): Epidemiology of psychiatric disorders in Edmonton. Acta Psychiatr Scand (Suppl 338) 77:1–80.

Blouin AG, Perez EL, Blouin JM (1987): Computerized administration of the Diagnostic Interview Schedule. Psychiatry Res 23:335–344.

Boyd JH, Burke JD, Gruenberg E, Holzer CE, Rae DS, George LK, Karno M, Stoltzman R, McEvoy L, Nestadt G (1984): Exclusion criteria of DSM-III: A study of co-occurrence of hierarchy-free syndromes. Arch Gen Psychiatry 41:983–989.

Breslau N, Kessler R, Peterson EL (1998): Post-traumatic stress disorder assessment with a structured interview: reliability and concordance with a standardized clinical interview. Int J Methods in Psychiatric Research 7:121–127.

Brodman K, Erdmann AJ, Lorge I, Deutschberger J, Wolff, HG (1954): The Cornell Medical Index–Health Questionnaire. VII. The prediction of psychosomatic and psychiatric disabilities in army training. Am J Psychiatry 111:37–40.

Brodman K, Erdman AJ, Lorge I, Irving C, Wolff H (1952): The Cornell Medical Index–Health Questionnaire. IV. The recognition of emotional disturbances in a general hospital. J Clin Psychol 8:289–293.

Brodman K, Erdmann AJ, Lorge I, Wolff HG (1949): The Cornell Medical Index: An adjunct to medical interview. JAMA 140:530–534.

Bromet EJ, Dunn LO, Connell MM, Dew MA, Schulberg HC (1986): Long-term reliability of diagnosing lifetime major depression in a community sample. Arch Gen Psychiatry 43:435–440.

Brown GW, Harris T (1978): "Social Origins of Depression: A Study of Psychiatric Disorder in Women." New York: The Free Press.

Bruce ML, Takeuchi DT, Leaf PJ (1991): Poverty and psychiatric status: longitudinal evidence from the New Haven Epidemiologic Catchment Area Study. Arch Gen Psychiatry 48:470–474.

Brugha TS, Jenkins R, Taub N, Meltzer H, Bebbington PE (2001): A general population comparison of the Composite International Diagnostic Interview (CIDI) and the Schedules for Clinical Assessment in Neuropsychiatry (SCAN). Psychol Med 31:1001–1013.

Campbell DT, Fiske DW (1959): Convergent and discriminant validation by the multitrait–multimethod matrix. Psychol Bull 56:81–105.

Cassano GB, Banti S, Mauri M, Dell'osso L, Miniati M, Maser JD, Shear MK, Frank E, Grochocinski V, Rucci P (1999): Internal consistency and discriminant validity of the Structured Clinical Interview for Panic Agoraphobic Spectrum (SCI-PAS). Int J Methods in Psychiatric Research 8:138–145.

Choi IC, Comstock GW (1975): Interviewer effect on responses to a questionnaire relating to mood. Am J Epidemiol 101:81–92.

Comstock GW, Helsing KJ (1976): Symptoms of depression in two communities. Psychol Med 6:551–563.

Cooper JE, Kendell RE, Gurland BJ, Sharpe L, Copeland JRM, Simon R (1972): "Psychiatric Diagnosis in New York and London." London: Oxford University Press.

Cooper JE, Oates M (2000): The principles of clinical assessment in general psychiatry. In Gelder MG, Lopez-Ibor JJ, Andreasen NC (eds): "New Oxford Textbook of Psychiatry." Oxford: Oxford University Press, pp. 71–87.

Coryell W, Endicott J, Reich T, Andreasen N, Keller M (1984): A family study of bipolar II disorder. Br J Psychiatry 145:49–54.

Cottler LB, Robins LN, Grant BF, Blaine J, Towle LH, Wittchen H-U, Sartorius N and Participants in the WHO/ADAMHA Field Trial (1991): The CIDI-core substance abuse and dependence questions: cross-cultural and nosological issues. Br J Psychiatry 159:653–658.

Covi L, Lipman RS, Pattison JH, Derogatis LR, Uhlenhuth EH (1973): Length of treatment with anxiolytic sedatives and response to their sudden withdrawal. Acta Psychiatr Scand 49:51–64.

Cronbach LJ (1951): Coefficient alpha and the internal structure of tests. Psychometrika 16:297–334.

Dahlstrom WG, Welsh GS, Dahlstrom LE (1972): "An MMPI Handbook," Vol.I. "Clinical Interpretation." Minneapolis: University of Minnesota Press.

Derogatis LR, Lipman RS, Covi L (1973): SCL-90: An outpatient psychiatric rating scale, preliminary report. Psychopharmacol Bull 9:13–28.

Derogatis LR, Lipman RS, Covi L, Rickels K (1971): Neurotic symptom dimensions: as perceived by psychiatrists and patients of various social classes. Arch Gen Psychiatry 24:454–464.

Derogatis LR, Lipman RS, Covi L, Rickels K (1972): Factorial invariance of symptom dimensions in anxious and depressive neuroses. Arch Gen Psychiatry 27:659–665.

Derogatis LR, Lipman RS, Rickels K, Uhlenhuth EH, Covi L (1974): The Hopkins symptom checklist (HSCL): A self-report symptom inventory. Behav Science 19:1–15.

Dinning WD, Evans RG (1977): Discriminant and convergent validity of the SCL-90 in psychiatric inpatients. J Pers Assess 41:304–310.

Dohrenwend BP, Crandell DL (1970): Psychiatric symptoms in community, clinic, and mental hospital groups. Am J Psychiatry 126:87–97.

Dohrenwend BP, Dohrenwend BS (1965): The problem of validity in field studies of psychological disorder. J Abnormal Psychol 70:52–69.

Dohrenwend BP, Dohrenwend BS (1969): "Social Status and Psychological Disorder: A Causal Inquiry." New York: Wiley-Interscience.

Dohrenwend BP, Dohrenwend BS (1982): Perspectives on the past and future of psychiatric epidemiology: The 1981 Rema Lapouse Lecture. Am J Public Health 72:1271–1279.

Dohrenwend BP, Dohrenwend BS, Gold MS, Link B, Neugebauer R, Wunsch-Hitzig R (1980a): "Mental Illness in the United States: Epidemiological Estimates." New York: Praeger Publishers.

Dohrenwend BP, Levav I, Shrout PE (1986): Screening scales from the Psychiatric Epidemiology Research Interview (PERI) In Weissman MM, Myers JK, Ross CE (eds): "Community Surveys of Psychiatric Disorders." New Brunswick, NJ: Rutgers University Press, pp 349–375.

Dohrenwend BP, Levav I, Shrout PE, Schwartz S, Guedalia N, Link BG, Skodol AE, Stueve A (1992): Socioeconomic status and psychiatric disorders: The causation–selection issue. Science 255:946–952.

Dohrenwend BP, Shrout PE, Egri G, Mendelsohn FS (1980b): Nonspecific psychological distress and other dimensions of psychopathology. Arch Gen Psychiatry 37:1229–1236.

Duncan-Jones P, Henderson S (1978): The use of a two-phase design in a prevalence survey. Soc Psych 13:231–237.

Eastwood MR, Trevelyan MH (1972): Relationship between physical and psychiatric disorder. Psychol Med 2:363–372.

Eaton WW, Holzer CE, Von Korff M, Anthony JC, Helzer JE, George L, Burnam MA, Boyd JH, Kessler LG, Locke BZ (1984): The design of the Epidemiologic Catchment Area surveys: The control and measurement of error. Arch Gen Psychiatry 41:942–948.

Eaton WW, Neufeld K, Chen LS, Cai G (2000): Comparison of self-report and clinical diagnostic interviews for depression: Diagnostic Interview Schedule and Schedules for Clinical Assessment in Neuropsychiatry in the Baltimore Epidemiologic Catchment Area Follow-up. Arch Gen Psychiatry 57: 217–222.

Endicott J, Spitzer RL (1978): A diagnostic interview: The Schedule for Affective Disorders and Schizophrenia. Arch Gen Psychiatry 35:837–844.

Eysenck HJ (1947): "Dimensions of Personality." London: Routledge and Kegan Paul Ltd.

Eysenck HJ, Eysenck SBG (1975): Eysenck Personality Questionnaire. San Diego, CA:: Educational and Industrial Testing Service.

Farmer AE, Katz, R, McGuffin P, Bebbington, P (1987): A comparison between the Present State Examination and the Composite International Diagnostic Interview. Arch Gen Psychiatry 44:1064–1068.

Feighner JP, Robins E, Guze SB, Woodruff RA, Winokur G, Munoz R (1972): Diagnostic criteria for use in psychiatric research. Arch Gen Psychiatry 26:57–63.

Fennig S, Bromet E (1992): Commentary: issues of memory in the Diagnostic Interview Schedule J Nerv Ment Dis 180:223–224.

First MB, Gibbon M, Spitzer RL, Williams JBW, Smith L (1997): "Structured Clinical Interview for DSM-IV Personality Disorders." Washington, DC: American Psychiatric Press.

Frank JD (1974): Psychotherapy: the restoration of morale. Am J Psychiatry 131:271–274.

Freedman DX (1978): The President's Commission: realistic remedies for neglect. Pragmatic next steps—not a trip. Arch Gen Psychiatry 35:675–676.

Furukawa TA, Goldberg DP, Rabe-Hesketh S, Üstün TB (2001): Stratum-specific likelihood ratios of two versions of the General Health Questionnaire. Psychol Med 31: 519–529.

Giuffra LA, Risch N (1994): Diminished recall and the cohort effect of major depression: a simulation study. Psychol Med 24:375–383.

Goering P, Lin E, Campbell D, Boyle MH, Offord DR (1996): Psychiatric disability in Ontario. Can J Psychiatry 41:564–571.

Goldberg DP (1972): "The Detection of Psychiatric Illness by Questionnaire: A Technique for the Identification and Assessment of Non-Psychotic Psychiatric Illness." London: Oxford University Press.

Goldberg DP, Cooper B, Eastwood MR, Kedward HB, Shepherd M (1970): A standardized psychiatric interview for use in community surveys. Br J Prev Soc Med 24:18–23.

Goldberg DP, Hillier VF (1979): A scaled version of the General Health Questionnaire. Psychol Med 9:139–145.

Goldberg DP, Rickels K, Downing R, Hesbacher P (1976): A comparison of two psychiatric screening tests. Br J Psychiatry 129:61–67.

Goldberg DP, Simpson N (1995): Personal Health Questionnaire, described in Rizzo et al., 2000.

Goodman WK, Price LH, Rasmussen SA, Mazure C, Fleischmann ML, Hill CL, Heninger GR, Charney DS (1989): The Yale-Brown Obsessive-Compulsive Scale, I: Development, use, and reliability. Arch Gen Psychiatry 46:1006–1011.

Gove WR, McCorkel J, Fain T, Hughes MD (1976): Response bias in community surveys of mental health: Systematic bias or random noise? Soc Sci Med 10:497–502.

Guilford S (1936): "Psychometric Methods." New York: McGraw-Hill.

Gurin G, Veroff J, Feld S (1960): "Americans View Their Mental Health: A Nationwide Interview Survey." Monograph No. 4, Joint Commission on Mental Illness and Health. New York: Basic Books.

Hambleton RK, Swaminathan H (1985): "Item Response Theory." Boston: Kluwer-Nijoff.

Hamilton M (1960): A rating scale for depression. J Neurol Neurosurg Psychiatry 23:57–62.

Hanley JA, McNeil BJ (1983): A method of comparing the areas under Receiver Operating Characteristic Curves derived from the same cases. Radiology 148:839–843.

Hare EH, Shaw GK (1965): "Mental Health on a New Housing Estate: A Comparative Study of Health in Two Districts in Croydon." London: Oxford University Press.

Healy D (1997): "The Antidepressant Era." Cambridge, MA: Harvard University Press.

Helzer JE (2000): President's Letter to the members of the American Psychopathological Association announcing the theme of the 1999–2000 annual meeting.

Helzer JE, Canino GJ (1992): "Alcoholism in North America, Europe, and Asia." New York: Oxford University Press.

Helzer JE, Robins LN, Croughan JL, Weiner A (1981): Renard Diagnostic Interview: Its reliability and procedural validity with physicians and lay interviewers. Arch Gen Psychiatry 38:393–398.

Helzer JE, Robins LN, McEvoy LT, Spitznagel EL, Stoltzman RK, Farmer A, Brockington IF (1985): A comparison of clinical and Diagnostic Interview Schedule Diagnoses: Physician reexamination of the lay-interviewed cases in the general population. Arch Gen Psychiatry 42:657–666.

Henderson S, Duncan-Jones P, Byrne DG, Scott R, Adcock S (1979): Psychiatric disorder in Canberra: A standardized study of prevalence. Acta Psychiatr Scand 60;355–374.

Hesbacher PT, Rickels K, Morris RJ, Newman H, Rosenfeld H (1980): Psychiatric illness in family practice. J Clin Psychiatry 41:6–10.

Hirschfeld RMA, Klerman GL, Andreasen NC, Clayton PJ, Keller MB (1986): Psycho-social predictors of chronicity in depressed patients. Br J Psychiatry 148:648–654.

Holzer CE, Shea BM, Swanson JW, Leaf PJ, Myers JK, George L, Weissman MM, Bednarski P (1986): The increased risk for specific psychiatric disorders among persons of low socioeconomic status. Am J Soc Psychiatry 6:259–271.

Horton NJ, Laird NM, Murphy JM, Monson RR, Sobol AM, Leighton AH (2001): Multiple informants: Mortality associated with psychiatric disorders in the Stirling County Study. Am J Epidemiol 154:649–656.

Hough RL, Landsverk JA, Jacobson GF (1990): The use of psychiatric screening scales to detect depression in primary care patients. In Attkisson CC, Zich JM (eds): "Depression in Primary Care: Screening and Detection." New York: Routledge.

Jablensky A, Schwarz R, Tomov T (1980): WHO collaborative study on impairments and disabilities associated with schizophrenic disorders. Acta Psychiatr Scand (Suppl 285) 62:152–163.

Jenkins R, Bebbington P, Brugha T, Farrell M, Gill B, Lewis G, Meltzer H, Petticrew M (1997a): The National Psychiatric Morbidity Survey of Great Britain—strategy and methods. Psychol Med 27:765–774.

Jenkins R, Lewis G, Bebbington P, Brugha T, Farrell M, Gill B, Meltzer H (1997b): The National Psychiatric Morbidity Surveys of Great Britain—initial findings from the Household Survey. Psychol Med 27:775–789.

Johnson PA, Goldman L, Orav EJ, Garcia T, Pearson SD, Lee TH (1995): Comparison of the Medical Outcomes Study Short-Form 36-Item Health survey in black patients and white patients with acute chest pain. Med Care 33:145–160.

Judd LL (1997): Commentary: The clinical course of unipolar major depressive disorders. Arch Gen Psychiatry 54:989–990.

Katz MM, Klerman GL (1979): The Psychobiology of Depression NIMH Clinical Research Branch Collaborative Program: Introduction: Overview of the clinical studies program. Am J Psychiatry 136:49–51.

Keller MM, Shapiro RW (1982): Double depression: superimposition of acute depressive episodes on chronic depressive disorders. Am J Psychiatry 139:438–442.

Keller MM, Shapiro RW, Lavori PW, Wolfe N (1982): Relapse in major depressive disorder: Analysis with the life table. Arch Gen Psychiatry 39:911–915.

Kendler KS, Roy MA (1995): Validity of a diagnosis of lifetime major depression obtained by personal interview versus family history. Am J Psychiatry 152:1608–1614.

Kessler R, Andrews G, Mroczek D, Üstün B, Wittchen H-U (1998b): The World Health Organization Composite International Diagnostic Interview Short-Form (CIDI-SF). Int J Methods in Psychiatric Research 7:171–185.

Kessler RC, Foster CL, Saunders WB, Stang PE (1995): Social consequences of psychiatric disorders, I: Educational attainment. Am J Psychiatry 152:1026–1032.

Kessler RC, Frank RG, Edlund M, Katz SJ, Lin E, Leaf P (1997): Differences in the use of psychiatric outpatient services between the United States and Ontario. N Engl J Med 336:551–557.

Kessler RC, McGonagle KA, Nelson CB, Hughes M, Swartz M, Blazer DG (1994b): Sex and depression in the National Comorbidity Survey, II: Cohort effects. J Affect Disord 30:15–26.

Kessler RC, McGonagle KA, Zhao S, Nelson CB, Hughes M, Eshleman S, Wittchen HU, Kendler KS (1994a): Lifetime and 12-month prevalence of DSM-III-R psychiatric disorders in the United States: results from the National Comorbidity Survey. Arch Gen Psychiatry 51:8–19.

Kessler R, Wittchen H-U, Abelson J, McGonagle K, Schwarz N, Kendler KS, Knäper B, Zhao S (1998a): Methodological studies of the Composite International Diagnostic Interview (CIDI) in the National Comorbidity Survey (NCS). Int J Methods in Psychiatric Research 7:33–55.

Klerman GL (1978): Affective Disorders. In Nicholi AM (ed): "The Harvard Guide to Modern Psychiatry." Cambridge, MA: The Belknap Press of the Harvard University Press.

Langner TS (1962): A twenty-two item screening score of psychiatric symptoms indicating impairment. J Health Hum Behav 3:269–276.

Lapouse R (1967): Problems in studying the prevalence of psychiatric disorder. Am J Public Health 57:947–954.

Leavitt HC (1946): A comparison between the Neuropsychiatric Screening Adjunct (NSA) and the Cornell Selectee Index (Form N). Am J Psychiatry 103:353–357.

Leighton AH (1959): "My Name Is Legion: The Stirling County Study of Psychiatric Disorder and Sociocultural Environment," Vol I. New York: Basic Books, Inc.

Leighton DC, Harding JS, Macklin DB, Hughes CC, Leighton AH (1963b): Psychiatric findings of the Stirling County Study. Am J Psychiatry 119:1021–1026.

Leighton DC, Harding JS, Macklin DB, Macmillan AM, Leighton AH (1963a): "The Character of Danger: The Stirling County Study of Psychiatric Disorder and Sociocultural Environment," Vol. III. New York: Basic Books, Inc.

Levav I, Arnon A, Portnoy A (1977): Two shortened versions of the Cornell Medical Index—A new test of their validity. Int J Epidemiol 6:135–141.

Lewis A (1970): The ambiguous word "anxiety." Int J Psychiatry 9:62–67.

Lewis G, Bebbington P, Brugha T, Farrell M, Gill B, Jenkins R, Meltzer H (1998): Socioeconomic status, standard of living, and neurotic disorder. Lancet 352:605–609.

Lewis G, Pelosi AJ, Araya R, Dunn G (1992): Measuring psychiatric disorder in the community: A standardized assessment for use by lay interviewers. Psychol Med 22:465–486.

Lewis G, Williams P (1989): Clinical judgement and the standardized interview in psychiatry. Psychol Med 19:971–979.

Li C, Johnson NP, Leopard K (2001): Risk factors for depression among adolescents living in group homes in South Carolina. J Health Soc Policy 13:41–59.

Link B, Dohrenwend BP (1980): Formulation of hypotheses about the true prevalence of demoralization in the United States. In Dohrenwend BP, Dohrenwend BS, Gould MS, Link B, Neugebauer R, Wunsch-Hitzig R: "Mental Illness in the United States: Epidemiological Estimates." New York: Praeger Press, pp 114–132.

Lipman RS, Cole JO, Park LC, Rickels K (1965): Sensitivity of symptom and nonsymptom: Focused criteria of outpatient drug efficacy. Am J Psychiatry 122:24–27.

Lipman RS, Rickels K, Covi L, Derogatis LR, Uhlenhuth EH (1969): Factors of symptom distress: Doctor ratings of anxious neurotic outpatients. Arch Gen Psychiatry 21:328–338.

Loranger AW, Sartorius N, Andreoli A, Berger P, Buchheim P, Channabasavanna SM, Coid B, Dahl A, Diekstra RFW, Ferguson B, Jacobsberg LB, Mombour W, Pull C, Ono Y, Regier DA (1994): "The International Personality Disorder Examination: The World Health Organization/Alcohol Drug Abuse, and Mental Health Administration Pilot Study of Personality Disorders." Arch Gen Psychiatry 51:215–224.

Lorr M, Jenkins RC et al. (1952): "The Multidimensional Scale for Rating Psychiatric Patients." Washington, DC, Hospital Form, Veterans Administration Technical Bulletin 43:10–507.

Lyketsos CG, Hoover DR, Guccione M, Dew MA, Wesch J, Bing EG, Treisman GJ (1996): Depressive symptoms over the course of HIV infection before AIDS. Soc Psychiatry Psychiatr Epidemiol 31:212–219.

Macmillan AM (1957): The Health Opinion Survey: Technique for estimating prevalence of psychoneurotic and related types of disorders in communities. Psychol Rep 3:325–339.

Manis JG, Brawer MJ, Hunt CL, Kercler LC (1964): Estimating the prevalence of mental illness. Am Sociol Rev 29:84–89.

Mari JJ, Williams P (1984): Minor psychiatric disorder in primary care in Brazil: A pilot study. Psychol Med 14:223–237.

Markush RE, Favero RV (1974): Epidemiologic assessment of stressful life events, depressed mood, and psychophysiological symptoms: A preliminary report. In Dohrenwend BS, Dohrenwend BP (eds): "Stressful Life Events: Their Nature and Effects." New York: Wiley, pp 171–190.

McDowell I, Newell C (1996). "Measuring Health: A Guide to Rating Scales and Questionnaires" 2nd ed. New York: Oxford University Press.

McHorney CA, Ware JE, Raczek AE (1993): The MOS 36-Item Short-Form Health Survey (SF-36): II. Psychometric and clinical tests of validity in measuring physical and mental health constructs. Med Care 31:247–263.

Meehl PE, Hathaway SR (1946): The K factor as a suppressor variable in the MMPI. J Appl Psychol 30:525–564.

Mellinger GD, Balter MB, Manheimer DI, Cisin JH, Parry HJ (1978): Psychic distress, life crisis, and use of psychotherapeutic medications: National household survey data. Arch Gen Psychiatry 35:1045–1052.

Meltzer H, Gill B, Petticrew M. Hinds K (1995): "Morbidity in Great Britain: The Prevalence of Psychiatric Morbidity among Adults Living in Private Households." London: Her Majesty's Stationery Office (HMSO).

Mollica RF, Wyshak G, de Marneffe D, Khuon F, Lavelle J (1987): Indochinese versions of the Hopkins Symptom Checklist-25: A screening instrument for the psychiatric care of refugees. Am J Psychiatry 144:497–500.

Mueller TI, Lavori PW, Keller MB, Swartz A, Warshaw M, Hasin D, Coryell W, Endicott J, Rice J, Akiskal H (1994): Prognostic effect of the variable course of alcoholism on the 10-year course of depression. Am J Psychiatry 151:701–706.

Muncie W (1963): Depression or depressions. Can Psychiatr Assoc J 8:217–224.

Murphy JM (1981): "Psychiatric Instrument Development for Primary Care Research: Patient Self-Report Questionnaire." Monograph prepared for National Institute of Mental Health Contract 80M014280101D, pp 1– 253.

Murphy JM (1986): Diagnosis, screening, and "demoralization": Epidemiologic implications. Psychiatr Develop 2:101–133.

Murphy JM (1990): Depression screening instruments: History and issues. In Attkisson CC, Zich JM (eds): "Depression in Primary Care: Screening and Detection." New York: Routledge, Chapman and Hall, pp 65–83.

Murphy JM (1993): The psychiatric survey in epidemiologic research: Some findings from the Stirling County Study. Presentation for the Rema Lapouse Award, Mental Health Section, American Public Health Association.

Murphy JM (1995): What happens to depressed men? Harvard Rev Psychiatry 3:47–49.

Murphy JM, Berwick DM, Weinstein MC, Borus JF, Budman SH, Klerman GL (1987): Performance of screening and diagnostic tests: Application of Receiver Operating Characteristic (ROC) analysis. Arch Gen Psychiatry 44:550–555.

Murphy JM, Laird NM, Monson RR, Sobol AM, Leighton AH (2000b): Incidence of depression in the Stirling County Study: Historical and comparative perspectives. Psychol Med 30:505–514.

Murphy JM, Monson RR, Laird NM, Sobol AM, Leighton AH (1998): Identifying depression in a forty-year epidemiologic investigation: The Stirling County Study. Int J Methods in Psychiatric Research 7:89–109.

Murphy JM, Monson RR, Laird NM, Sobol AM, Leighton AH (2000c): A comparison of diagnostic interviews for depression in the Stirling County Study: Challenges for psychiatric epidemiology. Arch Gen Psychiatry 57:230–236.

Murphy JM, Monson RR, Laird NM, Sobol AM, Leighton AH (2000a): A forty-year perspective on the prevalence of depression from the Stirling County Study. Arch Gen Psychiatry 57:209–215.

Murphy JM, Neff RK, Sobol AM, Rice JX, Olivier DC (1985): Computer diagnosis of depression and anxiety: The Stirling County Study. Psychol Med 15:99–12.

Murphy JM, Olivier DC, Monson RR, Sobol AM, Federman EB, Leighton AH (1991): Depression and anxiety in relation to social status: A prospective epidemiologic study. Arch Gen Psychiatry 48:223–229.

Murphy JM, Olivier DC, Monson RR, Sobol AM, Leighton AH (1988): Incidence of depression and anxiety: The Stirling County Study. Am J Public Health 78:534–540.

Murphy JM, Sobol AM, Neff RK, Olivier DC, Leighton AH (1984): Stability of prevalence: Depression and anxiety disorders. Arch Gen Psychiatry 41:990–997.

Murray CJL, Lopez AD (1996): "The Global Burden of Disease: A Comprehensive Assessment of Mortality and Disability from Diseases, Injuries, and Risk Factors in 1990 and Projected to 2020." Boston: Harvard School of Public Health, World Health Organization and the World Bank.

Myers JK, Lindenthal JJ, Pepper MP (1971): Life events and psychiatric impairment. J Nerv Ment Dis 152:149–157.

Nunnally JC, Bernstein IH (1994): "Psychometric Theory," 3rd ed. New York: McGraw-Hill.

Offord DR, Boyle MH, Campbell D, Goering P, Lin E, Wong M, Racine YA (1996): One-year prevalence of psychiatric disorder in Ontarians 15 to 64 years of age. Can J Psychiatry 41:559–563.

Overall JE, Gorham DR (1962): The Brief Psychiatric Rating Scale. Psychol Rep 10:799–812.

Parloff MB, Kelman HC, Frank JD (1954): Comfort, effectiveness, and self-awareness as criteria of improvement in psychotherapy. Am J Psychiatry 111:343–351.

Paykel ES (1971): Classification of depressed patients: A cluster analysis derived grouping. Br J Psychiatry 118:275–288.

Paykel ES, Abbott R, Jenkins R, Brugha TS, Meltzer H (2000): Urban–rural mental health differences in Great Britain: Findings from the National Morbidity Survey. Psychol Med 30: 269–280.

Peters L, Andrews G (1995): Procedural validity of the computerized version of the Composite International Diagnostic Interview (CIDI-Auto) in the anxiety disorders. Psychol Med 25:1269–1280.

Phillips DL (1966): The "true prevalence" of mental illness in a New England state. Community Ment Health J 2:35–40.

Piccinelli M, Bisoffi G, Bon MG, Cunico L, Tansella M (1993): Validity and test–retest reliability of the Italian version of the 12-item General Health Questionnaire in general practice: A comparison between three scoring methods. Compr Psychiatry 34:198–205.

Plake BS, Impara JC (eds) (2001): "The Fourteenth Mental Measurements Yearbook." Lincoln, Nebraska: Buros Institute of Mental Measurements.

President's Commission on Mental Health (1978): "Report to the President," Vol. I. Washington DC: United States Government Printing Office.

Prince RH, Miranda L (1977): Monitoring life stress to prevent recurrence of coronary heart disease episodes. Can J Psychiatry 22:161–169.

Prince RH, Mombour W, Shiner EV, Roberts J (1967): Abbreviated techniques for assessing mental health in interview surveys: An example from central Montreal. Laval Médical 38:58–62.

Radloff LS (1977): The CES-D Scale: A self-report depression scale for research in the general population. Appl Psychol Measurement 1:385–401.

Reed V, Gander F, Pfister H, Steiger A, Sonntag H, Trenkwalder C, Sonntag A, Hundt W, Wittchen H-U (1998): To what degree does the Composite International Diagnostic Interview (CIDI) correctly identify DSM-IV disorders? Testing validity issues in a clinical sample. Int J Methods in Psychiatric Research 7:142–154.

Regier DA, Kaelber CT, Rae DS, Farmer ME, Knauper B, Kessler RC, Norquist GS (1998): Limitations of diagnostic criteria and assessment instruments for mental disorders: Implications for research and policy. Arch Gen Psychiatry 55:109–115.

Regier DA, Myers JK, Kramer M, Robins LN, Blazer DG, Hough RL, Eaton WW, Locke BZ (1984): The NIMH Epidemiologic Catchment Area (ECA) Program: Historical context, major objectives and study population characteristics. Arch Gen Psychiatry 41:934–941.

Rickels K, Garcia CR, Fisher E (1971b): A measure of emotional distress in private gynecologic practice. Obstet Gynecol 38:139–146.

Rickels K, Lipman RS, Park LC, Covi L, Uhlenhugh EH, Mock JE (1971a): Drug, doctor warmth, and clinic setting in the symptomatic response to minor tranquilizers. Psychopharmacologia 20:128–152.

Rizzo R, Piccinelli M, Mazzi MA, Bellantuono C, Tansella M (2000): The Personal Health Questionnaire: A new screening instrument for detection of ICD-10 depressive disorders in primary care. Psychol Med 30:831–840.

Roberts RE, Forthofer RN, Fabrega H (1976): The Langner items and acquiescence. Soc Sci Med 10:69–75.

Robins LN (1978): Psychiatry epidemiology. Arch Gen Psychiatry 35:697–702.

Robins LN (1985): Epidemiology: Reflections on testing the validity of psychiatric interviews. Arch Gen Psychiatry 42:918–924.

Robins LN, Helzer JE, Croughan J, Ratcliff KS (1981): National Institute of Mental Health Diagnostic Interview Schedule: Its history, characteristics and validity. Arch Gen Psychiatry 38:381–389.

Robins LN, Regier DA (eds) (1991): "Psychiatric Disorders in America: The Epidemiologic Catchment Area Study." New York: The Free Press.

Robins LN, Wing J, Wittchen HU, Helzer JE, Babor TF, Burke J, Farmer A, Jablenski A, Pickens R, Regier DA, Sartorius N, Towle, LH (1988): The Composite International Diagnostic Interview. Arch Gen Psychiatry 45:1069–1077.

Rogers B, Mann SA (1986): The reliability and validity of PSE assessments by lay interviews: A national population survey. Psychol Med 16:689–700.

Rogler LH, Malgady RG, Tryon WW (1992): Evaluation of mental health: Issues of memory in the Diagnostic Interview Schedule. J Nerv Ment Dis 180:215–222.

Rorer LG (1965): The great response-style myth. Psychol Bull 63:129–156.

Rosenthal SH (1966): Changes in a population of hospitalized patients with affective disorders. Am J Psychiatry 6:671–681.

Rubio-Stipec M, Canino G, Robins LN, Wittchen HU, Sartorius N, Torres De Miranda C and Participants in the WHO/ADMHA Field Trials (1993): The somatization schedule of the Composite International Diagnostic Interview: The use of the probe flow chart in 17 different countries. Int J Methods in Psychiatric Research 3:129–136.

Salek S (1998): "Compendium of Quality of Life Instruments." New York: Wiley.

Sandanger I, Moum T, Ingebrigtsen G, Sorensen T, Dalgard OS, Bruusgaard D (1999b): The meaning and significance of caseness: The Hopkins Symptom Checklist-25 and the Composite International Diagnostic Interview II. Soc Psychiatry Psychiatr Epidemiol 34:53–59.

Sandanger I, Nygård JF, Ingebrigtsen G, Sørensen T, Dalgard OS (1999a): Prevalence, incidence rate and age at onset of psychiatric disorders in Norway. Soc Psychiatry Psychiatr Epidemiol 34:570–579.

Sartorius N, Üstün TB, Costa e Silva J-A, Goldberg D, Lecrubier Y, Ormel J, Von Korff M, Wittchen H-U (1993): An international study of psychological problems in primary care. Arch Gen Psychiatry 50:819–824.

Schmitz N, Kruse J, Tress W (1999): Psychometric properties of the General Health Questionnaire (GHQ-12) in a German primary care sample. Acta Psychiatr Scand 100:462–468.

Schwab JJ, Bell RA, Warheit GJ, Schwab RB (1979): "Social Order and Mental Health: The Flordia Health Study." New York: Brunner/Mazel.

Seiler LH (1973): The 22-Item Scale used in field studies of mental illness: A question of method, a question of substance, and a question of theory. J Health Soc Behav 14:252–264.

Shader RI, Ebert MH, Harmatz JS (1971): Langner's Psychiatric Impairment Scale: A short screening device. Am J Psychiatry 128:596–601.

Shepherd M, Cooper B, Brown AC, Kalton G (1966): "Psychiatric Illness in General Practice." London: Oxford University Press.

Simon GE, von Korff M, Rutter CM, Peterson DA (2001): Treatment process and outcomes for managed care patients receiving new antidepressant prescriptions from psychiatrists and primary care physicians. Arch Gen Psychiatry 58:395–401.

Simon GE, von Korff M, Üstün TB, Gater R, Gureje O, Sartorius N (1995): Is the lifetime risk of depression actually increasing? J Clin Epidemiol 48:1109–1118.

Singer E, Cohen SM, Garfinkel R, Srole L (1976): Replicating psychiatric ratings through multiple regression analysis: The Midtown Manhattan Restudy. J Health and Soc Behavior 17: 376–387.

Solomon DA, Keller MB, Leon AC, Mueller TI, Lavori PW, Shea T, Coryell W, Warshaw M, Turvey C, Maser JD, Endicott J (2000): Multiple recurrences of major depressive disorder. Am J Psychiatry 157:229–233.

Spitzer RL (1983): Psychiatric diagnosis: are clinicians still necessary? In Williams JBW, Spitzer RL (eds): "Psychotherapy Research: Where Are We and Where Should We Go?" New York: Guilford Press, pp 273–292.

Spitzer RL, Endicott J (1968): DIAGNO I: A computer program for psychiatric diagnosis utilizing the differential diagnostic procedure. Arch Gen Psychiatry 18:746–756.

Spitzer RL, Endicott J (1969): DIAGNO II: Further developments in a computer program for psychiatric diagnosis. Am J Psychiatry 125:12–21.

Spitzer RL, Endicott J, Fleiss JL, Cohen J (1970): The Psychiatric Status Schedule: A technique for evaluating psychopathology and impairment in role functioning. Arch Gen Psychiatry 23:41–55.

Spitzer RL, Endicott J, Robins E (1978): Research Diagnostic Criteria: Rationale and reliability. Arch Gen Psychiatry 35:773–782.

Spitzer RL, Fleiss JL, Endicott J, Cohen J (1967): Mental Status Schedule: Properties of factor-analytically derived scales. Arch Gen Psychiatry 16:479–493.

Spitzer RL, Kroenke K, Williams JBW (1999): Validation and utility of a self-report version of PRIME-MD: The PHQ Primary Care Study. JAMA 282:1737–1744.

Spitzer RL, Williams JBW (1980): Classification in psychiatry. In: Kaplan HL, Freedman AM, Sadock BJ (eds): "Comprehensive Textbook of Psychiatry." Baltimore, Williams & Wilkins, pp 1035–1050.

Spitzer RL, Williams JBW, Gibbon M, First MB (1992): The Structured Clinical Interview for DSM-III-R (SCID). 1: History, rationale, and description. Arch Gen Psychiatry 49:624–629.

Spitzer RL, Williams JBW, Kroenke K, Linzer M, deGruy FV, Hahn SR, Brody D, Johnson JG (1994): Utility of a new procedure for diagnosing mental disorders in primary care: The PRIME-MD 1000 Study. JAMA 272:1749–1756.

Srole L, Fischer AK (1980a): The Midtown Manhattan Longitudinal Study vs 'The Mental Paradise Lost' doctrine. Arch Gen Psychiatry 37:209–221.

Srole L, Fischer AK (1980b): To the editor: Debate on psychiatric epidemiology. Arch Gen Psychiatry 37:1421–1423.

Srole L, Fischer AK (1980c): To the editor. Arch Gen Psychiatry 37:1423–1426.

Srole L, Langner TS, Michael ST, Opler MK, Rennie TAC (1962): "Mental Health in the Metropolis: The Midtown Manhattan Study." New York: McGraw-Hill.

Star SA (1950): The screening of psychoneurotics in the army: Technical development of tests. In Stouffer SA, Guttman L, Suchman EA, Lazarsfeld PF: "Measurement and Prediction." Princeton: Princeton University Press, pp 486–547.

Stewart AL, Hays RD, Ware JE (1988): The MOS Short-form General Health Survey: Reliability and validity in a patient population. Med Care 26:724–732.

Stouffer SA, Guttman L, Suchman EA, Lazarsfeld PF, Star SA, Clausen JA (1950): "The American Soldier: Measurement and Prediction," Vol. IV. Princeton: Princeton University Press.

Surtees PG, Dean C, Ingham JG, Kreitman NB, Miller PM, Sashidaran SP (1983): Psychiatric disorder among women from an Edinburgh community: Associations with demographic factors. Br J Psychiatry 142:238–246.

Swartz MS, Blazer DG, Woodbury MA,George LK, Landerman R (1986): Somatization disorder in a US Southern community: Use of a new procedure for analysis of medical classification. Psychol Med 16:595–609.

Swets JA, Pickett RM, Whitehead SF, Getty DJ, Schnur JA, Swets JB, Freeman BA (1979): Assessment of diagnostic technologies: Advanced measurement methods are illustrated in a study of computed tomography of the brain. Science 205:754–759.

Swinson RP, Soulios C, Cox BJ, Kuch K (1992): Brief treatment of emergency room patients with panic attacks. Am J Psychiatry 149:944–946.

Tarlov AR, Ware JE, Greenfield S, Nelson EC, Perrin E, Zubkoff M (1989): The Medical Outcomes Study: An application of methods for monitoring the results of medical care. JAMA 262:925–930.

Taylor L, Chave S (1964): "Mental Health and Environment." London: Longmans Green.

Teitelbaum L, Mullen B (2000): The validity of the MAST in psychiatric settings: A meta-analytic integration. J Stud Alcohol 61:254–261.

Thompson C (ed) (1989): "The Instruments of Psychiatric Research." New York: Wiley.

Tousignant M, Denis G, Lachapelle R (1974): Some considerations concerning the validity and use of the Health Opinion Survey. J Health Soc Behav 15:241–252.

Tsuang MT, Winokur G (1975): The Iowa 500: Field work in a 35-year follow-up of depression, mania, and schizophrenia. Can Psychiatr Assoc J 20:359–365.

Tsuang MT, Woolson RF, Simpson JC (1980): The Iowa Structured Psychiatric Interview: Rationale, reliability and validity. Acta Psychiatr Scand (Suppl) 283:58pp.

Uhlenhuth EH, Lipman RS, Balter MB, Stern M (1974): Symptom intensity and life stress in the city. Arch Gen Psychiatry 31:759–764.

Uhlenhuth EH, Balter MB, Mellinger GD, Cisin IH, Clinthorne J (1983): Symptom checklist syndromes in the general population: Correlations with psychotherapeutic drug use. Arch Gen Psychiatry 40:1167–1173.

Üstün TB, Tien AY (1995): Recent developments for diagnostic measures in psychiatry. Epidemiol Rev 17:210–220.

Veroff J, Douvan E., Kulka RA (1981a): "The Inner American: A Self-Portrait from 1957 to 1976." New York: Basic Books.

Veroff J, Kulka RA, Douvan E (1981b): "Mental Health in America: Patterns of Help-Seeking from 1957 to 1976." New York: Basic Books.

Von Korff M, Shapiro S, Burke JD, Teitlebaum M, Skinner EA, German P, Turner RS, Klein L, Burns B (1987): Anxiety and depression in a primary care clinic: Comparison of Diagnostic Interview Schedule, General Health Questionnaire, and practitioner assessments. Arch Gen Psychiatry; 44:152–156.

Ware JE, Sherbourne CD (1992): The MOS 36-item short-form health survey (SF-36): 1. Conceptual framework and item selection. Med Care 30:473–483.

Washington University in St. Louis (2002): Diagnostic Interview Schedule for Diagnostic Statistical Manual, 4th rev. DIS-IV Innovations. Available at http://epi.wustl.edu/dis/dishome.htm.

Weich S, Lewis G, Jenkins SP (2001): Income inequality and the prevalence of common mental disorders in Britain. Br J Psychiatry 178: 222–237.

Weider A, Mittelmann B, Wechsler D, Wolff HG (1944): The Cornell Selectee Index: A method for quick testing of selectees for the armed forces. JAMA 124:224–228.

Weissman MM, Bland RC, Canino GJ, Faravelli C, Greenwald S, Hwu HG, Joyce PR, Karam EG, Lee CK, Lellouch J, Lépine JP, Newman SC, Rubio-Stipect M, Wells JE, Wickramaratne PJ, Wittchen HU, Yeh EK (1996): Cross-national epidemiology of major depression and bipolar disorder. JAMA 276:293–299.

Weissman MM, Klerman GL (1978): Epidemiology of mental disorders: Emerging trends in the United States. Arch Gen Psychiatry 35:705–712.

Weissman MM, Klerman GL (1980a): Letter to the editor: Psychiatric nosology and the Midtown Manhattan Study. Arch Gen Psychiatry 37:229–230.

Weissman MM, Klerman GL (1980b): In reply. Arch Gen Psychiatry; 37:1423–1424.

Weissman MM, Myers JK, Harding PS (1978): Psychiatric disorders in a US urban community: 1975-1976. Am J Psychiatry 135:459–462.

Weissman MM, Myers JK, Harding PS (1977): Assessing depressive symptoms in five psychiatric populations: A validation study. Am J Epidemiol 106:203–214.

Weissman MM, Sholomskas D, Pottenger M, Prusoff BA, Locke BH (1977): Assessing depressive symptoms in five psychiatric populations: A validation study. Am J Epidemiol 106:203–214.

Wells KB, Stewart A, Hays RD, Burnam A, Rogers W, Daniels M, Berry S, Greenfield S, Ware J (1989): The functioning and well-being of depressed patients: Results from the Medical Outcomes Study. JAMA 262:914–919.

Williams JBW, Gibbon M, First MB, Spitzer RL, Davies M, Borus J, Howes MJ, Kane J, Pope HG, Rounsaville B, Wittchen HU (1992): The Structured Clinical Interview for DSM-III-R (SCID): II. Multisite test–retest reliability. Arch Gen Psychiatry 49:630–636.

Wing JK, Babor T, Brugha T, Burke J, Cooper JE, Giel R, Jablenski A, Regier D, Sartorius N (1990): SCAN: Schedules for Clinical Assessment in Neuropsychiatry. Arch Gen Psychiatry 47:589–593.

Wing JK, Birley JLT, Cooper JE, Graham P, Isaacs A (1967): Reliability of a procedure for measuring and classifying "present psychiatric state." Br J Psychiatry 113:499–515.

Wing JK, Cooper JE, Sartorius N (1974): "Measurement and Classification of Psychiatric Symptoms: An Instruction Manual for the PSE and Catego Program." London: Cambridge University Press.

Wing JK, Mann SA, Leff JP, Nixon JM (1978): The concept of a "case" in psychiatric population surveys. Psychol Med 8:203–217.

Wing JK, Sartorius N, Üstün TB (eds) (1998). "Diagnosis and Clinical Measurement in Psychiatry: A Reference Manual for SCAN." New York, Cambridge University Press.

Wittchen H-U (1994): Reliability and validity studies of the WHO-Composite International Diagnostic Interview (CIDI): A critical review. J Psychiat Res 28:57–84.

Wittchen H-U, Burke JD, Semler G, Pfister H, Von Cranach M, Zaudig M (1989): Recall and dating of psychiatric symptoms: Test–retest reliability of time-related symptom questions in a standardized psychiatric interview. Arch Gen Psychiatry 46:437–443.

Wittchen H-U, Höfler M, Gander F, Pfister H, Storz S, Üstün B, Müller N, Kessler RC (1999): Screening for mental disorders: Performance of the Composite International Diagnostic Screener (CID-S). Int J Methods in Psychiatric Research 8:59–70.

Wittchen H-U, Robins LN, Cottler LB, Sartorius N, Burke JD, Regier D and Particpants in the Multicentre WHO/ADAMHA Field Trials (1991): Cross-cultural feasibility, reliability and sources of variance of the Composite International Diagnostic Interview (CIDI). Br J Psychiatry 159:645–653.

World Health Organization (1973): "International Pilot Study of Schizophrenia." Geneva: World Health Organization.

World Health Organization (1977): "Manual of the International Statistical Classification of Diseases, Injuries, and Causes of Death," 9th rev. Geneva: World Health Organization.

World Health Organization (1992): "International Statistical Classification of Diseases and Related Health Problems," 10th rev. (ICD-10). Geneva, World Health Organization.

World Health Organization (1997): "Composite International Diagnostic Interview," Version 2.1. Geneva: World Health Organization.

World Health Organization (2000): "The World Mental Health 2000 Study" (WMH2000). Geneva, World Health Organization.

Zimmerman M, McDermut W, Mattia JI (2000): Frequency of anxiety disorders in psychiatric outpatients with major depressive disorder. Am J Psychiatry 157:1337–1340.

Zubin J, Fleiss J (1971): Current biometric approaches to depression. in Fieve R (ed): "Depression in the 1970's: Modern Theory and Research." Princeton, Excerpta Medica, pp 7–19.

Zung WWK (1963): A self-rating depression scale. Arch Gen Psychiatry 12:63–70.

CHAPTER 13

DSM-IV and Psychiatric Epidemiology

MICHAEL B. FIRST
New York State Psychiatric Institute, New York, N.Y. 10032

INTRODUCTION

A major component of many (if not most) psychiatric epidemiological investigations is the psychiatric diagnosis of the population being studied. Clearly, the task of determining the prevalence of psychiatric illness in a population depends on having reliable well-operationalized definitions of the disorders. Furthermore, the task of gleaning associations between possible causative factors and illness is impossible without clear and consistent methods of classifying and diagnosing the psychiatric conditions. Before the introduction of DSM-III in 1980 (American Psychiatric Association, 1980), psychiatric epidemiology was severely constrained by the lack of a widely accepted and reliable system of diagnosis that could be applied in community studies. The availability of DSM-III, and the subsequent development of a fully structured diagnostic interview based on it [i.e., the Diagnostic Interview Schedule (Robins et. al., 1981)] was a critical component of the Epidemiological Catchment Area (ECA) Study (Regier et al., 1984) and for subsequent studies of the prevalence of psychiatric disorders in the community.The purpose of this chapter is to explore the ways in which the DSM-IV classification may impact on the methods and results of epidemiological studies. We first review the historical background behind the development the DSM-IV classification (American Psychiatric Association, 1994) and then describe its impact on psychiatric epidemiology.

HISTORICAL BACKGROUND

There are three aspects of the DSM that have proved most valuable to advancing the methodologies of psychiatric epidemiology. First is the widespread acceptance of the DSM classification among all sectors of the fields of psychiatry, psychology, and social work as the *de facto* standard for psychiatric diagnosis. Having in place a common language for classifying mental disorders allows for the direct comparison of data among studies and the application of results across various disciplines

Textbook in Psychiatric Epidemiology, Second Edition, Edited by Ming T. Tsuang and Mauricio Tohen.
ISBN 0-471-40974-X

and areas of interest. For example, the fact that all psychiatric researchers use the same standardized definitions of disorders (and often the same diagnostic instruments) can facilitate the integration of studies exploring potential pathophysiological mechanisms with epidemiologic investigations of apparent causal factors in order to generate new hypotheses and drive future research. Second, is the reliance of the DSM definitions on symptomatic descriptions rather than hypothesized but untested etiological assumptions. Third is its provision of operationalized definitions in order to facilitate the assignment of a particular psychiatric diagnosis (or set of diagnoses) to a particular case.

Prior to the publication of DSM-III by the American Psychiatric Association in 1980, none of these aspects of the DSM were in fact the case. The first two editions of the DSM, published in 1952 and 1968, respectively (Committee on Nomenclature and Statistics, American Psychiatric Association, 1952, 1968), included only brief glossary definitions of the disorders and garnered very little interest outside the field of psychiatry. Even within psychiatry, these classifications were primarily used by clinicians for the purpose of assigning diagnostic codes for reimbursement and by inpatient facilities for the collection of census statistics. Furthermore, although the glossary definitions in DSM-I and DSM-II were relatively descriptive, the choice of terms in the classification itself reflected certain etiological theories. For example, many of the DSM-I disorders were called "reactions" reflecting Adolph Meyers psychobiological view that mental disorders represented reactions of the personality to psychological, social, and biological factors, and the Freudian concept of "neurosis" figured prominently in the DSM-II. Finally, the glossary definitions themselves were not sufficiently operationalized to allow for reliable diagnostic judgments (Spitzer and Fleiss, 1974).

Two major innovations implemented in DSM-III greatly impacted its utility for psychiatric epidemiology: its descriptive approach and its inclusion of diagnostic criteria. A basic principle of DSM-III was to provide comprehensive descriptions of the manifestations of disorders without regard to etiology, the only exception being those disorders that included etiologic statements as part of their definitions (e.g., organic mental disorders, adjustment disorders) (Spitzer et al., 1980). This generally atheoretical approach was intended to allow DSM-III to be useful across all theoretical orientations and was largely responsible for its wide acceptance among mental health professionals from varied disciplines as the standard language for diagnostic communication. For example, while a biologically oriented researcher and a cognitive-behavioral psychologist might have two completely different understandings of the etiologic mechanism underlying a panic attack, both could agree to the descriptive features of a panic attack (e.g., a sudden onset of intense fear accompanied by somatic symptoms such as shortness of breath, sweating, choking sensations, and depersonalization, among others) and thus find the DSM-III criteria useful in classifying individuals with symptoms of anxiety. The result is that since its introduction in 1980, the DSM definitions have been adopted by all mental health professionals, institutions, governmental agencies, private organizations in the United States, as well as a number of researchers and clinicians working in other countries. Consequently, the DSM revision process includes the active participation of a broad range of individuals and organizations in order to ensure that it continues to represent the broad consensus of mental health professionals.

The second, innovation with direct relevance to psychiatric epidemiology is the inclusion of operationalized diagnostic criteria for each disorder. The need for diagnostic criteria was recognized long before their adoption in DSM-III. In a 1959 report for the WHO Expert Committee on Mental Health written in response to disappointingly low international adoption rates for the sixth edition of the International Classification of Diseases (ICD-6) (World Health Organization, 1948), Stengel, a British psychiatrist, proposed that future diagnostic classifications contain operational definitions for each of the disorders (Stengel, 1959). This need was echoed by researchers in the United States who, starting in the 1970s, proposed and published diagnostic criteria for certain mental disorders with the goal of encouraging uniform adoption of diagnostic definitions in research settings in order to facilitate comparisons of results across studies. The first group of researchers, led by Eli Robbins and Samuel Guze at the Washington University School of Medicine in St. Louis, published a set of diagnostic criteria in 1972 for 16 diagnostic categories called the "Feighner Criteria," after the senior author of the paper (Feighner, 1972). While the development of these criteria sets were based on a review of the research data, the diagnostic thresholds and duration requirements were arrived at through a consensus process that represented the best educated guesses of the research team. The expectation was that these diagnostic parameters would be refined by future research studies, resulting in incrementally more valid definitions as more data become available. A few years later, as part of the National Institute of Mental Health (NIMH) collaborative project on the psychobiology of depression, Robert L. Spitzer and colleagues modified the Feighner criteria and added criteria for several additional disorders and subtypes; the resulting classification was called the Research Diagnostic Classification (RDC) (Spitzer et al., 1978). These criteria formed the starting point for the DSM-III criteria. However, because DSM-III endeavored to have criteria sets available for each and every disorder, additional diagnostic criteria sets were developed. Thus, the DSM-III committees were given the charge to develop criteria sets *de novo* through empirically informed expert consensus, a process that continued through to DSM-III-R, which was published in 1987 (American Psychiatric Association, 1987).

Starting with the DSM-IV revision process, the DSM development process shifted from an exclusive reliance on expert consensus to a process more firmly based on a comprehensive review of the empirical literature. A three-stage process of empirical review served as the organizational backbone of the investigations of the DSM-IV Work Groups. The requirement that decisions have empirical support ensured that everyone was working from a common and consensually accepted database. This resulted in a less passionate and more objective discourse and facilitated the development of consensus among individuals who often started from quite opposite positions (Frances et al., 1989; Widiger et al., 1991).

The first stage consisted of comprehensive and systematic reviews of the published literature (Widiger et al., 1990). Each work group identified which questions were most pertinent regarding each diagnosis. The 150 literature reviews that resulted each made specific recommendations that were presented to the task force, and then to the field, in the DSM-IV Options Book (American Psychiatric Association, 1991). The literature reviews revealed that there were a number of diagnostic questions of considerable importance for which there were very few answers available in the published literature. Fortunately, for many of these questions, data had been collected by various investigators but had not been analyzed or reported in a fashion that would be informative to the work group deliberations. A method of data reanalysis was devised to allow the work groups to benefit from these collected, but unpublished, data. These analyses also helped to develop and refine suggested new criteria items that could then be studied in field trials (Widiger et al., 1991).

Twelve issue-focused field trials were conducted under the auspices of the DSM-IV revision process and were sponsored by the National Institute of Mental Health (NIMH) in conjunction with the National Institute on Drug Abuse (NIDA) and the National Institute on Alcohol Abuse and Alcoholism (NIAAA) (Frances et al., 1991a). The field trials were intended to give the DSM-IV Work Groups the chance to test the advantages and disadvantages of the different criteria sets that were being considered for inclusion in DSM-IV. The alternatives tested included the criteria sets presented in DSM-III, DSM-III-R, and ICD-10 and new criteria items that were recommended by the work groups based on their literature reviews and data reanalyses. To ensure generalizability, many different sites were chosen. They reflected geographic, socioeconomic, cultural, and ethnic diversity, and, in some instances, included randomly selected community samples. Each trial compared the options at 510 sites, using approximately 100 subjects at each site.

One important aspect of the DSM-IV revision process was its openness to outside review. During the DSM-IV revision itself, every attempt was made to solicit input from interested individuals and organizations. Drafts of potential options for criteria sets as well as a draft of the criteria were distributed along with a solicitation for comments and suggestions (American Psychiatric Association, 1993). After the publication of DSM-IV in 1994, the entire three-stage process was documented in a four volume DSM-IV Sourcebook that also documents the Work Groups rationale for making changes (Widiger et al., 1994, 1996, 1997, 1998).

IMPACT OF DSM-IV ON EPIDEMIOLOGICAL STUDIES

In psychiatric epidemiology, "caseness" is determined by whether the subjects current or past symptomatology meets the diagnostic criteria for a DSM-IV disorder. Thus, a close examination of the factors in the DSM-IV classification that impact "caseness" can help in interpreting epidemiological findings. It is important to understand, however, that in epidemiological surveys the DSM-IV criteria sets themselves are only partially responsible for setting the diagnostic threshold between case and noncase. In actual practice, someone has to apply the diagnostic criteria to a particular subject's current and past history, in order to determine whether that subject is considered a case. In order both to increase the reliability of such diagnostic judgments and to allow non-clinicians to make these diagnoses, fully structured diagnostic interviews [like the Diagnostic Interview Schedule and the Composite International Diagnostic Interview (Robins et al., 1988)] have been developed which further operationalize the diagnostic criteria into specific interview questions (see Chapter 10). Differences in the way different structured interviews (or even different implementations of the same structured interview) have operationalized the DSM criteria have led to marked differences in reported prevalence (Regier et al., 1998).

Impact of Symptom Counts

Most disorders in DSM-IV are diagnosed when a patient exhibits a certain proportion of the criteria listed. In this sense, most DSM-IV diagnoses are polythetic rather than monothetic. The threshold number of criteria required for the disorder to be diagnosed will determine its prevalence in epidemiological studies. The restrictiveness of a threshold depends on how many criteria are offered in the definition of the disorder and what fraction must be present to make the diagnosis. The particular cut-off number of criteria required for any DSM-IV diagnosis has been set in an effort to maintain an optimal balance between specificity and sensitivity. Setting a low threshold provides for good sensitivity and few false negatives, but at the expense of lower specificity and many false positives. In contrast, setting a high threshold provides good specificity (few false positives) but low sensitivity (many false negatives).

Of course, any discussion of sensitivity and specificity immediately raises the question of what a "true positive" is in psychiatry. Given the lack of laboratory findings or even a rudimentary understanding of the pathophysiology of most mental disorders, a gold standard for establishing a psychiatric diagnosis is not forthcoming. What standard then was applied in when constructing the diagnostic thresholds used in the DSM? For the most part, the thresholds initially used in the criteria sets were set by expert consensus with the goal of approximating a clinician's sense that a diagnosis is appropriate. The expectation has been that the validity of the DSM diagnostic thresholds will be increased over time by subjecting them to various external validators. Proposed external validators include treatment response, heritability, course and prognosis, functional impairment and disability, and service utilization (Robins and Guze, 1970). For example, the diagnostic threshold for a major depressive episode (currently five out of nine symptoms) could be adjusted to maximize antidepressant response, family history of major depression and other depressive disorders, or number of visits to mental health care or general medical practitioners. Unfortunately, as pointed out by Kendler (1990), external validators do not always operate in concert; that is, adjusting a diagnostic threshold to maximize the validity on the basis of one type of external validator may reduce validity based on another type of validator. For example, whereas setting a lower diagnostic threshold for major depressive disorder will maximize the odds of having a relative with a depressive disorder, it will also reduce the odds that an individual responds to somatic treatment as compared to placebo.

A further complication in adjusting diagnostic thresholds based on maximizing a particular type of validator is considering the population in which these validators is being applied. As discussed above, the initial thresholds were set in order to best-fit clinical judgment as to the presence or absence of disorder. Since these thresholds are based on clinician's experience seeing patients in mental health settings, they may have questionable validity when applied in general medical and community settings. Indeed, it has been postulated that the relatively low rates of major depressive disorder (and high rates of so-called subthreshold conditions such as minor depression and other "unspecified" depressions) in primary care setting is because the diagnostic threshold for major depressive disorder was set at an inappropriately high level (Pincus et al., 1999).

Impact of Specific Wording of Criteria

The specific wording of the criteria sets for the disorders in DSM-IV will likewise have an appreciable effect on the definition of caseness and therefore on the prevalence of disorders in community samples. In some cases these words indicate requirements for the occurrence of symptoms over time, covering constructs such as minimum (or maximum) required duration (e.g., "duration is more than one month" in Post-traumatic Stress Disorder, "more than one day but less than one month" in Brief Psychotic Disorder), degree of persistence ("more days than not" in Dysthymic Disorder) or extent of recurrence ("recurrent unexpected panic attacks" in Panic Disorder). Some times the wording instructs the user to consider how symptoms cluster together over time (e.g., "three or more of the following occurring at any time in the same 12-month period" in Substance Dependence). Often the wording attempts to convey a minimum level of symptom severity (e.g., "markedly diminished interest or pleasure in activities" in Major Depressive Disorder, "grossly disorganized or catatonic behavior" in Schizophrenia). In all of these cases, precise operationalization of these parameters in critical and variations in such operationalizations across studies can impact reported prevalence rates.

The challenge of operationalizing criteria sets is complicated, however, by a tension between the needs of researchers and the needs of clinicians. From a research perspective, the more specific and concrete the wording in criteria sets, the greater the reliability and the greater the ease in operationalizing criteria in structured interviews. However, from a clinical perspective, the imposition of precise but essentially arbitrary severity, duration, and other requirements in criteria sets limits clinical judgment in their application and greatly reduces their clinical utility. Thus, in order to balance these competing needs, the DSM has opted in favor of combining both specific symptom counts and duration requirements with the use of relatively imprecise terms such as "marked," "persistent," "excessive," "prominent," and "intense" that require the user to exercise clinical judgment. One solution to this problem of competing needs has been implemented in the mental disorders section of the *International Classification of Diseases*, tenth edition (ICD-10). Two different implementations of the ICD-10 definitions are available, one for clinicians ["Clinical Descriptions and Diagnostic Guidelines" (WHO, 1992)] and another for researchers ["Diagnostic Criteria for Research" (WHO, 1993)], the latter containing very specific (albeit arbitrary) cutoffs throughout. This approach was considered and ultimately rejected by the developers of the DSM-IV because it was felt that having two different sets of definitions would hamper the application of research findings to clinical practice.

Impact of Clinical Significance Requirement

Another strategy used by DSM in setting the threshold between case and noncase is the requirement in the definition of mental disorder that the disturbance be associated with "present distress (e.g., a painful symptom) or disability (i.e., impairment in one or more important areas of functioning) or with a significantly increased risk of suffering death, pain, disability, or an important loss of freedom" (American Psychiatric Association, 2000, p. xxxi). This requirement has been operationalized into a criterion known as the clinical significance criterion (i.e., "the symptoms cause clinically significant distress or impairment in social, occupational, or other important areas of functioning") that has been applied to a majority of the DSM-IV disorders. (It was not added to those criteria sets in which distress or impairment was an inevitable consequence of meeting the diagnostic criteria, such as schizophrenia).

This additional criterion was included in recognition of the fact that individuals may experience the symptoms included in certain of the DSM-IV criteria sets and yet not have a mental disorder (Frances, 1998). For example, an individual may meet the specific definitional criteria for a major depressive episode at the threshold level, but this would not be sufficient to make the diagnosis unless there is also significant psychiatric distress or functional impairment associated with the symptom presentation. To reiterate, one must evaluate not only the presence of items that define the criteria set but also whether they cause clinically significant distress or impairment in making a diagnosis.

The attention to clinically significant distress or impairment is especially crucial in determining the prevalence of those disorders that are at the boundary with normality, a boundary that has particular relevance to the epidemiological study of community samples. Patients presenting in clinical settings are usually more severely impaired or distressed and have self-identified themselves as distressed or impaired. Furthermore, clinicians working in these settings are trained to assess the amount of distress and impairment caused by the symptoms. The judgment about clinically significant impairment is inherently easier for clinicians to make in clinical settings than for lay interviewers evaluating community samples. However, for reasons of feasibility and cost, epidemiological studies generally cannot use clinical interviewers and must usually rely on lay interviewers. While fully structured interviews have attempted to operationalize the clinical significance criteria by including questions such as whether the subject sought treatment or missed work because of the symptoms, it remains uncertain whether the judgment that a particular symptom constellation meets the criteria for "clinical significance" in a particular subject can be sufficiently operationalized to compensate for a lack of clinical experience in lay interviewers.

Impact of Comorbidity

A strategic issue in the design of a classification system is placement on the "lumping" versus "splitting" continuum (Frances et al., 1991b). Diagnostic classifications based on a lumping strategy tend to include a fewer number of more complexly defined disorders whereas classifications that lean towards "splitting" favor a larger number of more narrowly defined disorders. DSM-IV and its predecessors come clearly down on the side of splitting, dividing the mental disorder construct into over 250 categories. A by-product of this splitting paradigm is the high rates of comorbidity that are the rule when performing a comprehensive DSM-IV diagnostic evaluation, as occurs when administering a structured diagnostic interview. This tendency toward splitting is largely a result of the descriptive atheoretical stance taken by the DSM. Given the limited understanding about the relationship between symptomatic presentation and underlying pathophysiology, the most conservative and neutral strategy is to split the symptom clusters into the smallest most diagnostically homogeneous entries possible rather than assuming that the symptoms fit together into a coherent whole. It is thus important to understand that the high rates of comorbidity often encountered during epidemiological surveys are almost certainly artificial and do not represent separate disease processes (Frances et al., 1990). For example, although a patient with binge eating/purging, depression, panic attacks, substance abuse, and a lifelong pattern of stormy relationships might have symptoms that meet the DSM-IV criteria for five disorders (i.e., Bulimia Nervosa, Major Depressive Disorder, Panic Disorder, Substance Dependence, and Borderline Personality Disorder), he or she certainly does not have five distinct illnesses. The DSM tendency toward comorbidity is best viewed as allowing for the description of the various facets and manifestations of psychiatric illness, rather than interpreting it as true comorbidity in the medical sense.

THE FUTURE

The period from DSM-III to DSM-IV was marked by revisions in the manual at seven-year intervals (i.e., DSM-III in 1980, DSM-III-R in 1987, and DSM-IV in 1994). Although this relatively brief interval between revisions has insured that the DSM criteria sets are kept up-to-date with regard to the literature, too frequent revisions have some significant disadvantages, especially for psychiatric epidemiology. Each revision of the diagnostic criteria sets requires a corresponding effort on the part of instrument developers to revise structured diagnostic interviews and for users of the revised instrument to retool their diagnostic efforts (Zimmerman et al., 1991). Furthermore, periodic changes force epidemiologists to decide which edition of the DSM criteria sets to use when assessing diagnosis. Although there are clear advantages in using the most current edition of the DSM when doing an epidemiological study in order to maximize its applicability to other current research findings, it makes comparisons with epidemiological data using earlier editions of DSM criteria problematic. In fact, one of the hypotheses explaining the often substantial differences in prevalence between the ECA and NCS studies is the fact that the ECA used DSM-III criteria and the NCS used DSM-III-R criteria (Regier et al., 1998).

Largely in response to these concerns, the American Psychiatric Association has decided to delay the development and implementation of DSM-V. As of the writing of this chapter (in Spring 2002), it is anticipated that DSM-V will be published *no earlier than* 2010. Although an interim text revision of the DSM-IV was published in 2000 (American Psychiatric Association, 2000), there was only a handful of changes to criteria sets and only for the purpose of correcting known errors from the DSM-IV process (First and Pincus, 2002) and thus should have minimal impact on epidemiological studies.

Prior to formally starting work on the DSM-V, the American Psychiatric Association has initiated a DSM-V Research Planning Process, in which six work groups were convened to draft proposed research agendas with the goal of stimulating research in certain areas in order to lay the empirical groundwork in advance of the DSM-V revision process (Kupfer et al., 2002). One of these work groups, examining the area of disability and impairment, is specifically relevant to some of the issues raised in this chapter (Lehman et al., 2002). In particular, noting the inadequacies in the operationalization of the DSM-IV clinical significance criterion, the group proposed that research be conducted to delineate specific thresholds of distress and impairment that might apply to individual disorders. Advances in this area would clearly benefit epidemiological studies that rely on this threshold to distinguish case from noncase.

REFERENCES

American Psychiatric Association (1980): "Diagnostic and Statistical Manual of Mental Disorders," 3rd ed. (DSM-III) Washington, DC: American Psychiatric Association.

American Psychiatric Association (1987): "Diagnostic and Statistical Manual of Mental Disorders," 3rd ed. revised (DSM-III-R), Washington, DC: American Psychiatric Association.

American Psychiatric Association (1991): "Diagnostic and Statistical Manual of Mental Disorders," 4th ed. Options Book. Washington, DC: American Psychiatric Association.

American Psychiatric Association (1993): DSM-IV Draft Criteria 3/1/93. Washington, DC: American Psychiatric Association.

American Psychiatric Association (1994): "Diagnostic and Statistical Manual of Mental Disorders," 4th ed. (DSM-IV), Washington, DC: American Psychiatric Association.

American Psychiatric Association (2000): "Diagnostic and Statistical Manual of Mental Disorders," 4th ed. text revision (DSM-IV-TR). Washington, DC: American Psychiatric Association.

Committee on Nomenclature and Statistics of the American Psychiatric Association (1952): "Diagnostic and Statistical Manual of Mental Disorders" (DSM-I). Washington, DC: American Psychiatric Association.

Committee on Nomenclature and Statistics of the American Psychiatric Association (1968): "Diagnostic and Statistical Manual of Mental Disorders," 2nd ed. (DSM-II). Washington, DC: American Psychiatric Association.

Feighner JP, Robins E, Guze SB, Woodruff RA, Jr, Winokur G, Munoz R (1972): Diagnostic criteria for use in psychiatric research. Arch Gen Psychiatry 26:57–63.

First MB, Pincus HA (2001): The DSM-IV text revision: Rationale and potential impact on clinical practice, Psychiatric Services.

Frances A (1998): Problems in defining clinical significance in epidemiological studies. Arch Gen Psychiatry 55:119.

Frances A, Davis WW, Kline M et al. (1991a): The DSM-IV field trials: Moving toward an empirically derived classification. Eur Psychiatry 6:307–314.

Frances A, First MB, Widiger TA, Miele G, Tilly S, Davis W, Pincus HA (1991b): An A to Z guide to DSM-IV conundrums. J Abnorm Psychol 100:407–412.

Frances A, Widiger T, Fyer M (1990): The influence of classification methods on comorbidity. In Maser JD, Cloninger CR (eds): "Comorbidity of Mood and Anxiety Disorders." Washington, DC: American Psychiatric Association, pp 41–59.

Frances A, Widiger T, Pincus H (1989): The development of DSM-IV. Arch Gen Psychiatry 46:373–375.

Kendler KS (1990): Toward a scientific psychiatric nosology: strengths and limitations. Arch Gen Psychiatry; 47:969–973.

Pincus HA, Davis WW, McQueen LE (1999): "Subthreshold" mental disorders. A review and synthesis of studies on minor depression and other brand names. Br J Psychiatry 174:288–296.

Regier DA, Kaelber CT, Rae DS, Farmer ME, Knauper B, Kessler RC, Norquist GS (1998). Limitations of diagnostic criteria and assessment instruments for mental disorders. Implications for research and policy. Arch Gen Psychiatry 55:109–115

Regier DA, Myers JK, Kramer M, Robins LN, Blazer DG, Hough RL, Eaton WW, Locke BZ (1984): The NIMH Epidemiologic Catchment Area program. Historical context, major objectives, and study population characteristics. Arch Gen Psychiatry 41:934–941.

Robins E, Guze SB (1970): Establishment of diagnostic validity in psychiatric illness: its application to schizophrenia. Am J Psychiatry 126:983–987.

Robins LN, Helzer JE, Croughan J, Ratcliff KS (1981): National Institute of Mental Health Diagnostic Interview Schedule. Its history, characteristics, and validity. Arch Gen Psychiatry 38:381–389.

Robins LN, Wing J, Wittchen HU, Helzer JE, Babor TF, Burke J, Farmer A, Jablenski A, Pickens R, Regier DA (1988): The Composite International Diagnostic Interview. An epidemiologic Instrument suitable for use in conjunction with different diagnostic systems and in different cultures. Arch Gen Psychiatry 45:1069–1077.

Spitzer RL, Fleiss JL (1974): A reanalysis of the reliability of psychiatric diagnosis. Br J Psychiatry 125:341–347.

Spitzer RL, Endicott J, Robins E (1978): Research diagnostic criteria: rationale and reliability. Arch Gen Psychiatry 35:773–782.

Spitzer RL, Williams JBW, Skodol AE (1980): DSM-III: The major achievements and an overview. Am J Psychiatry 137:151–164.

Stengel (1959): Classification of mental disorders. Bull. World Health Organization 601–603.

Widiger TA, Frances AJ, Pincus HA, Davis WW (1990): The DSM-IV literature reviews: Rationale, process, and limitations. J Psychopathol Behave Assess 12:189–202.

Widiger TA, Frances AJ, Pincus HA et al. (1991): Towards an empirical classification for the DSM-IV. J Abnorm Psychol 100:280–288.

Widiger TA, Frances AJ, Pincus HA, Ross R, First MB, Davis WW (1994): "DSM-IV Sourcebook," Vol I. Washington, DC: American Psychiatric Association.

Widiger TA, Frances AJ, Pincus HA, Ross R, First MB, Davis WW (1996): "DSM-IV Sourcebook," Vol II. Washington, DC: American Psychiatric Association.

Widiger TA, Frances AJ, Pincus HA, Ross R, First MB, Davis WW (1997): "DSM-IV Sourcebook," Vol III. Washington, DC: American Psychiatric Association.

Widiger TA, Frances AJ, Pincus HA, Ross R, First MB, Davis WW, Kline, M (1998): "DSM-IV Sourcebook," Vol IV. Washington, DC: American Psychiatric Association.

World Health Organization (1948): "Manual of the International Statistical Classification of Diseases, Injuries and Causes of Death, 6th revision, vol 1. Geneva: World Health Organization.

World Health Organization (1992): ICD-10 Classification of Mental and Behavioral Disorders: Clinical Descriptions and Diagnostic Guidelines." Geneva, World Health Organization.

World Health Organization (1993): ICD-10 Classification of Mental and Behavioral Disorders: Diagnostic Criteria for Research." Geneva, World Health Organization.

Zimmerman M, Jampala VC, Sierles FS, Taylor MA (1991): DSM-IV: A nosology sold before its time? Am J Psychiatry 148:463–467.

CHAPTER 14

The National Comorbidity Survey

RONALD C. KESSLER and ELLEN WALTERS
Harvard Medical School

INTRODUCTION

This chapter presents an overview of the research program associated with the U.S. National Comorbidity Survey (NCS). The baseline NCS, which was fielded in the fall of 1990 and completed in the spring of 1992, was the first nationally representative mental health survey in the United States to use a fully structured research diagnostic interview to assess the prevalences and correlates of DSM-III-R disorders. The baseline NCS respondents are being reinterviewed in 2001 and 2002 (NCS-2) in order to study patterns and predictors of the course of mental and substance use disorders and to evaluate the effects of primary mental disorders in predicting the onset and course of secondary substance disorders. An NCS Replication survey (NCS-R) is also being carried out in conjunction with NCS-2 in a new national sample of 10,000 respondents. The goals of NCS-R are to study trends in a wide range of variables assessed in the baseline NCS and to obtain more information about a number of topics either not covered in the baseline NCS or covered in less depth than we currently desire. A survey of 10,000 adolescents (NCS-A) is being carried out in parallel with the NCS-R and NCS-2 surveys. The goal of NCS-A is to produce nationally representative data on the prevalences and correlates of mental disorders among youth. NCS-R and NCS-A, finally, are being replicated in a number of countries around the world. Centralized cross-national analysis of these surveys is being carried out by the NCS data analysis team under the auspices of the World Health Organization (WHO) World Mental Health 2000 (WMH2000) Initiative (Kessler and Ustun, to appear). This chapter presents a brief overview of each of these phases in the evolution of the NCS research program.

Textbook in Psychiatric Epidemiology, Second Edition, Edited by Ming T. Tsuang and Mauricio Tohen.
ISBN 0-471-40974-X

THE BASELINE NCS: BACKGROUND AND DESIGN

The need for a national survey on patterns and predictors of psychiatric disorders was noted nearly two decades ago in the report of the President's Commission on Mental Health and Illness (1978). Such a survey could not be undertaken at that time, though, due to the absence of a structured research diagnostic interview capable of generating reliable psychiatric diagnoses in general population samples. Recognizing this need, the National Institute of Mental Health funded the development of the Diagnostic Interview Schedule (DIS) (Robins et al., 1981), a research diagnostic interview that can be used by trained interviewers who are not clinicians.

The DIS was first used in the Epidemiologic Catchment Area (ECA) Study, a landmark series of surveys that interviewed over 20,000 respondents in five local community samples. The ECA was the main source of data in the United States on the prevalence of psychiatric disorders and utilization of services for these disorders during the decade between the early 1980s and the early 1990s (Bourdon et al., 1992; Regier et al., 1993; Robins et al., 1991). The baseline NCS was designed to take the next step beyond the ECA (Kessler, 1994) by carrying out a nationally representative survey of mental disorders. This was done by administering a face-to-face structured diagnostic interview to a widely dispersed sample that was representative of all people living in households in the continental United States. The 8098 NCS respondents were selected from over 1000 neighborhoods in over 170 counties distributed over 34 states.

The NCS diagnostic interview was a modification of the Composite International Diagnostic Interview (CIDI; World Health Organization, 1990), a state-of-the-art structured diagnostic interview based on the DIS. We deleted diagnoses known to have low prevalences in the ECA (e.g., obsessive-compulsive disorder, somatization disorder). We also modified the CIDI in several ways based on extensive pilot tests (Kessler et al., 1998c, 1999b). The most important of these modifications involved the diagnostic stem questions. Almost all CIDI diagnostic sections begin with a small number of questions that assess core features of the disorder. If these questions are answered positively, the respondent is asked a detailed series of follow-up questions about the disorder. If the stem questions are answered negatively, in comparison, the respondent is skipped to the next section. Our pilot work showed clearly that respondents quickly catch on to this stem-branch logic and sometimes deny stem questions in order to get through the interview more quickly. We addressed this problem by moving the diagnostic stem questions for all disorders into a separate lifetime review section that was administered before any other sections of the CIDI. We prefaced the administration of the lifetime review section with a preamble designed to motivate serious and honest responding (Kessler et al., 1999a). A field experiment that randomized pilot test respondents to receive the CIDI either with or without this lifetime review section showed that use of this section resulted in a statistically significant and substantively important increase in the estimated prevalences of most DSM-III-R disorders. A separate clinical validity study showed that this increase was due to a decrease in false-negative diagnostic evaluations rather than to an increase in false-positives (Kessler et al., 1998c).

Another NCS innovation was the use of a two-phase clinical reinterview design for complex cases. WHO CIDI field trials showed that most CIDI diagnoses have good inter-rater reliability, test-retest reliability, and validity in comparison to blind clinician reinterviews in nonpatient samples (Wittchen, 1994). An important exception to this general pattern, however, is nonaffective psychosis, which is diagnosed with low reliability and validity in structured interviews like the CIDI. Based on this fact, and given the great public health importance of nonaffective psychosis, the NCS included clinical reinterviews with respondents who reported any evidence of schizophrenia or other nonaffective psychoses. These reinterviews were administered by experienced clinicians using an adapted version of the Structured Clinical Interview for DSM-III-R (SCID; Spitzer et al., 1992), an instrument with demonstrated reliability in the diagnosis of schizophrenia (Williams et al., 1992). The NCS diagnoses of schizophrenia and other nonaffective psychoses are based on these clinical reinterviews rather than on the UM-CIDI interviews (Kendler et al., 1996). As described below, this reliance on clinical reinterviews for diagnosis of complex cases was expanded in NCS-R.

A final noteworthy NCS innovation was the systematic evaluation of the relationship between survey nonresponse and diagnosis. Based on a concern that nonrespondents might have considerably higher rates of some mental disorders than respondents, we carried out a systematic nonrespondent survey in which a random subsample of nonrespondents was recontacted by specially trained refusal conversion interviewers and asked to complete a ten-minute screening interview. The screening interview was completed either face-to-face or over the telephone by approximately one-third of the nonrespondents who were selected into this special subsample. Propensity score weighting that made use of the information about diagnostic stem question profiles obtained in these screening interviews was then used to adjust the sample for the underrepresentation of these initial refusers (Rosenbaum and Rubin, 1983). Analysis of response bias showed, interestingly, that failure to adjust for differential nonresponse led most importantly to an underestimation of the prevalence of anxiety disorders (Kessler et al., 1995b). This occurred because anxious people were more reluctant than other people to allow a stranger into their homes, while they were willing to complete the screening once the option of telephone administration was offered.

THE BASELINE NCS: RESULTS

Lifetime and Recent Prevalences

As reported in more detail elsewhere (Kessler et al., 1994), the NCS found that DSM-III-R disorders are more prevalent than previously thought to be the case. The results in Table 1 show prevalence estimates for the 14 lifetime and 12-month disorders assessed in the core NCS interview. Lifetime prevalence is the proportion of the sample who ever experienced a disorder, while 12-month prevalence is the proportion who experienced the disorder at some time in the 12 months prior to the interview. The prevalence estimates in Table 1 are presented without

TABLE 1. Lifetime and 12-Month Prevalence of DSM-III-R Disorders

	Male				Female				Total			
	Lifetime		12-Month		Lifetime		12-Month		Lifetime		12-Month	
Disorders	%	(SE)	%	(SE)	%	(SE)	%	(SE)	%	(SE)	%	(SE)
A. Mood disorders												
Major depression	12.7	(0.9)	7.7	(0.8)	21.3	(0.9)	12.9	(0.8)	17.1	(0.7)	10.3	(0.6)
Mania	1.6	(0.3)	1.4	(0.3)	1.7	(0.3)	1.3	(0.3)	1.6	(0.3)	1.3	(0.2)
Dysthymia	4.8	(0.4)	2.1	(0.3)	8.0	(0.6)	3.0	(0.4)	6.4	(0.4)	2.5	(0.2)
Any mood disorder	14.7	(0.8)	8.5	(0.8)	23.9	(0.9)	14.1	(0.9)	19.3	(0.7)	11.3	(0.7)
B. Anxiety disorders												
Generalized anxiety disorder	3.6	(0.5)	2.0	(0.3)	6.6	(0.5)	4.3	(0.4)	5.1	(0.3)	3.1	(0.3)
Panic disorder	2.0	(0.3)	1.3	(0.3)	5.0	(1.4)	3.2	(0.4)	3.5	(0.3)	2.3	(0.3)
Social phobia	11.1	(0.8)	6.6	(0.4)	15.5	(1.0)	9.1	(0.7)	13.3	(0.7)	7.9	(0.4)
Simple phobia	6.7	(0.5)	4.4	(0.5)	15.7	(1.1)	13.2	(0.9)	11.3	(0.6)	8.8	(0.5)
Agoraphobia without panic	3.5	(0.4)	1.7	(0.3)	7.0	(0.6)	3.8	(0.4)	5.3	(0.4)	2.8	(0.3)
Any anxiety disorder	19.2	(0.9)	11.8	(0.6)	30.5	(1.2)	22.6	(0.1)	24.9	(0.8)	17.2	(0.7)
C. Substance use disorders												
Alcohol abuse	12.5	(0.8)	3.4	(0.4)	6.4	(0.6)	1.6	(0.2)	9.4	(0.5)	2.5	(0.2)
Alcohol dependence	20.1	(1.0)	10.7	(0.9)	8.2	(0.7)	3.7	(0.4)	14.1	(0.7)	7.2	(0.5)
Drug abuse	5.4	(0.5)	1.3	(0.2)	3.5	(0.4)	0.3	(0.1)	4.4	(0.3)	0.8	(0.1)
Drug dependence	9.2	(0.7)	3.8	(0.4)	5.9	(0.5)	1.9	(0.3)	7.5	(0.4)	2.8	(0.3)
Any substance use disorder	35.4	(1.2)	16.1	(0.7)	17.9	(1.1)	6.6	(0.4)	26.6	(1.0)	11.3	(0.5)
D. Other disorders												
Antisocial personality (ASP)[a]	4.8	(0.5)	—	—	1.0	(0.2)	—	—	2.8	(0.2)	—	—
Nonaffective psychosis[b]	0.3	(0.1)	0.2	(0.1)	0.7	(0.2)	0.4	(0.1)	0.5	(0.1)	0.3	(0.1)
E. Any NCS disorder	48.7	(0.2)	27.7	(0.9)	47.3	(1.5)	31.2	(1.3)	48.0	(1.1)	29.5	(1.0)

[a]ASP was only assessed on a lifetime basis.
[b]Nonaffective psychosis = schizophrenia, schizophreniform disorder, schizoaffective disorder, delusional disorder, and atypical psychosis.

exclusions for DSM-III-R hierarchy rules. Standard errors are reported in parentheses.

The most common disorders are major depression and alcohol dependence. The next most common are social and simple phobias. As a group, substance use disorders and anxiety disorders are somewhat more prevalent than affective disorders, with approximately one in every four respondents reporting a lifetime substance use disorder and a similar number a lifetime anxiety disorder. Approximately one in every five respondents reported a lifetime affective disorder. Anxiety disorders, as a group, were considerably more likely to occur in the 12 months prior to interview than either substance use disorders or affective disorders, suggesting that anxiety disorders are more chronic than affective or substance disorders. The prevalences of other NCS disorders are considerably lower.

As shown in the last row of Table 1, 48.0% of the sample reported at least one lifetime disorder and 29.5% at least one disorder in the 12 months prior to the interview. While there is no meaningful sex difference in these overall prevalences, there are sex differences in prevalences of specific disorders. Consistent with previous research, men were much more likely to have substance use disorders and ASPD than women, while women were much more likely to have anxiety disorders and affective disorders than men (with the exception of mania, for which there is no sex difference). The data also show, consistent with a trend found in the ECA (Keith et al., 1991), that women in the household population are more likely than men to have nonaffective psychosis.

There was a good deal of skepticism about these results when they were first published. The main criticism was that the NCS prevalence estimates were higher than those found in the ECA and other epidemiologic surveys based on the ECA methodology. However, clinical reappraisal studies in which clinicians blindly reinterviewed a sample of NCS respondents subsequently showed that the NCS estimates are accurate (Kessler et al., 1998c), suggesting that the ECA estimates are biased downwards. A later reanalysis of the ECA data found that ECA estimates can be adjusted for reporting bias to approximate the NCS estimates (Regier et al., 1998). Methodological studies suggest that the life review section, mentioned earlier, is largely responsible for the more accurate estimates in the NCS than the ECA (Kessler et al., 1998c).

Age at onset

The NCS collected retrospective data on the ages of first onset of each lifetime disorder. Consistent with previous evidence (Burke et al., 1991), simple and social phobia were found to have much earlier ages at onset than the other disorders (Magee et al., 1996)—with simple phobia often beginning during middle or late childhood and social phobia during late childhood or early adolescence. Substance abuse was found to have a typical age of onset during the late teens or early twenties. A substantial proportion of people with lifetime major depression and dysthymia also reported that their first episode occurred during the late teens or twenties. Some other disorders had later ages at onset, but the most striking overall impression from the data as a whole was that most psychiatric disorders have first onsets quite early in life.

Comorbidity

The ECA Study was the first survey to document that comorbidity is widespread not only among patients but also in the general population (Regier et al., 1990; Robins et al., 1991). Over 54% of ECA respondents with a lifetime history of at least one DSM-III disorder were found to have a second diagnosis. Fifty-two percent of persons with a lifetime history of alcohol abuse or dependence received a second diagnosis and 75% of persons with lifetime drug abuse or dependence had a second diagnosis. Respondents with a lifetime history of at least one mental disorder in the ECA had a 2.3 relative-odds of having a lifetime history of alcohol abuse or dependence and a relative-odds of 4.5 of some other drug use disorder compared to respondents with no lifetime mental disorder.

Very similar patterns were found in the NCS. Fifty-six percent of NCS respondents with a lifetime history of at least one DSM-III-R disorder also had one or more other disorders (Kessler et al., 1994). Fifty-two percent of respondents with lifetime alcohol abuse or dependence also had a lifetime mental disorder, while 36% had a lifetime drug use disorder. Fifty-nine percent of the respondents with a lifetime history of drug abuse or dependence also had a lifetime mental disorder and 71% had a lifetime alcohol use disorder.

More detailed analyses showed that lifetime comorbidities of specific pairs of disorders are very similar in the ECA and NCS surveys (Kessler, 1995). In both surveys, virtually all the odds-ratios (ORs) between each pair of lifetime disorders is greater than 1.0. This means that there is a positive association between the lifetime occurrences of almost all ECA and NCS disorders, demonstrating that comorbidity of psychiatric disorders is truly pervasive in the general population. There is considerable variation in the sizes of the ORs. This variation is systematic and quite consistent across the two surveys. For example, the results in both surveys show that major depression is most strongly comorbid with dysthymia and mania and least strongly comorbid with substance use disorders and antisocial personality disorder.

Pure and Comorbid Lifetime Disorders

It is of interest to look beyond simple two-variable associations for broader patterns of comorbidity among multiple disorders. The 48% of persons in the NCS who had a lifetime history of at least one DSM-III-R disorder was found to be made up of 21% with exactly one, 13% with exactly two, and 14% with three or more disorders. Thinking of disorders as the unit of analysis, we found that only 21% of all lifetime disorders occurred to the subsample of respondents who had no lifetime comorbidity. The other 79% occurred to respondents with lifetime comorbidity. The vast majority of lifetime disorders, then, were comorbid disorders (Kessler et al., 1994). Furthermore, we found that over 50% of all lifetime disorders occurred to the 14% of the population with a history of three or more disorders. This highly comorbid segment of the population also accounted for close to 60% of all 12-month disorders and close to 90% of severe 12-month disorders. These results show that while psychiatric disorders are widespread in the general population, the major burden of psychopathology is concentrated among people with high comorbidity.

Primary and Secondary Disorders

Given the importance of comorbidity, a question arises as to which disorders in comorbid sets have the earliest ages at onset. The results in Table 2 show that there was considerable variation across disorders in the NCS in the probability of being the first lifetime disorder. Simple phobia, social phobia, alcohol abuse, and conduct disorder were the only disorders considered in the NCS where the majority of lifetime cases were temporally primary. In general, anxiety disorders were most likely to be temporally primary, with 82.8% of NCS respondents having

TABLE 2. Percent and Distribution of Temporally Primary NCS/DSM-III-R Disorders[a]

Disorder	Percent Temporally Primary Among Those Having the Disorder		Distribution of Temporally Primary Disorder	
	%	(SE)	%	(SE)
I. Mood disorders				
Major depression	41.1	2.7	13.4	0.9
Dysthymia	37.7	3.1	4.8	0.5
Mania	20.2	6.0	0.7	0.2
Any mood disorder	43.8	2.4	16.4	0.9
II. Anxiety disorders				
Generalized anxiety disorder	37.0	2.9	3.6	0.4
Panic disorder	23.3	3.2	1.6	0.2
Social phobia	63.1	2.0	16.0	0.9
Simple phobia	67.6	2.7	14.5	1.0
Agoraphobia	45.2	4.0	5.9	0.7
Posttraumatic stress disorder	52.1	3.0	7.5	0.7
Any anxiety disorder	82.8	1.3	45.3	1.4
III Substance use disorders				
Alcohol abuse	57.0	2.3	10.2	0.6
Alcohol dependence	36.8	3.1	9.9	0.6
Drug abuse	39.7	3.0	3.4	0.3
Drug dependence	20.8	2.5	3.0	0.3
Any substance use disorder	48.1	1.6	24.5	1.0
IV. Other disorders				
Conduct disorder	71.1	2.0	17.7	1.0
Adult antisocial behavior	14.0	1.8	1.4	0.2
Nonaffective psychosis	28.8	5.6	0.4	0.1

[a]All disorders are operationalized using DSM-III-R criteria ignoring diagnostic hierarchy rules. (SE) = standard error; NCS = National Comorbidity Survey.

one or more anxiety disorders reporting that one of these was their first lifetime disorder compared to 71.1% of those with conduct disorder, 43.8% of those with an affective disorder, and 48.1% of those with a substance use disorder. Results in the third column of Table 2 show the percent of overall respondents who reported each disorder as temporally primary. Anxiety disorders, again, were more likely to be temporally primary (45.3% of all lifetime cases) than either affective disorders (26.4%), substance use disorders (24.5%), or other disorders (19.5%).

Information about age at onset was used to study the time-lagged effects of earlier disorders in predicting the subsequent onset of secondary disorders using a discrete-time survival analysis approach. This work showed clearly that early-onset anxiety disorders are the most important primary disorders in terms of predicting later disorders (Kessler, 1997). Interestingly, while most of these effects are only associated with active disorders, there are others that are also associated with remitted disorders. For example, respondents with a history of early-onset panic attacks have an elevated risk of secondary major depression throughout the majority of their adulthood even if their panic attacks occurred exclusively many years in the past (Kessler et al., 1998d). Results such as this suggest that some early-onset anxiety disorders are risk markers rather than direct causes of secondary disorders.

The Social Costs of Psychiatric Disorders

Epidemiologists have traditionally been much more concerned with the causes than with the consequences of the illnesses they study. However, the rise of cost-effectiveness analysis as a tool for allocating health care resources has led to a dramatic increase in research on the adverse consequences of untreated chronic conditions and the benefits of treatment (Gold et al., 1996). The NCS analyses consequently included an investigation of the adverse consequences of mental disorders. Consistent with the Rand Medical Outcome Study (Wells et al., 1996), we found that mental disorders have adverse effects on role functioning that equal or exceed the effects of most chronic physical conditions (Kessler et al., 2001a). Data from clinical trials on the reversibility of these role impairments, when combined with NCS data on the costs of work-related role impairments to employers, suggest that the cost savings due to increased work productivity might well make it cost-effective for employers to develop aggressive screening, outreach, and treatment programs for employees with some mental disorders (Kessler et al., 1999a). As described below, this is an issue that is being examined in much more detail in NCS-R and the other WMH2000 surveys.

NCS analyses also found that the early age at onset of mental disorders led them to have much greater effects than physical disorders on critical life course transitions such as educational attainment, teen childbearing, the timing and stability of marriage, and early career decisions (Kessler et al., 1995a, 1997a, 1998b). These adverse effects typically occur as part of a cascade of events as a result of the onset of serious early-onset mental disorders. People with this complex pile-up of emotional and psychosocial difficulties typically do not seek professional mental health treatment until at least a decade after the onset of their first mental disorder. It is consequently of great importance to develop aggressive outreach and treatment programs for young people with mental disorders. This is a topic of central importance in the NCS-A survey.

Utilization of Services

Although only four out of every ten NCS respondents with a lifetime history of at least one DSM-III-R disorder reported ever obtaining professional treatment, a survival analysis that compared age at onset with time to treatment suggested that the vast majority of people with persistent mental illness eventually seek treatment (Kessler et al., 1998a). Delays in initial help-seeking, however, are pervasive, with the median time between first lifetime onset of a mental illness and first treatment contact greater than a decade. Importantly, delays in seeking treatment are inversely related to age at onset, with child and adolescent onsets being associated with the lowest probabilities of ever seeking treatment. This is a critical finding because early-onset disorders are the ones most likely to promote comorbidity and adverse life course consequences. On a more positive note, analysis of retrospective NCS data suggests that rates of treatment-seeking increased over the four decades of historical time retrospectively assessed in the NCS. This presumably reflects a combination of increases in access to care, in awareness that mental illness is treatable, and in attitudes conducive to seeking care.

Primary Prevention of Secondary Disorders

One question suggested by the NCS results is whether early treatment of pure child-onset or adolescent-onset mental disorders would result in a reduction in the percentage of people who go on to develop comorbid mental disorders and, if so, a reduction in the persistence and adverse social consequences of primary mental disorders. We do not know the answer because no large-scale controlled study has ever attempted to screen and treat a representative sample of children or adolescents with mental disorders and then follow them over time to document the long-term effects of treatment. Given the high prevalences and enormous personal and societal costs of mental disorders, such an investigation should be undertaken.

An issue of special interest in the current social policy arena is the prevention of adolescent substance disorder. Current federal policy on substance abuse prevention emphasizes a combination of strategies that focus on reduction in access to drugs and unproven school-based primary prevention programs, such as DARE, that ignore the fact that the majority of adolescent substance abusers have a primary mental disorder (Kessler et al., 1996, 1997b). Policy simulations based on the NCS data suggest that a more cost-effective strategy would be to develop outreach and treatment programs for youngsters with early-onset mental disorders that predispose to substance abuse. In addition to sharply reducing the proportion of youth who become substance abusers, such an effort could have a powerful preventive effect on subsequent adult serious mental disorder.

NCS-2: DESIGN AND RATIONALE

NCS-2 was designed with the explicit purpose of providing an epidemiological foundation for early intervention programs of the sort just described. While the baseline NCS simulations suggested that early primary mental disorders are important predictors of the subsequent onset and course of secondary mental and substance disorders, these results are based on retrospective reports about age at onset. NCS-2 seeks to determine whether these results hold up prospectively. This is being done using a life chart approach to assess onset and course of disorders during the decade between the baseline NCS and the NCS-2 interview. The life chart method, pioneered by Freedman and her colleagues (Freedman et al., 1988), provides respondents with a paper calendar covering the recall period that includes notations of important historical events in an effort to create memory anchors. Respondents are also asked to include personal memory anchors in the calendar further to enhance the accuracy of dating.

Life charting is facilitated in NCS-2 by the use of laptop computerized interviews that include a customized preloaded data file for each respondent based on baseline NCS reports. Respondents with a history of a particular disorder as of the baseline NCS are asked to chart the course of that disorder during the decade since the baseline NCS, while respondents with no history of the disorder as of the baseline NCS are asked about subsequent onsets and, if onsets occur, about the course of the disorder after the time of onset. A similar procedure was used by Eaton and his associates in a thirteen-year follow-up of the Baltimore ECA sample (Lyketsos et al., 1994).

In addition to charting the course of mental disorders, NCS-2 charts major role transitions in education, marriage, childbearing, and work that might play a part in influencing the onset and course of mental and substance disorders. Major stressor events and difficulties are also charted using a structured version of the Brown and Harris (1978) Life Events and Difficulties system (Wethington et al., 1995). Charting is done separately for each year across the decade between the two interviews and for each month in the 12 months prior to the NCS-2 interview.

NCS-R: DESIGN AND RATIONALE

As noted above, NCS-R is being carried out to study trends in a wide range of variables assessed in the baseline NCS and to obtain more information about a number of topics either not covered in the baseline NCS or covered in less depth than we currently desire. A new sample of 10,000 adult respondents is being interviewed in the same nationally representative sampling segments as the baseline NCS. There will also be an update of new segments to adjust for population shifts over the past decade. The NCS-R interview will repeat many of the questions assessed in the baseline NCS for purposes of trending. New questions will also be asked to expand old topics as well as to add new topics of investigation. The recruitment procedures and materials will be identical to the baseline NCS. As in the baseline, interviews will be carried out face-to-face in the homes of respondents. Unlike the baseline NCS, though, as many as 1000 NCS-R respondents will be followed up by telephone with clinical reappraisal interviews using the Structured Clinical Interview for DSM-IV (SCID; First et al., 1997) in an effort to clarify diagnostic uncertainties in the CIDI interviews.

NCS-R trend analyses will focus on recent prevalences of disorders, attitudes and perceptions about mental illness and its treatment, patterns of help-seeking, and treatment adequacy. Although we have no hypotheses about trends in prevalences, we anticipate finding significant changes in attitudes and perceptions about mental illness and its treatment based on the unprecedented volume of mass media attention given to mental illness and psychotropic medications over the past decade. We also expect to find that rates of treatment have increased over the past decade due, at least in part, to changes in attitudes and perceptions. Structural changes in the financing and delivery of mental health services have also occurred over the decade that could promote changes in rates of treatment. We also anticipate finding that treatment adequacy has improved in the health care sector over the decade. This expectation is based on the fact that practice guidelines for the treatment of a number of mental disorders have been published and widely disseminated during this interval of time and the fact that a number of special disease management programs for the treatment of mental disorders have been created and implemented in managed care organizations. Another important development over the past decade has been the rise of alternative therapy. It is conceivable that an increase in self-medication with St.-John's-Wort and other alternative therapies has led to a decline in the use of conventional treatments (Kessler et al., 2001b). The NCS-R trend analysis will allow us to evaluate this possibility rigorously.

Alternative medicine is only one of a number of new topics in the NCS-R that were not covered in the baseline NCS. Another one of special importance is violence. Violence is an issue of increasing concern that is being assessed in the NCS-R in several ways. For one, we are evaluating the possibility that, as with the ICD and DSM criteria for depression among children and adolescents, irritability should be considered an alternative to dysphoria or anhedonia in evaluating the prevalence of depressive disorders among adults. Second, we are evaluating anger attacks in parallel with panic attacks in an assessment of intermittent explosive disorder. Third, we are assessing hostility as a personality characteristic and the use of violence (in interpersonal relationships as well as in broader interactions) as a strategy for resolving disagreements. We are also collecting data on the recent prevalences of carrying weapons and being involved in physical fights.

Another new topic of special importance in NCS-R is pathological gambling. The dramatic growth in the United States of state sponsorship of gambling (e.g., state lotteries) and legalization of gambling venues has led to a great deal of concern about government complicity in vice and the rise in problem gambling. We also know from a number of screening surveys that a substantial proportion of the population gamble regularly and that a meaningful number of these people have gambling problems (National Research Council, 1999). However, no national survey has yet carried out a detailed evaluation of the prevalence of pathological gambling in conjunction with a larger set of potentially comorbid underlying mental disorders. This is being done in NCS-R. Detailed information on gambling patterns and motivations for gambling is also being collected in order to study pathological gambling subtypes.

THE NCS-R ADOLESCENT SURVEY: DESIGN AND RATIONALE

The NCS-R adolescent survey (NCS-A) is designed to provide basic descriptive psychiatric epidemiological information on adolescents comparable to the information on adults obtained in the baseline NCS. In addition, the NCS-A interview schedule includes a detailed risk factor battery that we hope to use to study modifiable determinants of the onset and course of child and adolescent mental disorders. Furthermore, as a nationally representative sample of schools will be selected to help recruit the NCS-A sample (described below), the survey includes considerable detail on school and neighborhood environmental factors that might be important determinants of early detection, outreach, and treatment of child and adolescent mental disorders.

A number of important design decisions arose in planning NCS-A that deviate from the model used in the adult NCS-2 and NCS-R surveys. One of these concerned sampling. Because adolescents only reside in a small proportion of all households, a critical design decision concerned the sampling scheme. The scheme we settled on uses a dual-frame approach in which a representative sample of all schools in the country and a representative sample of all households in the country were both used to select adolescents for interview. The school sample is a probability sample of the schools in the communities used in the NCS-2 and NCS-R samples. A probability sample of students in the eligible age range (12–17) is selected in each sample school. The household sample is based on a random selection of one adolescent in each household contacted for the NCS-2 and NCS-R adult surveys. Information is recorded for each household sample respondent regarding whether or not they still attend school and, if so, the name of their school. This information is used to weight the data to adjust for the undersampling of school dropouts and of students who, along with their parents, agreed to participate in the survey as part of the household sample while the principal of the school they attend did not agree to include the school in the school sample. This dual frame approach is facilitated by the fact that the adult NCS-2 and NCS-R surveys are being carried out in parallel with the adolescent survey. Dual-frame sampling is much more efficient than other sample designs in a situation of this sort.

Another critical design decision concerned instrumentation. A number of research diagnostic interviews exist to assess mental disorders among children and adolescents (e.g., Shaffer et al., 2000; Angold and Costello, 2000; Reich, 2000). We were unable to achieve consensus among our advisors in selecting one of these instruments based on the simultaneous consideration of accuracy and ease of implementation. As a result, we elected to use a modified version of the NCS-2 and NCS-R diagnostic interview, the CIDI, in the adolescent survey. This decision was based, in part, on the fact that the CIDI was previously used successfully in a German adolescent sample (Wittchen et al., 1998) as well as among 15–17 year olds in the baseline NCS. An additional consideration was that the same interview staff that administers the NCS-2 and NCS-R adult interviews is also administering the adolescent interviews. We reasoned that it would be much easier for these interviewers if we maintained relative consistency in the instrument across samples rather than using a totally different instrument for the adolescents than for the adults.

The CIDI was expanded for NCS-A to include new sections on child and adolescent disorders derived from the DIS. These include oppositional-defiant disorder, conduct disorder, attention deficit hyperactivity disorder, and separation anxiety. We also modified existing CIDI diagnostic sections that have different criteria for adolescents than adults. In addition, the risk factor battery was expanded to include a more detailed assessment of childhood adversity, while the interview questions on treatment for emotional disorders were revised to blend relevant questions from NCS-R with questions in another instrument designed for use with children and adolescents (Stiffman et al., 2000). Once all these modifications were complete, revisions in question wording were made to improve comprehension among adolescent respondents. This work made use of recently developed cognitive interviewing methods to gain insights into areas of confusion in the instrument and into ways that these confusions might be resolved with modified questions (Kessler et al., 1998c, 1999b). Finally, a self-administered informant version of the instrument was developed to obtain information from the parents of respondents.

THE WHO WORLD MENTAL HEALTH SURVEYS

The World Health Organizations World Mental Health 2000 (WMH2000) Initiative is an outgrowth of the WHO Global Burden of Disease (GBD) study (Murray and Lopez, 1994, 1996), an investigation of the comparative prevalences and social costs of major diseases throughout the world. The first phase of the GBD study concluded that mental disorders are among the most burdensome of all diseases in the world today and that major depression will become the single most burdensome disease in the world within the next two decades. These striking conclusions are based on a unique combination of characteristics shared by depression and many other mental disorders: that they are very common diseases; that they typically have much earlier ages of onset than most chronic physical diseases; that they have high rates of chronicity in conjunction with high risks of impairment and disablement; and that they have low rates of treatment. It might be hoped that these results would influence health policy planners throughout the world to move mental disorders up in their priority list for prevention and treatment initiatives. However, this has not happened as yet. At least one reason for this is that the first phase of the GBD study relied entirely on panels of clinical experts to estimate comparative levels of disease-specific impairment and disablement. The validity of these ratings can be called into question, undercutting the persuasive power of the GBD results concerning the importance of mental disorders.

The WMH2000 Initiative is designed to address this limitation by carrying out a series of parallel community epidemiological surveys based on the interview schedule developed for the NCS-R in countries throughout the world in order to obtain objective estimates of the prevalences, impairments, and patterns of treatment for mental disorders. Over two dozen countries from all regions of the world are participating in WMH2000, with a combined sample size anticipated to be in excess of 200,000 respondents. Because of their emphasis on comparative disease burden, the WMH2000 surveys, including NCS-R, will differ from previous CIDI surveys in five important respects. Each of these will be briefly reviewed here.

Recent Prevalences and Severity

While the focus of almost all CIDI surveys up to now has been on lifetime disorders, WMH2000 will have an equal interest in past year and current (at the time of interview) disorders. All previous versions of CIDI, including the version used in the baseline NCS, provided only superficial information on recent disorders by focusing on lifetime symptoms and asking only one question, "How recently have you had (the disorder)?", to learn about recency. This makes it impossible to characterize the persistence of disorders over the recent past or to know whether respondents with a lifetime disorder meet full criteria during the recent past. The CIDI has been modified to correct these problems for use in WMH2000 by obtaining information about current symptoms and persistence of symptoms over the past year.

In addition to clarifying estimates of recent prevalence, WMH2000 also seeks to focus on recent prevalence to address a question raised by critics of the baseline NCS concerning the clinical significance of community cases (Regier et al., 2000).

These critics hypothesized that a substantial proportion of community cases of mental disorders are not clinically significant. We are addressing this concern by administering structured versions of standard clinical severity measures to all WMH2000 respondents with recent CIDI disorders. Included here are such measures as a structured version of the Inventory of Depressive Symptomatology to assess the severity of recent depression (Rush et al., 1996), a structured version of the Panic Disorder Severity Scale to assess the severity of panic (Shear et al., 1997), and a structured version of the Yale-Brown Obsessive-Compulsive Scale to assess the severity of OCD (Goodman et al., 1989a, 1989b). Our hope is that the use of standard clinical severity scales such as these will help provide a heretofore missing crosswalk between the findings in our epidemiological surveys and the findings in clinical studies.

Clinical Significant Impairment

Related to the issue of clinical significance is the issue of impairment. The CIDI asks only one dichotomous disorder-specific role impairment question for all disorders: "Did (the disorder) ever interfere a lot with your life or activities?" No questions about impairment are asked independent of disorders. This is inadequate for the purposes of WMH2000. Consequently, we have expanded the assessment of impairment in the CIDI to include more detailed disorder-specific questions about both lifetime and 12-month role impairments. All WMH2000 surveys also include the WHO Disability Assessment Schedule (World Health Organization, 1998) to assess overall role impairment and disablement independent of particular disorders.

It is of interest to note that both disorder-specific and global assessments of impairment are important to obtain. Disorder-specific assessments are important because they can be used to make direct comparisons among different mental and physical disorders. These direct comparisons are becoming increasingly central to health care resource allocation decisions as evidence-based medicine becomes the basis for more and more triage decisions. However, disorder-specific assessments are limited by the fact that they require respondents to make inferences about the cause of their impairments. This can be difficult, especially among the large number of people with serious mental disorders who have comorbidity (Kessler et al., 1994).

External assessments are important to obtain because they allow the researcher to overcome the limitation of disorder-specific assessments by empirically estimating the relative effects of different disorders from prediction equations in which information about the prevalences of these disorders and their comorbidities are included as predictors of global impairment. However, as it is not possible to make detailed assessments of all possible disorders for inclusion in such prediction equations, estimates of the impairments due to specific disorders based on analysis of such equations are necessarily imperfect. In the absence of any obvious way to overcome this problem, WMH2000 will collect data to make both direct (based on disorder-specific questions) and indirect (based on analysis of prediction equations) assessments of disorder-specific impairments.

Comparative Impairments of Mental and Physical Disorders

In order to provide comparative information on the impairments of mental and physical disorders, a checklist of chronic physical disorders is included in the WMH2000 assessment. The problem of under-reporting due to some people with chronic conditions not being aware of their disorders is dealt with for symptom-based condition by using symptom screening questions for a random subsample of physical diseases for each WMH2000 respondent. The random subsampling strategy is required because comprehensive screening for all possible physical disorders would be too time-consuming for a one-session survey devoted to mental disorders. However, by taking care to screen randomly to select a separate representative subsample of physical disorders for each respondent, we will guarantee that data will be collected for a representative subsample of people with each chronic disorder for purposes of comparative assessment of within-disorder role impairments.

Calibrating CIDI Diagnoses Based on Clinical Reassessments

There is little doubt but that carefully administered semistructured research diagnostic interviews administered by well-trained clinicians yield diagnostic data that are superior to the data obtained in the CIDI. However, it is infeasible both financially and logistically to use well-trained and experienced clinicians in large-scale surveys of the sort to be carried out in WMH2000. Fortunately, clinical validity studies show that diagnostic discrepancies between the CIDI and clinical interviews are within the bounds of acceptability for most of the disorders assessed in the CIDI (Wittchen, 1994). However, these results have been demonstrated only in Western countries. Legitimate concerns can be raised that these same high levels of validity do not apply across all the countries in which the WMH2000 surveys will be carried out. Based on these concerns, extensive clinical validation interviews are being carried out in WMH2000.

It is fairly common for CIDI surveys to include a small clinical validation component in which a representative subsample of respondents is blindly reinterviewed by a clinical rater using a semistructured research diagnostic interview like the SCID (Spitzer et al., 1992) or the SCAN (Wing et al., 1990). We plan to go beyond these conventional procedures of merely documenting the degree of validity of the CIDI in WMH2000. Based on the assumption that we will find significant between-country differences in validity, we plan to develop corrected estimates of the prevalences of CIDI diagnoses (Shrout and Newman, 1989) and estimates of the correlates of disorders (Spiegelman and Valantis, 1998) based on the results of these validation studies. A technical discussion of procedures involved in generating these corrected estimates is presented elsewhere (Kessler, 1999).

OVERVIEW

Descriptive studies like the NCS are of more importance in psychiatric epidemiology than in other branches of epidemiology because psychiatric epidemiology has traditionally been hampered by difficulties in conceptualizing and measuring disorders. The baseline NCS has been important mainly because it helped resolve these difficulties by providing accurate descriptive data on the prevalence and correlates of mental disorders. However, we have to remember, as we expand the NCS in the ways described in this chapter, that the ultimate goals of epidemiology are to understand and control disease by empirically studying associations between variation in exposure to disease-causing agents external to the individual, variation in the resistance of individuals exposed to the disease-causing agents, and variation in resistance resources in the environments of exposed individuals. Although these investigations are initially carried out by examining natural variations of the sort assessed in the NCS surveys, we have to move beyond this initial step to develop hypotheses that can be tested provisionally in naturalistic quasi-experimental situations with matching or statistical controls used to approximate the conditions of an experiment. If the hypotheses stand up to these preliminary tests, they then need to be evaluated in interventions aimed at preventing the onset or altering the course of the disorders. These evaluations cannot be carried out with the NCS data.

This perspective on the role of the NCS surveys suggests that they should be seen as a necessary step in the evolution of epidemiological research on mental disorders that provide a firm descriptive foundation for further analytic and experimental epidemiological research. The NCS surveys also can be used to provide provisional tests of a number of hypotheses about psychosocial risk factors for the onset and course of mental disorders as well as about barriers to seeking treatment. As multipurpose data collection efforts rather than focused investigations of single disorders, the NCS surveys lend themselves to a great many descriptive and analytic purposes. As such, they should be considered resources for the field. Because of this fact, all the NCS surveys are archived for public use as soon as they are ready for analysis. A public use data tape of the baseline NCS survey has been available for a number of years and similar public data files for the NCS-2, NCS-R, and NCS-A will be made available as soon as documented data files are created. Information about access to these public data file as well as about NCS technical reports can be obtained from the NCS webpage at http://www.hcp.med.harvard.edu/ncs.

ACKNOWLEDGMENTS

The baseline National Comorbidity Survey (NCS) was supported by National Institute of Mental Health (NIMH) grants MH46376, MH49098, and MH52861, with supplemental support from the W.T. Grant Foundation (Grant 90135190). Ronald Kessler was the Principal Investigator of the baseline NCS. His participation in the survey was supported by NIMH Research Scientist Award MH00507. NCS-2 is funded by National Institute of Drug Abuse (NIDA) grant DA12058, with supplemental support from NIMH. NCS-R is funded by NIMH grants MH60220 and MH54280-04. Ronald Kessler and Kathleen Merikangas are Co-Principal Investigators of NCS-2 and NCS-R. Centralized coordination and analysis of the WMH2000 surveys are funded by grants from the John D. and Catherine T. MacArthur Foundation and the Pfizer Foundation. Ronald Kessler and T. Bedirhan Ustun are Co-Directors of WMH2000. A complete list of NCS publications along with information about NCS-2, NCS-R, and WMH2000 can be obtained from the NCS home page at http://www.hcp.med.harvard.edu.ncs. Address comments to RC Kessler, Department of Health Care Policy, Harvard Medical School, 180 Longwood Avenue, Boston, MA 02115.

REFERENCES

Angold A, Costello EJ (2000): The child and adolescent psychiatric assessment (CAPA). J American Acad Child Adoles Psychiatry 39:39–48.

Bourdon KH, Rae DA, Locke BZ, Narrow WE, Regier DA (1992): Estimating the prevalence of mental disorders in U.S. adults from the Epidemiologic Catchment Area Study. Public Health Reports, 107:663–668.

Brown GW, Harris TO (1978): "Social Origins of Depression: A Study of Psychiatric Disorders in Women." New York: Free Press.

Burke KC, Burke JD, Rae DS, Regier DA (1991): Comparing age at onset of major depression and other psychiatric disorders by birth cohorts in five U.S. community populations. Arch Gen Psychiatry 48:789–795.

First MB, Spitzer RL, Gibbon M, Williams JBW (1997): "Structured Clinical Interview for DSM-IV Axis I Disorders, Research Version, Non-patient Edition (SCID-I/NP)." New York: Biometrics Research, New York State Psychiatric Institute.

Freedman D, Thornton A, Camburn D, Alwin D, Young-DeMarco L (1988): The life history calendar: a technique for collecting retrospective data. In Clogg CC (ed): "Sociological Methodology," vol. 18 San Francisco: Jossey-Bass, pp. 37–68.

Gold MR, Siegel JE, Russell LB, Weinstein MC (1996): "Cost-Effectiveness in Health and Medicine." Oxford: Oxford University Press.

Goodman W, Price L, Rasmussen S, Mazure C, Fleischmann R, Hill C, Heninger G, Charney D (1989a): The Yale-Brown obsessive compulsive scale. I. Development, use, and reliability. Arch Gen Psychiatry 46:1006–1011.

Goodman W, Price L, Rasmussen S, Mazure C, Delgado P, Heninger G, Charney D (1989b): The Yale-Brown obsessive compulsive scale. II. Validity. Arch Gen Psychiatry 46:1012–1016.

Keith SJ, Regier DA, Rae DS (1991): Schizophrenic disorders. In "Psychiatric Disorders in America: The Epidemiologic Catchment Area Study." New York: Free Press, pp 33–52.

Kendler KS, Gallagher TJ, Abelson JM, Kessler RC (1996): Lifetime prevalence, demographic risk factors, and diagnostic validity of nonaffective psychosis as assessed in a US community sample. Arch Gen Psychiatry 53:1022–1031.

Kessler RC (1994): Building on the ECA: The National Comorbidity Survey and the Children's ECA. Int J Methods Psychiatric Res 4:81–94.

Kessler RC (1995): The epidemiology of psychiatric comorbidity. In Tsaung MT, Tohen M, Zahner GEP (eds): "Textbook in Psychiatric Epidemiology." New York: Wiley, pp 179–197.

Kessler RC (1997): The prevalence of psychiatric comorbidity. In Wetzler S, Sanderson WC (eds): "Treatment Strategies for Patients with Psychiatric Comorbidity." New York: Wiley, pp 23–48.

Kessler R (1999): The World Health Organization International Consortium in Psychiatric Epidemiology (ICPE): Initial work and future directions—the NAPE lecture 1998. Acta Psychiatrica Scand 99:2–9.

Kessler RC, Berglund PA, Foster CL, Saunders WB, Stang PE, Walters EE (1997a): The social consequences of psychiatric disorders: II. Teenage childbearing. Am J Psychiatry 154:1405–1411.

Kessler RC, Birnbaum HG, Greenberg PE, Simon GE, Barber C, Frank RG, Rose RM, Wang P (1999a): Depression in the workplace: effects on short-term work disability. Health Affairs 18:163–171.

Kessler RC, Crum RM, Warner LA, Nelson CB, Schulenberg J, Anthony JC (1997b): The lifetime co-occurrence of DSM-III-R alcohol abuse and dependence with other psychiatric disorders in the National Comorbidity Survey. Arch Gen Psychiatry 54:313–321.

Kessler RC, Foster CL, Saunders WB, Stang PE (1995a): The social consequences of psychiatric disorders: I. Education attainment. Am J Psychiatry 152:1026–1032.

Kessler RC, Greenberg PE, Mickelson KD, Meneades LM, Wang PS (2001a): The effects of chronic medical conditions on work loss and work cutback. J Occupational Environ Medicine 43 (suppl 3):218–225.

Kessler RC, Little RJA, Groves RM (1995b): Advances in strategies for minimizing and adjusting for survey nonresponse. Epidemiologic Rev 17:192–204.

Kessler RC, McGonagle KA, Zhao S, Nelson CB, Hughes M, Eshleman S, Wittchen HU, Kendler KS (1994): Lifetime and 12-month prevalence of DSM-III-R psychiatric disorders in the United States: Results from the National Comorbidity Survey. Arch Gen Psychiatry 51:8–19.

Kessler RC, Mroczek DK, Belli RF (1999b): Retrospective adult assessment of childhood psychopathology. In Shaffer D, Lucas CP, Richters JE (eds): "Diagnostic Assessment in Child and Adolescent Psychopathology." New York: Guilford Press, pp 256–284.

Kessler RC, Nelson CB, McGonagle KA, Edlund MJ, Frank RG, Leaf PJ (1996): The epidemiology of co-occurring addictive and mental disorders: Implications for prevention and service utilization. Am J Orthopsychiatry 66:17–31.

Kessler RC, Olfson M, Berglund PA (1998a): Patterns and predictors of treatment contact after first onset of psychiatric disorders. Am J Psychiatry 155:62–69.

Kessler RC, Soukup J, Davis RB, Foster DF, Wilkey SA, Van Rompay MI, Eisenberg DM (2001b): The use of complementary and alternative therapies to treat anxiety and depression in the United States. Am J Psychiatry 158:289–294.

Kessler RC, Walters EE, Forthofer MS (1998b): The social consequences of psychiatric disorders: III. Probability of marital stability. Am J Psychiatry 155:1092–1096.

Kessler RC, Wittchen HU, Abelson JM, McGonagle KA, Schwarz N, Kendler KS, Knauper B, Zhao S (1998c): Methodological studies of the Composite International Diagnostic Interview (CIDI) in the U.S. National Comorbidity Survey. Int J Methods Psychiatric Res 7:33–55.

Kessler RC, Wittchen HU, Ustun B, Roy-Byrne PP, Walters EE (1998d): Lifetime panic-depression comorbidity in the National Comorbidity Survey. Arch Gen Psychiatry 55:801–808.

Kessler RC, Ustun TB (2000): Editorial: The World Health Organization World Mental Health 2000 (WMH2000) Initiative. Hospital Management International, pp 195–196.

Lyketsos CG, Nestadt G, Cwi J, Heithoff K, Eaton WW (1994): The Life-Chart Interview: A standarzied method to describe the course of psychopathology. Int J Methods Psychiatric Res 4:143–155.

Magee WJ, Eaton WW, Wittchen HU, McGonagle KA, Kessler RC (1996): Agoraphobia, simple phobia, and social phobia in the National Comorbidity Survey. Arch Gen Psychiatry 53:159–168.

Murray CJ, Lopez AD (1994): "Global Comparative Assessments in the Health Sector." Geneva: World Health Organization.

Murray CJ, Lopez AD (1996): "The Global Burden of Disease: A Comprehensive Assessment of Mortality and Disability from Diseases, Injuries, and Risk Factors in 1990 and Projected to 2020." Cambridge: Harvard University Press.

National Research Council, Committee on the Social and Economic Impact of Pathological Gambling (1999): "Pathological Gambling: A Critical Review." Washington, DC: National Academy Press.

President's Commission on Mental Health and Illness (1978): "Report to the President from the President's Commission on Mental Health, vol I. Washington, DC: U.S. Government Printing Office.

Regier DA, Farmer ME, Rae DS, Locke BZ, Keith SJ, Judd LL, Goodwin FK (1990): Comorbidity of mental disorders with alcohol and other drug abuse. J Am Med Assoc 264:2511–2518.

Regier DA, Kaelber CT, Rae DS, Farmer ME, Knauper B, Kessler RC, Norquist GS (1998): Limitations of diagnostic criteria and assessment instruments for mental disorders. Implications for research and policy [see comments]. Arch Gen Psychiatry 55:109–115.

Regier DA, Narrow WE, Rae DS, Manderscheid RW, Locke BZ, Goodwin FK (1993): The de facto U.S. Mental and Addictive Disorders Service System: Epidemiologic Catchment Area prospective 1-year prevalence rates of disorders and services. Arch Gen Psychiatry 50:85–94.

Regier D, Narrow W, Rupp A, Rae D, Kaelber C (2000): The epidemiology of mental disorder treatment need: community estimates of medical necessity. In Andrews G, Henderson S (eds): "Unmet Need in Psychiatry." Cambridge: Cambridge University Press, pp 41–58.

Reich W (2000): Diagnostic interview for children and adolescents (DICA). J Am Acad Child Adoles Psychiatry 39:59–66.

Robins LN, Helzer JE, Croughan JL, Ratcliff KS (1981): National Institute of Mental Health Diagnostic Interview Schedule: Its history, characteristics and validity. Arch Gen Psychiatry 38:381–389.

Robins LN, Locke BZ, Regier DA (1991): An overview of psychiatric disorders in America. In Robins LN, Regier DA (eds): Psychiatric Disorders in America: the Epidemiologic Catchment Area Study. New York: Free Press, pp 328–366.

Rosenbaum PR, Rubin DB (1983): The central role of the propensity score in observational studies for causal effects. Biometrika 70:41–55.

Rush A, Gullion C, Basco M, Jarrett R, Trivedi M (1996): The Inventory of Depressive Symptomatology (IDS): psychometric properties. Psychological Medicine 26:477–486.

Shaffer D, Fisher P, Lucas CP, Dulcan MK, Schwab-Stone ME (2000): NIMH Diagnostic Interview Schedule for Children Version IV (NIMH DISC-IV): description, differences from previous versions, and reliability of some common diagnoses. J Am Acad Child Adoles Psychiatry 39:28–38.

Shear M, Brown T, Barlow D, Money R, Sholomskas D, Woods S, Gorman J, Papp L (1997): Multicenter collaborative panic disorder severity scale. Am J Psychiatry 154:1571–1575.

Shrout P, Newman S (1989): Design of two-phase prevalence surveys of rare disorders. Biometrics 45:549–555.

Spiegelman D, Valantis B (1998): Correcting for bias in relative risk estimates due to exposure measurment error: A case study of occupational exposure to antineoplastics in pharmacists. Am J Pub Health 36:1–37.

Spitzer RL, Williams JBW, Gibbon M, First MB (1992): The Structured Clinical Interview for DSM-III-R (SCID). I. History, rationale, and description. Arch Gen Psychiatry 49:624–629.

Stiffman A, Horwitz S, Hoagwood K, Compton WR, Cottler L, Bean D, Narrow W, Weisz J (2000): The Service Assessment for Children and Adolescents (SACA): Adult and child reports. J Am Acad Child Adoles Psychiatry 39:1032–1039.

Wells KB, Sturm R, Sherbourne CD, Meredith L (1996): Caring for Depression. Cambridge: Harvard University Press.

Wethington E, Brown GW, Kessler RC (1995): Interview measurement of stressful life events. In Cohen S, Kessler RC, Gordon LU (eds): "Measuring Stress: A Guide for Health and Social Scientists." New York: Oxford University Press, pp 59–79.

Williams JBW, Gibbon M, First MB, Spitzer RL, Davies M, Borus J, Howes MJ, Kane J, Harrison GP, Jr, Rounsaville B, Wittchen HU (1992): The structured clinical interview for DSM-III-R (SCID). II. Multisite test-retest reliability. Arch Gen Psychiatry 49:630–636.

Wing J, Babor T, Brugha T, Burke J, Cooper J, Giel R, Jablenskii A, Regier D, Sartorius N (1990): SCAN. Schedules for clinical assesment in neuropsychiatry. Arch Gen Psychiatry, 47:589–593.

Wittchen H-U (1994): Reliability and validity studies of the WHO Composite International Diagnostic Interview (CIDI): A critical review. J Psychiatric Res (Oxford) 28:57–84.

Wittchen H-U, Perkonigg A, Lachner G, Nelson CB (1998): Early developmental stages of psychopathology study (EDSP): objectives and design. Eur Addiction Res 4:18–27.

World Health Organization (1990): Composite International Diagnostic Interview (CIDI), version 1.0. Geneva: World Health Organization.

World Health Organization (1998): WHO Disablements Assessment Schedule II (WHO-DAS II). Geneva: World Health Organization.

PART III

Epidemiology of Major Psychiatric Disorders

CHAPTER 15

Epidemiology of Psychosis with Special Reference to Schizophrenia

EVELYN J. BROMET, MARY AMANDA DEW, and WILLIAM W. EATON

State University of New York at Stony Brook (E.J.B.); University of Pittsburgh (M.A.D.); Johns Hopkins University (W.W.E.)

INTRODUCTION

Psychotic disorders, such as schizophrenia, schizoaffective disorder, psychotic depression, bipolar disorder with psychotic features, and delusional disorder, are among the most debilitating and persistent diseases known to humankind. Psychotic disorders are associated with increased mortality (Allebeck and Wistedt, 1986) and are costly and uniquely distressing for patients and their families (Brown and Birtwistle, 1998). Estimates of the annual direct and indirect cost in the United States of schizophrenia alone range from $30 billion (American Psychiatric Association, 2001) to $65 billion (Wyatt et al., 1995). To date, epidemiologic research on psychosis has focused primarily on the incidence, prevalence, and risk factors associated with schizophrenia, as well as its etiology, course, and outcome. Indeed, Häfner (2000) described the field as a thriving discipline at the turn of the century. Many comprehensive reviews of this body of research have appeared, including contributions by the current authors (e.g., Bromet et al., 1988, 1995; Eaton, 1999; Eaton et al., 1988) and other eminent investigators (e.g., Beiser and Iacono, 1990; Cooper, 1978; Jablensky, 1986, 1995, 1997, 2000; Jones and Cannon, 1998). This chapter builds on these reviews, considering both descriptive research on rates and risk factors and analytic findings on etiology and course. We begin with a brief overview of the methodological approaches encompassed by epidemiologic research on schizophrenia and other psychotic disorders and then review recent descriptive and analytic findings. Last, we delineate some target areas for future research.

Textbook in Psychiatric Epidemiology, Second Edition, Edited by Ming T. Tsuang and Mauricio Tohen. ISBN 0-471-40974-X

TABLE 1. Types of Research Methods Applied to Epidemiologic Studies of Schizophrenia and Related Disorders

	Source of Case Ascertainment and Classification	
Target Population	Medical Record/Informant/ Case Registry	Structured Diagnostic Interview
Patients	A	B
Community residents	N/A	C

METHODOLOGICAL APPROACHES

Three approaches to investigating the rates and risk factors for schizophrenia can be found in the literature. The first type of study (A in Table 1) relies on key informant reports, clinical records, or registry data for case ascertainment. One of the earliest prevalence studies of this sort was the classic census of the "insane" conducted in Massachusetts in the nineteenth century. This survey enumerated approximately 3,600 "lunatics" and "idiots" in family, private, or public care (Jarvis, 1971). Another classic contribution was the Faris and Dunham (1939) ecological investigation of risk factors for mental disorders. Using Illinois state mental hospital records, they showed that, unlike patients with other diagnoses, individuals with schizophrenia were most likely to come from inner-city, socially disintegrated urban areas and least likely to have lived in suburban areas with better socioeconomic conditions. This study provided strong evidence that rates of schizophrenia were inversely related to social class, although whether this association was attributable to social selection, environmental stress, or a combination of the two could not be tested from the aggregated data at hand.

Recent studies of rates and risk factors have taken advantage of psychiatric case registries, including linking them with birth and medical registries to examine, for example, temporal changes in rates, patterns of urban–rural birth, season of birth, family history of schizophrenia, age of onset, age and sex-specific morbid risk, and patterns of treatment (e.g., Eaton et al., 2000; Mortensen et al., 1999). In settings like Denmark, the quality of the registry diagnoses is enhanced by the uniformity of training in psychiatry throughout the country and the relatively narrow definitions of disorders that are employed. Moreover, Jablensky (1997) argued that in some parts of Europe, the diagnosis of dementia praecox in 1908 is comparable to ICD schizophrenia in the 1970s, thus facilitating the analysis of temporal trends in rates of schizophrenia. The registries are comprehensive (in Denmark, all hospitals report to the registry, and since 1995, all specialty clinics as well), and the analysis of registry data has contributed immeasurably to our understanding of the epidemiology of schizophrenia as well as other psychiatric and medical disorders (Mortensen, 1995).

However, in many countries, including the United States, diagnostic practices are variable, and record-based diagnoses are not reliable sources of information on diagnosis. Moreover, Cooper et al. (1978) argued that differences in diagnostic practices, amplified by the absence of explicit operational criteria, were major impediments to progress in research on the epidemiology of schizophrenia. The issue reached a crescendo with the publication of the findings of the landmark

U.S.–U.K. project (Cooper et al., 1972). Prior to this project, higher rates of schizophrenia were reported in hospitalized patients in the United States compared to England, while relatively more patients were diagnosed with affective disorders, such as manic depressive disorder, in the United Kingdom. The U.S.–U.K. project for the first time trained psychiatrists in both countries in a structured diagnostic interview (the Present State Examination) and applied a common set of diagnostic criteria. The results showed that the proportions of patients with schizophrenia and affective disorder were similar, indicating that previously observed variations in the distributions were a function of diagnostic practices rather than of true differences in morbidity patterns.

The introduction of modern nosologic systems that followed on the heels of the U.S.–U.K. study led to renewed interest in epidemiologic research on schizophrenia using research methods that incorporated structured interviews and formal diagnostic systems, such as the Research Diagnostic Criteria (RDC) (Spitzer et al., 1978) and DSM-III (American Psychiatric Association, 1980). Thus, the second type of study (B in Table 1) is characterized by a focus on treated populations using psychometric advances in diagnosis. The most noteworthy epidemiologic undertaking in this category is the World Health Organization's (WHO's) program of research on schizophrenia, particularly the Determinants of Outcome of Severe Mental Disorders (DOSMED) conducted in catchment areas in ten countries. In this project, 1,379 psychotic individuals aged 15–54 years were identified at the point of their first lifetime mental health service contact (including with traditional healers in developing countries) and followed annually over a two-year period (Jablensky et al., 1992). The DOSMED findings on incidence rates are reported below. In North America, several first-admission studies also focused on incidence rates (Beiser et al., 1988), as well as etiology (Pulver et al., 1981) and illness course (Beiser et al., 1989; Bromet et al., 1992; Tohen et al., 1992) in systematically diagnosed patient populations. These studies are distinct from other clinical studies of psychotic disorders in their attention to representative sampling, use of structured diagnostic interview schedules, and focus on first-admission patients, as opposed to consecutive admissions with varying treatment histories.

The third type of epidemiologic study of schizophrenia combines modern community sampling techniques with structured diagnostic interviews (C in Table 1). The earliest such studies were conducted by psychiatrists in Europe starting before World War II (Jablensky, 1986). The first large-scale community study in the United States to administer a diagnostic interview in the community was the Epidemiologic Catchment Area (ECA) study, in which lay interviewers were trained to administer the Diagnostic Interview Schedule (DIS) (Robins and Regier, 1991). Unfortunately, the DIS diagnosis of schizophrenia was not congruent with psychiatrists' classification. For example, in the Baltimore ECA site, the DIS identified only 20% of the cases of schizophrenia that a psychiatrist diagnosed in an independent examination (Anthony et al., 1985). As a consequence, ten years later, when Kessler et al. (1994) conducted the National Comorbidity Survey, a two-stage procedure for case identification was implemented. The first stage involved a lay-administered structured interview, the Composite International Diagnostic Interview, or CIDI. In the second stage, respondents who endorsed psychotic symptoms (and a random sample of those who did not) were reinterviewed by a clinician on the telephone with a modified version of the Structured

Clinical Interview for DSM-III-R (SCID; Spitzer et al., 1992; Williams et al., 1992). Classification was thus based on the additional clinical information rather than on the lay interviews alone.

In the next sections, we summarize findings on the incidence and prevalence of schizophrenia, factors associated with the occurrence of the disorder, and variables linked to better or worse courses.

PREVALENCE AND INCIDENCE RATES

Definition of Disorder

Since almost all prevalence and incidence studies to date have focused on schizophrenia, we begin with a definition of this disorder. The essential features of schizophrenia are the presence of specific psychotic symptoms (delusions, hallucinations, thought disorder, grossly disorganized or catatonic behavior, negative symptoms); social or occupational dysfunction (functioning below the level achieved before onset); and a six-month duration of illness, including the prodromal and residual phases and one month of psychotic symptoms (American Psychiatric Association 1994).

Rates

Prevalence. Prior to the introduction of the DSM-III and recent revisions of the ICD, the prevalence of schizophrenia was estimated to range from 1–7 percent. In a review of more recent studies, Jablensky (2000) placed the prevalence rate in the range of 1.4–4.6 per thousand. This downward shift is largely due to the narrowing of the criteria for schizophrenia in nosological systems published after 1980.

In the Eaton et al. (1988) review of 25 treated prevalence studies involving samples of at least 2,500 persons and study diagnosis formulated by a psychiatrist, the median point prevalence rate was 3.2 per 1,000 (range 0.6–8.3), the median lifetime prevalence rate was 2.7 per 1,000 (range 0.9–3.8), and the median period prevalence rate was 4.4 per thousand (range 1.7–7.0).

Four community-based sources of data on psychotic disorders have reported rates based on clinician-based diagnoses using recent diagnostic criteria (Table 2). The first is the Baltimore ECA clinical reinterview study, noted above, in which a subsample of respondents were evaluated by psychiatrists with an expanded version of the Present State Examination; the lifetime prevalence rate of DSM-III schizophrenia was 6.4 per 1000, and the "active" case rate was 4.6 per 1000 (Von Korff et al., 1985). The second source is the two-phase study of mental disorders conducted with a cohort born in Israel between 1949 and 1958 (Dohrenwend et al., 1992); they were assessed with the Schedule for Affective Disorders and Schizophrenia and diagnosed using the Research Diagnostic Criteria (Endicott and Spitzer, 1978). The lifetime prevalence rates of definite schizophrenia for the North African and European members of the cohort were 5.7 and 8.9 per thousand, respectively. In 1990, the US National Comorbidity Survey (NCS) was conducted with approximately 8,000 individuals aged 15–55; based on a subsample reinterviewed by psychiatrists with the Structured Clinical Interview for DSM-III-R

TABLE 2. Lifetime Prevalence Rates from Two-Stage Community Studies with Clinical Reinterview Information

Source	Diagnostic System	Disorder	Rate per 1,000
Baltimore ECA clinical reinterview subsample (von Korff et al., 1985)	DSM-III	Schizophrenia	6.4
Israeli cohort born 1948–1959 (Dohrehwend et al., 1992)	RDC	Schizophrenia (definite)	5.7 (North Africans) 8.9 (Europeans)
U.S. National Comobidity Survey (Kendler et al., 1996)	DSM-III-R	Schizophrenia Nonaffective psychosis	1.4 6.9
Dutch national survey (van Os et al., 2001)	DSM-III-R	Schizophrenia, schizo-affective disorder, schizophreniform disorder Affective psychoses	3.7 11.4

(SCID), the lifetime prevalence rates were 1.4 per thousand for DSM-III-R schizophrenia, and 6.9 per thousand for five nonaffective psychoses combined, e.g., schizophrenia, schizophreniform disorder, schizoaffective disorder, delusional disorder, and atypical psychosis (Kendler et al., 1996). The fourth study is the Dutch national morbidity survey of approximately 7,000 individuals aged 18–64 (van Os et al., 2001). Applying a similar methodology to the NCS, this study estimated a lifetime prevalence rate of 3.7 per thousand for DSM-III-R schizophrenia, schizoaffective disorder, and schizophreniform disorder combined, and 11.4 per thousand for affective psychosis.

Clearly, the rates are not perfectly consistent across the studies. Jablensky (2000) noted that demographic differences, particularly age-specific mortality and migration, will influence the specific rates. It is worth emphasizing, however, that compared to prevalence findings for other multifactorial diseases, such as heart disease, diabetes, and autoimmune disorders like Sjogrens syndrome, the magnitude of the differences in rates of schizophrenia across studies is relatively small.

Incidence. In his landmark review of incidence studies published between 1950 and 1986, Eaton et al. (1988) reported a median annual incidence rate per thousand of 0.20 for 11 case register studies, 0.22 for the 8 sites participating in the WHO DOSMED study, and 0.35 for four community studies. More recently, Eaton (1999) presented data from 27 incidence studies of schizophrenia published in English since 1985. Only studies involving diagnosis by psychiatrist and samples drawn from both outpatient as well as inpatient facilities were included. Not surprisingly, given the narrowing of the diagnostic criteria, the median incidence rate, 0.16 per thousand, was lower than reported previously. The lowest rate was found in Vancouver (0.04 per thousand per year) and the highest in Madras (0.58 per thousand per year). However, Eaton did not find an effect of region on the magnitude of the incidence rate.

A related and controversial question concerns the temporal stability of the incidence rate over the past 100 years. There is some suggestion that the rate has declined (e.g., Eagles and Whalley, 1985; Woogh, 2001), while other evidence

TABLE 3. Risk and Protective Factors

Demographic Characteristics	Predisposing Characteristics	Precipitating Factors
Social class	Family history, genetics	Stress: life events, expressed emotion
Race, ethnicity	Autoimmunity	Substance abuse
Age	Season of birth	
Gender	Urban vs. rural birth	
Marital Status	Obstetric, birth, and early childhood complications	

indicates that it has remained stable (Ösby et al., 2001). As Ösby et al. (2001) note, it will be important for future studies to clarify the temporal trends both to enhance our understanding of the causes of schizophrenia and to plan appropriately for mental health services.

RISK AND PROTECTIVE FACTORS

Cooper (1978) grouped the risk factors for schizophrenia into three categories: demographic characteristics (social class, ethnicity, gender and age, marital status), predisposing factors (familial and genetic background, season of birth, pregnancy and birth complications, rheumatic or autoimmune disease), and precipitating factors (stress, substance abuse) (Table 3). We briefly review the findings in each of these areas.

Demographic Characteristics

Social Class. One of the most consistent epidemiologic findings is the inverse relationship between social class and schizophrenia (Dohrenwend and Dohrenwend, 1969). Eaton et al. (1988) concluded that there is a three to one difference in rates between the lowest and highest class. Since the publication of the Faris and Dunham study in 1939 described above, two sets of hypotheses have been tested to explain this association. One hypothesis is that environmental exposures that are more common in lower social class populations are responsible in large part for the elevated rate of schizophrenia found in these populations. These exposures include infectious agents, noxious workplace conditions (Link et al., 1986; Muntaner et al., 1991), poor quality maternal and obstetric care leading to higher risk of fetal injury, inadequate nutrition early in life, and social factors (isolation, trauma exposure, paternal alcoholism, daily stress). A recent analysis of incident cases in Maastricht, Holland, extended and refined the social causation argument by suggesting that there may be an interaction between neighborhood environmental characteristics and premorbid vulnerability (van Os et al., 2000). The evidence linking these environmental risk factors to the occurrence of schizophrenia is reviewed below.

The second hypothesis, termed the *selection-drift hypothesis*, is that schizophrenia-prone individuals are either prevented from attaining higher social class levels (selection) or move progressively downward (drift). Both the failure to be upwardly mobile and downward mobility are believed to occur because the onset of schizophrenia is insidious and begins during adolescence, when social and occupational skills are learned. In support of the selection-drift hypothesis, Turner and Wagenfeld (1967) showed that in Monroe County, New York, males with schizophrenia were less upwardly mobile from their father than were their peers in the general population. Similarly, in a classic study of young, male patients with schizophrenia, Goldberg and Morrison (1963) found both less than expected upward mobility from their fathers' socio-economic level as well as downward drift after the initial appearance of psychotic symptoms. More recently, Jones et al. (1993) confirmed both patterns in schizophrenia and most important, showed that patients with affective psychosis suffered a decline in occupational performance after diagnosis but were not downwardly mobile compared to their fathers.

One of the most elegant tests of the causation versus selection hypotheses was the birth cohort study in Israel. This study was designed specifically to test these two competing hypotheses by contrasting effects of minority status with socioeconomic status. The findings for schizophrenia strongly supported the selection hypothesis (Dohrenwend et al., 1992).

Since one of the cardinal features of schizophrenia is the failure to achieve one's potential, or once diagnosed, to return to one's best premorbid level of functioning, the selection-drift hypothesis has the most adherents. On the other hand, if schizophrenia is a heterogeneous disease (Bellack and Blanchard, 1993), then both hypotheses may have merit in different subgroups of individuals carrying this diagnosis.

Race and Ethnicity. These associations with schizophrenia have been evaluated from a number of points of view, including race differences in prevalence and incidence rates, cross-national comparisons, and comparisons of immigrant groups to rates in their home countries (Eaton and Harrison, 2000).

Using medical record diagnoses, both early (e.g., Malzberg, 1940; Khuri and Wood, 1984) and more recent studies of hospitalized patients (Lawson et al., 1994; Snowden and Cheung, 1990; Strakowski et al., 1995, 1993) report that blacks are more frequently diagnosed with schizophrena while whites are disproportionately diagnosed with affective disorders. One important exception is the Suffolk County study which did not find evidence of race differences in clinical discharge diagnoses (Sohler and Bromet, 2001). Craig et al. (1982), however, found that when diagnosis was based on systematic assessment of symptoms, race differences in rates of schizophrenia and depression were small and nonsignificant, suggesting that the observed race difference in medical record diagnosis reflects racial bias in the assignment of unstructured clinical diagnoses (Adebimpe, 1994). In a similar vein, two large community surveys using standardized diagnostic procedures reported no racial differences in the prevalence of schizophrenia (Robins and Regier, 1991; Kessler et al., 1994). In the absence of any reasonable hypotheses other than racial bias, and the consensus that the rate of schizophrenia is similar in countries around the world (Eaton, 1999), it seems reasonable to conclude that there are no systematic differences in the rates of schizophrenia by race and that observed differences in treatment samples are largely attributable to bias.

There have been isolated reports of unusually high or low prevalence rates in specific geographic areas. For example, elevated rates were found in the Istrian peninsula in the former Yugoslavia (Lemkau et al., 1980) and the western coast of Ireland (Walsh et al., 1980). Conceivably, these differences can be explained by other extraneous factors. Torrey et al. (2001) noted that the geographic differences in rates of schizophrenia in Denmark could be accounted for by age, gender, and urbanicity of place of birth. The presumed low treated prevalence rate of the Hutterites in North Dakota and western Canada was the subject of an early study by Eaton and Weil (1955) who found that the Hutterites took care of their mentally ill members without using outside mental health services.

While the rate of schizophrenia in Caribbean countries is similar to the rate for the white population in England, an excess in the relative risk of psychosis ranging from 1.7 to 13.2 has been reported in the British-born children of immigrants from African-Caribbean countries (Bhugra, 2000; Eaton and Harrison, 2000). Similar findings have appeared for immigrants who came to Holland from Surinam and the Netherlands Antilles (Selten et al. 1997). A considerable body of research has emerged, but little support has been found for explanations involving misclassification or biological, social, genetic, or cultural risk factors. The search for potential confounding variables, that is, variables associated with both schizophrenia and disadvantaged ethnic status, has also failed to identify any obvious candidates (Sharpley et al. 2001). Eaton and Harrison (2000) have proposed that the excess may be due to the developmental challenge of fomulating a life plan, which may be more difficult in disadvantaged ethnic minorities.

Gender and Age. Early studies of treatment samples diagnosed with less systematic criteria concluded that the prevalence of schizophrenia was equal in males and females (Dohrenwend et al., 1980). It is instructive that the lifetime prevalence rate for schizophrenia in the Israeli community cohort was twice as high in men (10.2 per thousand) compared to women (5.3 per thousand) (Dohrenwend et al., 1992). This cohort was not biased by treatment seeking or chronicity (Angermeyer et al., 1989; Munk-Jorgensen, 1985), and the diagnosis was based on a modern classification system. Recent findings based on incidence data indicate a male excess in first-episode schizophrenia (e.g., Murray and van Os, 1998), especially in populations with onset under age 35 (Beiser and Iacono, 1990; Jablensky, 1986; Jones et al., 1998; Riecher et al., 1991). In the Suffolk County sample, where consensus-based DSM-IV diagnoses were applied, the male:female ratios were 3:1 for schizophrenia, 1:1 for bipolar disorder with psychotic features, and 2:5 for major depressive disorder with psychotic features.

Males develop schizophrenia at an earlier age than females (Murray and van Os, 1998), with onset occurring in the early 20s in males and in the late 20s to early 30s in females, a 5–10 year difference. This finding is typically based on studies that use age at first hospitalization to define age of onset (Riecher et al., 1991) although in the Suffolk County first-admission sample, the age at first psychotic symptom (as opposed to first admission) was also significantly younger in males with schizophrenia (mean 24.8; SD = 7.5) than females (mean 27.1; SD = 8.0) ($p < 0.05$). However, the gender difference in age of onset may not be as striking in samples ascertained at the time of their first episode. In the Vancouver cohort, for example, the age of onset was comparable for males and females (early 20s) across three definitions of onset, namely, age at first noticeable symptom, age of first prominent psychotic symptom, and age at initiation of treatment (Beiser et al., 1993).

Examination of age and gender effects continues to be an important topic of research. To the extent that there are gender differences in age of onset, questions arise about the disease process itself. If schizophrenia has an earlier onset in males, and this onset tends to be more insidious than in females, then what biologic factors might account for this? For example, some studies have shown that the gender difference in age of onset is more often found in "sporadic" cases rather than familial schizophrenia (e.g., DeLisi et al., 1994). Another hypothesis tested by the Mannheim research program was that an "elevated vulnerability threshold for women until menopause" could be due to "the sensitivity-reducing effect of estrogen on D_2 receptors in the central nervous system" (Häfner et al., 1998). Identification of these factors might provide clues about disease-promotion mechanisms.

Marital Status. The findings for marital status are as consistent as those for social class. Eaton et al. (1988) previously noted that the ratio of nomarried to married persons varied from 2.6 to 7.2. Several studies have found that females with schizophrenia are more likely to marry than males. Riecher et al. (1991) found that in Mannheim and Denmark, 31% and 29% of first-admission females with schizophrenia were married, respectively, compared with 13% and 9% of males. In the Suffolk sample age 25 and older at admission, twice as many females (49%) had ever married compared to males (24%). These findings are consistent with studies showing that females have better premorbid social competence than males. It may also be the case that females have a milder form of the disease, that they are better able to adapt to their illness than males, or as Seeman (2001) and others have suggested, that estrogen exerts a protective effect by neutralizing the neurotoxic effects of stress.

PREDISPOSING FACTORS

Family History and Genetics. Schizophrenia aggregates strongly in families (Jones and Cannon, 1998). Over the past two decades, there have been numerous reviews of the genetic epidemiology of schizophrenia (cf. Murray et al., 1986). In their classic book on this topic, Gottesman and Shields (1982) calculated that the morbid risk in first-degree relatives was 5.6% in the parents of schizophrenics, 12.8% in the children of one schizophrenic parent, and 46.3% in the children of two schizophrenic parents. In dizygotic twins and siblings, the rate is about 15%, and in monozygotic twins reared together or apart, the rate is over 50% (Jones and Cannon, 1998; Murray et al., 1986). Kendler (1988) concluded that in family studies using blind diagnoses, control groups, personal interviews and operationalized diagnostic criteria, the risk for schizophrenia in close relatives of patients with schizophrenia is 5–15 times greater than in the general population. In the Roscommon Family Study, the risk for schizophrenia was 6.5% in relatives who were directly interviewed (Kendler et al., 1993). Of special interest is the similar risk of schizophrenia in relatives of patients with other psychotic diagnoses: 6.7% for relatives of probands with schizoaffective disorder, 6.9% for schizotypal personality disorder, and 5.1% for other nonaffective psychoses. The exception was psychotic affective disorder, where the risk for schizophrenia in first degree relatives was considerably lower, 2.8%. The rate of schizophrenia in the relatives of patients with all diagnoses was significantly higher than the rate in controls (Kendler et al., 1993).

Given the accumulated evidence from genetic epidemiologic research, and an overall heritability estimate for the liability to schizophrenia of 60–70% (Kendler, 1988; Jones and Cannon, 1998), it is not surprising that considerable effort has focused on identifying the genes responsible for schizophrenia. Although some progress has been made (e.g., replications have now been reported for loci on chromosomes 6p, 8p, 10p, 13q, 15q, and 22q), Tsuang et al. (2001) among others have concluded that we are a long way from discovering the genes that cause schizophrenia.

While the findings from genetic studies demonstrate the unequivocal importance of heritability, they have also been used to imply that 20–30% of the variance in the liability to schizophrenia is attributable to environmental or other nongenetic factors. However, the precise contribution of such variables cannot be ascertained from genetic studies. An obvious issue raised by genetic epidemiology findings is the extent to which the effects of genetic predisposition to schizophrenia are mediated by other vulnerability factors, such as prenatal or perinatal exposure (Cooper, 2001). No doubt, the interconnections are complicated both by the heterogeneity of schizophrenia itself and by the multiplicity of exposures that co-occur in the population.

Autoimmune Disease. Rheumatoid arthritis rarely occurs in patients with schizophrenia (Jablensky, 1986; Eaton et al., 1992) and hence has been conceptualized as a protective factor. Eaton et al. reviewed the 14 published studies on this topic. The median prevalence of rheumatoid arthritis was 0.047% in schizophrenia compared to 0.16% in people with other psychiatric diagnoses. In spite of the consistency of this association across the 14 studies, the methodologies were found to be wanting. On the other hand, there is evidence for an increased rate of thyroid disease and insulin-dependent diabetes mellitus in the first degree relatives of individuals with psychosis compared to normal controls, suggesting that heritability of psychosis might be associated with heritability of autoimmune diseases (e.g., Gilvarry et al., 1996). A recent study of 121 DSM-III-R diagnosed patients with schizophrenia found, based on interviews with the mothers, that among the 30 patients with a first degree relative with schizophrenia, 60% had a parent or sibling with an autoimmune disease compared to 20% of the 91 nonfamilial schizophrenia patients (Wright et al., 1996). Overall, the frequency of insulin-dependent diabetes was higher in the relatives of patients compared to relatives of healthy controls. Thus, if confirmed in other studies, these findings suggest that at least in some cases, schizophrenia may be a variant of an autoimmune disease.

Season of Birth. The proportion of people with schizophrenia born during the winter months is about 5–15% higher than at other times of the year (Torrey, 1993). Similar seasonal differences have been reported in Down's syndrome and certain cardiovascular diseases although not in other psychiatric diagnoses (Jablensky, 1986). This differential has been found to be greater in females with schizophrenia (Pulver et al., 1991) and in patients without a family history of schizophrenia (O'Callaghan et al., 1991). However, Angst (1991) argued that, statistical significance aside, the contribution of this variable to explaining the occurrence of schizophrenia is very weak. Moreover, season of birth may be a proxy for several underlying factors, such as viral infections, diet, or other variables affecting fetal development.

Urban versus Rural Place of Birth. Several studies suggest that being raised in an urban environment is a direct, or at least indirect, risk factor for schizophrenia (e.g., David et al., 1992; Eaton et al., 2000; Haukka et al., 2001; Takei et al., 1992) and for psychosis and psychotic symptoms (van Os et al., 2001). Using data from a cohort of close to 50,000 Swedish conscripts, Lewis et al (1992) found that individuals raised in an urban area had a 1.65 times greater risk of schizophrenia than those raised in rural areas. More recently, Mortensen et al. (1999) compared the risk for schizophrenia associated with three factors, urban place of birth, family history of schizophrenia, and season of birth; family history had the strongest relative risk, but place of birth yielded the largest attributable risk. Moreover, in some studies the effects were specific to schizophrenia rather than psychotic disorders in general. For example, by linking the Danish Medical Birth Register with the Danish Psychiatric Case Register, Eaton et al. (2000) showed that in individuals born after 1972 and hospitalized in Denmark before 1994, the risk of hospitalization for schizophrenia and other non-affective psychoses (mostly paranoid psychoses) was 4.2–5.9 times higher for those born in Copenhagen compared to rural areas, but there was no urban–rural difference in risk of hospitalization for affective psychosis. Using prevalence data, Widerlov et al. (1997) also found an urban–rural gradient for schizophrenia but not for other diagnostic groups suffering from "long-term functional psychoses."

Of course, urban–rural comparisons combine a host of differences in morbidity, comorbidity, service availability, selective migration, and social and physical environmental parameters that must be incorporated into hypotheses explaining the mechanisms underlying the urban–rural findings. In one of the few studies to adjust for such variables, Eaton et al. (2000) noted that the urban–rural relationship for schizophrenia was not mediated by obstetric complications. Thus, given the strength of the findings for urban birth, and the trend toward urbanization over the past two centuries, it is important to continue to try to understand why the rate of schizophrenia is higher in urban areas.

Obstetric, Birth and Early Childhood Complications. Several complications of pregnancy and fetal development have been studied as risk factors for schizophrenia, including maternal stress, pre-eclampsia, low maternal weight, rhesus incompatibility, small head circumference, fetal distress, and low birth weight. A meta-analysis of 18 schizophrenia studies reported an odds ratio of 2.0 (95% confidence interval 1.6–2.4) for obstetric complications of all kinds although the authors cautioned that both selection and publication bias could have inflated the association (Geddes and Lawrie, 1995). Nevertheless, the odds ratio is impressive since these events are relatively common in the general population and may themselves be associated with risk factors such as low social class.

The findings on maternal stress during pregnancy come primarily from two studies of pregnant women exposed to war. One study focused on mothers exposed to the bombing in the Netherlands during World War II and found an increase in schizophrenia among children who were *in utero* during the first trimester (van Os and Selten, 1998). In the other study, Meijer (1985) suggested that the offspring of mothers exposed during pregnancy to the six-day Arab–Israeli war displayed developmental delays and behavioral deviance. Of course, the interpretation of this relationship is complicated because stress is associated with both biological changes (e.g., elevations in epinephrine and norepinephrine), changes in health behavior (increased smoking, alcohol, or other substance abuse, dietary changes), and/or preterm delivery, and these variables were not studied directly.

The three specific classes of variables with the most compelling evidence to date are exposure to prenatal nutritional deprivation, prenatal brain injury, and prenatal influenza. The evidence regarding nutritional deprivation comes from both case–control and cohort studies. For example, Kendell et al. (1996) compared the obstetric records of 115 patients born in Scotland in 1971–1974 and later hospitalized with schizophrenia to controls matched on place and date of birth, sex, maternal age, maternal parity, parental social class, and twin status. Significant differences were found for pregnancy complications in general, and for preeclampsia in particular. Susser and colleagues conducted a cohort study of effects of nutritional deprivation during the Dutch Hunger Winter of 1944–1945 (Susser and Lin, 1992; Susser et al., 1996). A twofold increase in the risk for schizophrenia was found in both male and female offspring of nutritionally deprived mothers compared to unexposed controls. Recent findings from more than 500,000 children in the Swedish National Birth Register born between 1973 and 1977 also support the increased risk for schizophrenia associated with malnutrition, particularly early onset schizophrenia (Dalman et al., 1999). The latter finding is consistent with the suggestion that pre- or perinatal complications confer a somewhat younger age of onset (Verdoux et al., 1997). Finally, a recent review of the world literature concluded that low birthweight (< 2500 g) is a "modest but definite" risk factor for schizophrenia (Kunugi et al., 2001).

Children exposed *in utero* to viral infection (Jones and Cannon, 1998) have also been found to be at increased risk for developing schizophrenia. Most of the evidence on viral infection is circumstantial (inferences drawn from populations who were *in utero* during a flu epidemic compared to controls) rather than direct (fetal exposure to influenza confirmed by analysis of blood samples). Current research is underway to confirm and extend these findings in birth cohorts in which blood samples obtained *in utero* were preserved.

Early childhood data also suggest that some individuals who go on to develop schizophrenia had prenatal brain damage or were impaired as children (Jones et al., 1998; Jones and Tarrant, 200; Kremen et al., 1998). Compelling evidence from the 1946 British birth cohort shows that the 30 (out of 4,746) children who went on to develop schizophrenia were more likely to have delayed motor development, speech problems, lower educational test scores in childhood, and a preference for solitary play (Jones and Cannon, 1998).

While the predictive power of prenatal and birth complications and early childhood performance is modest and not necessarily specific to schizophrenia per se, the results have generally been viewed as providing support for the neurodevelopmental model of schizophrenia. Some convergent evidence is available from a nested case–control study showing that impairments during high school in social functioning, organizational ability, and intellectual functioning significantly predicted being diagnosed with schizophrenia after induction into the army (Davidson et al., 1999). From a public health standpoint, the significance of this general area of research rests not only with discovering clues about etiology but also for providing avenues for identification of risk factors that can inform the design of prevention and intervention programs (Jones et al., 1998; Jones and Tarrant, 2000; McNeil, 1995).

PRECIPITATING FACTORS

Stress

Earlier we noted that environmental stress was seen as one possible explanation for the relationship between social class and schizophrenia. Two lines of research have addressed the role of stress as an etiologic factor in schizophrenia: exposure to adverse life events and expressed emotion in the family.

Stressful Life Events. Although there is continued interest in the contribution of life events stressors to the onset of mental disorders, their role in increasing the risk of onset of psychotic disorders appears to be weak. With a few exceptions, such as the Chung et al. (1986) finding of an association between life event stressors and first lifetime onset of schizophreniform disorder (Chung et al., 1986), most studies find small and nonsignificant effects of life event stressors (e.g., Dohrenwend and Egri, 1981). At best, it has been suggested that social environmental stressors trigger psychotic episodes in individuals already diagnosed with a psychotic disorder (Bromet et al., 1995). As noted above, Dohrenwend et al. (1992) concluded from their classic study of the social determinants of mental illness in Israel that social selection rather than social causation (e.g., stress) was responsible for the social class differences in schizophrenia.

Expressed Emotion. Since the classic papers by Brown and colleagues (1972) and Vaughn and Leff (1976), many studies have confirmed that people with schizophrenia (and with other psychiatric disorders) who live in family settings characterized by high levels of "expressed emotion" (critical and over-protective behavior and verbalizations toward the family member with schizophrenia) have higher rates of relapse after discharge from the hospital (Falloon 1986). However, there is no evidence that this form of stress is associated with first lifetime onset of schizophrenia (Butzlaff and Hooley, 1998). Thus, there is no strong evidence from current research that psychosocial stress or strain plays a role in precipitating first lifetime onset of schizophrenia or other psychotic disorders.

Substance Abuse

While substance use or abuse can provoke a psychotic episode in vulnerable individuals, the question of whether it is a risk factor for schizophrenia or lowers the age of onset is unresolved. The most compelling evidence comes from the 15-year follow-up of 45,570 Swedish army recruits showing that those consuming cannabis on more than 15 occasions were six times more likely to develop schizophrenia than less frequent users and nonusers (Andreasson et al., 1987). On the other hand, the opposite interpretation of the data is equally plausible—namely, that preschizophrenic individuals were more likely to abuse cannabis. As Jones and Cannon (1998) argue, given the increase in consumption of cannabis over the past three decades, one would expect to see an increase in schizophrenia if cannabis played a causal role in the etiology of schizophrenia, and this has simply not occurred.

In general, the epidemiologic evidence suggests that certain drugs, such as cannabis, can exacerbate symptoms of schizophrenia (Hall and Degenhardt, 2000). This raises the issue about whether patients with schizophrenia who have comorbid substance abuse are clinical different from those without such comorbidity. Many clinical investigators report that patients with both schizophrenia and substance abuse are more difficult to manage than patients without comorbid substance abuse (Lieberman and Bowers, 1990). However, both Mueser et al. (1990) and Kovasznay et al. (1993) found that substance abusers did not differ clinically at admission from nonabusing schizophrenia patients.

COURSE AND ITS PREDICTORS

Although one of the major functions of epidemiology is to describe the natural history of illness, the perception that schizophrenia has a chronic, deteriorating course is based primarily on nonepidemiologic studies of patients who stay in or return to treatment (Cohen and Cohen, 1984). Indeed, with some notable exceptions, most longitudinal studies of schizophrenia and other psychoses, especially affective disorders, focus on the course and outcome of samples consecutively admitted to treatment facilities rather than first-admission patients. Thus the cohorts being followed typically are not homogeneous with respect to stage of illness at the start of the study, a basic element of a cohort study. Morever, most follow-up studies of severely mentally ill people identify their samples from single hospitals or clinics (usually academic facilities), exclude patients with serious substance abuse histories, use chart diagnoses or cross-sectional research diagnosis, and have low baseline response rates and substantial attrition (Bromet and Fennig, 1999). Thus, it is not surprising that findings have been inconsistent regarding the proportions who do well or poorly over time, and the predictors of better or worse outcomes.

Ram et al. (1992) reviewed three sets of follow-up studies of first-admission patients: statistical reports from state hospitals, long-term follow-back (historical cohort) studies, and prospective studies. The latter are distinguished from the statistical reports and follow-back studies by the use of research diagnoses formulated using structured diagnostic procedures. They concluded that over a two-year period, about one-third of patients with schizophrenia had a benign course, while two-thirds either relapsed, failed to recover, or were readmitted to the hospital. In the Vancouver first-episode study, 40/72 psychotic patients were incapacitated at 18-month follow-up (Beiser et al., 1988). However, the longer the follow-up extends, the smaller the proportion with "good outcome" and the larger the proportion with social disability. For example, a study of 82 first-contact cases in the Netherlands found that after 15 years, only 12% had had a single episode followed by complete remission although another 15% had multiple episodes with complete remission in between (Wiersma et al., 1998). In the 13-year follow-up of a small cohort in Nottingham, only 17% were classified as recovered at follow-up, that is, alive, without symptoms or disability and receiving no treatment (Mason et al. 1995).

Many studies find that younger patients, males, and those with a family history of schizophrenia have the poorest course. As noted above, the evidence on substance abuse has been particularly inconsistent, with some studies finding that substance abuse predicts better outcome, others reporting that it predicts poorer outcome, and still others finding no association (Rabinowitz et al., 1998). Other prognostic variables that were confirmed across a number of studies include premorbid intelligence, premorbid social competence, duration between onset of psychosis and effective neuroleptic treatment, severity of positive symptoms, severity of negative symptoms, and non-adherence with medication treatment (Westermeyer and Harrow, 1988; Wyatt et al., 1998). Of all these variables, the failure to adhere to medication treatment is regarded as the strongest predictor of relapse (Ayuso-Gutiérrez and Vega, 1997). However, most of the evidence comes from clinical trials, and clinical trials do not contain representative samples of patients. Future naturalistic follow-up studies of representative samples of first-admission patients are needed to document and evaluate the relative contribution of medication adherence to course and outcome.

We noted earlier that the World Health Organization conducted one of the few epidemiologically based longitudinal studies of psychotic patients. One of the most widely cited findings was that patients in developing countries had a more benign course than patients in developed countries (Leff et al., 1992). A recent reanalysis by Craig et al. (1997) confirmed the original finding but also suggested that two developed centers (Prague and Nottingham) had outcome results at two-year follow-up that were similar to developing countries.

There have been very few first-admission follow-up studies of patients with affective psychosis, and those that exist are primarily studies of patients in academic medical centers. Coryell et al. (1990a, b) published two parallel studies on psychotic depression and psychotic bipolar disorder, finding similar predictors of poorer outcome as is seen in schizophrenia, namely, poorer adolescent social functioning and longer duration of index episode. For bipolar disorder, both Coryell et al. (1990b) and Tohen et al. (1992) reported that the presence of mood-incongruent delusions also predicted poorer outcome. More recently, Strakowski et al. (1998) assessed the 12-month course of first-admission patients with affective psychosis and found that the sample had great difficulty recovering from their illness, and that delayed recovery was significantly predicted by low socioeconomic status, poor premorbid functioning, treatment noncompliance, and substance abuse.

The patterns of illness course in schizophrenia and other psychoses have rarely been directly compared (Vetter and Köller, 1996). However, the available evidence indicates that people with schizophrenia have poorer short- and long-term outcomes than individuals with other psychosis diagnoses (Bromet et al., 1996; Harrow et al., 1997; Vetter and Köller, 1996). On the other hand, while people with schizophrenia function more poorly over time than other patients, the existing data do not support the notion of either an inevitable progressive deterioration in schizophrenia or a uniformly rosy outcome in affective disorder (Huber, 1997).

TARGET AREAS FOR FUTURE EPIDEMIOLOGIC RESEARCH

In this chapter, we attempted to highlight some of the important findings and new insights from research on the epidemiology of psychosis. In so doing, it becomes clear that a number of areas either have received relatively little attention or are poised to take advantage of new methodologies. These avenues of research include:

1. Investigating the prevalence and incidence of all psychoses besides schizophrenia and of psychotic symptoms using modern interviewing techniques and instruments;
2. Examining the frequency, distribution and course of abnormal brain morphology and brain processes (Häfner, 2000);
3. Clarifying the neurodevelopmental, pathophysiologic, biologic, and genetic antecedents of specific psychiatric disorders using cohort and modern case–control approaches and making use of tissue banks (Jones and Tarrant, 2000);
4. Specifying the environmental factors in research on gene-environment interactions and testing for age, cohort, and gender effects;
5. Exploring the relationship of psychosis to physical diseases, including autoimmune conditions, in patients and their families;
6. Examining potential biological markers and psychosocial risk factors for course and outcome of different psychotic disorders using large, multicenter cohort studies of first-episode patients

Epidemiology opens the possibility of identifying interventions tailored to reduce the risk of developing an illness or minimizing the morbidity associated with an illness. Enthusiasm for continued research on the epidemiology of psychosis has run parallel with advances in epidemiology more generally, particularly the expanded use of nested case–control designs, the study of gene–environment interactions, and the evaluation of biological markers derived from archived tissue samples. The Zubin and Spring (1977) vulnerability framework remains a compelling conceptual model from which to launch epidemiologic research on schizophrenia and related disorders. This model highlights six etiologic pathways: genetic, internal environment, ecological. neurophysiologic, developmental, and learning theory. Explicit testing of this, and similar, models continues to represent the challenge for epidemiologic research on psychotic disorders.

REFERENCES

Adebimpe VR (1994): Race, racism, and epidemiological surveys. Hosp Comm Psychiatry 45:27–31.

Allebeck P, Wistedt B (1986): Mortality in schizophrenia: a ten-year follow-up based on the Stockholm County Inpatient Register. Arch Gen Psychiatry 43:650–653.

American Psychiatric Association (1980): "Diagnostic and Statistical Manual of Mental Disorders," 3rd ed. Washington, DC: American Psychiatric Association Press.

American Psychiatric Association (1994): "Diagnostic and Statistical Manual of Mental Disorders," 4th ed. Washington, DC: American Psychiatric Association Press.

American Psychiatric Association (2001): www.psych.org/public_info/schizo.

Andreasson S, Allebeck P, Engstrom A, Ryberg U (1987): Cannabis and schizophrenia: A longitudinal study of Swedish conscripts. Lancet 2(8574):1483–1486.

Angermeyer M, Goldstein J, Kuehn L (1989): Gender differences in schizophrenia: Rehospitalization and community survival. Psychol Med 19:365–382.

Angst J (1991): Epidemiology of schizophrenia: Discussion. In Häfner H, Gattaz WF (eds): Search for the Causes of Schizophrenia. Berlin: Springer, pp 48–53.

Anthony JC, Folstein M, Romanoski AJ, Von Korff M, Nestadt G, Chahal R, Merchant A, Brown H, Shapiro S, Kramer M, Gruenberg E (1985): Comparison of lay DIS and a standardized psychiatric diagnosis: Experience in Eastern Baltimore. Arch Gen Psychiatry 42:667–675.

Ayuso-Gutiérrez JL, Vega JMR (1997): Factors influencing relapse in the long-term course of schizophrenia. Schizophr Res 28:199–206.

Beiser M, Erickson D, Fleming UJ, Iacono W (1993): Establishing the onset of psychotic illness. Am J Psychiatry 150:1349–1354.

Beiser M, Iacono W (1990): An update on the epidemiology of schiozphrenia. Can J Psychiatry 35:657–668.

Beiser M, Iacono WG, Erickson D (1989): Temporal stability in major mental disorders. In Robins LN, Barrett JE (eds): The Validity of Psychiatric Diagnosis. New York: Raven Press, pp 77–98.

Beiser M, Jonathan AE, Fleming MB, Iacono WG, Lin T (1988): Refining the diagnosis of schizophreniform disorder. Am J Psychiatry 145:695–700.

Bellack A, Blanchard JJ (1993): Schizophrenia: Psychopathology. In Bellack A, Hersen M (eds): Psychopathology in Adulthood. Boston: Allyn and Bacon, pp 216–233.

Bhugra D (2000): Migration and schizophrenia. Acta Psychiatr Scand (Supp) 102:68–73.

Bromet E, Davies M, Schulz SC (1988): Basic principles of epidemiologic research in schizophrenia. In Tsuang MT, Simpson JC (eds): "Handbook of Schizophrenia, vol 3. Nosology, Epidemiology and Genetics." Amsterdam: Elsevier Science, pp 151–168.

Bromet EJ, Dew MA, Eaton W (1995): Epidemiology of psychosis with special reference to schizophrenia. In Tsuang M, Tohen M, Zahner G (eds): "Textbook in Psychiatric Epidemiology." New York: Wiley-Liss, pp 283–300.

Bromet EJ, Fennig S (1999): Epidemiology and natural history of schizophrenia. Biol Psychiatry 46:871–881.

Bromet EJ, Jandorf L, Fennig S, Lavelle J, Kovasznay B, Ram R, Tanenberg-Karant M, Craig T (1996): The Suffolk County Mental health project: demographic, pre-morbid and clinical correlates of 6 month outcome. Psychol Med 26:953–962.

Bromet E, Schwartz J, Fennig S, Geller L, Jandorf L, Kovasznay B, Lavelle J, Miler A, Pato C, Ram R, Rich C (1992): The epidemiology of psychosis: The Suffolk County Mental Health Project. Schizophr Bull 18:243–255.

Brown GW, Birley JLT, Wing JK (1972): Influence of family life on the course of schizophrenic disorders: A replication. Br J Psychiatry 121:241–258.

Brown S, Birtwistle J (1998): People with schizophrenia and their families. Br J Psychiatry 173:139–144.

Butzlaff RL, Hooley JM (1998): Expressed emotion and psychiatric relapse: a meta-analysis. Arch Gen Psychiatry 55:547–552.

Chung RK, Langeluddecke P, Tennant C (1986): Threatening life events in the onset of schizophrenia, schizophreniform psychosis and hypomania. Br J Psychiatry 148:680–685.

Cohen P, Cohen J (1984): The clinicians illusion. Arch Gen Psychiatry 41:1178–1182.

Cooper B (1978): Epidemiology. In Wing JK (ed): Schizophrenia: Towards a New Synthesis. New York: Grune and Stratton, pp 31–51.

Cooper B (2001): Nature, nurture and mental disorder: Old concepts in the new millennium. Br J Psychiatry 178(suppl 40):s91–s101.

Cooper JE, Kendell RE, Gurland BJ, Sharpe L, Copeland JRM, Simon R (1972): "Psychiatric Diagnosis in New York and London: A Comparative Study of Mental Hospital Admissions." Institute of Psychiatry, Maudsley Monographs, No. 20. London: Oxford University Press.

Coryell W, Keller M, Lavori P, Endicott J (1990a): Affective syndromes, psychotic features, and prognosis, I: Depression. Arch Gen Psychiatry 47:651–657.

Coryell W, Keller M, Lavori P, Endicott J (1990b): Affective syndromes, psychotic features, and prognosis. I: Mania. Arch Gen Psychiatry 47:658–662.

Craig TJ, Goodman AB, Haugland G (1982): Impact of DSM-III on Clinical Practice. Am J Psychiatry 139:922–925.

Craig TJ, Siegel C, Hopper K, Lin S, Sartorius N (1997): Outcome in schizophrenia and related disorders compared between developing and developed countries. Br J Psychiatry 176:229–233.

Dalman C, Allebeck P, Cullberg J, Grunewald C, Kster M. (1999): Obstetric complications and the risk of schizophrenia. Arch Gen Psychiatry 56:234–240.

David AS, Lewis GH, Allebeck P, Andreasson S (1992): Urban-rural differences in place of upbringing and later schizophrenia. Schizophr Res 6:101–107.

Davidson M, Reichenberg MA, Rabinowitz J, Weiser M, Kaplan Z, Mordehai M (1999): Behavioural and intellectual markers for schizophrenia in apparently healthy male adolescents. Am J Psychiatry 156:1328–1335.

DeLisi LE, Bass N, Boccio A, Shields G, Morganti C, Vita A (1994): Age of onset in familial schizophrenia. Arch Gen Psychiatry 51:334–335.

Dohrenwend BP, Dohrewnwend BS (1969): "Social Status and Psychological Disorder: A Causal Inquiry." New York: Wiley.

Dohrenwend BP, Dohrewnwend BS, Gould MS, Link B, Neugebauer R, Wunsch-Hitzig R (eds) (1980): "Mental Illness in the United States: Epidemiological Estimates." New York: Praeger.

Dohrenwend BP, Egri G (1981): Recent stressful life events and episodes of schizophrenia. Schizophr Bull 7:12–23.

Dohrenwend BP, Levav I, Shrout PE, Schwartz S, Naveh G et al. (1992): Socioeconomic status and psychiatric disorders: the causation-selection issue. Science 255:946–952.

Eagles JM, Whalley LJ (1985): Decline in the diagnosis of schizophrenia among first admissions to Scottish mental hospitals from 1969–1978. Br J Psychiatry 146:151–154.

Eaton JW, Weil RJ (1955): Culture and Mental Disorders. New York: Free Press of Glencoe.

Eaton WW (1999): Evidence for universality and uniformity of schizophrenia around the world: assessment and implications. In Gattaz WF and Häfner H. (eds): "Search for the Causes of Schizophrenia." Vol IV. "Balance of the Century." New York: Springer, pp 21–33.

Eaton WW, Day R, Kramer M (1988): The use of epidemiology for risk factor research in schizophrenia: An overview and methodologic critique. In Tsuang MT, Simpson JC (eds):"Handbook of Schizophrenia," vol 3. "Nosology, Epidemiology and Genetics." Amsterdam: Elsevier Science, pp 169–204.

Eaton WW, Harrison G (2000): Ethnic disadvantage and schizophrenia. Acta Psychiatr Scand 102(Suppl 407):1–6.

Eaton WW, Hayward C, Ram R (1992): Schizophrenia and rheumatoid arthritis: A review. Schizophr Res 6:181–192.

Eaton WW, Mortensen PB, Frydenberg M (2000): Obstetric factors, urbanization and psychosis. Schizophr Res 43:117–123.

Endicott J, Spitzer R (1978): A diagnostic interview: The Schedule for Affective Disorders and Schizophrenia. Arch Gen Psychiatry 35:837–855.

Falloon IRH (1986): Family stress and schizophrenia. The Psychiatric Clinics of North America 9:165–182.

Faris R, Dunham H (1939): "Mental Disorders in Urban Areas: An Ecological Study of Schizophrenia and Other Psychoses." Chicago: University of Chicago Press.

Geddes JR, Lawrie SM. (1995): Obstetric complications and schizophrenia: a meta-analysis. Br J Psychiatry 167:786–793.

Gilvarry CM, Sham PC, Jones PB, Cannon M, Wright P, Lewis SW, Bebbington P, Toone BK, Murray RM (1996): Family history of autoimmune diseases in psychosis. Schizophr Res 19:33–40.

Goldberg E, Morrison S (1963): Schizophrenia and social class. Br J Psychiatry 109:785–802.

Gottesman I, Shields J (1982): "Schizophrenia: The Epigenetic Puzzle." Cambridge: Cambridge University Press.

Häfner H (2000): Epidemiology of schiozphrenia. A thriving discipline at the turn of the century. Eur Arch Psychiatry Clin Neurosci 250:271–273.

Häfner H, an der Heiden W, Behrens S, Gattaz WF, Hambrecht M, Löffler W et al. (1998): Causes and consequences of the gender difference in age at onset of schizophrenia. Schizophr Bull 24:99–113.

Hall W, Degenhardt L (2000): Cannabis use and psychosis: a review of clinical and epidemiological evidence. Aust N Z J Psychiatry 34:26–34.

Harrow M, Sands JR, Silverstein ML, Goldberg JF (1997): Course and outcome for schizophrenia versus other psychotic patients: a longitudinal study. Schizophr Bull 23:287–303.

Haukka J, Suvisaari J, Varilo T, Lönnqvist J (2001): Regional variation in the incidence of schizophrenia in Finland: a study of birth cohorts born from 1950 to 1969. Psychol Med 31:1045–1053.

Huber G. (1997): The heterogeneous course of schizophrenia. Schizophr Res 28:177–185.

Jablensky A (1986): Epidemiology of schizophrenia: a European perspective. Schizophr Bull 12:52–73.

Jablensky A, Sartorius N, Ernberg G, Anker M, Korten A, Cooper JE, Day R, Bertelsen A (1992): Schizophrenia: manifestations, incidence and course in different cultures. A World Health Organization ten-country study. Psychol Med Monogr (Supp) 20:1–97.

Jablensky A (1995): Schizophrenia: Recent epidemiologic issues. Epidemiol Rev 17:11–20.

Jablensky A (1997): The 100-year epidemiology of schizophrenia. Schizophrenia Res 28:111–125.

Jablensky, A (2000): Epidemiology of schizophrenia: the global burden of disease and disability. Eur Arch Psychiatry Clin Neurosci 250:274–285.

Jarvis E (1971): Insanity and Idiocy in Massachusetts. Cambridge, MA: Harvard University Press.

Jones PB, Bebbington P, Foerster A, Lewis S, Murray R, Russell A, Sham P, Toone B, Wilkins S (1993): Premorbid social underachievement in schizophrenia: Results from the Camberwell Collaborative Psychosis Study. Br J Psychiatry 162:65–71.

Jones P, Cannon M (1998): The new epidemiology of schizophrenia. The Psychiatric Clinics of North America 21:1–25.

Jones PB, Rantakallio P, Hartikainen AL, Isohanni M, Sipila P (1998): Schizophrenia as a longterm outcome of pregnancy, delivery, and perinatal complications: A 28year followup of the 1966 North Finland general population birth cohort. Am J Psychiatry 155:355–364.

Jones PB, Tarrant CJ (2000): Developmental precursors and biological markers for schizophrenia and affective disorders: Specificity and public health implications. Eur Arch Psychiatry Clin Neurosci 250:286–291.

Kendell RE, Juszczak E, Cole SK (1996): Obstetric complications and schizophrenia: a case control study based on standardised obstetric records. Br J Psychiatry 168:556–561.

Kendler KS (1988): The genetics of schizophrenia. In Tsuang MT, Simpson JC (eds): "Handbook of Schizophrenia," vol 3. "Nosology, Epidemiology and Genetics." Amsterdam: Elsevier Science, pp 437–462.

Kendler KS, Gallagher TJ, Abelson JM, Kessler RC (1996): Lifetime prevalence, demographic risk factors, and diagnostic validity of nonaffective psychosis as assessed in a US community sample. Arch Gen Psychiatry 53:1022–1031.

Kendler KS, McGuire M, Gruenberg AM, OHare A, Spellman M, Walsh D (1993): The Roscommon Family Study: I. Methods, diagnosis of probands, and risk of schizophrenia in relatives. Arch Gen Psychiatry 50:527–539.

Kessler R, McGonagle K, Zhao S, Nelson C, Hughes M, Eshleman S, Wittchen H-U, Kendler K (1994): Lifetime and 12-month prevalence of DSM-III-R psychiatric disorders in the United States: Results from the National Comorbidity Survey. Arch Gen Psychiatry 51:8–19.

Khuri R, Wood K (1984): The Role of Diagnosis in a Psychiatric Emergency Setting. Hosp Community Psychiatry 135:715–718.

Kovasznay B, Bromet E, Schwartz J, Ram R, Lavelle J, Brandon L (1993): Substance abuse and onset of psychotic illness. Hosp Comm Psychiatry 44:567–571.

Kremen WS, Buka SL, Seidman LJ, Goldstein JM, Koren D, Tsuang MT (1998): IQ decline during childhood and adult psychotic symptoms in a community sample: a 19-year longitudinal study. Am J Psychiatry 155:672–677.

Kunugi H, Nanko S, Murray RM (2001): Obstetric complications and schizophrenia: prenatal underdevelopment and subsequent neurodevelopmental impairment. Br J Psychiatry 178(suppl 40):s25–s29.

Lawson WB, Hepler N, Holladay J, Cuffel B (1994): Race as a factor in inpatient and outpatient admissions and diagnosis. Hosp Community Psychiatry 45:72–74.

Leff J, Sartorius N, Jablensky A, Korten A, Ernberg G (1992): The International Pilot Study of Schizophrenia: Five-year follow-up findings. Psychol Med 22:131–145.

Lemkau PV, Kulcar Z, Kesic B, Kovacic L. (1980): Selected aspects of the epidemiology of psychoses in Croatia, Yugoslavia. IV. Representative sample of Croatia and results of the survey. Am J Epidemiol 112:661–674.

Lewis G, David A, Andreasson S, Allebeck P (1992): Schizophrenia and city life. Lancet 340:137–140.

Lieberman JA, Bowers JB (1990): Substance abuse comorbidity in schizophrenia. Schizophr Bull 16:29–30.

Link BG, Dohrenwend BP, Skodol AE (1986): Socio-economic status and schizophrenia: noisome occupational characteristics as a risk factor. Am Soc Rev 51:242–258.

Malzberg B (1940): "Social and Biological Aspects of Mental Disease." New York: State Hospitals Press.

Mason P, Harrison G, Glazebrook C, Medley I, Dalkin T, Broudace T (1995): Characteristics of outcome in schizophrenia at 13 years. Br J Psychiatry 167:596–603.

McNeil TF (1995): Perinatal risk factors and schizophrenia: Selective review and methodological concerns. Epidemiol Rev 17:107–112.

Meijer A (1985): Child psychiatric sequelae of maternal war stress. Acta Psychiatrica Scand 72:505–511.

Mortensen PB (1995): The untapped potential of case registers and record-linkage studies in psychiatric epidemiology. Epidemiol Rev 17:205–209.

Mortensen PB, Pedersen CB, Westergaard T, Wohlfahrt J, Ewald H, Mors O, Andersen PK, Melbye M (1999): Effects of family history and place and season of birth on the risk of schizophrenia. N Eng J Med 340:603–608.

Mueser K, Yarnold P, Levinson D, Singh H, Bellack A, Kee K, Morrison R, Yadalam K (1990): Prevalence of substance abuse in schizophrenia: Demographic and clinical correlates. Schizophr Bull 16:31–56.

Munk-Jorgensen P (1985): The schizophrenia diagnosis in Denmark. A register-based investigation. Acta Psychiatr Scand 72:266–273.

Muntaner C, Tien AY, Eaton WW, Garrison R (1991): Occupational characteristics and the occurrence of psychotic disorders. Soc Psychiatry Psychiatr Epidemiol 26:273–280.

Murray RM, Reveley A, McGuffin P (1986): Genetic vulnerability to schizophrenia. The Psychiatric Clinics of North America 9:3–16.

Murray RM, van Os J (1998): Predictors of outcome in schizophrenia. J Clin Psychopharm 18:2S–4S.

O'Callaghan E, Gibson T, Colohan H, Walshe D, Buckley P, Larkin C, Waddington JL (1991): Season of birth in schizophrenia: evidence for confinement of an excess of winter births to patients without a family history of mental disorder. Br J Psychiatry 158:764–769.

Ösby U, Hammar N, Brandt L, Wicks S, Thinsz Z, Ekbom A, Sparén P (2001): Time trends in first admissions for schizophrenia and paranoid psychosis in Stockholm County, Sweden. Schizophr Res 47:247–254.

Pulver A, Sawyer JW, Childs B (1981): The association between season of birth and the risk of schizophrenia. Am J Epidemiol 114:73–749.

Rabinowitz J, Bromet EJ, Lavelle J, Carlson G, Kovasznay B, Schwartz JE (1998): Prevalence and severity of substance use disorders and onset of psychosis. Psychol Med 28:1411–1419.

Ram R, Bromet E, Eaton W, Pato C, Schwartz J (1992): The natural course of schizophrenia: A review of first-admission studies. Schizophr Bull 18:185–207.

Riecher A, Maurer K, Loffler W, Fatkenheuer B, An Der Heiden W, Munk-Jorgensen P, Stromgren E, Hafner H (1991): Gender differences in age of onset and course of schizophrenic disorders. In Hafner H, Gattaz WF (eds): Search for the Causes of Schizophrenia. Berlin: Springer, pp 14–33.

Robins LN, Regier DA (eds) (1991): "Psychiatric Disorders in America. The Epidemiologic Catchment Area Study." New York: The Free Press.

Seeman MV (2001): Schizophrenia in women. Presented at the 1st World Congress on Women's Mental Health, Berlin, Germany.

Selten JP, Slaets J, Kahn RS (1997): Schizophrenia in Surinamese and Dutch Antillean immigrants to the Netherlands: Evidence of an increased incidence. Psychol Med 27:807–811.

Sharpley M, Hutchinson G, McKenie K, Murray RM (2001): Understanding the excess of psychosis among the African-Caribbean population in England: Review of current hypotheses. Br J Psychiatry 178(suppl 40):s60–s68.

Snowden LR, Cheung FK (1990): Use of inpatient mental health services by members of ethnic minority groups. Am Psychologist 45:347–355.

Sohler N, Bromet EJ (2002): Does racial bias influence psychiatric diagnoses? Under review.

Spitzer R, Endicott J, Robins E (1978): Research diagnostic criteria: Rationale and reliability. Arch Gen Psychiatry 35:773–782.

Spitzer RL, Williams J, Gibbon M, Rirst MB (1992): The Structured Clinical Interview for DSM-III-R (SCID): History, rationale, and description. Arch Gen Psychiatry 49:624–629.

Strakowski SM, Keck PE, McElroy SL, West SA, Sax KW, Hawkins JM, Kmetz GF, Upadhyaya VH, Tugrul KC, Bourne ML (1998): Twelve-month outcome after a first hospitalization for affective psychosis. Arch Gen Psychiatry 55:49–55.

Strakowski SM, Lonczak HS, Sax KW, West SA, Crist A, Mehta R, Thienhaus OJ (1995): The effects of race on diagnosis and disposition from a psychiatric emergency service. J Clin Psychiatry 56:101–107.

Strakowski SM, Shelton RC, Kolbrener ML (1993): The effects of race and comorbidity on clinical diagnosis in patients with psychosis. J Clin Psychiatry 54:96–102.

Susser E, Lin S (1992): Schizophrenia after prenatal exposure to the Dutch hunger winter of 1944–1945. Arch Gen Psychiatry 49:983–988.

Susser E, Neugebauer R, Hoek HW, Brown AS, Lin S, Labovitz D, Gorman JM (1996): Schizophrenia after prenatal famine: further evidence. Arch Gen Psychiatry 53:25–31.

Takei N, OCallaghan E, Sham P, Glover G, Murray RM (1992): Winter birth excess in schizophrenia: Its relationship to place of birth. Schizophr Res 6:102–108.

Tohen M, Tsuang M, Goodwin D (1992): Prediction of outcome in mania by mood-congruent or mood-incongruent psychotic features. Am J Psychiatry 149:1580–1584.

Torrey EF, Bowler AE, Rawlings R, Terrazas A (1993): Seasonability of schizophrenia and stillbirths. Schizophr Bull 19:557–562.

Torrey EF, Mortensen PB, Pedersen CB, Wohlfahrt J, Melbye M (2001): Risk factors and confounders in the geographical clustering of schizophrenia. Schizophr Res 49:295–299.

Tsuang MT, Stone WS, Faraone SV (2001): Genes, environment and schizophrenia. Br J Psychiatry 178(suppl 40):s18–s24.

Turner RJ, Wagenfeld MO (1967): Occupational mobility and schizophrenia: an assessment of the social causation and social selection hypotheses. Am Soc Rev 32:104–113.

van Os J, Driessen G, Gunther N, Delespaul P (2000): Neighbourhood variation in incidence of schizophrenia. Evidence for person-environment interaction. Br J Psychiatry 176:243–248.

van Os J, Hanssen M, Bijl RV, Vollebergh W (2001): Prevalence of psychotic disorder and community level of psychotic symptoms: an urban-rural comparison. Arch Gen Psychiatry 58:663–668.

van Os J, Selten J-P (1998): Prenatal exposure to maternal stress and subsequent schizophrenia. Br J Psychiatry 172:324–326.

Vaughn CE, Leff JP (1976): The influence of family and social factors on the course of psychiatric illness: A comparison of schizophrenic and depressed neurotic patients. Br J Psychiatry 129:125–137.

Verdoux H, Geddes JR, Takei N, Lawrie SM, Bovet P, Eagles JM, Heun R, McCreadie RG, McNeil TF, O'Callaghan E, Stober G, Willinger MU, Wright P, Murray RM (1997): Obstetric complications and age of onset in schizophrenia: an international collaborative meta-analysis of individual patient data. Am J Psychiatry 154:1220–1227.

Vetter P, Köller O (1996): Clinical and psychosocial variables in different diagnostic groups: their interrelationships and value as predictors of course and outcome during a 14-year follow-up. Psychopathology 29:159–168.

Von Korff M, Nestadt G, Romanoski A, Anthony J, Eaton W, Merchant A, Chahal R, Kramer M, Folstein M, Gruenberg E (1985): Prevalence of treated and untreated DSM-III schizophrenia: results of a two-stage community survey. J Nerv Ment Dis 173:577–581.

Walsh D, O'Hare A, Blake B, Halpenny JV, O'Brien PF (1980): The treated prevalence of mental illness in the Republic of Ireland--the three county case register study. Psychol Med 10:465–470.

Westermeyer JF, Harrow M (1988): Course and outcome in schizophrenia. In: Tsuang MT, Simpson JC (eds) "Handbook of Schizophrenia." vol 3. Nosology, Epidemiology and Genetics. Amsterdam: Elsevier Science, pp 205–244.

Widerlov B, Lindstrom E, von Knorring L (1997): One-year prevalence of long-term functional psychosis in three different areas of Uppsala. Acta Psychiatr Scand 96:452–458.

Wiersma D, Nienhuis FJ, Slooff CJ, Giel R (1998): Natural course of schizophrenic disorders: a 15-year followup of a Dutch incidence cohort. Schizophr Bull. 24:75–85.

Williams JBW, Gibbon M, First MB, Spitzer RL, Davies M, Borus J, Howes MJ, Kane J, Pope HG, Rounsaville B, Wittchen H-U (1992): The structured clinical interview for DSM-III-R (SCID): II. Multisite test-retest reliability. Arch Gen Psychiatry 49:630–636.

Woogh C (2001): Is schizophrenia on the decline in Canada? Can J Psychiatry 46:61–67.

Wright P, Sham PC, Gilvarry CM, Jones PB, Cannon M, Sharma T, Murray RM (1996): Autoimmune diseases in the pedigrees of schizophrenic and control subjects. Schizophr Res 20:261–267.

Wyatt RJ, Henter I, Leary MC, Taylor E (1995): An economic evaluation of schizophrenia, 1991. Soc Psychiatry Psychiatr Epidemiol 30:196–205.

Wyatt RJ, Damiani M, Henter I (1998): First-episode schizophrenia: Early intervention and medication discontinuation in the context of course and treatment. Br J Psychiatry 72 (suppl 33):77–83.

Zubin J, Spring B (1977): Vulnerability—a new view of schizophrenia. J Abnorm Psychol 86:103–126.

CHAPTER 16

Epidemiology of Depressive and Anxiety Disorders

EWALD HORWATH, ROSE S. COHEN, and MYRNA M. WEISSMAN

College of Physicians and Surgeons of Columbia University and Acute Inpatient Unit, Washington Heights Community Service, New York State Psychiatric Institute, New York 10032 (E.H.); College of Physicians and Surgeons of Columbia University (R.S.C.); College of Physicians and Surgeons of Columbia University; and Division of Clinical and Genetic Epidemiology; New York State Psychiatric Institute (M.M.W.).

INTRODUCTION

The epidemiologic study of mood and anxiety disorders spans greater than six decades of history. The community surveys of the 1950s and 1960s are relevant to our current understanding of depression and anxiety insofar as they adopted the methodology of direct interview in the community, paid close attention to psychosocial variables, and documented significant levels of functional impairment caused by psychiatric symptoms. However, these studies defined mental health and illness along a continuum and intentionally failed to establish rates of specific psychiatric disorders. They also assumed the social etiology of mental illness as a given. Therefore, the findings of these studies had limited applications as research on the genetics, neuroscience and psychopharmacology of psychiatric disorders emerged in the 1970s and 1980s.

We will limit our review to epidemiologic studies of the 1980s and 1990s that used *standardized interview instruments*, operationalized diagnostic criteria, and reported data on widely agreed-upon diagnostic categories, such as those in the *Diagnostic and Statistical Manual of Mental Disorders*, third edition (DSM-III), (American Psychiatric Association [APA], (1980), DSM-III-R, (third edition, revised APA 1987); DSM-IV (fourth edition, revised), APA (1994); and *International Classification of Diseases*, ninth revision (ICD-9), World Health Organization, (1978). We will focus on two *categories of mood disorder*: *major depression and dysthymia* and on five anxiety disorders: *panic disorder*, *agoraphobia*, *social phobia*, *generalized anxiety disorder and obsessive–compulsive disorder*. Readers interested in the epidemiological survey data prior to 1980 are referred to reviews by Boyd and Weissman (1982) and Charney and Weissman (1988).

Textbook in Psychiatric Epidemiology, Second Edition, Edited by Ming T. Tsuang and Mauricio Tohen.
ISBN 0-471-40974-X

MAJOR DEPRESSION

Definition

The DSM-III diagnosis of major depression requires a persistent period of dysphoric mood or loss of interest or pleasure and at least two weeks of four other symptoms, which may include significant weight loss or gain, appetite disturbance, insomnia or hypersomnia, psychomotor agitation or retardation, fatigue or loss of energy, feelings of worthlessness, inappropriate guilt, impaired concentration, recurrent suicidal ideas or a suicide attempt (APA, 1980). The DSM-III-R criteria are similar, but specify a two-week period of at least five symptoms, one of which must be depressed mood or loss of interest or pleasure (APA, 1987).

Rates

Table 1 shows the sample sizes and Table 2 shows the 6-month, 1-year and lifetime prevalence rates per 100 of major depression based on community surveys in the United States; Edmonton, Canada; Puerto Rico; Florence, Italy; Seoul, Korea; Taiwan; and Zurich, Switzerland, using DSM-III or DSM-III-R criteria. The highest annual prevalence rate was 10.3 from the U.S. National Comorbidity Study (NCS). The one-year five-site prevalence in the ECA study was 2.7, with a range from 1.7 in Durham to 3.4 in New Haven. The lowest annual and lifetime rates were reported from Taiwan.

As with annual prevalence rates, the highest lifetime prevalence estimates for major depression came from the National Comorbidity Survey (17.1 per 100). The

TABLE 1. Epidemiological Community Surveys of Psychiatric Disorders Using DSM-III (or DSM-III-R) Diagnostic Criteria

Place	No.	Age (years)	Investigator
USA-NCS (DSM-III-R)	8,098	15–54	Kessler et al. (1994)
USA-ECA	18,572	18 +	Weissman et al. (1988a, b)
New Haven, CT	5,034		
Baltimore, MD	3,481		
St. Louis, MO	3,004		
Durham, NC	3,921		
Los Angeles, CA	3,132		
Edmonton, Canada	3,258	18 +	Bland et al. (1988)
Puerto Rico	1,551	17–64	Canino et al. (1987)
Florence, Italy	1,110	15 +	Faravelli et al. (1989, 1990)
Seoul, Korea	5,100	18–65	Lee et al. (1987, 1990a, b)
Taiwan	11,004	18 +	Hwu et al. (1989)
Urban	5,005		
Small towns	3,004		
Rural villages	2,995		
New Zealand	1,498	18 +	Joyce et al. (1989, 1990)
Zurich, Switzerland	6,193	19–24	Angst and Dobler, Mikola (1984, 1985)

Source: Adapted from Tsuang et al. (1995).

TABLE 2. Prevalence Rates per 100 for Major Depression Based on Community Surveys Using DSM-III (or DSM-III-R) Diagonsis

Place	Rate/100[a]		
	6 month	1 year	Lifetime
USA-NCS (DSM-III-R)	—	10.3	17.1
USA-ECA	2.2	2.6	4.4
New Haven, CT	2.8	3.4	5.8
Baltimore, MD	1.7	1.9	2.9
St. Louis, MO	2.3	2.7	4.4
Durham, NC	1.5	1.7	3.5
Los Angeles, CA	2.6	3.2	5.6
Edmonton, Canada	3.2	—	8.6
Puerto Rico	3.0	—	4.6
Florence, Italy	—	5.2	—
Seoul, Korea	—	—	3.4
Taiwan			
Urban	—	0.6	0.9
Small towns	—	1.1	1.7
Rural villages	—	0.8	1.0
New Zealand	5.3	5.3	12.6
Zurich, Switzerland	—	7.0	—

[a] Rates rounded off to 1 decimal place in most cases.

Source: Adapted from Tsuang et al. (1995).

most comparable survey, in terms of location (U.S.) and magnitude of sample size, was the ECA, which reported much lower rates. The surveys in Edmonton, Canada, and New Zealand reported rates intermediate between those of the ECA and NCS. The NCS prevalence rates, however, are quite similar to estimates from an earlier epidemiologic study of depression in New Haven (Weissman and Myers, 1978; Myers et al., 1984), which used the Schedule for Affective Disorders and Schizophrenia/Research Diagnostic Criteria (SADS/RDC) for case finding. The higher rates reported in the New Haven study may reflect more complete case finding based upon the use of a clinical interview like the SADS/RDC.

Blazer et al. (1994) and Kessler et al. (1994) have suggested several methodologic explanations for the substantially higher rates in the NCS compared to the ECA. First, the survey instrument used in the NCS, the University of Michigan Composite International Diagnostic Interview (UM-CIDI) was different from that used in the ECA study, the Diagnostic Interview Schedule (DIS). The UM-CIDI used techniques of memory probing quite different from those used in the DIS. The UM-CIDI presented stem questions leading into a diagnostic category in a life review section, which occurred early in the interview prior to extensive follow-up questions which might discourage the endorsement of other stem diagnostic questions. Second, the UM-CIDI used three separate stem questions probing for major depression, including probes for periods of feeling "sad, blue or depressed," feeling "down in the dumps or gloomy," and "losing interest in most things like work, hobbies, or things you usually like to do for fun." The DIS, in contrast, used only one stem question. The memory probes used in the UM-CIDI may have resulted in additional case finding, similar to the results of the New Haven survey, which used a clinical interview, the SADS/RDC.

A significant question is whether these cross-national differences are related to true cross-cultural variation in risk factors or to methodologic differences across studies. By far the lowest rates of major depression were reported in Taiwan even though, on the basis of diagnostic criteria, measurement and sampling methods, the Taiwanese studies are comparable to the ECA and other cited studies. This suggests that the reported differences may represent true differences in rates of major depression or that there is a culturally mediated tendency to experience or report depression differently in Taiwan than in the West. This interpretation of the data is suggested by the fact that substance abuse or dependence and major depression are the most prevalent disorders in the ECA study, while psychophysiologic disorders are most prevalent in Taiwan. In Seoul, Korea, which is more westernized than Taiwan, the lifetime prevalence per 100 of major depression was 3.4, more comparable to the 5-site ECA rate of 5.4 than the low Taiwanese rates.

Several investigators have reported on incidence data from the ECA study (Eaton et al. 1989; Anthony and Petronis, 1991; Horwath et al., 1992a). Annual incidence of first onset major depression was 1.6 per 100 across 4 sites (New Haven was excluded) (Eaton et al., 1989). *Although incidence data are particularly valuable in studying risk factors which may improve our understanding of disease etiology, community epidemiological surveys rarely provide such data because large prospectively observed samples are required in order to generate accurate estimates of incidence*. We will comment further on the ECA incidence data in the discussion of specific risk factors for major depression.

Table 3 shows sample sizes and Table 4 shows point prevalence rates of depression based on community surveys using PSE, CATEGO (D, R, N) and ICD-9 (296.2/300.4). The rates range from a low of 4.6 per 100 in Finland to a high of 7.4

TABLE 3. Recent Epidemiological Studies Using PSE and ICD-9

Place	No. Sampled	*n* interviewed 2nd Stage	Age (years)	Investigator
Nijmegen-Netherlands	3245	775	18–64	Hodiamont et al. (1987)
Camberwell, UK	800	310	18–64	Bebbington et al. (1981)
Canberra, Australia	756	170	18 +	Henderson et al. (1979)
Santander, Spain	1223	452	18 +	Vazguez-Barquero et al. (1986)
Two districts Finland	747	—	30 +	Lehtinen et al. (1990)
Athens, Greece	487	—	18 +	Mavreas and Bebbington (1988)
Greek Cypriots in UK	285	—	18 +	Mavreas and Bebbington (1988)

Source: Adapted from Tsuang et al. (1995).

TABLE 4. Point Prevalence Rates per 100 for Depression by Sex Based on Community Surveys Using PSE, CATEGO (D, R, N) and ICD-9 (296.2/300.4)

Place	Female	Male	Total
Nijmegen, Netherlands	7.7	4.3	5.4
Camberwell, UK	9.2	4.9	7.1
Athens, Greece	10.2	4.3	7.4
Greek Cypriots in Camberwell	7.1	4.2	5.6
Canberra, Australia	7.7	4.3	6.1
Santander, Spain	5.5	4.3	4.6
Two districts Findland	5.5	3.6	4.6
Edinburgh, Scotland	—	4.3	—

Source: Adapted from Tsuang et al. (1995).

per 100 in Athens, Greece. The rates for these ICD-9 depression categories tend to be higher than the six-month and one-year prevalence rates reported in the DSM-III studies, but not as high as the DSM-III-R rates in the NCS.

Subtypes of Major Depression

Several studies of the ECA data have found evidence supportive of the validity of major depression with psychotic features and major depression with atypical features as subtypes. Johnson et al. (1991) found that 14% of major depressions were accompanied by psychotic features and that these cases, when compared with nonpsychotic depression, had a more severe course, as reflected in increased risk of relapse, persistence over one year, suicide attempts, hospitalization, comorbidity, and financial dependency. These findings, based on a community sample, are consistent with reports from clinical samples and provide epidemiologic support for the validity and clinical significance of psychotic depression.

Horwath et al. (1992b), also reporting on ECA data, found that major depression with atypical features (defined as overeating and oversleeping) when compared to major depression without atypical features was associated with a younger age of onset, more psychomotor slowing, and more comorbid panic disorder, drug abuse or dependence, and somatization disorder. These differences could not be explained by differences in demographic characteristics or symptom severity. Prior treatment studies by Quitkin and colleagues (1991) found that atypical depression preferentially responds to monoamine oxidase inhibitors. Together, the evidence from epidemiologic and treatment studies suggests that major depression with atypical features constitutes a distinct and valid subtype of major depression.

ECA Follow-up

During the period 1993–1996, a follow-up at the 1981 Baltimore site of the Epidemiologic Catchment Area Study found an incidence of DIS/DSM-IV major depression to be 3.0 per 1000 per year, with incidence peaks occurring when subjects were in their 30s and in their 50s. The gender distribution reflected true differences in new cases, rather than chronicity of major depression. Women were at higher risk of new onset major depression, but had neither higher rates of recurrence nor longer episodes of major depression than men (Eaton et al., 1997). Prodromal periods were assessed in this follow-up study ($n = 71$) for the various symptoms of depression. The prodromal period for symptoms of anhedonia, slowness or restlessness, tiredness, feelings of worthlessness, difficulty concentrating, and sleep disturbance was found to be one year. The prodromal period for appetite disturbance, suicidal thoughts or behavior was found to be two years. The longest prodromal period occurred for the symptoms of dysphoria at five years (Eaton et al., 1997).

Depression as a Disabling Disease: Shifting Paradigms

It has been known for some time that depression can cause substantial impairment in overall functioning. However, it was not until recently that large scale studies with appropriate measures of disability and adequate comparison groups have provided systematic, reliable data on the issue of disability due to depression. These studies have highlighted the extensive disability caused by depression, comparable in magnitude to that associated with a number of other chronic medical disorders.

The Global Burden of Disease Study conducted by WHO in 1990 (Murray et al., 1997) investigated the worldwide prevalence and disability due to mental disorders, including unipolar major depression and panic disorder. This study developed a measurement index, the Disability-Adjusted Life Years (DALYs) to be used to compare the burden of disease from premature mortality and years lived with disability across various types of disease and injury in global populations. The DALYs consists of two classes, the YLL (years of life lost to premature mortality) and the YLD (years lived with disability, adjusted for severity of disability). Using these two measures, depression was found to be one of the most disabling diseases in the world and ranked as the fourth most disabling disease after lower respiratory infections, diarrheal diseases, and perinatal diseases (Murray et al., 1997)

In the Rand Medical Outcomes Study (MOS), 1790 adult outpatients at a general medical clinic with various diagnoses including depression, diabetes, hypertension, recent myocardial infarction, or congestive heart failure were followed for changes in functional status and well-being. Limitations in functioning and well-being were found to be comparable to or worse than the limitations related to chronic medical illnesses (Hays et al., 1995).

The Rand MOS also assessed the course of depression during a two-year period among outpatients with current major depression, dysthymia, or double depression (Wells et al., 1992). The functional status of each subject was assessed, with measures aimed at well-being, rating energy or fatigue, general health, bodily pain, number of bedridden days in the past month, social, physical, emotional functional status. The worst functional outcomes were found in patients with dysthymia, intermediate outcomes were found in patients with current major depression, and the best outcomes were found in patients with subthreshold depressive symptoms. Notably, severity of symptoms and baseline functional status contributed more to the explained variance in functional outcomes than the particular type of depressive disorder (Wells et al., 1992).

Depressive symptoms in the absence of a full DSM-IV diagnosis have also been linked to increased physical disability, as measured by physical decline among the elderly. In the geriatric population, major depression has been found to occur in 1 to 2% of the population. However, 12 to 20% of seniors suffer from depressive symptoms that do not meet full diagnostic criteria for DSM-IV major depression. A four-year prospective study of patients aged 71 years and older demonstrated that increasing levels of depressive symptoms were predictive of greater decline in physical performance (i.e., standing balance, timed 8-ft. walk, and timed test of five repetitions of rising from a chair and sitting down), with an OR 1.55 (95% CI 1.0–1.08) (Pennix et al., 1998).

Risk Factors

Gender Ratios. Clinical and epidemiological studies in the Western world have consistently documented an increased risk for major depression in women. Studies reporting differential rates of major depression by sex and proposed explanations for this difference have been reviewed by Weissman and Klerman (1977, 1985), who concluded that the difference is not simply due to a tendency for women to report distress or to seek help more readily than men. This conclusion is supported by the observation that rates of bipolar disorder are similar in men and women, and by the fact that rates of major depression are elevated for women even in community studies which report on both treated and untreated cases.

Consistently higher rates of major depression in women were reported in community studies using DSM-III and DSM-III-R (Table 5) and in all the ICD-9 surveys (Table 4). The ratios of rates of major depression in females to males were about 2:1, with a range from 1.4:1 in urban Taiwan to 2.7:1 in the ECA.

Simply relying upon prevalence rates would leave open the possibility that this sex ratio could be explained, in part, by women having more persistent or recurrent courses of major depression, accounting for more active cases at any one point in time or better recall for lifetime rates. However, the increased risk of major depression was also seen in the incidence data from four sites of the ECA, in which the annual incidence rate was almost twice as great in women as in men. This suggests that the higher prevalence rates in women reflect a truly increased risk of first onset of major depression.

In a large-scale community study of Asian Americans (Chinese American Psychiatric Epidemiological Study) lifetime and twelve month prevalence rates were reported for DSM-III-R major depressive episodes and dysthymia. Lifetime prevalences for major depressive episodes and dysthymia were 6.9% and 5.2%, respectively. Twelve month rates of major depressive episode and dysthymia were 3.4% and 0.9%, respectively (Takeuchi et al., 1998). While the rates of major

TABLE 5. Rates of Major Depresion by Sex in Community Surveys Using DSM-III (or DSM-III-R) Diagnosis

	Lifetime Rates/100		
Place	Female	Male	Sex Ratios Female/Male
USA-NCS (DSM-III-R)	21.3	12.7	1.7
USA-ECA[a]	7.0	2.6	2.7
Edmonton, Canada	11.4	5.9	1.9
New Zealand	16.3	8.8	1.9
Taiwan			
Urban	1.0	0.7	1.4
Small towns	2.5	1.0	2.6
Rural villages	1.4	0.6	2.3
Seoul, Korea	4.1	2.4	1.6
Puerto rico	5.5	3.5	1.6
		Annual incidence rate/100	
USA-ECA[a]	1.98	1.10	1.8

[a]Four sites: New Haven excluded.

Source: Adapted from Tsuang et al. (1995).

depressive episodes for Chinese Americans were much lower than those found in the NCS, the most striking finding was the absence of association between gender and major depression or dysthymia (Takeuchi et al., 1998).

The first community-based study of major and minor depression with a seasonal pattern, found a prevalence of 1%. Women and respondents with higher income were more likely to have minor depression with a seasonal pattern. Notably, among study respondents with major depression, male gender as well as older age was associated with a higher prevalence of seasonal pattern (Blazer et al., 1997).

The reports of a higher risk of major depression in women are remarkably consistent across cultures and persistent over time. The elevated rates for women appear in studies with a variety of sampling and measurement methods. Several recent studies have suggested a decreasing sex difference in rates among those persons born after World War II (see the following section on secular changes for further discussion of this). Although the increased risk of major depression in women is a firmly established and widely accepted finding, the reason for this increased risk remains unclear.

Secular changes. Recently, evidence from both epidemiologic and family studies has suggested that important temporal changes are occurring in the rates of major depression. Whereas previously depression was viewed as an illness of middle-aged and elderly persons, it is increasingly evident that this is no longer accurate. In a review of studies relevant to temporal trends in depression, Klerman and Weissman (1989) found evidence for an increase in the rates of major depression in cohorts born after the Second World War, a decrease in the age of onset, and an increase in rates of depression for all ages during the period between 1960 and 1975. Although a persistent gender effect was observed, with a two to three times greater risk for women than men across all ages, there was evidence for a narrowing of this differential risk to men and women due to a greater increase in the risk of depression among young men than young women.

Secular or temporal effects on rates of major depression are variations in rates over time, and can be separated into age, period, or cohort effects. *Age effects* refer to age-specific stages in life during which persons are at higher risk of illness onset. The risk of schizophrenia onset, for example, rises sharply during late adolescence and young adulthood. *Period effects* refer to variations in rates of illness associated with a specific time period. The epidemic of AIDS during the 1980s is an example. *Cohort effects* usually refer to changes in rates of illness among groups of people born in the same year or decade. These temporal changes may occur separately or may interact with one another.

Evidence has been found of both period and birth-cohort effects for major depression. Hagnell (1986), in a 25-year follow-up of 2500 inhabitants of Lundby, Sweden, found an increased risk for depression among both sexes in cohorts born after 1937. Lavori et al. (1987) described both a post-1930 birth cohort effect among siblings of depressed patients and a strong 1965–975 period effect for all birth cohorts. In an analysis of the ECA data, Wickramaratne et al. (1989) found a similar combination of a 1935–1945 birth cohort effect and a 1960-1980 period effect.

More recently, the Cross-National Collaborative Group (1992) reported similar changes in the rate of major depression based upon evidence from approximately 39,000 subjects in 9 community surveys and 4,000 relatives from 3 family studies conducted in the 1980s in North America, Puerto Rico, Western Europe, the Middle East, Asia, and the Pacific Rim. Analyses of data from these studies showed an increase in the cumulative lifetime rates of major depression with each successive younger birth cohort at all sites with the exception of the Hispanic samples. Although the overall trend was toward increasing rates of depression over time over all countries, there were significant variations in the magnitude of the increase and in short-term fluctuations by country.

Klerman and Weissman (1989) have reviewed various explanations for these period and cohort effects, including potential artifactual causes, such as memory loss with increasing age, selective mortality or institutionalization, selective migration, and reporting bias of subjects. Although several studies have failed to support a diminishing recall hypothesis (Farrer et al., 1989; Lavori et al., 1987), the explanation for these secular trends remains controversial. Various environmental causes, including biological, cultural and economic factors, have been proposed as mediators of these temporal rate changes. The Cross-National Collaborative Group concluded that the variations in short-term trends for major depression by country was evidence that these rates were sensitive to changing historical, social, economic, or biological environmental conditions.

Geriatric Depression. Data on the prevalence and incidence of depression in the older adult population is incomplete. Available data include the ECA study, which found that while major depression decreased with age, particular depressive symptoms increased with age (Gallo et al., 1999). Most community studies using DSM-IV criteria for major depression have found major depression prevalence rates to be less than 5% in the geriatric population (Gallo et al., 1999). Several large epidemiologic studies using standardized psychiatric interviews such as the National Comorbidity Study did not include adults aged 55 and older (Gallo et al., 1999). While major depression has been estimated between 1 to 2% of the elderly population, and no more than 5%, a much greater proportion of the older community dwelling population, 12 to 20%, suffer from depressive symptoms. A recent prospective cohort study clearly describes a relationship between depressive symptoms and risk of physical decline in the elderly (Penninx et al., 1998).

The prognosis of depressive disorders in the community dwelling elderly aged 65 and older has been studied using the GMS-AGECAT (Geriatric Mental State-Automated Geriatric Examination for Computer Assisted Taxonomy) as well as psychiatrist confirmed DSM-IV criteria for depressive disorders (Denihan et al., 2000). At three-year follow-up 30.2% of depressed subjects had died, 34.9% had persistent or relapsed depression, and 10.4% had recovered completely. Degree of physical illness, bereavement, and positive family history were associated with poorer outcome.

Adolescent Depression. Depending on the specific community study, estimated lifetime prevalence rates for DSM-IV major depressive disorder in the adolescent age group (usually 14–19 years of age) range from 4% to 17% (Oldehinkel et al., 1999). In a recent study of 1228 adolescents aged 14–17 at baseline; with 20-month follow-up, lifetime prevalence of any depressive disorder was found to be 20%, major depressive disorder 12.2%, dysthymia 3.5%, subthreshold major depressive disorder 6.3%. In this cohort, few depressive disorders started before age 13. Consistent with the gender distribution of depressive disorders in adults, females were approximately twice as likely as males to develop a depressive disorder (Oldehinkel et al., 1999). These results were similar to those found by Kessler et al. (1994) in a cohort of individuals aged 15–24 in the National Comorbidity Study, where 12-month prevalence of major depressive episode was 12.8%, and lifetime prevalence was 15.3% for major depression and 9.9% for minor depression (Kessler et al., 1998).

Predictors of recurrence of major depressive disorder were investigated in a community sample of subjects with adolescent onset major depressive disorder, followed up at ages 19–23. Risk factors identified in this cohort included female gender, multiple major depressive disorder episodes in adolescence, higher proportion of family members with recurrent major depressive disorder, elevated symptoms of borderline personality disorder, and conflict with parents (in female respondents) (Lewinsohn et al., 2000).

Comorbidly occurring psychiatric disorders are quite common and disabling in adolescent populations. A community sample of 1507 adolescents aged 14–18 with single and comorbid forms of depression, anxiety, substance use, and disruptive behavior was compared on six clinical outcome measures (Lewinsohn et al., 1995). Comorbidity had the greatest impact on academic performance, mental health treatment usage, and past suicide attempts. Adolescents with comorbid disorders had the poorest academic performance, the highest mental health treatment usage, and highest rate of past suicide attempts.

Race and Ethnicity. In comparing rates of major depression by race and ethnic group, both the similarities and differences are of interest. In the five ECA study sites, prevalence rates of major depression showed no consistent differences between African-American and white subjects (Somervell et al., 1989). In the NCS, nonblack race or ethnicity was found to be one potential risk factor for major depression, but only among persons who had "pure" major depression, and not in those with comorbid disorders. More specifically, blacks in the NCS had a lower risk for pure major depression than whites, but a similar risk for comorbid major depression (Blazer et al., 1994).

Rates of major depression in Puerto Rico did not differ significantly from the rates in the ECA study, except that no significant birth-cohort differences were found in Puerto Rico (Canino et al., 1987; Cross-National Collaborative Group, 1992). The results for Hispanics at the Los Angeles site of the ECA were somewhat inconsistent. Lifetime prevalence of major depression was lower among Hispanics in Los Angeles (Burnam et al., 1987), while the incidence rate was higher (Horwath et al., 1992a). A birth-cohort effect was not found for the Hispanic sample in Los Angeles (Cross-National Collaborative Group, 1992). In the NCS, Hispanics were found to be at higher risk for comorbid major depression than whites, but the risk for pure depression was similar (Blazer et al., 1994). The reason for these differences is not clear.

The study from Taiwan (Hwu et al., 1989) showed much lower rates of major depression than did the Western studies. This finding is interesting in light of the work of Kleinman (1977), who suggests that depression may take on a different, more somatic and less psychologic, form in Chinese culture. Based on collaborative research with the Hunan Medical College in the People's Republic of China, Kleinman (1982) found that Chinese psychiatrists diagnosed a third of their patients with "neurasthenia," which is thought of as a functional disorder of the neurological system characterized by weariness, irascibleness, difficulty in concentrating, and unstable and depressed mood. When 100 Chinese neurasthenic patients were interviewed using the Schedule for Affective Disorders and Schizophrenia (SADS), 87% were found to meet DSM-III criteria for major depressive disorder.

This cross-cultural research suggests that culturally mediated values and views of symptoms may influence the expression of psychiatric disorder. Although the use of standard interview techniques and methodologies across cultures may mitigate these effects to some extent, the sharply lower rates of depression in Taiwan as compared to the West suggest that cultural factors may play an important role in the expression of depression.

That culturally mediated factors may exert differential effects across diagnoses is suggested by the fact that psychophysiologic disorders were most common in Taiwan, while rates of depression were much lower than in the West. Similarly, comparisons between Greeks living in Athens and British Greek Cypriot immigrants living in Camberwell showed higher rates of anxiety disorders among both Greek groups as compared with native Camberwell subjects, while rates of depression were comparable (Mavreas and Bebbington, 1988).

Socioeconomic Status. The NCS found that a lower level of education and employment classification as homemaker or "other" (which included unemployed) were significant risk factors for major depression, even after controlling for the effects of other variables associated with depression (such as age, sex, and marital status). The finding of an increased risk for depression among homemakers is in accord with the work of Brown and Harris (1978), who found elevated rates of depression among homemakers with small children when compared to other women in Camberwell, England.

No association was found between socioeconomic status and major depression in the ECA study, although rates of major depression were higher among the unemployed. Men and women who had been unemployed at least six months in the last five years had a three fold higher risk for an episode of major depression in the past year. The causal direction of this association is unclear. Certainly, job loss and inability to find a job contribute to psychological, social, and economic stress, which may predispose to depression. On the other hand, depressed individuals may be impaired in their ability to find or hold a job.

The New Haven survey by Weissman and Myers (1978) found current rates of major depression to be higher among lower social classes and lifetime rates higher among the upper classes. It was hypothesized that these differences reflected a longer persistence of symptoms in the lower social class as compared to the upper social class.

Urban–Rural Residence. The secular trend of increasing rates of major depression in successive birth cohorts raises questions about potential environmental causes of this effect. One hypothesis is that living in urban and suburban areas, where populations have been growing steadily since World War II, may be associated with factors which predispose to major depression. Community studies in the United States, Puerto Rico, Taiwan, and South Korea permitted urban–rural comparisons which could test such a hypothesis. In fact, some differences were found.

The ECA study found significant differences between urban and rural rates of major depression at the Durham, NC and at the St. Louis, MO sites. The urban–rural relationship was different in these two sites, however. In Durham, the one-year prevalence of major depression was more than twice as high in the urban as compared to the rural sample, while in St. Louis major depression was more prevalent in the rural sample. These sites were different in that the Durham rural area sampled was remote and isolated from the urban center, while in St. Louis the large urban center was more transitionally connected by suburban sprawl to the rural area. These contrasting ECA findings from two different geographical locations, as well as the lack of urban–rural differences in the nationwide sample of the NCS, suggest that the effects of urban versus rural residence on rates of depression are complex and not subject to generalization.

In Taiwan, the small town samples showed trends toward higher major depression rates than the "rural village" or "metropolitan Taipei" samples (Hwu et al., 1989). The Puerto Rico study found trends toward higher prevalence rates among urban as compared to rural residents. The cause of these differences is unclear, but one may hypothesize that factors in urban or transitional places of residence may predispose to depression. Hwu and colleagues suggested conflicts in values between industrialized metropolitan areas and traditional rural areas might account for the rural–urban contrasts in their study.

Marital Status. Marital status was associated with rates of major depression in all of the North American studies (the ECA, NCS, and Edmonton studies). Married and never-married persons had a significantly lower risk of depression when compared to those who were separated, divorced or widowed, even after controlling for sex, age, and other variables associated with depression.. Persons who were currently separated or divorced had a risk for major depression two or three times higher than those in another marital status.

Causal inferences regarding the nature and direction of the association between rates of major depression and separation and divorce are problematic. Episodes of major depression are often followed by marital maladjustment, which can persist for years after the acute depressive episode (Bothwell and Weissman, 1977; Rounsaville et al., 1980). On the other hand, the stresses of separation and divorce may predispose to the onset of depression.

Other Psychiatric Disorder. As a study with a large community sample and a longitudinal design, the ECA provided diagnostic and other data on predictors of first-onset major depression. Using a logistic regression model controlling for the effects of age, race, marital status, sex, and ECA site, Horwath and colleagues (1992a) found that DSM-III dysthymic disorder was associated with a five-fold increase and schizophrenia was associated with an almost three-fold increase in the risk for first-onset major depression. Moreover, persons with a history of two symptoms of major depression of two weeks duration at any time in their lives had a greater than four-fold increased risk for a first episode of major depression.

Although the occurrence of dysthymic disorder and schizophrenia prior to onset of major depression had been observed previously in clinical settings, clinical studies of comorbidity are often skewed by the tendency of persons with more than one illness to preferentially seek treatment, a phenomenon referred to as Berkson's bias (Berkson, 1946). The ECA findings were based upon community respondents and prospectively observed first episodes of major depression. Therefore, case identification was not confounded with treatment status or comorbidity, suggesting that dysthymic disorder and schizophrenia may be true risk factors for the development of first-onset major depression.

The National Comorbidity Study was specifically designed to investigate the comorbidity of psychiatric disorders and to study variations in risk factors based upon comorbidity. As a result, the NCS did find that younger age and lower education were associated with major depression only among those with comorbid psychiatric disorders. In contrast, nonblacks were found to be at higher risk than blacks for pure, but not comorbid, major depression (Blazer et al., 1994). Blazer and colleagues speculated that comorbid major depression may be a more environmentally driven disorder and that psychosocial adversity may play a lesser or at least a different role in pure major depression.

Approximately 50–60% of individuals with a lifetime history of major depression (MDD) have a lifetime history of one or more anxiety disorders (Kessler et al., 1998; Fava et al., 2000). Among respondents of the National Comorbidity Study, 56% of those with a history of at least one disorder were found to have two or more disorders (Kessler et al., 1994). The majority of those with anxiety disorder had comorbid major depression. Comorbidity with major depression was greatest among panic disorder cases (56–73%), followed by generalized anxiety (62–67%), and social phobia (15–21%) (Kaufman et al., 2000).

The NCS found strong associations between lifetime prevalences of panic and major depressive episode with OR 6.2 for panic attacks with depression, and OR 6.8 for panic disorder with depression (Kessler et al., 1998). Moreover, DSM-III-R Generalized Anxiety Disorder has been found to be strongly associated with major depression, with 30-day GAD, and lifetime GAD odds ratios of 13.86 (95% CI 7.93–24.25), and 9.72 (95% CI 6.68–14.12) (Wittchen et al., 1994).

A predictable timeline of the comorbidity of anxiety and depression has not been validated by epidemiological studies. In a study of 255 depressed outpatients, comorbid anxiety disorders with major depression were found in 50.6%, and included social phobia (27%), simple phobia (16.9%), panic disorder (14.5%), generalized anxiety disorder (10.6%), obsessive-compulsive disorder 6.3%, and agoraphobia (5.5%). Both social phobia and generalized anxiety tended to precede the first onset of major depression, by 65% and 63%, respectively. On the other hand, panic disorder (21.6%) and agoraphobia (14.3%) were much more likely to have an onset after a first episode of major depression (Fava et al., 2000).

Recent analyses of the National Comorbidity Study (NCS) have shown a strong association between lifetime and 12-month comorbid panic and depression with symptom severity, impairment, disease course, and help-seeking from health care professionals (Roy-Byrne et al., 2000). This analysis underscores the disabling effect of comorbid panic and depression as compared to either disorder alone. Notably, comorbidity (both 12 month and lifetime) was strongly linked to impairment, measured by help-seeking from health care professionals, taking medication, perceived role impairment, suicide attempts, recency of active disorders, frequency of lifetime depressive disorders or panic attacks.

Role impairment was also assessed using the average number of lost work days, which was 4.5 days in comorbid cases, 4 times higher than respondents with a single disorder and 20 times higher than those with no disorder.

Apart from impairment, comorbidity is associated with greater severity of disease course. Respondents with panic attack and comorbid lifetime depression were found to experience a significantly higher quantity of physiological symptoms (9.1) during a panic attack than respondents without comorbid lifetime major depression (7.9) (Roy-Byrne et al., 2000). A relationship between comorbidity and number of DSM-III-R Criterion A depressive symptoms were also found (7.1 compared to 6.5, $p < 0.001$).

Family History. Investigators have noted for some time the tendency of major depression to cluster in families. Family studies have shown a two to threefold increased risk of major depression among first-degree relatives of probands with major depression as compared with relatives of normal controls (Winokur and Morrison 1973; Winokur 1969; Weissman et al., 1982, 1993; Maier et al., 1991). A genetic contribution to this increased risk of major depression among relatives is suggested by twin studies, which have shown higher concordance rates of major depression among monozygotic than dizygotic twin pairs (27% vs. 12%, Torgersen 1986).

Attributable Risk. While estimates of relative risk have often been used in epidemiologic studies, the attributable risk, a useful measure to document the burden of risk to a community, has been used infrequently in published psychiatric studies. Attributable risk depends both on the magnitude of relative risk and on the prevalence of the risk factor in the population. Using longitudinal data from the ECA study, Horwath and colleagues (1992a) found that more than 50% of cases of first-onset major depression were associated with the earlier presence of two concurrent depressive symptoms for two weeks. This population attributable risk of greater than 50% was due to the substantial relative risk (5.5%) associated with prior depressive symptoms and because of their high prevalence in the community.

The high attributable risk of depressive symptoms for first-onset major depression has implications for the development of preventive interventions for major depression. Heuristically, attributable risk may be thought of as the proportion of disease occurrence that would be prevented if exposure to a given risk factor were prevented. For example, the proportion of cases of lung cancer attributable to smoking is approximately 90% (Chyou et al., 1992). This implies that 90% of cases of lung cancer could be prevented if smoking were totally eliminated.

In a public health effort outside of psychiatry, the finding that *carcinoma in situ* of the cervix was predictive of more advanced and invasive stages of cervical carcinoma led to mass screening of cervical cytology in young women, and the virtual elimination of invasive cervical carcinoma in regularly screened women. With additional study and public education, early identification of depressive symptoms may be a first step toward the prediction and prevention of major depression.

Any preventive intervention program that seeks to identify cases with depressive symptoms prior to the onset of the full syndrome would need to take into account the fact that most early cases will be false positives, that is, will not develop major depression. Similarly, most smokers do not develop lung cancer, and most women with abnormal cervical cytology do not develop invasive cervical carcinoma, yet public health interventions, such as education about the risks of smoking and cervical cytologic screening, have been enormously successful in reducing morbidity and mortality from lung and cervical carcinoma. Hopefully, similar preventive efforts could be developed for major depression.

Summary

Rates of major depression are considerably higher than for bipolar disorder and somewhat more variable by site. The lifetime prevalence of DSM-III/DSM-III-R major depression varied from 2.9 per 100 to 17.1 per 100. As with bipolar disorder, prevalence rates of major depression in Taiwan were considerably lower. The more variable rates of major depression, as compared to the narrower range of rates for bipolar disorder, may be due to greater clinical heterogeneity of major depression or a stronger association between rates of major depression and psychosocial factors, which may vary considerably between different study samples and sites.

The ECA study has provided evidence supportive of the validity of major depression with psychotic features and major depression with atypical features (overeating and oversleeping) as subtypes. This epidemiological evidence is consistent with clinical findings.

The community studies provided data on a number of risk factors for major depression. Female gender was a clear and consistent risk factor across all community studies, using either DSM-III, DSM-III-R or ICD-9 diagnosis, and for the first time incidence data showed that the increased risk for women applied to first-onset cases. There is convincing evidence from the cross-national data of an increase in the cumulative lifetime rates of major depression with each successive younger birth cohort.

The ECA study showed few racial differences in rates of major depression when education and social class were controlled. In contrast, the NCS found that nonblacks were at higher risk than blacks for pure, but not comorbid, major depression. The Taiwan study found substantially lower rates of major depression than other community studies.

The ECA, NCS and Edmonton studies found that marital status was strongly associated with rates of major depression, with married persons showing the lowest prevalence and separated or divorced persons showing the highest rates.

The ECA longitudinal data showed that a prior history of other psychiatric disorder or depressive symptoms was strongly predictive of the first-onset of major depression. Dysthymic disorder increased the relative risk of first-onset major depression five-fold; a two-week period of 2 concurrent depressive symptoms increased the risk more than four-fold; and schizophrenia increased the risk almost three-fold.

The ECA study found that depressive symptoms have significant public health implications for the onset of major depression. More than 50% of cases of first-onset major depression were attributable to a prior episode of two weeks of two concurrent depressive symptoms. These findings may have implications for the prediction and prevention of major depression.

Family studies have shown a clear and consistent increased risk for major depression among first-degree relatives of probands with major depression. This increased familial risk appears to be limited to cases of early onset major depression.

DYSTHYMIC DISORDER

Definition

The essential features of dysthymic disorder in both DSM-III and DSM-III-R are a chronically depressed mood associated with appetite disturbance, insomnia or hypersomnia, low energy or fatigue, low self-esteem, impaired concentration or indecisiveness, or feelings of hopelessness. The symptoms cannot meet criteria for major depression during the first two years of disturbance, cannot be superimposed on a chronic psychotic disorder, and may not be comorbid with mania or hypomania.

Rates

Lifetime rates of DSM-III or DSM-III-R dysthymic disorder are shown in Table 6. As with major depression, the rates of dysthymic disorder were higher in the NCS data than in the other studies. The NCS found a lifetime rate of 6.4 per 100, while the 5-site rate of dysthymic disorder in the ECA study was 3.0 per 100, similar to

TABLE 6. Rates of Dysthymic Disorder by Sex in Community Surveys Using DSM-III (or DSM-III-R) Diagnosis

	Lifetime Rates/100			
Place	Female	Male	Total	Sex Ratios Female/Male
USA-NCS (DSM-III-R)	8.0	4.8	6.4	1.7
USA-ECA	4.1	2.2	3.0	1.9
New Haven, CT	—	—	3.2	—
Baltimore, MD	—	—	2.1	—
St. Louis, MO	—	—	3.8	—
Durham, NC	—	—	2.3	—
Los Angeles, CA	—	—	4.2	—
Edmonton, Canada	5.2	2.2	3.7	2.4
Puerto Rico	7.6	1.6	4.7	4.8
Florence, Italy	—	—	2.3	—
Taiwan				
Urban	1.1	0.7	0.9	1.6
Small towns	1.6	1.4	1.5	1.1
Rural villages	1.4	0.6	0.9	2.6
Seoul, Korea	2.8	1.6	2.2	1.7

Source: Adapted from Tsuang et al. (1995).

the prevalence of 3.7 per 100 in Edmonton, Canada. Apart from Taiwan, other studies found fairly comparable rates per 100, ranging from 2.2 in Korea to 4.7 in Puerto Rico. As with other disorders, Taiwan had the lowest rates of dysthymic disorder, ranging from 0.9 to 1.5 per 100 in the different sites.

Risk Factors

The study of risk factors for dysthymic disorder is somewhat complicated by the unresolved question of whether it is a mood disorder distinct from major depression. The ECA data showed that almost half (42%) of cases of dysthymia had a history of major depression as well. Clinical observation of depressed patients over time suggests that dysthymic disorder may be prodromal to or a residual state of major depression. Epidemiological evidence indicates that individuals with dysthymic disorder, when compared to controls, are at a greater than fourfold increased risk for major depression (Horwath et al., 1992a). However, even those persons with the uncomplicated form of dysthymic disorder, when compared to individuals with no psychiatric disorder, have significantly elevated rates of medical and psychiatric treatment utilization, and suicide thoughts and attempts (Weissman et al., 1988b). Therefore, although the boundary between dysthymic disorder and major depression remains unclear, the evidence that uncomplicated dysthymic disorder predicts psychosocial morbidity and first-onset major depression suggests its continued utility as a separate diagnostic category.

Sex. All of the community studies reporting separate male and female rates of dysthymic disorder found an excess of cases among women. With the exception of small towns in Taiwan, where rates were similar, the ratios of female:male rates of dysthymic disorder ranged from 1.6:1 in urban Taiwan to a high of 4.8:1 in Puerto Rico. As with major depression, and unlike bipolar disorder, dysthymic disorder is associated with an excess risk among women.

Age. Unlike the situation for major depression, in which the highest prevalence was found in younger groups, the lifetime rates of dysthymic disorder in the ECA tended to increase in the 30–65 age group and then drop dramatically in those over 65 years of age. South Korea and Edmonton, Canada, also found an increasing prevalence with age. As in the ECA, Edmonton showed a steep drop in prevalence over 65, but Korea did not sample those over 65. Data from the NCS regarding the association between age and rates of dysthymic disorder have not yet been published.

It is not clear why the age effects are different for major depression and dysthymic disorder. The variations by age may reflect true differences between these disorders, but an understanding of these differences is complicated by the high comorbidity between major depression and dysthymic disorder and by the fact that these are comparisons between the chronic disorder, dysthymia, and major depression, which may range in duration from a brief to a chronic condition.

Race. The ECA study showed no significant differences in rates of dysthymic disorder when comparing African-Americans and whites. However, rates of dysthymic disorder were higher among Hispanics than those of African-Americans or whites, which is consistent with the higher rate in Puerto Rico. As with major depression, rates of dysthymic disorder were markedly lower in Taiwan than in the West, while the prevalence in Korea was comparable to that in the West.

Marital Status. Dysthymic disorder was more prevalent among unmarried than married persons under the age of 65 in the ECA study. In Edmonton, divorced or widowed persons had higher rates compared with married persons, who had higher rates than the never married. As is the case with major depression, the direction of causality in these associations between age and prevalence of dysthymic disorder is not clear.

Urban–Rural. Puerto Rico showed a significantly higher rate of dysthymic disorder among urban when compared to rural dwellers (5.5 vs. 3.3 per 100). In Taiwan, urban and rural rates were similar, but the small town rates were somewhat higher, as was the case for major depression.

Summary

Dysthymic disorder, a milder but more chronic form of depression than major depression, appears to share some of the characteristics of major depression. In terms of risk factors, dysthymic disorder, like major depression, had higher rates among women than men, and higher rates among divorced than married persons. Although almost half of persons with dysthymic disorder also had episodes of major depression, those persons with uncomplicated dysthymic disorder, when compared to individuals with no psychiatric disorder, had substantial evidence of morbidity, such as treatment-seeking and suicide attempts. Whether dysthymic disorder is distinct from major depression remains unclear.

ANXIETY DISORDERS

Anxiety has been recognized as a symptom ever since the writings of Freud. However, it was only recently, with the incorporation into DSM-III and DSM-III-R of Klein's conceptualization of panic disorder as a separate entity, that anxiety states began to be subdivided into distinct disorders such as panic, phobias, and generalized anxiety disorders.

In a review of five population studies conducted in the United States, the United Kingdom and Sweden prior to the development of specified diagnostic criteria, Marks and Lader (1973) found that anxiety states were fairly common (about 2.0 to 4.7 per 100 point prevalence) and more prevalent in women, particularly younger women between 16 and 40 years of age. In a separate epidemiologic review, Weissman (1985) identified nine additional community studies of anxiety states which showed rates in the range reported by Marks and Lader (1973), and also showed that rates were higher in women than in men. Our focus in this section is on the more recent epidemiologic studies in which anxiety disorders are subdivided on the basis of DSM-III or DSM-III-R criteria.

In a cross-national study of 10 independently conducted community surveys in 10 different countries (United States, Canada, Puerto Rico, France, West Germany, Italy, Lebanon, Taiwan, Korea, New Zealand), lifetime prevalence rates for DIS/DSM-III panic disorder were found to range from 1.4 per 100 to 2.9 per 100 in Florence Italy with a much lower prevalence rate in Taiwan of 0.4 per 100 (Weissman et al., 1997). These findings underscore the relative consistence of panic disorder in its prevalence and distribution across diverse cultures. Women were found to have higher prevalence rates than males in all countries, and age of onset was found to be early to middle 20s (Weissman et al, 1997.) Consistent with previous epidemiologic studies, across all countries included in the study, panic disorder was found to be strongly associated with increased risk of major depression and agoraphobia.

Anxiety as a Disabling Disease

Anxiety disorders cause substantial disability in mental and role functioning. The degree of disability was shown in the Medical Outcomes Study, in which the health related quality of life of patients with panic disorder was compared to patients with other chronic medical illnesses (hypertension, diabetes, heart disease, arthritis, chronic lung problems) as well as other psychiatric disorders (major depression) (Sherbourne et al., 1996). Patients with panic disorder had levels of role functioning that were substantially lower than patients with other major medical illnesses but were higher or comparable to patients with depression. In contrast, physical functioning and self-perception of current health in panic patients were similar to that of patients with hypertension and the general population (Sherbourne et al., 1996).

PANIC DISORDER

Definition

The key feature of panic disorder in DSM-III is the occurrence of three or more panic attacks within a three week period. These attacks cannot be precipitated only by exposure to a feared situation, cannot be due to a physical disorder, and must be accompanied by at least four of the following symptoms: dyspnea, palpitations, chest pain, smothering or choking, dizziness, feelings of unreality, paresthesias, hot and cold flashes, sweating, faintness, trembling or shaking (APA, 1980). In DSM-III-R, the definition was revised to require four attacks in four weeks or one or more attacks followed by a persistent fear of having another attack. In DSM-III-R, the list of potential symptoms was revised to include nausea or abdominal distress and to exclude depersonalization or derealization (APA, 1987).

More important, DSM-III-R changed the diagnostic hierarchy so that panic disorder could be diagnosed as a primary disorder with or without agoraphobia and dropped the category of agoraphobia with panic attacks. This change placed the emphasis on identifying panic disorder as a discrete entity and reflected the clinical experience that panic attacks tended to occur prior to the development of agoraphobia, which was increasingly viewed as a phobic avoidance response to the frightening experience of spontaneous panic attacks, near panic experiences or limited symptom attacks.

TABLE 7. Prevalence Rates per 100 of Panic Disorder Using DSM-III (or DSM-III-R) Criteria

	Rate/100[a]		
Place	6 month	1 year	Lifetime
USA-NCS (DSM-III-R)		2.3	3.5
USA-ECA (5 sites)			1.6
ECA New Haven, CT	0.6		
Baltimore, MD	1.0		
St. Louis, MO	0.9		
Piedmont, NC	0.7		
Los Angeles, CA	0.9		
Zurich survey		3.1	
Edmonton, Canada	0.7		1.2
Puerto Rico	1.1		1.7
New Zealand			1.4
Florence, Italy			1.4
Korea			1.7
Taiwan			
Urban			0.20
Small towns			0.34
Rural			0.13

[a]Rates rounded off to one decimal place in most cases.

Source: Adapted from Tsuang et al. (1995).

Rates. Table 7 shows prevalence rates of panic disorder from community studies using DSM-III or DSM-III-R criteria. For studies using DSM-III, the 6-month prevalence of panic disorder ranged from 0.6 per 100 in New Haven, CT, to 1.1 per 100 in Puerto Rico, representing a remarkable level of consistency across sites. The annual prevalence rate of 3.1 per 100 from the Zurich survey was based upon a definition of panic which only approximated that of DSM-III. The NCS reported a 1-year prevalence of 2.3 per 100 for DSM-III-R panic disorder.

Lifetime rates of DSM-III panic disorder showed good agreement, with prevalence varying from 1.2 per 100 in Edmonton, Canada, to 2.2 per 100 in New Zealand. The exception to this narrow range of lifetime rates was Taiwan, where panic disorder occurred at rates from 0.13 per 100 rural areas to 0.34 per 100 in small towns. The only study that reported on lifetime DSM-III-R panic disorder was the NCS, which found a rate of 3.5 per 100, considerably higher than the lifetime rates based upon DSM-III. This may be due to the broadening of the concept of panic disorder in DSM-III-R or to the differences in memory probes used in the UM-CIDI, as compared to those used in the DIS..

Risk Factors

Gender. Comparing lifetime prevalence rates, all of the studies reporting on panic disorder showed higher rates for women than for men. With the exception of Puerto Rico and Taiwan, the higher lifetime risk for women was statistically significant in all of the community studies. In an analysis of the NCS data, Eaton and colleagues (1994) found uniformly higher rates of panic attacks and panic disorder for women compared to men within every age group. Of interest, Keyl and Eaton (1990) analyzed incidence rates from the ECA study and found two fold increased odds of incident panic disorder in women compared to men. This finding is analogous to the increased incidence and prevalence rates for major depression in women compared to men and suggests that for both panic disorder and major depression the higher rates in women reflect a true increase in the risk for new onset panic and depression rather than a greater tendency to seek treatment or have longer episodes of illness.

Age. In both the NCS and the ECA data, a bimodal distribution of age of onset was reported (Eaton et al., 1994; Anthony and Aboraya, 1992). The NCS found an early mode for panic disorder in the 15–24 year age range for both men and women, and a later mode in the 45–54 range (Eaton et al., 1994).

Few studies have investigated anxiety disorders among adolescents. Data from the Bremer Adolescent Study reveal that among 1035 adolescents, age 12–17 years, the prevalence of DSM-IV panic disorder was 0.5%. However, 18% of adolescents reported having had at least one panic attack, with girls experiencing slightly more panic attacks than their male adolescent counterparts, and the peak age range of both panic attack and panic disorder occurring between 14 and 15 year of age (Essau et al., 1999).

In the ECA and Edmonton studies, older persons (65 and over) had the lowest lifetime prevalence rates of panic disorder. This pattern was quite different for Hispanics in the ECA and in the Puerto Rican study. In Puerto Rico and in Hispanic women in the ECA, the lifetime prevalence tended to increase with age. For Hispanic men in the ECA, the lifetime rate dropped with each age group, reaching 0 in the group over 65 years of age.The NCS reported no significant ethnic differences for young adults, but did find lower rates in nonwhite compared to white older age groups. The reason for these differences is not clear.

Race and Ethnicity. In the ECA study, there were no significant differences in prevalence rates between African-American, Hispanic, and white groups (Horwath et al., 1993; Eaton et al., 1991). Similarly, the NCS found no main effects of race or ethnicity, but did report an age by race or ethnicity interaction effect (see above). Comparisons of other studies are more remarkable for the cross-cultural similarities in rates of panic disorder, with the exception of the Taiwan study, which had the lowest rates of panic. As with major depression, Korean prevalence rates of panic disorder were comparable to those in the West, while Taiwan's were much lower.

Family History. Panic disorder appears to have an associated familial risk related to the type of symptoms experienced by an individual. Symptoms of smothering appear to incur greater familial risk, and may be a marker for a subtype of panic disorder worthy of further genetic study. In a family study of 104 panic disorder probands and 247 of their first-degree relatives, it was found that first-degree relatives of individuals with panic disorder with smothering symptoms were at greater risk for panic [OR 2.7 (95% CI 1.2-6.1)] and for panic with smothering symptoms [OR 5.7 (95% CI 1.3-25.1)] than relatives of individuals with panic disorder without smothering symptoms (Horwath et al., 1997.)

Summary

The prevalence of panic disorder was fairly uniform, with higher risks for women and persons under the age of 65. The NCS and ECA data suggested a bimodal distribution in the ages of onset. As with other disorders, the NCS reported higher lifetime rates while Taiwan found much lower rates of panic disorder.

AGORAPHOBIA

Definition

DSM-III agoraphobia is defined as a fear and avoidance of being in places or situations from which escape might be difficult or in which help might not be available in the event of sudden incapacitation (APA, 1980). As a result of such fears, the agoraphobic person avoids travel outside the home or requires the accompaniment of a companion when away from home. Moderate cases may cause some constriction in lifestyle, while severe cases of agoraphobia may result in the person being completely housebound or unable to leave home unaccompanied.

As outlined in the panic disorder section above, DSM-III-R revised the diagnosis of agoraphobia to a condition accompanying panic disorder (panic disorder with agoraphobia). Although the diagnosis of agoraphobia without history of panic disorder was retained, this category emphasized the avoidance behavior as a

TABLE 8. Prevalence Rates per 100 of Agoraphobia Using DSM-III (or DSM-III-R) Criteria

Place	Rate/100[a]		
	6 month	1 year	Lifetime
USA-NCS (DSM-III-R)		2.8	5.3
USA-ECA (4 sites)			5.6
ECA New Haven, CT	2.8		
Baltimore, MD	5.8		
St. Louis, MO	2.7		
Piedmont, NC	5.4		
Los Angeles, CA	3.2		
Puerto Rico	3.9		6.9
Zurich survey	2.5		
New Zealand			3.8
Florence, Italy			1.3
Edmonton, Canada			2.9
Korea			2.7
Taiwan			
Urban			1.1
Small towns			1.5
Rural			1.3

[a]Panic with agoraphobia.

Source: Adapted from Tsuang et al. (1995).

response to the sudden development of anxiety or somatic symptoms (APA 1987). DSM-IV has further emphasized that the agoraphobic avoidance behavior occurs specifically in response to situationally predisposed panic attacks or panic-like symptoms (APA 1994).

Rates

Table 8 shows prevalence rates of agoraphobia from community studies using DSM-III or DSM-III-R criteria. In the ECA study, 6-month prevalence rates ranged from 2.7 per 100 in St. Louis to 5.7 per 100 in Baltimore. Comparable 6-month and 1-year prevalence rates were found in Zurich and Puerto Rico. Lifetime rates of agoraphobia showed considerable variation, from a low of 1.1 per 100 in urban Taiwan to a high of 6.9 per 100 in Puerto Rico. Some of this variation may have been due to the use of a translated Diagnostic Interview Schedule (DIS) (Robins et al 1981). If one considers only the studies carried out in primarily English-speaking countries, the lifetime prevalence rates vary over a narrower range, from 2.9 per 100 in Edmonton, Canada, to 5.6 per 100 in the ECA data from 4 sites. In spite of the changes in the diagnostic definition between DSM-III and DSM-III-R, the lifetime rates from the ECA and NCS studies (5.6 vs. 5.3 per 100, respectively) show remarkable consistency.

Risk factors

Lifetime rates of agoraphobia were significantly higher for women than for men in each of the community studies. This is consistent with the gender differences found for panic disorder and major depression.

In a community study of 3021 adolescents and young adults aged 14–24 years, the lifetime prevalence of DSM-IV agoraphobia was found to be 8.5%, higher than panic attack (4.3%) or panic disorder with (0.8%) or without (0.8%) agoraphobia (Wittchen et al., 1998). A clinical analysis of community cases of agoraphobia from the ECA found that most cases were misidentified (Horwath et al., 1993). This raises questions about the validity of this high rate of agoraphobia.

In the ECA study, lifetime prevalence of agoraphobia was higher among African-Americans than among whites or Hispanics. The effects of race or ethnicity and gender combined to produce a considerable range in lifetime prevalence, from 2.9 per 100 in white males to 12 per 100 in African-American women (Eaton et al., 1991). In the NCS, current agoraphobia (past month) was associated with an increased risk in African-Americans compared to whites, and in homemakers compared to those working outside the home (Magee et al., 1996). Current agoraphobia was inversely related to income and education in a bivariate analysis of the NCS data (Magee et al., 1996).

Two studies reported significant urban–rural differences in rates of agoraphobia, but they were in opposite directions. Puerto Rico found a significantly higher lifetime prevalence for the urban area, while Korea reported a higher rural rate. The NCS found no significant urban–rural differences in rates of agoraphobia.

Relationship Between Agoraphobia and Panic

In DSM-III, agoraphobia was considered a separate phobic disorder which may or may not be accompanied by panic attacks. Largely due to the influence of Klein's argument that agoraphobia is a conditioned avoidance response to the aversive stimulus of spontaneous panic attacks, the diagnostic view of agoraphobia changed considerably in DSM-III-R, in which panic disorder is viewed as primary, with or without the secondary development of agoraphobia. An important factor in this change was the observation by Klein and others that, in clinic settings, agoraphobia rarely occurs without preceding spontaneous panic attacks or limited symptom attacks.

Considerable controversy continues regarding the nature of the relationship between agoraphobic avoidance and panic attacks. Marks (1987) and other European investigators have questioned the temporal precedence and causal role of panic attacks in the development of agoraphobia.

Contributing to the controversy are the large differences between clinic and community studies in their estimates of the relative prevalence of agoraphobia with and without panic attacks. Table 9 shows the results of published community and clinical studies that have reported data permitting calculation of the proportion of agoraphobics with a history of panic attacks.

The population based surveys found that a substantial proportion of subjects with agoraphobia reported no history of panic attacks. In these studies, 80% of the subjects were interviewed by lay persons using the Diagnostic Interview Schedule

TABLE 9. Reported Frequency of Agoraphobia Without Panic Attacks

Author	Date	No. Agoraphobia w/o Panic Attacks	Total No. Agoraphobia	%
Community studies				
Thompson et al.	1998[a]	88	104	85
Angst and Dobler-Mikala	1985	15	22	68
ECA		656	961	68
Wittchen	1986	13	26	50
Joyce et al.	1989	35[b]	76	46
Faravelli et al.	1989	4	14	29
Clinic studies				
Torgersen	1983[c]	8	26	31
Thyer and Himle	1985	20[d]	115	17
Argyle and Roth	1986	5	42	12
Garvey and Tuason	1984	1	13	8
Aronson and Logue	1987	2	36	6
Pollard et al.	1989	61[e]	993	6
Uhde et al.	1985	1	32	3
Barlow	1988	1[f]	42	2
DiNardo	1983	0	23	0
Breier	1986	0	54	0
Noyes	1986	0	67	0
Kleiner	1987	0	50	0
Thyer et al.	1985	0	28	0

[a]Thompson study reported on agoraphobia without panic disorder.
[b]Joyce study: 10 of 35 subjects reported limited symptom attacks.
[c]Torgersen study reported on agoraphobia without panic disorder.
[d]Thyer study: These subjects "often suffered from unpredictable somatic symptoms... functional equivalent to panic attacks."
[e]Pollard study: Some subjects had limited symptom attacks.
[f]Barlow study: Subject had linited symptom attacks.
Source: Adapted from Horwath et al. (1993).

(DIS). In contrast, clinic-based studies, using less structured interviews administered by clinicians, almost invariably found much lower rates of agoraphobia without panic.

Several explanations for this discrepancy have been suggested. One explanation is that treated samples of persons with any illness have high rates of comorbidity (Berkson, 1946). An alternative explanation is that population studies may have overestimated the rate of agoraphobia without panic disorder.

In a reanalysis of the ECA data on agoraphobia without panic (Horwath et al., 1993), 22 community cases of agoraphobia without panic were clinically reappraised and only a single case of probable agoraphobia without panic was found. The diagnostic reappraisal found that 19 (87%) of the cases had simple or social phobias rather than agoraphobia, or had no DSM-III phobia at all. The reappraisal also identified six cases of panic disorder, panic attacks or limited symptom attacks which had been missed by the DIS interview. The authors concluded that community studies using the DIS may have overestimated the prevalence of agoraphobia without panic attacks in the community. Similar to the ECA, an initial analysis of the NCS data found that only about one-third of NCS agoraphobics reported a history of a panic attack. More detailed analyses of the NCS data are underway to determine whether agoraphobia without panic is in fact as common as the initial analyses suggest (Magee et al., 1996).

Summary

Prevalence rates of agoraphobia based upon the DIS and DSM-III varied considerably. These rates and their variations by study are difficult to interpret for two reasons. First, the diagnostic view of agoraphobia has changed considerably since these studies were done. Second, a clinical reappraisal study of ECA cases of agoraphobia without panic attacks suggested that studies using the DIS may have overestimated rates of agoraphobia without panic. This overestimate may have been due to missed cases of panic disorder, panic attacks and limited symptom attacks and due to difficulty differentiating the boundary between agoraphobia and simple phobias.

In spite of the problems suggested above, the community studies consistently found higher rates of agoraphobia among women than men, and the ECA and NCS studies found higher rates among African-Americans than among whites.

SOCIAL PHOBIA

Definition

The central feature of DSM-III social phobia is a persistent, irrational fear accompanied by a compelling desire to avoid situations in which a person may act in a humiliating or embarrassing way while under the scrutiny of others (APA, 1980). DSM-III-R allowed for the phobic situation to be avoided or endured with intense anxiety and added the requirement that the avoidant behavior interferes with occupational or social functioning or that there is marked distress about having the fear (APA, 1987). Common social phobias involve fears of speaking or eating in public, urinating in public lavatories, writing in front of others, or saying foolish things in social situations.

Rates

Table 10 shows the lifetime prevalence of social phobia from studies using DSM-III or DSM-III-R criteria. Lifetime rates of DSM-III social phobia varied considerably, with a low of 0.4 per 100 in rural Taiwan and a high of 3.9 per 100 in New Zealand. It is not clear whether these contrasting rates reflect true cross-cultural differences or are due to differences in methodology or translation of the DIS. The lifetime prevalence rates of social phobia vary over a somewhat narrower range: from 1.7 per 100 in Edmonton, Canada, to 3.9 per 100 in New Zealand when comparing rates from English-speaking countries.

The rate of lifetime DSM-III-R social phobia from the NCS was considerably higher (13.3 per 100) than in any of the DSM-III studies. Magee and colleagues

TABLE 10. Lifetime Prevalence Rates per 100 of Social Phobia Using DSM-III (or DSM-III-R) Criteria

Community Survey	Rates/100
USA-NCS (DSM-III-R(	13.3
USA-ECA (4 sites)	2.4
Baltimore, MD	3.1
St. Louis, MO	1.9
Durham, NC	3.2
Los Angeles, CA	1.8
Edmonton, Canada	1.7
Puerto Rico	1.6
New Zealand	3.9
Florence, Italy	1.0
Korea	0.6
Taiwan	
Urban	0.6
Small towns	0.5
Rural	0.4

Source: Adapted from Tsuang et al. (1995).

(1996) attributed the higher prevalence to differences between the DIS and UM-CIDI. The UM-CIDI uses a stem question based on the broader DSM-III-R criteria allowing either avoidance of a feared situation or endurance with intense anxiety, and it also asks about six specific social-phobic fears (compared to three in the DIS), including the high prevalence fears of using a public toilet, writing in front of others, or talking to people and sounding foolish or having nothing to say.

Risk Factors

In an analysis of the ECA data from four sites (the New Haven site used a version of the DIS which did not include social phobia items), Schneier et al. (1992) found that lifetime prevalence rates of social phobia were highest among women and persons who were younger (age 18 to 29 years), less educated, single, and of lower socioeconomic class. In the NCS, higher rates were found in women, those with less education or income, the never married, students, and those who live with their parents (Magee et al., 1996). A significantly higher prevalence of lifetime social phobia was also found among women in Korea and urban Taiwan, while no significant gender differences were found in Edmonton, Puerto Rico, or small town or rural areas of Taiwan.

GENERALIZED ANXIETY DISORDER

Definition

The DSM-III criteria for generalized anxiety disorder (GAD) require the presence of unrealistic or excessive anxiety and worry, accompanied by symptoms from three of four categories: (1) motor tension, (2) autonomic hyperactivity, (3) vigilance and scanning, and (4) apprehensive expectation. The anxious mood must continue for at least a month, and the diagnosis is not made if phobias, panic disorder, or obsessive–compulsive disorder are present, or if the disturbance is due to another physical or mental disorder, such as hyperthyroidism, major depression, or schizophrenia (APA, 1980). By this definition, generalized anxiety disorder is treated primarily as a residual category after the exclusion of the other major anxiety disorders. DSM-III-R narrowed the definition further by requiring a minimum of six symptoms and a duration of six months (APA 1987).

Rates

Table 11 shows the prevalence of generalized anxiety disorder from community studies using DSM-III or DSM-III-R criteria. In the ECA study, hierarchical diagnostic exclusion of panic disorder and major depression yielded the 1-year prevalence of 2.7 per 100, while dropping the exclusions resulted in a rate of 3.8 per 100 (Blazer et al., 1991). Lifetime prevalence of GAD in the ECA study was quite consistent across three study sites, varying from 4.1 per 100 in Los Angeles to 6.6 per 100 in Durham and St. Louis. In spite of differences in diagnostic criteria, the ECA and NCS rates of GAD were quite similar. Lifetime prevalence varied considerably more in the Taiwan study, from 3.7 per 100 in Taipei to 10.5 per 100 in small town areas of Taiwan.

TABLE 11. Prevalence Rates per 100 of Generalized Anxiety Disorder Using DSM-III (or DSM-III-R) Criteria

	Rate/100[a]	
Place	1 year	Lifetime
USA-NCS (DSM-III-R)	3.1	5.1
USA-ECA (3 sites)		
(no exclusions)	3.8	
(no panic, no MDD)	2.7	
USA-ECA (3 sites) (no panic, no MDD)		
Durham, NC		6.6
St. Louis, MO		6.6
Los Angeles, CA		4.1
Zurich survey	5.2	
Florence, Italy		5.4
Florence, Italy (DSM-III-R)		3.9
Taiwan		
Urban		3.7
Small towns		10.5
Rural		7.8
Korea		3.6

[a]Rates rounded off to one decimal place in most cases.

Source: Adapted from Tsuang et al. (1995).

The Florence study provides an interesting example of the effects of requiring the longer 6-month duration of DSM-III-R. For DSM-III, the lifetime rates were 5.4 per 100, while the narrower DSM-III-R definition resulted in the lower rate of 3.9 per 100. In the NCS, which used a different interview, the UM-CIDI, the changes in criteria did not yield changes in prevalence.

Risk Factors

Based upon data combined from three ECA study sites, the one-year prevalence of GAD, with or without diagnostic exclusions, was significantly higher in females, in African-Americans, and in persons under 30 years of age, but the differences were significant for age only without diagnostic exclusions and for race only when panic and depression were excluded (Blazer et al., 1991). The Taiwan study reported significantly higher rates for women than for men, but no gender differences were found in Korea.

OBSESSIVE—COMPULSIVE DISORDER

Definition

DSM-III obsessive–compulsive disorder (OCD) requires the presence of obsessions or compulsions which are sources of significant distress or impairment and are not due to another mental disorder. Obsessions are defined as recurrent, persistent thoughts, images or impulses that are experienced as senseless and repugnant. Compulsions are excessively repetitive, stereotyped behaviors, such as repeatedly checking locked doors or gas jets or washing hands (APA, 1980).

Rates

Table 12 shows prevalence rates of OCD from community studies using DSM-III criteria. Six-month prevalence of OCD varied from 0.7 per 100 in Los Angeles to 2.1 per 100 in Piedmont, North Carolina. Lifetime prevalence of OCD varied from 0.3 per 100 in rural Taiwan to 3.2 per 100 in Puerto Rico. The studies in English language sites showed excellent agreement, with lifetime prevalence of 2.6 per 100 in the ECA and 3.0 per 100 in Edmonton, Canada. Most remarkable about these rates is that they contradict the previous traditional view of OCD, on the basis of published clinical reports, as a rare disorder.

Risk Factors

As with other anxiety disorders, prevalence rates of OCD were higher among women than men in the ECA study. However, when gender comparisons were controlled for marital status, employment status, job status, ethnicity and age, there were no remaining differences in prevalence rates for women compared to men (Karno et al., 1987).

TABLE 12. Prevalence Rates per 100 of Obsessive–Compulsive Disorder Using DSM-III Criteria

	Rate/100[a]	
Place	6 month	Lifetime
ECA		
New Haven, CT	1.4	
Baltimore, MD	2.0	
St. Louis, MO	1.3	
Piedmont, NC	2.1	
Los Angeles, CA	0.7	
Puerto Rico	1.8	
Edmonton, Canada	1.6	
ECA (5 sites)		2.6
Florence, Italy		0.7
Korea		2.1
Edmonton, Canada		3.2
Puerto Rico		3.2
Taiwan		
Urban		0.94
Small towns		0.54
Rural		0.30

[a]Rates rounded off to one decimal place in most cases.

Source: Adapted from Tsuang et al. (1995).

SUMMARY

Affective Disorders

The epidemiologic data on rates of bipolar disorder is most notable for its similarities across cultures rather than differences. Rates of bipolar disorder are similar in men and women, but higher in divorced individuals when compared to married persons. Rates of bipolar disorder are substantially lower than for unipolar major depression.

Epidemiological data support the validity of two subtypes of major depression: (1) MDD with psychotic features, and (2) MDD with atypical features (overeating and oversleeping). The community studies found that female gender, divorce, and prior histories of dysthymic disorder, schizophrenia or depressive symptoms were risk factors for major depression. From a public health perspective, depressive symptoms were associated with a more than 50% population attributable risk of major depression.

Cross-national data showed an increase in the cumulative lifetime rates of major depression with each successive younger birth cohort, and substantially lower rates in Taiwan than in the West. Family studies showed an increased risk for major depression among relatives, apparently limited to cases of early onset major depression.

Dysthymic disorder, like major depression, had higher rates among women than men, and higher rates among divorced than married persons. There is evidence for psychiatric morbidity in uncomplicated dysthymia, but the boundary between dysthymic disorder and major depression remains unclear.

Anxiety Disorders

Lifetime prevalence rates of panic disorder were remarkably consistent across the community studies and across cultural, racial and ethnic boundaries, with the exception of the higher rates in the NCS and much lower rates in Taiwan. Panic disorder was more common among women.

The epidemiological data on agoraphobia show considerable variation in rates across studies and cross-culturally. A recent clinical reappraisal of the ECA data on agoraphobia without panic suggests that community studies relying upon the DIS and DSM-III may have overestimated the prevalence of agoraphobia without panic. Therefore, the prevalence estimates from studies such as these should be regarded with caution until the accuracy of their prevalence figures on agoraphobia can be more thoroughly tested.

Analyses of relative risks showed higher rates of agoraphobia for women than men, just as with panic disorder. Unlike panic disorder, however, agoraphobia was associated with higher rates for African-Americans than whites, and higher rates among those with less education or income. The differential effects of race and socioeconomic factors on panic disorder and agoraphobia suggest that the factors which cause panic disorder may not be the same as the factors which lead to the subsequent development of agoraphobia.

The ECA and NCS studies found that prevalence rates of social phobia were highest among women, those with less education or income, and the never married. Generalized anxiety disorder was also more prevalent among women. Based on community data, obsessive—compulsive disorder turned out to be a much more prevalent disorder than suggested by previous clinical studies.

FUTURE DEVELOPMENTS

A number of major epidemiologic studies have cross-sectionally examined the prevalence and nature of mood and anxiety disorders. Certain consistent findings have emerged, but the answers to major questions remain elusive. Although women have been found to consistently have higher rates of major depression and panic disorder, for example, no satisfactory scientific explanation has been found for this difference. Similarly, several studies have shown secular trends for increasing rates of depression, but no good understanding of this trend has yet been achieved. Substantial questions remain regarding the comorbidity between psychiatric disorders, such as the nature of the interaction between panic disorder and agoraphobia. The National Comorbidity Survey has addressed some of these comorbidity issues. Future epidemiologic studies will need to address questions regarding the nature, etiology, changing character, and interactions of mood and anxiety disorders. Considerable progress needs to be made in integrating the rapidly growing biological understanding of mood and anxiety disorders into epidemiological approaches which may clarify the complex interactions between biologic and psychosocial variables in the etiology and course of these disorders.

ACKNOWLEDGMENTS

This manuscript has been updated from chapters in *Textbook in Psychiatric Epidemiology*. Tsuang MT, Tohen M, Zahner GEP (eds.): New York: Wiley, 1995, pp 317–344.

The authors acknowledge the support of NIMH grant MH 28274 "Genetic Studies of Depressive Disorders"; NIMH grant MH 36197 "Children at High and Low Risk for Depression" and a NARSAD Established Investigator Award, "The Continuity between Childhood and Adult Depression: A Longitudinal Study of Children as Depressed Adults."

REFERENCES

American Psychiatric Association, (1980): "Diagnostic and Statistical Manual of Mental Disorders," 3rd ed. Washington, DC: American Psychiatric Association Press.

American Psychiatric Association (1987): "Diagnostic and Statistical Manual of Mental Disorders," 3rd ed. revised. Washington, DC: American Psychiatric Association Press.

American Psychiatric Association, (1994): "Diagnostic and Statistical Manual of Mental Disorders," 4th ed. Washington, DC: American Psychiatric Association Press.

Angst J, Dobler-Mikola A (1985): The Zurich study: V. Anxiety and phobia in young adults. Eur Arch Psychiatr Neurol Sci 235:171–178.

Angst J, Dobler-Mikola A (1984): The Zurich study: III. Diagnosis of depression. Euro Arch Psychiatry and Neurological Sci 234:30–37.

Anthony JC, Aboraya A (1992): The epidemiology of selected mental disorders in later life. In Birren JE, Sloane RB, Cohen GD. (eds):. "Handbook of Mental Health and Aging," 2nd ed. San Diego: Academic Press.

Anthony JC, Petronis KR (1991): Suspected risk factors for depression among adults 18–44 years old. Epidemiology 2:123–132.

Argyle N, Roth M (1986): The relationship of panic attacks to anxiety states and depression. In Shagass C (ed): "Abstracts of the World Congress of Biological Psychiatry," New York: Elsevier Science, pp 460–462.

Armenian, HK, Pratt, LA, Gallo J, et al. (1998): Psychopathology as a Predictor of Disability: A Population-based Follow-up Study in Baltimore, Maryland. Am J Epidemiology 148: 269–275.

Aronson TA, and Logue CM (1987): On the longitudinal course of panic disorder. Compre Psychiatry 28:344–355.

Barlow DH (1988): "Anxiety and Its Disorders: The Nature and Treatment of Anxiety and Panic." New York: Guilford Press.

Bebbington P, Hurry J, Tennant C, Sturt E, Wing JK (1981): Epidemiology of mental disorders in Camberwell. Psychological Med 11:561–579.

Beekman, ATF, de Beurs, E, et. al. (2000): Anxiety and Depression in Later Life: Co-Occurrence and Communality of Risk Factors. Am J Psychiatry 157: 89–95.

Berkson J. (1946): Limitations of the application of fourfold table analysis to hospital data. Biomet Bull 2:47–53.

Bland RC, Newman SC, Orn H (eds) (1988): Epidemiology of psychiatric disorders in Edmonton. Acta Psychiatr Scand 77 (supp 338).

Blazer DG, Hughes D, George LK, Swartz M, Boyer R (1991): Generalized anxiety disorder. In Robins LN, Regier DA (eds): "Psychiatric Disorders in America. The Epidemiologic Catchment Area Study." New York: The Free Press.

Blazer DG, Kessler RC, McGonagle KA, Swartz MS (1994): The prevalence and distribution of major depression in a national community sample: The National Comorbidity Study. Am J Psychiatry 151:979–986.

Blazer, DG, Kessler, RC, Swartz MS. (1997): Epidemiology of recurrent major and minor depression with a seasonal pattern. The National Comorbidity Survey. Br J Psychiatry :164–167

Bothwell S, Weissman MM (1977): Social impairments 4 years after an acute depressive episode. Am J Orthopsychiatry 47:231–237.

Boyd JH, Weissman MM (1982): Epidemiology. In Paykel ES (ed): "Handbook of Affective Disorders," New York: Guilford Press, pp 109–125.

Brown GW, Harris T (1978): "Social Origins of Depression: A Study of Psychiatric Disorder in Women." New York: Free Press.

Brunello, N, den Boer, JA, Judd, LL, et al. (Kornstein, SG, Schatzberg, AF, et al. (2000): Social Phobia: diagnosis and epidemiology, neurobiology and pharmacology, comorbidity and treatment. J of Aff Disorders 60: 61–74.

Burnam MA, Hough RL, Escobar JI, Karno M (1987): Six-month prevalence of specific psychiatric disorders among Mexican Americans and non-hispanic whites in Los Angeles. Arch Gen Psychiatry 44:687-691.

Canino GJ, Bird HR, Shrout PE, Rubio-Stipec M, Bravo M, Martinez R, Sesman M, Guevara LM (1987): The prevalence of specific psychiatric disorders in Puerto Rico. Arch Gen Psychiatry 44:727–735.

Charney EA, Weissman MM (1988): Epidemiology of depressive and manic syndromes. In: Georgotas A, Cancro R (eds): "Depression and Mania." New York: Elsevier, pp 45–74.

Chyou PH, Nomura AM, Stemmermann GN (1992): A prospective study of the attributable risk of cancer due to cigarette smoking. Am J Public Health 82:37–40.

Cross-National Collaborative Group (1992): The changing rates of major depression. Cross-national comparisons. JAMA 268:3098–3105.

Denihan, A, Michael, Kirby, M, et al. (2000): Three-year prognosis of depression in the community-dwelling elderly. Br J Psychiatry 176: 453–457.

Dinardo PA, O'Brien GT, Barlow DH, et al. (1983): Reliability of DSM-III anxiety disorder categories using a new structural interview. Arch Gen Psychiatry 40:1070–1074.

Eaton, WW, Anthony, JC et al. (1997): Natural History of Diagnostic Interview Schedule/DSM-IV Major Depression. The Baltimore Epidemiologic Catchment Area Follow-up. Arch Gen Psychiatry 54: 993–991.

Eaton, WW, Anthony, JC et al. (1998): Onset and recovery from panic disorder in the Baltimore Epidemiologic Catchment Area. Br J Psychiatry 501–507.

Eaton WW, Dryman A, Weissman MM (1991): Panic and phobia. In Robins LN, Regier DA (eds): "Psychiatric Disorders in America. The Epidemiologic Catchment Area Study." New York: The Free Press.

Eaton WW, Kessler RC, Wittchen HU, Magee WJ (1994): Panic and panic disorder in the United States. Am J Psychiatry 151:413–420.

Eaton WW, Kramer M, Anthony JC, Dryman A, Shapiro S, Locke BZ (1989): The incidence of specific DIS/DSM-III mental disorders: Data from the NIMH epidemiologic Catchment Area Program. Acta Psychiatr Scand 79:163–168.

Essau, CA, Conradt, J, et al. (1999): Frequency of Panic Attacks and Panic Disorder in Adolescents. Depression and Anxiety 9: 19–26.

Faravelli C, Deggl'Innocenti BG, Aiazzi L, Incerpi G, Pallanti S. (1990): Epidemiology of mood disorders: a community survey in Florence. J Affect Dis 20:135–141.

Faravelli C, Degl'Innocenti BG, Giardinelli L. (1989): Epidemiology of anxiety disorders in Florence. Acta Psychiatr Scand 79:308–312.

Faris REL, Dunham HW (1967): "Mental disorders in urban areas: An ecological study of schizophrenia and other psychoses." Cicago: University of Chicago Press.

Farrer LA, Florio LP, Bruce ML, Leaf PJ, Weissman MM (1989): Reliability and consistency of self-reported age at onset of major depression. J Psychiatric Res 23:35–47.

Fava, M, Rankin, MA, Wright EC, et al. (2000): Anxiety Disorders in Major Depression. Comprehensive Psychiatry 41: 97–102.

Gallo, JJ, Lebowitz, BD. (1999): The Epidemiology of Common Late-Life Mental Disorders in the Community: Themes for the New Century. Psychiatric Services 50: 1158–1166.

Gammon GD, John K, Rothblum ED, Mullen K, Tischler GL, Weissman MM (1983): Use of a structured diagnostic interview to identify bipolar disorder in adolescent inpatients: Frequency and manifestations of the disorder. Am J Psychiatry 140:543–547.

Garvey M, and Tuason V (1984): The relationship of panic disorder to agoraphobia. Compre Psychiatry 25 529–531.

Geerlings, SW, Beekman, ATF, et al. (2000): Physical Health and the onset and persistence of depression in older adults: an eight-wave prospective community based study. Psychological Medicine 30: 369–380.

Gershon E, Hamovit J, Gurroff J, et al. (1987): Birth-cohort changes in manic and depressive disorders in relatives of bipolar, and schizoaffective patients. Arch Gen Psychiatry 44:314–319.

Hagnell O (1986): The 25-year follow-up of the Lundby study: Incidence and risk of alcoholism, depression, and disorders of the senium. In Barret J, Rose RM (eds): "Mental Disorders in the Community: Findings from Psychiatric Epidemiology." New York: Guilford Press, pp 89–110.

Hays, RD, Wells, KB, Sherbourne, CD, et al. (1995): Functioning and Well-being Outcomes of Patients With Depression Compared With Chronic General Medical Illnesses. Arch Gen Psychiatry 52: 11–19.

Henderson S, Duncan-Jones P, Byrne DG, Scott R, Adcock S (1979): Psychiatric disorder in Canberra. Acta Psychiatr Scanda 60:355–374.

Hodiamont P, Peer N, Syben N (1987): Epidemiological aspects of psychiatric disorder in a Dutch health area. Psychological Med 17:495–505.

Horwath, E, Adams, P, Wickramaratne, P et al. (1997): Panic Disorder with Smothering Symptoms: Evidence for Increased Risk in First-Degree Relatives. Depression and Anxiety61:147–153.

Horwath E, Johnson J, Klerman GL, Weissman MM (1992a): Depressive symptoms as relative and attributable risk factors for first-onset major depression. Arch Gen Psychiatry 49:817–823.

Horwath E, Johnson J, Weissman MM, Hornig CD (1992b): The validity of major depression with atypical features based on a community study. J Affect Dis 26:117–126.

Horwath E, Lish J, Johnson J, Hornig CD, Weissman MM (1993): Agoraphobia without panic: Clinical re-appraisal of an epidemiologic finding. Am J Psychiatry 150:1496–1501.

Hwu H-G, Yeh E-K, Chang L-Y (1989): Prevalence of psychiatric disorders in Taiwan defined by the Chinese Diagnostic Interview Schedule. Acta Psychiatry Scandin 79:136–147.

Janzing, J, Teunisse, R, et al. (2000): The course of depression in elderly subjects with and without dementia. J of Aff Disorders 57: 49–54.

Johnson J, Horwath E, Weissman MM (1991): The validity of major depression with psychotic features based on a community study. Arch Gen Psychiatry 48:1075–1081.

Joyce PR, Oakley-Browne MA, Wells JE, Bushnell JA, Hornblow AR (1990): Birth cohort trends in major depression: Increasing rates and earlier onset in New Zealand. J Affect Dis 18:83–90.

Joyce PR, Bushnell JA, Oakley-Brown MA, Wells JE, Hornblow AR (1989): The epidemiology of panic symptomatology and agoraphobic avoidance. Comp Psychiatry 30:303–312.

Kandel, DB, Johnson, JG, Bird, HR et al. (1999): Psychiatric Comorbidity Among Adolescents With Substance Use Disorders: Finding from the MECA Study. J Am Acad Child Adolesc Psychiatry 38: 693–699.

Karno M, Hough RL, Burnam MA, Escobar JI, Timbers DM, Santan F, Boyd JH (1987): Lifetime prevalence of specific psychiatric disorders among Mexican Americans and non-Hispanic whites in Los Angeles. Arch Gen Psychiatry 44:695–701.

Karno M, Golding JM, Burnam MA, Hough RL, Escobar JI, Wells KM, Boyer R (1989): Anxiety disorders among Mexican Americans and non-Hispanic whites in Los Angeles. J Nerv Men Dis 177:202–209.

Kaufman J, Charney, D. (2000): Comorbidity of Mood and Anxiety Disorders. Depression and Anxiety 12, Supplement 1: 69–76.

Kessler RC, McGonagle KA, Zhao S, Nelson CB, Hughes M, Eshleman S, Wittchen H-U, Kendler KS (1994): Lifetime and 12-month prevalence of DSM-III-R Psychiatric disorders in the United States. Results from the National Comorbidity Study. Arch Gen Psychiatry 51:8–19.

Kessler RC, Foster, CL, Saunders, WB et al. (1995): Social Consequences of Psychiatric Disorders, I: Educational Attainment. Amer J Psychiatry 152:1026–1032.

Kessler RC, Nelson, CB, et al. (1996): Comorbidity of DSM-III-R Major Depressive Disorder in the General Population: Results from the US National Comorbidity Survey. Br J Psychiatry 168: 17–30.

Kessler RC, Zhao S, et al. (1997): Prevalence, correlates, and course of minor depression and major depression in the national comorbidity survey. J of Aff Disorders 45: 19–30.

Kessler RC, Davis, CG, et al. (1997): Childhood adversity and adult psychiatry disorder in the US National Comorbidity Survey. Psychological Medicine 27: 1101–1119.

Kessler RC, Berglund, PA, et al. (1997): Social Consequences of Psychiatric Disorder, II: Teenage Parenthood. Am J Psychiatry 154: 1405–1411.

Kessler RC, Stang, PE, Wittchen, HU et al. (1998): Lifetime Panic-Depression Comorbidity in the National Comorbidity Survey. Arch Gen Psychiatry 55: 801–808.

Kessler RC, Walters, EE, et al. (1998): The Social Consequences of Psychiatric Disorders, III: Probability of Marital Stability. Am J Psychiatry 155: 1092–1096.

Kessler RC, DuPont, RL, Berglund, P, et al. (1999): Impairment in Pure and Comorbid Generalized Anxiety Disorder and Major Depression at 12 Months in Two National Surveys. Am J Psychiatry 159: 1915–1923.

Kessler RC, Stang, P, et al. (1999): Lifetime co-morbidities between social phobia and mood disorders in the US National Comorbidity Survey. Psychological Medicine 29: 555–567.

Keyl PM, Eaton WW (1990): Risk factors for the onset of panic disorder and other panic attacks in a prospective, population-based study. Am J Epidemiology 131:301–311.

Kleiner L, Marshall WL (1987): The role of interpersonal problems in the development of agoraphobia with panic attacks. J Anxiety Disorders 1:313–323.

Kleinman A. (1982): Neurasthenia and depression: A study of somatization and culture. Culture Med Psychiatry 6:117.

Kleinman A. (1977): Depression, somatization, and the "new cross-cultural psychiatry." Soc Sci Med 11:3.

Klerman GL, Weissman MM (1989): Increasing rates of depression. JAMA 261:2229–2235.

Kornstein, SG, Schatzberg, AF, et al. (2000): Gender differences in chronic major and double depression. J of Aff Disorders 60: 1–11.

Lavori PW, Klerman GL, Keller MB, Reich T, Rice J, Endicott J (1987): Age-period-cohort analysis of secular trends in onset of major depression: Findings in siblings of patients with major affective disorder. J Psychiatric Res 21:23–36.

Lee C-K, Han J-H, Choi J-O (1987): The epidemiological study of mental disorders in Korea IX: Alcoholism anxiety and depression. Seoul J Psychiatry 12:183–191.

Lee CK, Kwak YS, Yamamoto J, Rhee H, Kim YS, Han JH, Choi JO, Lee YH (1990a): Psychiatric epidemiology in Korea. Part I: Gender and age differences in Seoul. J Nerv Ment Dis 178: 242–246.

Lee CK, Kwak YS, Yamamoto J, Rhee H, Kim YS, Han JH, Choi JO, Lee YH. (1990b): Psychiatric epidemiology in Korea. Part II: Urban and rural differences. J Nerv Ment Dis 178:247–252.

Lehtinen V, Lindholm T, Veijola J, Vaisanen E (1990): The prevalence of PSE-CATEGO disorders in a Finnish adult population cohort. Soc Psychiatry and Psychiatric Epidemiol 25:187–192.

Lewinsohn, PM, Rohde P, et al. (1995): Adolescent Psychopathology: III. The Clinical Consequences of Comorbidity. J Am Child Adolesc Psychiatry 34: 510–519.

Lewinsohn PM, Rohde P, Seeley JR, et al. (2000): Natural course of adolescent major depressive disorder in a community sample: predictors of recurrence in young adults. Am J Psychiatry 157:1584–1596.

Loranger AW, Levine PM (1978): Age at onset of bipolar affective illness. Arch Gen Psychiatry 35:1345–1348.

Magee WJ, Eaton WW, Wittchen HU, McGonagle KA, Kessler RC. (1996): Agoraphobia, simple phobia and social phobia in the National Comorbidity Survey. Arch Gen Psychiatry 53:159–168.

Maier W, Hallmayer J, Lichtermann D, et al. (1991): The impact of the endogenous subtype on the famial aggregation of unipolar depression. Eur Arch Psychiatry Clin Neurosci 240:355–362.

Marks, I. M. (1987): "Fears, Phobias and Rituals." New York: Oxford University Press.

Marks I, Lader M (1973): Anxiety states (anxiety neurosis): A review. J Nerv Ment Dis 156:3.

Masi, G, Letizia, F, et al. (2000): Depressive Comorbidity in Children and Adolescents with Generalized Anxiety Disorder. Child Psychiatry and Human Development 20: 205–215.

Mavreas VG, Bebbington PE (1988): Greeks, British Greek Cypriots and Londoners: A comparison of morbidity. Psychological Med 18:433–442.

Murray, CJL, Lopez, AD. (1997): Regional patterns of disability-free life expectancy and disability-adjusted life expectancy: Global Burden of Disease Study. The Lancet 349: 1347–1352.

Myers JK, Weissman MM (1980): Screening for depression in a community sample: The use of a self-report scale to detect the depressive syndrome. Am J Psychiatry 137:1081–1084

Myers JK, Weissman WW, Tischler GL, et al. (1984): Six-month prevalence of psychiatric disorders in three communities 1980 to 1982. Arch Gen Psychiatry 41:959–967.

Noyes R, Crowe RR, Harris EL (1986): Relationship between panic disorder and agoraphobia. Arch Gen Psychiatry 43:227–232.

Oldehinkel, AJ, Wittchen, HU, et al. (1999): Prevalence, 20-month incidence and outcome of unipolar depressive disorders in a community sample of adolescents. Psychological Medicine 29: 655–668.

Penninx, BWJH, Guralnik, JM, Ferucci, L et al. (1998): Depressive Symptoms and Physical Decline in Community-Dwelling Older Persons. JAMA 279: 1720–1726.

Pollard CA, Bronson SS, Kenney MR (1989): Prevalence of agoraphobia without panic in clinical settings. Am J Psychiatry 146:559.

Quitkin F, Harrison W, Stewart J, et al. (1991): Response to phenelzinc and imipramine in placebo non-responders with atypical depression. Arch Gen Psychiatry 48:319–323.

Rende, R, Warner, V. et al. (1999): Sibling aggregation for psychiatric disorders in offspring at high and low risk for depression: 10-year follow-up. Psychological Medicine 29: 1291–1298.

Robins LN, Helzer JE, Croughan J, Ratcliff KS (1981): National Institute of Mental Health Diagnostic Interview Schedule. Arch Gen Psychiatry 38:381–389.

Rounsaville BJ, Prusoff BA, Weissman WW (1980): The course of marital disputes in depressed women: a 48-month follow-up study. Compr Psychiatry 21:111–118.

Roy-Byrne, PP, Stang, P, Wittchen HU et al. (2000): Lifetime panic-depression comorbidity in the National Comorbidity Survey. Associations with symptoms, impairment, course and help-seeking. Brit J Psychiatry 176:229–235.

Sartorius, N, Ustun, TB, et al. Depression Comorbid with Anxiety: Results from the WHO Study on Psychological Disorders in Primary Health Care. Br J Psychiatry 168: 38–43.

Schneier FR, Johnson J, Hornig CD, Liebowitz MR, Weissman MM (1992): Social Phobia: Comorbidity and Morbidity in an Epidemiological Sample. Arch Gen Psychiatry 49:282–288.

Schoevers, RA, Beekman, ATF, et al. (2000): Risk factors for depression in later life; results of a prospective community based study (AMSTEL). J of Aff Disorders 59: 127–137.

Sherbourne, CD, Wells, KB, Judd, LL (1996): Functioning and Well-Being of Patients With Panic Disorder. Am J Psychiatry 153: 213–218.

Somervell PD, Leaf PJ, Weissman MM, Blazer DG, Bruce ML (1989): The prevalence of major depression in black and white adults in five United States communities. Am J Epidemiology 130:725–735.

Steffens, DC, Skoog, I, Norton, MS et al. (2000): Prevalence of Depression and Its Treatment in an Elderly Population. The Cache County Study. Arch Gen Psychiatry 57: 601–607.

Takeuchi, DT, Chung, RC-Y, Lin, KM et al. (1998): Lifetime and Twelve-Month Prevalence Rates of Major Depressive Episodes and Dysthymia Among Chinese Americans in Los Angeles. Am J Psychiatry 155: 1407–1998.

Thompson AH, Bland RC, Orn HT (1989): Relationship and chronology of depression, agoraphobia, and panic disorder in the general population. J Nerv Ment Dis 177:456–463.

Thyer BA, Himle J (1985): Temporal relationship between panic attack onset and phobic avoidance in agoraphobia. Behav Res Ther 23:607–608.

Thyer BA, Parrish RT, Curtis GC, Nesse RM, Cameron OG (1985): Ages of onset of DSM-III anxiety disorders. Compre Psychiatry 26:113–122.

Torgersen S. (1983): Genetic factors in anxiety disorders. Arch Gen Psychiatry 40:1085–1089.

Torgersen S (1986): Genetic factors in moderately severe and mild affective disorders. Arch Gen psychiatry 43:222–226.

Tsuang MT, Tohen M, Zahner GEP (eds) (1995): "Textbook in Psychiatric Epidemiology." New York: Wiley.

Uhde TW, Boulenger JP, Roy-Byrne PP, Geraci MF, Vittone BJ, Post RM (1985): Longitudinal course of panic disorder. Prog Neuropsychopharmacol Biol Psychiatry 9:39–51.

Vazquez-Barquero JF, Diez-Manriqe JF, Pena C, Quintanal G, Lopez LM (1986): Two stage design in a community survey. Br J Psychiatry 149:88–97.

Weissman MM (1985): The epidemiology of anxiety disorders: rates, risks, and familial patterns. In Tuma AH, Maser JD (eds.): "Anxiety and the Anxiety Disorders," Hilldale, NJ: Lawrence Erlbaum Associates, pp 275–296.

Weissman MM, Adams PA, Lish J, Wickramaratne P Horwath E, Charney D, Wood S, Leeman E, Frosch E. (1993): The relationship between panic disorder and major depression: a new family study. Arch Gen Psychiatry 50:767–780.

Weissman, MM, Bland RC et al. (1997): The cross-national epidemiology of panic disorder. Arch Gen Psychiatry 54: 305–309.

Weissman MM, Bruce ML, Leaf PJ, Florio LP, Holzer C (1991): "Psychiatric disorders in America." In Robins L, Regier D (eds). Free Press. New York pp 53–81.

Weissman MM, Klerman GL (1977): Sex differences in the epidemiology of depression. Arch Gen Psychiatry 34:98–111.

Weissman MM, Klerman GL (1985): Gender and depression. Trends in the Neurosciences 8:416–420.

Weissman MM, Leaf PJ, Bruce ML, Florio L (1988b): The epidemiology of dysthymia in five communities: Rates, risks, comorbidity; and treatment. Am J Psychiatry 145:815–819.

Weissman MM, Leaf PJ, Tischler GL, Blazer DG, Karno M, Bruce ML, Florio LP (1988a): Affective disorders in five United States communities. Psychological Med 18:141–153.

Weissman MM, Myers JK (1978): Affective disorders in a US urban community. Arch Gen psychiatry 35:1304–1311.

Weissman MM, Olfson, M. (1995): Depression in Women: Implications for Health Care Research. Science 269: 799–801.

Wells KB, Burman MA, Rogers W, et al. (1992): The course of depression in adult outpatients. Results from the Medical Outcomes Study. Arch Gen Psychiatry 49:788–794.

Wickramaratne PJ, Weissman MM, Leaf PJ, Holford TR (1989): Age, period and cohort effects on the risk of major depression: Results from five United States communities. J Clin Epidemial 42:333–343.

Winokur G, Morrison J (1973): The Iowa 500: Follow-up of 225 depressives. Br J Psychiatry 123:543–548.

Wittchen H-U (1986): "Natural Course and Spontaneous Remissions of Untreated Anxiety Disorders: Results of the Munich Follow-up Study (MFS)." "Panic and Phobias." Hand I and Wittchen H-U (eds): Berlin: Vol 2, Springer-Verlag.

Wittchen HU Reed, V, et al. (1998): The Relationship of Agoraphobia and Panic in a Community Sample of Adolescents and Young Adults. Arch Gen Psychiatry 55: 1017–1024.

Wittchen HU, Zhao, S et al. (1994): DSM-III-R Generalized Anxiety Disorder in the National Comorbidity Survey. Arch Gen Psychiatry 51: 355–364.

World Health Organization (1978): Mental disorders: Glossary and Guide to Their Classification in Accordance with the 9th Revision of the International Classification of Diseases. Geneva: WHO.

CHAPTER 17

Epidemiology of Bipolar Disorder

MAURICIO TOHEN and JULES ANGST

Lilly Research Laboratories, Indianapolis IN; Department of Psychiatry, Harvard Medical School McLean Hospital, Belmont, MA (M.T.); Zurich University Psychiatric Hospital, Switzerland (J.A.)

INTRODUCTION

Disease in human populations develops through complex interactions of competing factors, including genetics, demographic variables, and psychosocial factors. Epidemiologic observational studies are conducted with large groups of individuals. This chapter will focus on the epidemiology of bipolar disorder. Epidemiology is the study of the causes and distribution of illnesses. To understand bipolar disorder, we count its incidence and prevalence, observe its course, and identify putative risk factors.

To count, it is necessary to first observe and describe. To describe and compare findings from time to time and from place to place, case definition must be established. Since case definition in bipolar disorder has been an ongoing evolution, the identification of cases represents a challenge. Not unlike other psychiatric disorders, diagnostic criteria in bipolar illness have changed across different time periods, significantly affecting the case definition. In addition, until recently, the definition of a case was not clearly operationalized, causing a great degree of variability in the assessment of cases.

Three decades ago, the U.S./U.K. diagnostic study (Cooper et al., 1972) highlighted the variability of diagnosis in patients with psychotic disorders. The study demonstrated that when clear operational criteria are not utilized, the differential diagnosis of manic-depressive illness or schizophrenia may be uncertain. However, in spite of the use of operationalized diagnostic criteria, inconsistencies of diagnosis may persist due to poor reliability in the method of assessment or in the collection of symptoms.

To diminish such variability, standardized diagnostic instruments have been developed for different diagnostic classifications. The limitation of most epidemiologic studies of bipolar disorder conducted prior to 1980 is that the failure to use a structured instrument or diagnostic criteria make their results difficult to interpret.

Textbook in Psychiatric Epidemiology, Second Edition, Edited by Ming T. Tsuang and Mauricio Tohen.
ISBN 0-471-40974-X

NOSOLOGY

Bipolar disorder appears to have been first described by Aretaeus of Cappadocia in A.D. 30 (Adams, 2000). In contemporary history, it was Falret (1854) in the mid-nineteenth century who first described the condition as a new separate disorder and called it *folie circulaire*. Kraepelin (1921) further defined the concept by separating it from *dementia praecox* or schizophrenia. According to Kraepelin, manic-depressive illness is characterized by a periodic course with good prognosis and mood symptoms in the acute phase. For Kraepelin, course of illness was the major distinction. He, therefore, included under the category of manic-depressive illness mild and severe, single episode and periodic affective disorders, including involutional melancholia. This classification resulted in an overestimation of the disorder in the early literature. However, there has also been an underestimation, as most studies have not included Bipolar II disorder (hypomania and depression) cases as part of the bipolar spectrum.

During the last 50 years there has been considerable interest in psychiatric nosology. The advent of new treatments, especially psychopharmacologic, has invigorated the field's interest in differentiating the diagnoses of manic-depressive illness and schizophrenia (Cade 1949; Delay et al., 1952; Lambert et al., 1966; Pope et al., 1983; Tohen et al., 2000). Baldessarini (1970) emphasized that the appearance of phenothiazines in the early 1950s biased the diagnosis of schizophrenia over manic-depressive illness. More recently, investigators from McLean Hospital (Stoll et al., 1994) reported that in six major North American teaching hospitals from 1972 to 1991 the rate of admissions for affective disorder increased as the rate of admission of schizophrenic disorders decreased. Several factors have influenced this change, including the more narrow definition of schizophrenia and parallel broadening of the category of affective disorders. Also, as new drugs for the treatment of affective disorders have been developed, clinicians may have been influenced toward the diagnosis of affective disorders, causing a treatment-oriented diagnostic bias. The authors also speculate that third-party reimbursement rates may have favored patients with the diagnosis of an affective disorder. A number of reports (Klerman and Weissman, 1989; Cross National Collaborative Group, 1992; Kessler et al., 1994) have suggested that the incidence of affective disorders has increased worldwide.

CASE DEFINITIONS OF BIPOLAR DISORDER

According to the *Diagnostic and Statistical Manual of Mental Disorder*, fourth edition, revised (DSM-IV) (American Psychiatric Association [APA], 1994), the essential feature of mood disorders is disturbance of mood that is defined as a sustained emotion that colors the perception of the world. Although elevated mood may be considered the characteristic of a manic episode, the predominant mood may also be irritability. Patients with mania have inflated self-esteem, which may range from unusual self-confidence to grandiose delusions. Decreased need to sleep is associated with hyperactivity, where the individual remains awake during long periods of the night, involved in new projects, or making numerous telephone calls. The speech is usually pressured and at times difficult to interrupt. Flight of ideas may be present. Other symptoms include hypersexuality and impulsivity. The disturbance must be severe enough to cause marked impairment in social activities, occupational functioning, and interpersonal relationships or to require hospitalization.

According to DSM-IV, to meet Bipolar I disorder criteria there must have been at least one manic episode. Hypomania is a less severe presentation of mania without impairment of social or occupational functioning or the need for hospitalization. Bipolar II disorder is characterized by the history of hypomanic and full major depressive episodes. A manic episode may be subclassified as mild, moderate, or severe with or without psychotic features. Psychotic features may also be specified as mood congruent or mood incongruent. Mood congruent psychotic features are defined as being consistent with typical manic themes of inflated worth, power, knowledge, identity, or special relationship to a deity or famous person. Mood-incongruent psychotic features are delusions or hallucinations whose content does not involve the typical manic themes (APA, 1994). Psychotic features considered to be mood incongruent include persecutory delusions (not directly related to grandiose) and the so-called schneiderian first-rank symptoms (Schneider, 1959).

A controversial DSM-IV criterion (APA, 1994) is that manic episodes precipitated by somatic antidepressant treatment such as electroconvulsive therapy or medication are not considered part of a Bipolar I disorder but instead would be classified as substance induced mood disorder. DSM-IV includes specific criteria for hypomanic episodes and for cyclothymic disorder. A cyclothymic disorder is characterized by hypomanic episodes interspersed with mild symptoms of depression. In addition, DSM-IV provides criteria for subtypes of Bipolar I disorder, including the single manic episode where there should be the presence of only one manic episode and no past major depressive episodes. It also includes bipolar disorder not otherwise specified (NOS); examples include a history of recurrent hypomanic episodes without any recurrent depressive symptoms or manic episodes superimposed on psychotic disorder NOS, residual schizophrenia, or a delusional disorder. DSM-IV also includes the category "mood disorder due to a general medical condition."

Another feature of DSM-IV is cross-sectional symptom features, which includes melancholic features, atypical features, or catatonic features. In addition, the course of mood disorders may be defined with course specifiers, which include (1) rapid cycling, (2) seasonal pattern, and (3) postpartum onset. Furthermore, DSM-IV provides a description for the longitudinal course for Bipolar I disorder, which includes (1) with full interepisode recovery, defined as "if no prominent mood symptoms between two most recent manic or major depressive episodes," and (2) without full interepisode recovery, defined as "if prominent mood symptoms between two most recent manic or major depressive episodes." There are, also a number of options to define the longitudinal course, which include (1) single episode with no cyclothymic disorder; (2) single episode superimposed on cyclothymic disorder; (3) recurrent with full inter-episode recovery with no cyclothymic disorder; (4) recurrent without full interepisode recovery with no cyclothymic disorder; (5) recurrent with full interepisode recovery superimposed on cyclothymic disorder; and (6) recurrent without full interepisode recovery superimposed on cyclothymic disorder.

A major limitation of the DSM-IV classification is the lack of empirical validity of the different categories. It is therefore important that different validity predictors such as response to treatment or the prediction of outcome be tested empirically in order to determine their clinical and theoretical value. It is of course desirable that empirical studies be considered when new editions of the DSM classification are produced. Due to space limitations this chapter will not review the International Classification of Diseases (ICD) nosology.

MAJOR EPIDEMIOLOGIC STUDIES

Population-Based Studies

In the last two decades, a number of population-based studies were conducted that have estimated the lifetime prevalence of bipolar disorder to be approximately 1% (see Table 1). In 1978, Weissman and Myers published the first epidemiologic survey using research diagnostic criteria. The authors utilized the Schedule for Affective Disorders and Schizophrenia and the Diagnostic Research Criteria (SADS-RDC) (Spitzer et al., 1978). Weissman and Myers sampled 1,095 households and identified a lifetime prevalence rate of 0.8% for mania and 0.8% for hypomania. They found that bipolar disorders cluster in the higher socioeconomic classes, with 4.6% in Hollingshead and Redlichs classes 1 and 2 (1958), 1% in class 3, 0.9% in class 4, and no cases in class 5.

TABLE 1. Lifetime Prevalence of Bipolar Disorder across Different Countries

Author	Publication Date	Location	Diagnostic Instrument	Lifetime Prevalence (%)
Weissman and Myers	1978	New Haven, CT	SADS[a]	0.6–1.2
Robins et al.	1984	New Haven, CT	DIS[b]	1.1
		Baltimore, MD		0.6
		St. Louis, MO		1.1
Canino et al.	1987	Puerto Rico	DIS	0.5
Karno et al.	1987	Los Angeles, CA	DIS	1.0
Bland et al.	1988	Edmonton	DIS	0.6
Wells et al.	1989	New Zealand	DIS	0.7
Lee et al.	1990	Korea	DIS	0.4
Stefansson et al.	1991	Iceland	DIS	0.7
Wittchen et al.	1992	Munich	DIS	0.2
Kessler et al.	1994	48 U.S. states	CIDI[c]	1.6
Weissman et al.	1996	10 counties	DIS	0.3–1.5
Kessler et al.	1997	48 U.S. states[b]	SCID[d]	0.4

[a]SADS: Schedule for Affective Disorders and Schizophrenia;
[b]DIS: Diagnostic Interview Schedule;
[c]Structured SCID: Clinical Interview for DSM-III-R;
[d]CIDI: Composite International Diagnostic Interview.

The Amish Study

Almost two decades ago, Egeland and Hostetter (1983) reported their epidemiologic study of affective disorders among the Amish. It was a six-year study of affective disorders among the Old Order Amish, an ultraconservative Protestant religious sect. This study was conducted in one of their settlements in Lancaster County, Pennsylvania, with approximately 11,000 residents. The investigators have stressed that the Amish are a culturally and genetically homogenous group where alcohol and drug abuse are essentially not found. One of the major goals of the Amish study was to explore the genetic aspects of affective disorders. The prevalence of Bipolar I and II disorders in the population aged 15 years and older was 0.46%.

Epidemiologic Catchment Area (ECA) Program

In this chapter, we only review the findings related to bipolar disorder. The ECA program collected data on bipolar disorder according to the DSM-III criteria with the use of the Diagnostic Interview Schedule (DIS) (Robins et al., 1981). With the exception of the study conducted by Weissman and Myers (1978), it was the first study in the United States that obtained prevalence rates for bipolar disorder utilizing structured diagnostic instruments. Using a probability sample, the ECA project obtained prevalence data for Bipolar I and Bipolar II disorders, but did not obtain information on cyclothymic disorder. In addition to obtaining prevalence rates of Bipolar I and II disorders, an estimate of specific manic symptoms was also obtained (Weissman et al., 1991). The criteria for a manic episode consisting of elevated, expansive, or irritable mood for at least 1 week duration had a lifetime prevalence of 2.7%. The most frequent manic symptom reported was hyperactivity (9.3%), followed by decreased need for sleep (7.5%), and distractibility (7.2%). Not surprisingly, manic symptoms were more frequent in the age group 18–29 years and also in men more than in women. African-Americans were also more likely to present manic symptoms, especially hyperactivity, in 12.3% compared with 9% in whites and 1% in Latinos; and decreased need for sleep, with 9.8% in African-Americans, 7.3% in whites, and 6.2% in Latinos. Men were more likely than women to present hyperactivity, inflated self-esteem, distractibility, and involvement in risky activities; females were more likely to experience racing thoughts and distractibility. For all symptoms, the ages 18–29 had the highest prevalence rate.

The lifetime prevalence rate of a manic episode was 0.8% (Robins et al., 1984). The age group with the highest lifetime prevalence rate was 30–44 years old, in contrast to manic symptoms for which the highest prevalence was in the 18–29 year old group. There was no difference by sex or ethnic group. Bipolar II disorder was present in 0.5% of the population. Table 2 presents data on lifetime prevalence for Bipolar I and Bipolar II disorders stratified by age group, gender, and ethnicity. It demonstrates that all age groups show a difference in prevalence rates, but there was no difference in gender or ethnicity. There was also a difference for Bipolar I across different sites, with New Haven showing a 1.2% and St. Louis 1.0% in contrast to 0.6% for Baltimore and Los Angeles and 3.4% for Durham. The rates for Bipolar II disorders were also inconsistent across sites, ranging from

TABLE 2. ECA Lifetime Prevalence (Percent) of Bipolar Disorder Subtypes by Age, Sex, and Ethnicity[a]

	Bipolar I	Bipolar II
Total	0.8	0.5
Age (years)		
18–29	1.1***	0.7**
30–44	1.4	0.6
45–64	0.3	0.2
65 +	0.1	0.1
Sex		
Male	0.7	0.4
Female	0.9	0.5
Ethnicity		
White	0.8	0.4
Black	1.0	0.6
Hispanic	0.7	0.5

[a]Variation within groups, controlling for age, sex, or ethnicity; $^{**}p < 0.01$, $^{***}p(< 0.001$.

Source: Weissmann et al. (1991).

0.4% in Durham to 0.6% in Baltimore. The 1-year prevalence of Bipolar I disorder showed, again, only a difference in age, with the highest rate (1.2%) in the age group 30–44 years old.

One-month prevalence for manic episodes (Regier et al., 1988) ranged in the five sites from as low as 0.1% in Los Angeles to 0.6% in St. Louis. The highest prevalence for males concentrated in the 25–44 year old age group, where it was 0.5%, and for females in the 18–24 year old age group, where it was 0.8%. Regier et al. (1993) estimated a 1-year prevalence of 1.2%, which translates to 1,908,000 people suffering from bipolar disorder in the United States.

Weissman et al. (1988) reported that the mean age of onset of bipolar disorder in the ECA data was 21 years. The mean age of onset across the 5 sites was 21.2 years, adjusting for the age distribution at each site. The range was 17.9 years for the Los Angeles site compared with 26.3 for the Baltimore site.

The National Comorbidity Survey

The National Comorbidity Survey (NCS) (Kessler et al., 1994) was based on a probability sample of individuals aged 15 to 54 years from noninstitutionalized populations from 48 states. It utilized the University of Michigan version of the Composite International Diagnostic Instrument (UM-CIDI). A total of 8,098 individuals were interviewed. It built upon the experience of the ECA but expanded into a more comprehensive assessment on risk factors (Kessler et al., 1994).

The NCS reported a lifetime prevalence of 1.6% for a manic episode compared with only 0.6% for nonaffective psychosis (schizophrenia, schizophreniform disorder, schizoaffective disorder, delusional disorder, and atypical psychosis). The

1-year prevalence for a manic episode was 1.3% (Kessler et al., 1994). Of note, the diagnosis of nonaffective psychosis was based on a clinical interview using the SCID while the diagnosis for mania was based only on the UM-CIDI.

In a more recent clinical reappraisal study, Kessler and collaborators (1997) reported that the only manic symptoms that could be assessed with validity were euphoria, grandiosity and decreased need to sleep. The lifetime prevalence of bipolar disorder estimated considering the validated symptom profile was 0.4%. This study was conducted by reinterviews conducted by trained clinical interviewers and final diagnoses determined using a best estimate approach. The correspondence of the initial NCS diagnoses and the clinical reinterviews was low with a high degree of false-positive cases diagnosed in the initial NCS assessment. The investigators concluded that the true lifetime prevalence of bipolar disorder was not as high as the originally reported value of 1.6%, but it also was not as low as determined by the narrow definition of the clinical reappraisal. They estimated that the lifetime prevalence of bipolar disorder is approximately 0.9%. Of note, all cases were found to have at least one other DSM-III-R disorder with close to 60% manifesting the comorbid disorder before meeting criteria for bipolar disorder. At the time of the assessment, 44.7% were receiving treatment, but almost all (93.2%) had received treatment at some point during their illness. Another interesting finding was related to course of illness, specifically that 20% of cases had never manifested a depressive episode, with men (38.9%) having a larger proportion of unipolar mania than women (4.1%).

The Cross-National Epidemiology of Major Depression and Bipolar Disorder

Weissman and collaborators (1996) estimated the rates and patterns of bipolar disorder based on population-based studies that had used similar methodology. Studies from 10 different countries (United States, Canada, Puerto Rico, France, West Germany, Italy, Lebanon, Taiwan, South Korea, and New Zealand) were included. Lifetime prevalence rates for bipolar disorder were consistent among countries. The lowest rate was found in Taiwan (0.3 per 100) and the highest in New Zealand (1.5 per 100). Gender ratios did not differ across countries. Due to the relatively small sample size, risk factors were not explored.

Studies Outside the United States

In addition to the ECA study, a number of population-based prevalence studies using structured diagnostic instruments and modern diagnostic criteria have recently been conducted outside the United States that have included the assessment of individuals with bipolar disorder.

In Florence, Italy, Faravelli et al. (1990) obtained DSM-III diagnoses with interviews conducted by psychiatrists in a community sample of 1,000 people. The 1-year prevalence for Bipolar I disorder was 1.86% for females and 0.65% for males. For Bipolar II disorder, the overall prevalence was 0.2%. In a study in Taiwan, Hwu and collaborators (1989) conducted a multistage random sampling of 5,005 residences from metropolitan Taipei, 3,004 from small towns, and 2,995 from rural villages. They utilized the DIS and found a prevalence for manic episode of 1.6% for Taipei, 0.7% for small towns, and 1.0% for rural villages. Another study that utilized the DIS was conducted in Puerto Rico by Canino and collaborators (1987). The lifetime prevalence for manic episode was 0.7% for males and 0.4% for females. The 6-month prevalence was 0.3% for males and 0.3% for females. Bland et al. (1988) conducted a prevalence study in Alberta, Canada from a community sample of 3,258, also utilizing the DIS. The lifetime prevalence for manic episode was 0.7% for males and 0.4% for females.

A study conducted in the Netherlands (Hodiamont et al., 1987) utilized the Present State Examination (PSE) instrument, which uses the International Classification of the Diseases (ICD) system. For manic episodes, the prevalence was 0.1% for both genders.Levav et al. (1993) conducted a prevalence study in Israel in a population defined as a ten-year cohort born between 1949 and 1958. Cases were defined using the clinician-administered SADS instrument and reported relatively low rates. The 6-month prevalence rate for manic episode was 0.1%. In contrast, Szadoczky et al. (1998) in a study conducted in Hungary found a lifetime prevalence rate of 2.4% of bipolar disorder.

The Netherlands Mental Health Survey and Incidence Study (NEMESIS) of 7976 subjects aged 18–64 used the CIDI and found a lifetime prevalence rate of DSM-III-R bipolar disorder of 1.8%, a 12-month rate of 1% and a 1-month rate of 0.6% (Bijl et al., 1998).

In Munich (Germany) Wittchen et al. (1998) administered the CIDI in a longitudinal cohort study to 3021 adolescents and young adults (aged 14 to 24) with DSM-IV diagnoses and identified the following lifetime prevalence rates: single episode mania, 0.1% and 1.4% for Bipolar I disorder.

Incidence Data

Incidence is the measure of new cases over a specified period of time. Incidence rates are more difficult to estimate than prevalence rates, as they require a longitudinal assessment. Boyd and Weissman (1981) reported incidence data for bipolar disorders in Scandinavian countries. The annual incidence rate for bipolar disorders varied from 9.2 to 15.2 cases per 100,000 subjects in males and from 7.4 to 32.5 cases per 100,000 in females. Leff and collaborators (1976), using the PSE, obtained first-admission rates for patients hospitalized with mania in London, England, and Aarhus, Denmark. The incidence rate was 2.6 per 100,000 individuals in both sites. The ECA Project also provided incidence data (Eaton et al., 1989; Regier et al., 1993). Regier et al. (1993) reported new cases during a 1-year period (annual incidence rates).

The project, known as Wave 2 of the ECA study, was conducted on approximately 20% of the initial population. This prospective follow-up permitted the estimation of new cases as well as of relapses. For bipolar disorder, the annual cumulative rate was 0.5% $\pm$ 0.1%.

Daly et al. (1995) in a treatment-based study conducted in Dublin, Ireland, found that the incidence rate of mania in the age group 18–60 was 4.5/100,000 per year. Previously Leff et al. (1976) had reported that the incidence in Aarhus, Denmark, and London, England, was 2.6 per 100,000 per year. Daly and collaborators (1995) speculated that the higher rates found in Dublin were not likely to be explained by higher community incidence rates as just secondary to different admission patterns.

OTHER BIPOLAR DISORDER SUBTYPES

Bipolar II Disorder

Bipolar II disorder has been less widely studied than Bipolar I. In a review conducted by Angst (1998) prevalence rates for Bipolar II disorder ranged from 0.5% to 2.0%. However, considering only studies that have utilized the DIS or the SADS, the lifetime prevalence range is 0.2%–0.9% (see Table 2). Angst pointed out that is likely that rates for Bipolar II disorder are underestimated as hypomania is at times not recognized. In a recent study, Angst and Hantouche (2002) found rates of 4.8%. Simpson et al. (1993) have suggested that Bipolar II is perhaps the most common bipolar phenotype and emphasized the importance of their identification in genetic studies. Szadoczky et al. (1998) in their study conducted in Hungary reported a prevalence rate of 2.0% for Bipolar II disorders and 5.1% for the total bipolar spectrum. Wittchen et al. (1998) found a lifetime prevalence of 0.4% and a 12-month prevalence rate of 1.3%.

Cyclothymia

Epidemiologic rates on cyclothymia have been estimated for the last two decades (Table 3). Studies have been small but for the most part have utilized clinician-administered diagnostic instruments. Prevalence rates have ranged from 0.3% to 2.8%.

Full Bipolar Spectrum

The overall prevalence of bipolar disorders if all subtypes are included may be as high as 10%. It is, therefore, likely that the full bipolar spectrum may be one of the most prevalent psychiatric conditions. Studies conducted at the end of last century

TABLE 3. Prevalence Rates of Cyclothymi

Author	Publication Date	Diagnostic Instrument	Period	Prevalence (%)
Weissman and Myers	1978	SADS-L[a]	Lifetime	2.8
Faravelli and Incerpi	1985	SADS-L	1 year	1.4
Heun and Maier	1993	SADS-L/RDC[b]	Lifetime	1.4
Levav	1993	SADS-L	6 months	0.5

[a]SADS-L: Schedule for Affective Disorders and Schizophrenia—Lifetime version.
[b]RDC, Research Diagnostic Criteria.

TABLE 4. Prevalence Rates of Bipolar Spectrum Disorders

Author	Publication Date	Diagnostic Instrument	Period	Prevalence (%)
Weissman and Myers	1978	SADS-L[b]	Lifetime	3.0
Oliver and Simmons	198	DIS[c]	Lifetime	3.3
Faravelli and Incerpi	1985	SADS-L	1 year	3.4
Levav et al.	1993	SADS-L	6 month	2.6
Heun and Maier	1993	SADS-L	Lifetime	6.5
Angst	1995[a]	SPIKE[d]	Lifetime	5.5
Lewinsohn et al.	1995[a]	DIS	Lifetime	1.0–5.7
Wittchen et al.	1998[a]	CIDI[e]	Lifetime	3.4
Angst	1998[a]	SPIKE	Lifetime	7.8
Szádáczky et al.	1998	CIDI	Lifetime	5.1
Angst and Hantouche	2002[a]	SPIKE	Lifetime	7.2–10.8

[a]Adolescents or young adults;
[b]SADS-L: Schedule for Affective Disorders and Schizophrenia—lifetime version;
[c]DIS: Diagnostic Interview Schedule;
[d]SPIKE: Semi-structured interview
.[e]CIDI: Composite International Diagnostic Interview;

and beginning of the twenty-first century have found rates that range between 1% to 10% (see Table 4). Angst and Hantouche (2002) recently estimated the rate to be as high as 10.8%.

Comorbidity and Bipolar Disorders

Kessler (1994) reported the comorbidity of different psychotic disorders in the NCS and in the ECA. In both surveys, mania was accompanied by a comorbid disorder in more than 50% of the cases. Goodwin and Jamison (1990) argued that comorbidity in bipolar patients has not been studied as comprehensively as it has in major depressive disorder and stressed the importance of studying the effects of comorbidity in illness course. They summarized the existing literature and estimated a 35% prevalence of Bipolar Illness and alcohol abuse. They also raised the issue of determining the chronologic sequence of the onset of each disorder and the lack of much needed empirical information in this area.

The ECA study (Regier et al., 1990) reported that the Bipolar I group had a prevalence of substance abuse of 60.7%. The ECA investigators suggested that a high degree of comorbidity in bipolar disorders greatly complicates treatment. Interestingly, the ECA Study (Helzer and Pryzbeck, 1988) reported that the prevalence of comorbid alcoholism in mania was three times that in major depression. Furthermore, the likelihood (odds ratio) of an individual with bipolar disorder having a substance use disorder was 6.6 times greater than that of the general population. The only diagnosis that had a higher ratio than mania was antisocial personality disorder. Tohen et al. (2000) found in a treatment-based sample that the comorbidiy of substance use disorder in a cohort of first episode mania patient to be 17.3%. This finding suggests that in most cases the sequence of comorbid substance use disorder appears after the onset of bipolar disorder.

Comorbidiy of anxiety disorder has also been found to be frequent in bipolar disorder. Cosoff and Hafner (1998) found, in a treatment-based study conducted in Australia, a comorbidity prevalence of 17% for social phobia, 13% for generalized anxiety disorder, 30% of obsessive–compulsive disorder, and 15% for panic disorder.

RISK FACTORS

Age

Goodwin and Jamison (1990) estimated that the mean age of onset for bipolar disorder was 30 years of age. There is some evidence in some recent studies that the age of onset in bipolar disorder may be lower. This finding may be due in part to an increased awareness of the diagnosis among child psychiatrists in recent years. The range of age of onset goes as low as 12 or 13 years, but may also be present in the over-65 age group. A study by Tohen and collaborators (1994) suggested that first-episode mania cases in the elderly might be associated with a comorbid cerebrovascular disorder.

Secular trends may also play a role in the incidence of bipolar disorder. Klerman and Weissman (1989) noted an increased rate for major depression in cohorts born after 1940. The same observation has been noted for bipolar disorder (Gershon et al., 1987). Gershon and collaborators (1987) published birth cohort changes in patients with mania in a cohort of relatives of bipolar and schizoaffective patients. Utilizing life table analysis, the investigators also reported higher rates of bipolar disorder in the cohorts born after 1940, suggesting that the cumulative hazard for bipolar disorder in a given age group was greater in those born after 1940. The authors found that for individuals born in the 1940s, the prevalence for Bipolar I was 6.0%, and for those born in the 1950s it was 8.6%, in contrast to individuals born in the 1920s, for whom the rate was 3.4%, and for those born in the 1930s, at 2.5%. The authors speculate that the cohorts with high rates of affective illness seem to have been born in decades during which there was a major war, accompanied by extensive use of alcohol and illicit drugs. Lasch et al. (1990) reported birth cohort changes in prevalence rates for mania utilizing data from the ECA study. The authors identified 17,827 individuals and divided them into different cohorts separated by decades. They found a high risk of developing mania in those born after 1935. The authors also suggested that environmental and historical events might have increased the rates, suggesting a gene–environment interaction.

Urban Versus Rural

In the ECA St. Louis site (Weissman et al., 1991), the rate in the urban population was 1.5% compared with 0.5% in the rural population, with an odds ratio of 2.25 adjusted for sex, age, and ethnicity ($p = 0.001$). For the Durham site (Blazer et al., 1985), again there was a higher rate in the urban population, with 0.8% compared with 0.2% in the rural population and an adjusted odds ratio of 3.78 ($p = 0.05$). Not surprisingly, the rate of Bipolar Illness was higher in institutionalized individuals living in prisons or nursing homes, with a 9.7% prevalence rate for individuals living in nursing homes and 5.4% for those living in prisons. The odds ratio comparing nursing home residents with those living in households was 10.8, adjusted for sex, age, and ethnicity and 5.75 for those living in prison.

Gender

Most studies have noticed no gender difference in the prevalence of bipolar disorder. Both the ECA and NCS studies found a one-to-one female–male ratio. Hendrick and collaborators (2000) have suggested that treatment-based samples show larger prevalence for females because women are more likely to be hospitalized than men. Akiskal et al. (1998), reporting data from the French national multisite collaborative study on the clinical epidemiology of mania (EPIMAN), found that mixed mania is more frequent in female patients.

Social Class

Most studies published before 1980 found a higher prevalence in the upper socioeconomic classes. This finding may be attributed to a bias assessment of researchers and clinicians in diagnosing subjects from lower socioeconomic status as schizophrenic and psychotic subjects from upper socioeconomic status as bipolar. In contrast, more recent epidemiologic studies have not found a significant difference of bipolar disorder related to social class. However, the New Haven Community Sample (Weissman and Myers, 1978) found higher rates in upper socioeconomic groups. On the other hand, the ECA program found higher rates of mania in adults with fewer years of education (Weissman et al., 1991). Individuals with less than 12 years of education had a prevalence of 1.1% compared with 0.9% in those with more than 12 years of education. The odds ratio after adjusting for sex, age, and ethnicity was 1.93.

Race

The ECA program found no significant race difference. Jones et al. (1981) suggested that in previous studies where an ethnic difference was reported, African-Americans were more likely to be diagnosed as schizophrenic and whites as bipolar, with a consequent under diagnosing of Bipolar Illness in African-Ameicans patients. Levav and collaborators (1993) in a study conducted in Israel identified higher rates in individuals of European descent compared to those of North African descent. Kirov and Murray (1999) in a treatment-based study conducted in South London found that patients of African descent were more likely to present manic episodes with mood incongruent psychotic features than those of European descent. Similarly Strakowski et al. (1996) suggested that African-Americans suffering from mania are more likely to be misdiagnosed as suffering from schizophrenia due to their higher rate of presenting with hallucinations compared to their counterparts of European descent.

Marital Status

The ECA study (Weissman et al., 1991) found that individuals who are cohabiting, divorced, or never married are more likely to suffer from bipolar disorder than married individuals. The ECA data estimated that the 1-year prevalence of suffering from bipolar disorder was 3.2% in subjects who are cohabitating compared with 1.3% in those never married and 0.2% in those subjects married. The odds ratio for those cohabitating compared with the married/never divorced was 8.3 adjusting for sex, age, and race. Similarly, Boyd and Weissman (1981) found that more single and divorced individuals suffer from manic-depressive illness.

Cultural Factors

Since the turn of the century, Kraepelin noted that certain cultures may show high rates of manic-depressive illness. Whether this is secondary to the genetic load or to cultural factors still needs to be determined. Specifically, Kraepelin noted a higher incidence of manic-depressive illness in some Indonesian groups. Other societies in which manic-depressive illness appears to be particularly high include the Hutterities in North American (Eaton and Weil, 1955). Similarly, higher rates of manic depressive illness have been identified in Jews of European background than in those of North African background (Miller, 1967; Gershon and Liebowitz, 1975). Emigration has also been considered a risk factor of Bipolar Illness (Hemsi, 1967; Pope et al., 1983). It is not clear if individuals predisposed to a Bipolar Illness are more likely to emigrate or if the migration process in itself precipitates the condition in otherwise predisposed individuals.

Homelessness

Koegel et al. (1988), utilizing the DIS, found very high rates for manic episode among the homeless across different ethnic groups. Prevalence rates were 10.7% for whites, 11.7% for African-Americans, and 8.5% for Latinos.

UTILIZATION OF MENTAL HEALTH SERVICES

The ECA study (Weissman et al., 1991) reported that individuals suffering from bipolar disorder are high users of health services; 38.5% will receive outpatient psychiatric treatment within a one-year period, and 9.6% will receive inpatient treatment within a six-month period. Approximately 79.2% received treatment in a medical outpatient facility, and 29.5% received treatment in a medical inpatient facility (six-month period).

Regier et al. (1993) described the *de facto* U.S. mental and addictive disorders service system as composed by general medical physicians, other human services professions, and the voluntary support sector; the latter includes self-support groups, family and friends. For bipolar disorder, 60.9% received one of those services with overlap among sectors. Professional services were received by 58.9% of Bipolar (I and II) patients. Specialty mental health was provided by general medical (32.4%) and other human service (10%) professionals. The voluntary support network provided 9.6% of services. Narrow et al. (1993) reported use of services by individuals with different disorders. Of the 1.9 million individuals suffering from bipolar disorder, 1.1 million received care during a 1-year period. The services included 16 million outpatient visits including 23.7% of them by mental health specialists in private practice and 19% by a general medical physician. The average number of visits per treated person per year in ambulatory services was 14.7 including 13.9 by mental health specialists and 16.3 by the voluntary support network. Bipolar patients received inpatient treatment in a variety of settings, including 34.4% in a VA hospital psychiatric unit and 33.4% in a general hospital psychiatric unit.

FAMILIAL AND GENETIC TRANSMISSION

The NIMH Collaborative Program on the Psychobiology of Depression (Rice et al., 1987) estimated the morbid risk of bipolar disorder in family members of bipolar patients. Rates varied depending on the familial relationship. For children, the risk was 1.5%, with 6% for siblings, 4.1% for mothers, and 6.4% for fathers.

Genetic Studies

The evidence that many psychiatric conditions are genetically based appears solid. However, the field is not yet advanced to the point of unraveling the web of psychiatric genetics. The hope is that at some point genetics will help to develop new strategies for prevention and treatment of psychiatric disorders. The evidence from family, adoption, and twin studies clearly supports the evidence that bipolar disorder is genetically transmitted (Blehar et al., 1988). However, the mode of transmission and its genetic relationship to other affective disorders remains unclear.

Craddock and Jones (1999) recently reviewed the lifetime risk of suffering bipolar disorder in relatives of bipolar probands 40%–70% in monozygotic co-twins, 5%–10% in first-degree relatives, and 0.5%–1.5% in nonblood-related individuals.

In recent years, molecular genetics has made progress in mapping the entire genome. In spite of this, the search continues. In addition to issues in molecular genetics, other aspects of genetic epidemiology require close attention, including the identification of informative families, the precision of diagnostic methods, and the criteria utilized in studying family members. Other aspects that still need to be resolved are the relationships between bipolar and other conditions such as schizophrenia, unipolar depression, and personality disorders. It is possible that there may be families where the etiology may be a single gene, but most likely it is the interaction of multiple genes and complex genetic mechanisms. To date there has been no clear evidence of any particular gene in bipolar disorder. Studies conducted in the last two decades have suggested a possible X-linkage as initially suggested by Baron et al. (1990) and chromosome 11 as suggested by the Amish studies. Other candidate chromosomes include 18 (Berritini et al., 1997). Most genetic studies have focused on neurotransmitter systems that have shown affinity to mood stabilizing drugs. It is likely that new targets will be identified over the coming years. The identification of susceptible genes will most likely have major implication in our understanding of the pathophysiology and treatment response of this devastating condition.

REFERENCES

Adams F (2000): "The Extant Works of Aretaeus, the Cappadocian." London: The Syndenham Society, 1856. Reprinted in the Classics of Medicine Library Series. Birmingham, AL: Gryphon Editions, Inc.

Akiskal HS, Hantouche EG, Bourgeois ML, Azorin J-M, Sechter D, Allilaire J-F, Lancrenon S, Fraud J-P, Chatenet-Duchene L (1998): Gender, temperament, and the clinical picture in dysphoric mixed mania: Findings from a French National Study (EPIMAN). J Aff Disord. 50:175–186.

American Psychiatric Association (1994): "Diagnostic and Statistical Manual of Mental Disorders," 4th ed. Washington, DC: The American Psychiatric Association.

Angst J (1998): The emerging epidemiology of hypomania and Bipolar II disorder. J Aff Disord 50:143–151.

Angst J (1995): Epidémiologie des troubles bipolaires. In Bourgeois ML, Verdoux H (eds): "Les Troubles Bipolaires de lHumeur." Mason Médecine et Psychothérapie: Paris, pp 29–42.

Angst J, Hantouche EG (2002): The epidemiology of minor bipolar disorder and hypomania: New territory. In Vieta E and Angst J (ed): "Hypomania." Madrid, Grupo Aula Medica.

Baldessarini RJ (1970): Frequency of diagnoses of schizophrenia versus affective disorders from 1944 to 1968. Am J Psychiatry 127:759–763.

Baron M, Endicott J, Ott J (1990): Genetic linkage in mental illness: Limitations and prospects. Br J Psychiatry 157:645–655.

Berrettini WH, Ferraro TN, Goldin LR, Detera-Wadleigh SD, Choi H, Muniec D, Guroff JJ, Kazuba KM, Nurnberger JI Jr., Hsieh W-T, Hoehe MR, Gershon ES (1997): A linkage study of Bipolar Illness. Arch Gen Psychiatry 54:27–35.

Bijl RV, van Zessen G, Ravelli A, de Rijk C, Langendoen Y (1998): The Netherlands Mental Health Survey and Incidence Study (NEMESIS): Objectives and design. Soc Psychiatry Psychiatr Epidemiol 33:581–586.

Bland RC, Newman SC, Orn H (eds) (1988): Epidemiology of psychiatric disorders in Edmonton. Acta Psychiatr Scand 77(Suppl 338).

Blazer DG, George LK, Landerman R, Pennybacker M, Melville ML, Woodbury M, Manton KG, Jordan K, Locke B (1985): Psychiatric disorders: A rural/urban comparison. Arch Gen Psychiatry 42:651–656.

Blehar MC, Weissman MM, Gershon ES, Hirschfeld MA (1988): Family and genetic studies of affective disorders. Arch Gen Psychiatry 44:289–292.

Boyd JH, Weissman MM (1981): Epidemiology of affective disorders: A re-examination and future directions. Arch Gen Psychiatry 38:1039–1046.

Cade JFJ (1949): Lithium salts in the treatment of psychotic excitement. Med J Aust 36:349–352.

Canino GJ, Bird HR, Shrout PE, Rubio-Stipec M, Bravo M, Sesman M, Guevara LM (1987): Prevalence of specific psychiatric disorders in Puerto Rico. Arch Gen Psychiatry 44:727–735.

Cooper JE, Kendell RE, Gurland BJ, Sharpe L, Copeland JRM, Simon R (1972): "Psychiatric Diagnosis in New York and London." London: Oxford University Press.

Casoff, Hafner (1998):

Craddock N, Jones I (1999): Genetics of bipolar disorder. J Med Genet 36, 585–594.

Cross-National Collaborative Group (1992): The changing rates of major depression. Cross-national comparisons. JAMA 268:3098–3105.

Daly I, Webb M, Kaliszer M (1995): First admission incidence study of mania, 1975–1981. Br J Psychiatry 167:463–468.

Delay J, Deniker P, Harl J (1952): Utilization thérapeutique psychiatrique d'une phénothiazine d'action cetrale élective. Ann Med Psychol 110:112–117.

Eaton JW, Weil RJ (1955): "Culture and Mental Disorders: A Comparative Study of the Hutterites and Other Populations." New York: Free Press.

Eaton WW, Kramer M, Anthony JC, Dryman A, Shapiro S, Locke BZ (1989): The incidence of specific DIS/DSM-III mental disorders: Data from the NIMH Epidemiologic Catchment Area Program. Acta Psychiatr Scand 79:163–178.

Egeland JA, Hostetter AM (1983): Amish study, I: Affective disorders among the Amish, 1976–1980. Am J Psychiatry 140:56–61.

Falret JP (1854): Memoire sur la folie circulaire, forme de maladie mentale caracterisée per la reproduction successive et regulière de l'etat maniaque, de l'etat melancolique, et d'un intervalle lucide plus ou moins prolongé. Bull Acad Med 19:382–415.

Faravelli C, DeglInnocenti BG, Aiazzi L, Incerpi G, Pallanti S (1990): Epidemiology of mood disorders: A community survey in Florence. J Aff. Disord 20:135–141.

Faravelli C, Incerpi G (1985): Epidemiology of affective disorders in Florence. Preliminary results. Acta Psychiatr. Scand. 72:331–333.

Gershon ES, Hamovit JH, Guroff JJ, Nurnberger JI (1987): Birth-cohort changes in manic and depressive disorders in relatives of bipolar and schizoaffective patients. Arch Gen Psychiatry 44:314–319.

Gershon ES, Liebowitz JH (1975): Sociocultural and demographic correlates of affective disorders in Jerusalem. J Psychiatr Res 12:37–50.

Goodwin FK, Jamison KR (1990): "Manic-Depressive Illness." New York: Oxford University Press.

Helzer JE, Pryzbeck TR (1988): The co-occurrence of alcoholism with other psychiatric disorders in the general population and its impact on treatment. J Study Alcohol 49:219–224.

Hemsi LK (1967): Psychiatric morbidity of West Indian immigrants. Soc Psychiatry 2:95–100.

Hendrick V, Altshuler L, Gitlin MJ, Delrahim S, Hammen C (2000): Gender and Bipolar Illness. J Clin Psychiatry 61: 393–396.

Heun R, Maier W (1993): The distinction of Bipolar II disorder from Bipolar I and recurrent unipolar depression: results of a controlled family study. Acta Psychiatr Scand 87:279–284.

Hodiamont P, Peer N, Syben N (1987): Epidemiological aspects of psychiatric disorder in a Dutch health area. Psychol Med 17:495–505.

Hwu HG, Yeh EK, Chang LY (1989): Prevalence of psychiatric disorders in Taiwan defined by the Chinese Diagnostic Interview Schedule. Acta Psychiatr Scand 79:136–147.

Jones BE, Gray BA, Parson EB (1981): Manic-depressive illness among poor urban blacks. Am J Psychiatry 138:654–657.

Karno M, Jenkins JH, de la Selva A, Sanatan F, Telles C, Lopez S, Mintz J (1987): Expressed emotion and schizophrenic outcome among Mexican-American families. J Nerv Ment Dis 175:143–151.

Kessler RC, McGonagle KA, Zhao S, et al. (1994): Lifetime and 12-month prevalence of DSM-III-R psychiatric disorders in the United States. Arch Gen Psychiatry 51:8–19.

Kessler RC (1995): Epidemiology of psychiatric comorbidity. In Tsuang MT, Tohen M, and Zahner GEP (eds): Textbook in Psychiatric Epidemiology. New York: Wiley-Liss, pp 179–197.

Kessler RC, Rubinow DR, Holmes C, Abelson JM, Zhao S (1997): The epidemiology of DSM-III-R Bipolar I disorder in general population survey. Psychological Med 27:1079–1089.

Kirov G, Murray RM (1999): Ethnic differences in the presentation of bipolar affective disorder. Eur Psychiatry 14:199–204.

Klerman GL, Weissman MM (1989): Increasing rates of depression. JAMA 261:2229–2235.

Koegel P, Burnam A, Farr RK (1988): The prevalence of specific psychiatric disorders among homeless individuals in the inner city of Los Angeles. Arch Gen Psychiatry 45:1085–1092.

Kraepelin E (1921): "Manic-depressive insanity and paranoia." Edinburgh: E & S Livingstone.

Lambert PA, Cavaz G, Borselli S, Carrel S (1966): Action neuro-psychotrope dun nouvel anti-épileptique: Le dépamide. Ann Med Psychol 1:707–710.

Lasch K, Weissman MM, Wickramaratne PJ, Bruce ML (1990): Birth cohort changes in the rates of mania. Psychiatry Res 33:31–37.

Lee CK, Kwak YS, Yamamoto J, Rhee H, Kim YS, Han JH, Choi JO, Lee YH (1990): Psychiatric epidemiology in Korea. Part I. Gender and age differences in Seoul. J Nerv Ment Disord 178:242–246.

Leff JP, Fischer M, Bertelsen A (1976): A cross-national epidemiological study of mania. Br J Psychiatry 129:428–442.

Levav I, Kohn R, Dohrenwend BP, Shrout PE, Skodol AE, Schwartz S, Link BG, Naveh G (1993): An epidemiological study of mental disorders in a 10-year cohort of young adults in Israel. Psychological Med. 23:691–707.

Lewinsohn PM, Klein DN, Seeley JR (1995): Bipolar disorders in a community sample of older adolescents: prevalence, phenomenology, comorbidity, and course. J Am Acad Child Adolesc Psychiatry 34:454–463.

Miller L (1967): The social psychiatry and epidemiology of mental ill health in Israel. Top Prob Psychiatr Neurol 6:96–137.

Narrow WE, Regier DA, Rae DS, Manderscheid RW, Locke BZ (1993): Use of services. Findings from the National Institute of Mental Health Epidemiologic Catchment Area Program. Arch Gen Psychiatry 50:95–107.

Oliver JM, Simmons ME (1985): Affective disorders and depression as measured by the Diagnostic Interview Schedule and the Beck Depression Inventory in an unselected adult population. J Clin Psychol 41:496–576.

Pope HG Jr, Ionescu-Pioggia M, Yurgelun-Todd D (1983): Migration and manic-depressive illness. Comp Psychiatry 24:158–165.

Regier DA, Boyd JH, Burke JD, Rae DS, Myers JK, Kramer M, Robins LN, George LK, Karno M, Locke BZ (1988): One month prevalence of mental disorders in the US based on the five epidemiologic catchment area sites. Arch Gen Psychiatry 45:977–986.

Regier DA, Farmer ME, Rae DS, et al. (1990): Comorbidity of mental health disorders with alcohol and other drug abuse. JAMA 264:2511–2518.

Regier DA, Narrow WE, Rae DS, Manderscheid RW, Locke BZ, Goodwin FK (1993): The de Facto U.S. Mental and Addictive Disorders Service System. Epidemiologic Catchment Area prospective 1-year prevalence rates of disorders and services. Arch Gen Psychiatry 50:85–94.

Rice J, Reich T, Andreasen NC, Endicott J, Van Eerdewegh M, Fishman R, Hirschfeld RMA, Klerman GL (1987): The familial transmission of Bipolar Illness. Arch Gen Psychiatry 44:441–447.

Robins LN, Helzer JE, Croughan J, Ratcliff KS (1981): National Institute of Mental Health Diagnostic Interview Schedule: Its history, characteristics, and validity. Arch Gen Psychiatry 38:381–389.

Robins LN, Helzer JE, Weissman MM, Orvaschel H, Gruenberg E, Burke JD Jr, Regier DA (1984): Lifetime prevalence of specific psychiatric disorders in three sites. Arch Gen Psychiatry 41:949–958.

Schneider K (1959): "Clinical psychopathology." (Hamilton MW ,translator.) New York: Grune and Stratton.

Simpson SG, Folstein SE, Meyers DA, McMahon FJ, Brusco DM, DePaulo JR (1993): Bipolar II: The most common bipolar phenotype? Am J Psychiatry 150:901–903.

Spitzer RL, Williams JBW, Gibbon M (1990): Structured Clinical Interview for DSM-III. New York: Biometric Research, New York State Psychiatric Institute.

Stoll AL, Tohen M, Baldessarini RJ, Goodwin DC, Stein SM, Katz SM, Swinson RP, McGlashan T (1994): Shifts in the diagnostic frequencies of schizophrenia and affective disorders from 1972 through 1988: A combined analysis from four North American Psychiatric Hospitals. Am J Psychiatry 151:1642–1645.

Stefansson JG, Lindal E, Bjornsson JK, Guomundsdottir A (1991): Lifetime prevalence of specific mental disorders among people born in Iceland in 1931. Acta Psychiatr Scand. 84:142–149.

Strakowski SM, McElroy SL, Keck PE, West SA (1996): Racial influence on diagnosis in psychotic mania. J Aff Disord 39:157–162.

Szadoczky E, Papp ZS, Vitrai J, Rihmer Z, Furedi J (1998): The prevalence of major depressive and bipolar disorders in Hungary: Results from a national epidemiologic survey. J Aff Disord 50:153–162

Tohen M, Shulman KI, Satlin A (1994): First-episode mania in late life. Am J Psychiatry 151:130–132.

Tohen M, Hennen J, Zarate C, Baldessarini R, Strakowski S, Stoll A, Faedda G, Suppes T, Gebre-Medhin P, Cohen B (2000): The McLean/Harvard First Episode Project: Two-year syndromal and functional recovery in 219 cases of major affective disorders with psychotic features. Am J Psychiatry 57:220–228.

Weissman MM, Bland RC, Glorisa MB et al. (1996): Cross-national epidemiology of major depression and bipolar disorder. JAMA 276:293–299.

Weissman MM, Bruce ML, Leaf PJ, Florio LP, Holzer C (1991): Psychiatric disorders in America. In Robins L, Regier D (eds). New York: Free Press, pp 53–81.

Weissman MM, Leaf PJ, Tischler GL, Blazer DG, Karno M, Bruce ML, Florio LP (1988): Affective disorders in five United States communities. Psychol Med 18:141–153.

Weissman MM, Myers JK (1978): Affective disorders in a U.S. urban community: The use of Research Diagnostic Criteria in an epidemiological survey. Arch Gen Psychiatry 35:1304–1311.

Wells JE, Bushnell JA, Hornblow AR, Joyce PR, Oakley-Browne MA (1989): Christchurch Psychiatric Epidemiology Study: Methodology and lifetime prevalence for specific psychiatric disorders. Aus N Z J Psychiatry 23:315–326.

Wittchen HU, Essau CA, von Zerssen D, Krieg JC, Zaudig M (1992): Lifetime and six-month prevalence of mental disorders in the Munich Follow-up Study. Eur Arch Psychiatry Clin Neurosci 241:247–249.

Wittchen HU, Nelson CB, Lachner G (1998): Prevalence of mental disorders and psychosocial impairments in adolescents and young adults. 38:109–126.

CHAPTER 18

The Epidemiology of First-Onset Mania

T. LLOYD and P. B. JONES

University of Nottingham, Duncan Macmillan House, Porchester Road, Nottingham, NG3 6AA, UK (T.L.); University of Cambridge, Addenbrooke's Hospital, Cambridge, CB2 2QQ. (P.B.J.)

INTRODUCTION

The past twenty years have seen much research into affective disorders, reflecting advances in both pharmacological and psychological treatments, and our understanding of its occurrence, mechanisms and causes. However, first episodes of mania remain relatively uncharted in terms of the descriptive epidemiology of what can be a devastating event in terms of individuals and families; first-episode mania is less familiar than its more mature, affective siblings of depression and bipolar disorder. In this chapter we attempt to synthesize the available evidence regarding the basic epidemiology (other than genetic epidemiology) of mania and point to areas where further research is needed.

DEFINITIONS AND DIAGNOSIS

The origins of the idea that mania might be a distinct clinical entity within mental illness has been attributed to the French clinicians, Falret (1854) and Baillarg, (1854; see reviews by Krauthammer and Klerman, 1979; Roth, 2001). However, it was Kraepelin (translation 1921) who developed the notion that manic-depressive insanity is different from *dementia praecox*, the latter called schizophrenia by others. Kraepelin considered that the predominance of affective features, the periodic course and ultimate good prognosis were sufficient to differentiate it from *dementia praecox* in terms of cross-sectional phenomenology and long-term course. Although his ideas on schizophrenia were relatively specific, identifying subjects that would be familiar today as having severe schizophrenia, Kraepelin's category of manic-depressive insanity included all forms of serious and recurrent affective illness, though he believed there was a common and fundamental core. Concepts of manic-depression have evolved steadily (Goodwin and Jamison, 1990),

Textbook in Psychiatric Epidemiology, *Second Edition*, Edited by Ming T. Tsuang and Mauricio Tohen. ISBN 0-471-40974-X

and its place within the spectrum of affective disorders remains uncertain despite having become less controversial over the past century (Roth, 2001). However, the current importance of polarity within a long-term affective syndrome (Leonhard, 1957) as being the defining feature of a bipolar–unipolar distinction is almost beyond dispute, gaining early validation in terms of family history studies (Angst, 1966; Perris, 1966) and now rooted in modern diagnostic criteria described below.

This chapter touches on the epidemiology of the concept of unipolar mania. This is a most problematic nosological category. We agree with Goodwin and Jamison (1990, p. 66) when they concluded that "as the evidence now stands ... the existence of true unipolar mania as a separate entity is questionable." Indeed, the careful, long-term follow-up of large numbers of subjects (Angst, 1998) employing broad criteria indicates that the existence of polarity in mood disorder may be much more widespread than Leonhard originally thought; another example of the truism that the risk of anything generally increases with time. However, we think it justifiable to consider the occurrence and risk factors for what is likely to be, in essence, a part-syndrome; first-episode mania is an entity that patients and clinicians will face before the full story unfolds over their lifetime. In addition to heralding bipolar disorder, mania can evolve into other disorders, most notably schizophrenia; this aspect of diagnostic stability is also discussed below.

Krauthammer and Klerman (1979) wrote that, "Nosology logically precedes epidemiology; in practice, however, epidemiology does not and cannot wait." We are guilty of not waiting, although we have concentrated on more recent studies that use definitions familiar today. We suggest that this chapter be read in conjunction with other epidemiological reviews such as that by Boyd and Weissman (1981) and Angst (1998), and Angst's chapter concerning bipolar disorder in this volume; the present review is a comment on but one aspect of the disorder that he has done so much to define.

Case definition remains at the core of epidemiological study. The major classificatory systems now dominate the field, although the "edges" of conventional phenotypes, such as ultra-brief episodes or rapid cycling disorder (Dunner and Fiere, 1974; Maj et al., 1994) and the bipolar spectrum (Akiskal, 1992; Marneros, 2001) remain of considerable nosological interest and influential regarding therapy. Modern classifications have, as noted above, taken on the concept of polarity as central to the classification of affective disorders. However, the importance of mania in ICD-10 (World Health Organization, 1992) and DSM-IV (American Psychiatric Association, 1980) is somewhat different. In ICD-10, a single episode of mania is classed as a manic episode without assumptions of subsequent course or polarity. Similarly, a single episode of hypomania is classified as hypomanic episode. At least two separate episodes of an affective disorder must be present for the diagnosis of bipolar affective disorder. One of these episodes should be hypomania, mania or mixed, but the other episode may be depression.

In DSM-IV the minimum criteria for Bipolar I disorder is a single episode of mania; the expectation of bipolarity is explicit and probably correct (Angst, 1998). Patients who experience recurrent major depressive episodes with hypomanic episodes only are classified under Biploar II disorder. The current affective episode must be classified in both systems, and the definitions of mania are similar. For completeness, the definition of manic syndrome is shown in Table 1.

TABLE 1. Criteria for Manic Episode in DSM-IV

A. A distinct period of abnormally and persistently elevated, expansive, or irritable mood, lasting at least 1 week (or any duration if hospitalization is necessary).
B. During the period of mood disturbance, three (or more) of the following symptoms have persisted (four if the mood is only irritable) and have been present to a significant degree:
   (1) Inflated self-esteem or grandiosity
   (2) Decreased need for sleep (e.g., feels rested after only 3 hours of sleep)
   (3) More talkative than usual or pressure to keep talking
   (4) Flight of ideas or subjective experience that thoughts are racing
   (5) Distractibility (i.e., attention too easily drawn to unimportant or irrelevant external stimuli)
   (6) Increase in goal-directed activity (either socially, at work or school, or sexually) or psychomotor agitation
   (7) Excessive involvement in pleasurable activities that have a high potential for painful consequences (e.g., engaging in unrestrained buying sprees, sexual indiscretions, or foolish business investments)
C. The symptoms do not meet criteria for a Mixed Episode
D. The mood disturbance is sufficiently severe to cause marked impairment in occupational functioning or in usual social activities or relationships with others, or to necessitate hospitalization to prevent harm to self or others, or there are psychotic features.
E. The symptoms are not due to the direct physiological effects of a substance (e.g., a drug of abuse, a medication, or other treatment) or a general medical condition (e.g., hyperthyroidism).

Manic-like episodes that are clearly caused by somatic antidepressant treatment (e.g., medication, electroconvulsive therapy, light therapy) should not count toward a diagnosis of Bipolar I disorder.

Source: American Psychiatric Association (1994).

INCIDENCE OF THE MANIC SYNDROME

We have noted that we are really referring to the incidence of the manic syndrome as the likely first manifestation of a disorder that will, in time, usually have bipolar features. Indeed, many of those that are considered to be first episodes of mental illness may, in fact, have been preceded by episodes of depression or subthreshold mania that have been forgotten or subject to the many vagaries of information bias.

Estimates of the incidence of mania from various studies that define population-at-risk and diagnostic criteria are summarized in Table 2. We have adopted a convention of annual rates per hundred-thousand population-at-risk because these are immediately interpretable at the public health or routine service level.

The estimates show wide variation, party due to differences in methodology and definitions. Der and Bebbington reported an overall incidence rate of 20.8 per 10^5. The Camberwell case register included all first contacts with psychiatric services in this area of inner city, South London (Der and Bebbington, 1987), with diagnoses based upon ICD-9 (World Health Organization, 1992), a classification that put severe, uni- and bipolar affective disorder into a single broad category, with

TABLE 2. Incidence of First-Episode Mania

Investigators	Study Location	Dates	Contact	Criteria	Incidence per 100,000 per year		
					Male	Female	All
Der and Bebbington	Camberwell, S. London	1964–1982	All referrals	Modified ICD-9	4.5	4.8	20.8
Spicer et al.	England and Wales	1965–1966	First admission	DHSS	3.0	3.9	3.5
Leff et al.	Camberwell, S. London	1965–1974	First admission	PSE	3.1	2.3	2.6
	Aarhus, Denmark	1969–1973	First admission	PSE	3.1	2.0	2.6
Van Os et al.	Camberwell, S. London	1965–1969	All referrals	RDC criteria	—	—	1.7
		1970–1974	All referrals	RDC criteria	—	—	2.0
		1975–1979	All referrals	RDC criteri	—	—	3.8
		1980–1984	All referrals	RDC criteria	—	—	3.4
Veijola	Northern Finland	1982–1993	First admission	DSM-III-R	—	—	1.7
Daly et al.	Dublin	1975–1981	First admission	PSE	4.1	4.9	4.5
Brewin et al.[b]	Nottingham	1992–1994	All psychosis referrals	ICD-10/PSE	1.5	4.1	2.8
AESOP study	Nottingham	1997–1999	All referrals	ICD-10/PSE	2.6	2.3	2.5

[b]Calculated from published data.

specifiers below that. All cases over the age of 15 with a diagnosis of mania or hypomania were used to calculate the incidence rates.

As might be expected, the reported incidences based on first admission (rather than contacts) rates are lower, ranging from 3.0 to 4.1 per 10^5 per year for men and from 2.0 to 4.9 per 10^5 per year for women. These probably systematically exclude more mild illness and concentrate on Bipolar I disorder, those with psychotic affective features and people who are at risk of suicide. Similarly, the reported incidences in the remaining studies, which were based on first contact rates, excluded cases with hypomania.

The incidence rates reported in the studies by Spicer and others (1973) and Veijola and colleagues (1996), were based on first hospital admissions of mania. Spicer (1973) collected data from the now defunct British Mental Health Enquiry that was, effectively, a case register for England and Wales, again based upon the ICD. All cases of manic-depressive illness, manic or circular were assumed to be manic. Veijolas study was based on a prospective 27-year follow up of the Northern Finland birth cohort (Veijola et al., 1996) and so can be interpreted as a morbid risk as well as a true incidence study. The Finnish Hospital Discharge Register was used together with supplementary, clinical information in order to make DSM-III-R diagnoses. The relatively low incidence needs to be interpreted against the upper age limit imposed by the cohort methodology and a high incidence of schizophrenia in the same sample. This latter is particularly interesting as the diagnostic criteria (DSM-III-R) were narrow for both sets of disorders.

Leff et al. (1976), conducted a prospective study of first admission manic patients as well as a retrospective study of the case notes in both London and Aarhus, Denmark. The motivation was to investigate previously documented differences in the incidence of mania in these two centers. The study population was restricted to patients aged between 18 and 60, and ICD diagnoses were based upon phenomenology from the Present State Examination (Wing et al., 1974). The annual incidence of mania, so defined, was found to be virtually identical in both centers. This is unlikely to have been an artefact of methodology. Daly and colleagues (1995) conducted their study in Dublin using the same methods as Leff and others (1976) and confirmed the hypothesized higher rate of mania in Ireland. The study of Van Os et al. (1996) is included in the Table 2 but discussed later when we consider geography.

Brewin and colleagues (1997) identified all people aged 16–64 with first-onset psychosis seen by the general adult psychiatric services in Nottingham, United Kingdom. The ICD-10 criteria were used. We have recently been part of a large, multicenter study known as "AESOP," funded by the U.K. Medical Research Council and the Stanley Foundation to investigate the intimate link between aetiology and ethnicity in schizophrenia and other psychoses. The study compares first-onset psychoses with controls, both cases and controls drawn from three defined populations in England; the full study has yet to report. The Nottingham center ascertained first onset cases, including all with psychotic and nonpsychotic manic syndrome, in a very similar fashion to Brewin and colleagues, such that the results from the same city separated by five years are broadly comparable; both incidence studies ran for two years.

Our preliminary finding for the overall incidence rate for first-episode mania is similar to that of Brewin et al. (1997). From an overall sample of 208 patients with first onset psychosis, 19 subjects fulfilled the ICD-10 criteria for manic episode. Six subjects who presented with mania at the time of inception had been diagnosed with a previous nonpsychotic depression and, therefore, received the ICD-10 diagnosis of bipolar affective disorder. We excluded them from the incidence figures for the initial manic syndrome, although acknowledge, as noted above, that recall biases may have been operating throughout and that more people may have had previous depression.

AGE AT ONSET

The reported median age of onset for mania appears to show a degree variation but is generally accepted as unimodal with the onset of mania or Bipolar I disorder being in the early adult years (Goodwin and Jamison, 1990). Variation between studies may be due to differences in the definition of onset and to sampling techniques and perhaps to cohort effects with earlier expression of disorder in younger cohorts. A recently reported investigation by Kessler et al. (1997) found the average age at onset of Bipolar I disorder to be 21 years. This is consistent with the median age of onset of 19 years reported by Burke et al. (1990) who found that rates for the onset of mania were highest between the ages of 15 and 19 for both men and women.

Daly et al. (1995) found the overall average ages at onset for Dublin and London to be 28.8 and 32.2 years, respectively. However, these values could be "older" estimates due to methodological issues as incidence rates were only established in the 18–60 year age range. In the Nottingham AESOP study mentioned above, we have found the mean age of onset of mania to be 31 years which is comparable to Daly et al. (1995), although, again, the age range was restricted between 16 and 65 years. We found the mean age at onset of first-episode mania for women to be higher than for men with values of 33 years and 29 years, respectively.

Loranger and Levine (1978) determined the age of onset for 200 patients who met DSM-III criteria for mania. They found the peak period of onset to be in the early twenties. Twenty percent of all their subjects had shown some evidence of illness in adolescence, 48.5% by the time they were 30 and 99% by 60 years of age. Onset after age 60 was rare in this and other recent studies.

Contrary to the above findings, some studies show that a large proportion of new cases of mania arise after the age of 60 (Wertham, 1929; Roth, 1955). Glasner and Rabins (1984) found that 4.6% of patients who were admitted for the first time to an old-age psychiatry ward presented with mania. Eagles and Whalley (1985) found an increase in the incidence of mania with age in a study of incidence from first admissions to hospital in Scotland. The authors found little difference in clinical presentation of these late-onset patients compared with early-onset cases and little evidence to suggest the aetiology was organic.

MANIA IN CHILDREN AND ADOLESCENTS

Currently, and certainly in Europe, the existence of prepubertal mania is thought to be rare. However, some emerging evidence suggests that mania in childhood is perhaps not so much rare as difficult to diagnose. Considerable overlap between the symptoms of mania and ADHD, oppositional disorder or conduct disorder, with the added complication of comorbid substance misuse, makes differentiation of mania from these disorders, and therefore diagnosis, difficult.

Weller et al. (1986) searched the literature of case reports describing children with severe psychiatric symptoms and identified 19 cases (12%) out of 157 with a diagnosis of mania in the original report. They rediagnosed another 12% of cases previously diagnosed as psychotic or schizophrenic as having DSM-III mania. In a retrospective study by Loranger and Levine (1978), 0.5% of adult patients with an established diagnosis of bipolar disorder reported an age of onset between 5 and 9 years and 7.5% between the ages of 10 and 14 years.

Furthermore, Biedermen and others (1995) have diagnosed children of 12 years or younger with DSM-III-R mania and differentiated this group from children with ADHD using a Child Behavior Checklist (CBCL). In contrast, Biedermen and colleagues, (1999) could find no evidence to support this in a European sample; the issue of possible U.S.–European differences in diagnostic practice remains unresolved.

Compared with children, manic disorder in adolescents is more widely accepted. An age of onset before 21 is thought to occur in 20–30% of patients, perhaps with a peak just after puberty (Goodwin and Jamison, 1990). Carlson and Kashani (1988) in the United States interviewed 150 randomly selected 14–16 year olds and their parents and identified 20 subjects who experienced four or more manic symptoms of at least two days duration, thereby meeting DSM-III criteria for the disorder. Verhulst and colleagues (1997) found the six-month prevalence of DSM-III-R (hypo)mania to be 1.8% in a national sample of Dutch adolescents. The prevalence rose to 2.8% when the parents were also interviewed.

GENDER

Overall, the evidence in Table 2 indicates that mania is rather more common in women. Recent studies using operational criteria, such as that by Brewin et al. (1997) indicate the greatest disparity. The incidence rates for mania in this study confirmed a considerable difference between men and women (rate ratio 2.7; 95% c.i. 1.0, 8.4; $p < 0.04$; higher for women). This is in contrast to schizophrenia where men predominate in studies that use narrowly defined criteria. Interestingly, in our study, the incidence rate for women was lower than for women (rate ratio 0.9; 95% c.i. 0.3, 2.4) but this is consistent with other studies, including Brewins, once sampling error is taken into account.

GEOGRAPHY AND MIGRATION

Findings from the first *International Pilot Study of Schizophrenia* (World Health Organization, 1973) suggested that the incidence of mania in Aarhus, Denmark might be higher than in London. This prompted a cross-national epidemiological study of the first admission rates in the two centers (Leff et al., 1976). The annual incidence of mania was, in fact, found to be virtually identical in the two countries although the London sample was found to contain 45% of immigrants, in contrast to the Aarhus sample, in which the proportion born outside Denmark was negligible. There were high rates of mania and hypomania among the African-Caribbean population living in Camberwell, United Kingdom.

Harrison and colleagues (1997) mentioned similar findings in their prospective Nottingham study that aroused so much attention concerning high risk of schizophrenia in the African-Caribbean population. Van Os and colleagues (1996), who established first contact rates for mania in Camberwell between 1965 and 1984, have confirmed the finding. There was some evidence for an increase over time in the first contact rate of mania, especially in women. Drawing on the earlier study (Leff et al., 1976) the authors suggested that the rise might be associated with the migration into Camberwell of individuals of African-Caribbean origin. This group showed significantly higher rates than the white group (adjusted rate ratio 3.1; 95% c.i. 1.4–6.9) and more often displayed mixed manic and schizophrenic symptoms.

Der and Bebbington (1987) reported a similar high rate of mania and hypomania in both sexes of those born in the Caribbean, whereas Irish males were found to have a low rate. The increased incidence of affective disorder in those of Caribbean origin may be explained by a propensity of individuals who are predisposed to bipolar disorder being more likely to migrate, an unlikely explanation similar to that proposed in schizophrenia and with as little empirical support (Bogers et al., 2000). However, it could also be a result of social or environmental factors related to urban living. Both acute and chronic social adversity may operate across first and second generation, African-Caribbean populations. Some components (e.g., limited opportunity) may be intensified in the British-born, second generation, where they may act as precipitating factors. Thus, we consider it vital to disentangle the differences between concepts of race, ethnicity, migration, and socioeconomic status, all of which may have confounding and otherwise attenuating effects.

Studies of populations with relative ethnic homogeneity and no inward migration merit consideration. In the classic investigation of the Amish in the United States, Egeland and Hostetter (1983) noted a low rate of all psychiatric disorders, including affective disorders, although the relative proportion of manic episodes and so bipolar disorder was high. On the contrary, Daly et al. (1995) found the crude incidence rate of mania in Dublin to be higher than expected for both men and women. Incidence rates of mania in Finland appear to be considerably lower than expected (Veijola et al., 1996). The reason for these discrepant findings is not obvious although evidence suggests a genetic basis for bipolar disorder, with wide variations in its incidence in specific populations perhaps reflecting genetic stratification or gene–environment interactions (Morell, 1996), as well as cultural discrepancies between clinician and subject.

CLINICAL FEATURES

In our recent small sample of nineteen subjects described above, sixteen patients (84%) had first episode mania with psychotic symptoms and three patients (16%) had mania without psychotic symptoms. Of the six patients who had experienced a previous episode of nonpsychotic depression and were excluded from the incidence figures, three subjects had a manic episode with psychotic features at the time of

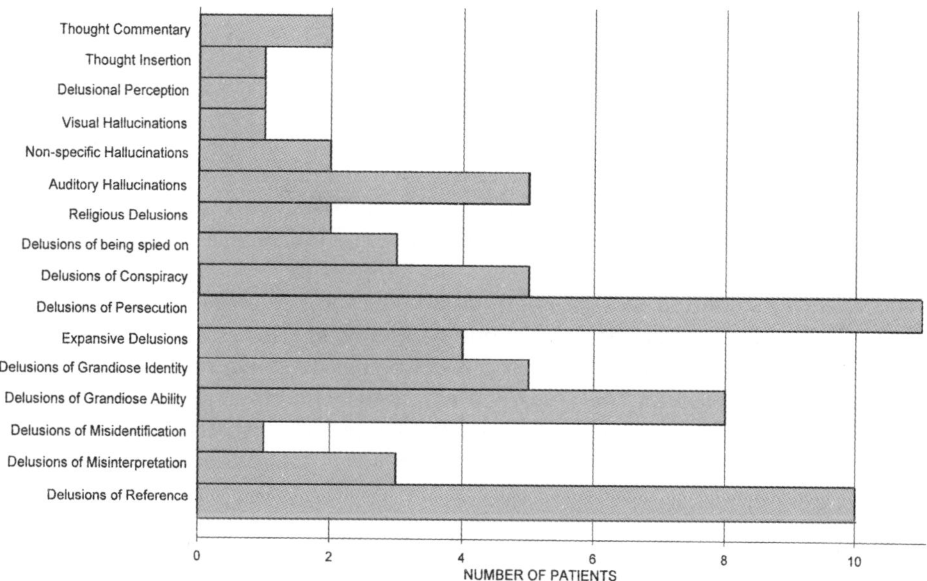

Figure 1. Clinical features of mania in the Nottingham Aesop Study of first onset psychosis.

inception and two had a mixed episode. Figure I shows the range of psychotic symptoms experienced by the patients in our sample.

First-rank symptoms of schizophrenia were present in four subjects or 25% of the sample with psychotic features, and 21% of the overall sample of nineteen patients. These included delusional perception, thought insertion, and voices commenting on the subjects actions. Our findings are in keeping with studies that have quoted a rate of 10–20% of first-rank symptoms of schizophrenia in manic patients (Mellor, 1982), that are summarized by Goodwin and Jamison (1990).

MANIA AND SUBSTANCE MISUSE

Population-based studies have shown the rates of comorbid substance abuse and dependence to be greater in patients with bipolar illness compared with other psychiatric disorders (Tohen et al., 1998). A comprehensive literature review revealed that early age of onset, gender, a family history of substance misuse disorders, and the presence of mixed mania were associated with comorbidity of these two disorders (Tohen et al., 1998). Winokur and colleagues (1998) explored the relationship between alcohol and drug abuse in Bipolar I disorder, unipolar disorder and a comparison group. The rates of alcohol and stimulant abuse and ever having abused a drug were higher in Bipolar I patients compared with unipolar patients and controls. Within the bipolar group, subjects who abused drugs had a significantly younger age of onset and a significantly greater family history of mania and schizoaffective mania.

Strakowski et al. (1996), examined the effects of antecedent substance abuse on the development of first-episode mania in a sample of 59 inpatients. Within this sample of manic or mixed episode patients with psychotic features, 32% had antecedent drug abuse and 20% had abused alcohol. Patients with antecedent substance abuse required hospital admission sooner than patients without. Alcohol abuse was, however, associated with a later age of onset of illness.

In the Aesop sample eleven subjects denied any present history of illicit drug use although two of these subjects had tried cannabis on one occasion in the past. Eight subjects were regular users of cannabis or a particularly strong form of the drug termed "skunk weed" in the United Kingdom. One subject had used cocaine on seven occasions in the past but not in the year of presentation. Of these eight patients, three admitted to consuming excess amounts of cannabis in the period immediately preceding the onset of manic symptoms and one subject took Ecstasy tablets for the first time prior to symptoms emerging. Although the role of drugs in the aetiology and presentation of psychosis remains controversial, all the patients in this sample fulfilled ICD-10 criteria for manic disorder and the duration of the symptoms exceeded a time period where they could not be explained by the use of drugs alone.

COURSE AND DURATION OF EPISODES

We have already discussed the nosological issue of mania most likely being best seen in the context of a broader, bipolar affective syndrome that has sometimes yet to unfold. In this context, it is the manic-depressive cycle that is often the subject of investigation. However, manic episodes themselves have a definable course. Most patients experience more than one episode of mania and the interval from one episode to the next tends to decrease during the first five episodes (Cookson, 1998). However, the length between episodes shows an appreciable amount of individual variation, tending to cluster around stressful life events (Cutler and Post, 1982). The duration of manic episodes before the availability of effective treatments was on average six months, something that is, thankfully, amenable to treatment.

DIAGNOSTIC STABILITY

We are aware that the clinical characteristics that we referred to above occurred in manic syndromes that may subsequently evolve into schizophrenia, rather than classic bipolar disorder; this is something that does not rest easily with the DSM approach. Amin and colleagues (1999) followed up the cohort of 168 patients with first episode psychosis described by Brewin et al. (1997) in order to determine the relative stability of 3-year ICD-10 and DSM-III-R diagnoses. Manic psychoses showed the highest positive predictive value at 91%. Women with first onset psychotic mania showed the greatest stability with all 15 subjects retaining this diagnosis at 3-year follow-up. This is in contrast to schizophrenia where over a third of cases with ICD-10 diagnoses at 3 years had diagnoses other than schizophrenia at onset.

Schwartz and colleagues (2000) demonstrated diagnostic movement over two years in an even larger sample of all psychosis. Once again, mania was relatively stable. There was some instability within this category, in schizophrenia and much in categories with short duration criteria. This confirms that the longitudinal view is essential to understand phenotypic variation.

CONCLUSIONS

Mania is an established clinical entity, the occurrence and causes of which are amenable to investigation and description. It is presently conceived mainly as a part of a more long-term nosological category of affective disorder that may evolve in individuals, predominately, though not entirely, over adult life. Thus, its epidemiology needs to be seen in that context. Only in a proportion of cases is there evidence of psychosis, although its evolution may occasionally involve other psychotic syndromes such as schizophrenia and schizoaffective disorder. Its associated, or risk factors also show intriguing similarities and differences with these disorders and other psychiatric disease, as do putative endophenotypic characteristics such as neuropsychological function (Murphy et al., 2001) that are beyond the scope of this review.

As with much epidemiology, the study of mania is aimed at illuminating causes as well as describing a target for clinical and public health services. Concentrating on the causes and precipitants of the manic syndrome, be they environmental (Paykel, 1982), genetic (Bradbury, 2001; Potash and DePaulo, 2000), or interactions (Mundo et al., 2001), may provide clues to the determinants of several aspects of the mind in normal and abnormal states.

REFERENCES

Akiskal H (1992): The distinctive mixed states of bipolar I, II and III. Clin Neuropharm 15(1):632–633.

American Psychiatric Association (1980): "Diagnostic and Statistical Manual of Mental Disorders" (DSM-III), 3rd ed. Washington, DC: American Psychiatric Association.

American Psychiatric Association (1994): "Diagnostic and Statistical Manual of Mental Disorders (DSM-IV), 4th ed. Washington, DC: American Psychiatric Association.

Amin S, Singh SP, Brewin J, Jones PB, Medley I, Harrison G (1999): Diagnostic stability of first-episode psychosis. Comparison of ICD-10 and DSM-II-R systems. Br J Psych 175:537–543.

Angst J (1966): Zur Aetiologie und Nosologie Endogener Depression Psychosen. Monogr Neurol Psychiatr 112:1–118.

Angst J (1966): "Zur Atiologie und nosologie endogener depressiver Psychosen. Eine genetische, soziologische und klinische Studie." Springer, Berlin.

Angst J (1998): The emerging epidemiology of hypomania and Bipolar II disorder. J Affect Disord 50:143–151.

Baillarger J (1854): De folie a double forme. Ann Med-psychol 6:369–389.

Biedermen J, Wozniak J, Keily (1995): CBLC clinical scales discriminate prepubertal children with structured interview-derived diagnoses of mania from those with ADHD. J Am Acad Child Adolesc Psychiatry 34:454–463.

Biederman J, Faraone SV, Chu MP, Wozniak J (1999): Further evidence of a bidirectional overlap between juvenile mania and conduct disorder in children. J Am Acad Child Adolesc Psychiatry 38:468–476.

Bogers JP, de Jong JT, Komproe IH (2000): Schizophrenia among Surinamese in the Netherlands: High admission rates are not explained by high emigration rates. Psychol Med 30:1425–1431.

Boyd JH, Weissman MM (1981): Epidemiology of affective disorders: a reexamination and future directions. Arch Gen Psychiatry 38:1039–1046.

Boyd JH, Weissman MM (1981): The epidemiology of affective disorders: a reexamination and future directions. Arch Gen Psychiatry 38:1039–1046.

Bradbury J (2001): Teasing out the genetics of bipolar disorder. Lancet 357 (9268):1596.

Brewin J, Cantwell R, Dalkin T, Fox R, Medley I, Glazebrook C, Kwiecinski R, Harrison G (1997): Incidence of schizophrenia in Nottingham. A comparison of two cohorts, 1978–80 and 1992–94. Br J Psychiatry 171:140–144.

Burke KC, Burke JD, Regier DA, Rae DS (1990): Age at onset of selected mental disorders in five community populations. Arch Gen Psychiatry 47:511–518.

Carlson GA, Kashani JH (1988): Manic symptoms in a non-referred adolescent population. J Affect Disord 15:219–226.

Cookson J (1998) : Mania, bipolar disorder and treatment. In Stein G, Wilkinson G (eds). "Seminars in General Adult Psychiatry." Glasgow: Gaskell, p 61.

Cutler NR, Post RM (1982): Life course of illness in untreated manic depressive patients. Compre Psychiatry 23:101–115.

Daly I, Webb M, Kaliszer M (1995): First admission incidence study of mania, 1975–1981. Br J Psychiatry 167:463–468.

Der G, Bebbington PE (1987): Depression in inner London: a register study. Soc Psychiatry 22:73–84.

Dunner DL, Fiere RR (1974): Clinical factors in lithium carbonate prophylaxis failure. Arch Gen Psychiatry 30:229–233.

Eagles JM, Whalley LJ (1985): Ageing and affective disorders: the age at first onset of affective disorders in Scotland, 1969–1978. Br J Psychiatry 147:180–187.

Egeland JA, Hostetter AM (1983): Amish Study I: Affective disorders among the Amish, 1976–1980. Am J Psychiatry 140:56–61.

Falret JP (1854): Mémoire sur la folie circulaire, forme de maladie mentale caractérisée par la production successive et régulière de l'état maniaque, de l'état mélancolique, et d'un intervalle lucide plus our moins prolongué. Bull Acad Med 19:382–415.

Glasser M, Rabins P (1984): Mania in the elderly. Age Ageing 13:210–213.

Goodwin FK, Jamison KR (1990). Manic Depressive Illness. New York: Oxford University Press.

Harrison G, Glazebrook C, Brewin J, Cantwell R, Dalkin T, Fox R, Jones P, Medley I (1997): Increased incidence of psychotic disorders in migrants from the Caribbean to the United Kingdom. Psychol Med 27:799–806.

Kessler RC, Rubinow DR, Holmes C, Abelson JM, Zhao S (1997): The epidemiology of DSM-III-R bipolar I disorder in a general population survey. Psychol Med 27:1079–1089.

Kraepelin E (1921): Manic-depressive insanity and paranoia. Translated by RM Barcley, edited by GM Robertson. Edinburgh: E & S Livingstone. Reprinted New York: Arno Press, 1976.

Krauthammer C, Kleman GL (1978): Secondary mania: manic syndromes associated with antecedent physical illness or drugs. Arch Gen Psychiatry 35(11):1333–1339.

Leff JP, Fischer M, Bertelsen A (1976): A cross-national epidemiological study of mania. Br J Psychiatry 129:428–437.

Leonhard K (1979): "The Classification of Endogenous Psychoses," 5th Robins E (ed.). Trans Berman, R. New York: Irvington Publishers. (Aufteilung der Endogenen Psychosen, 1st ed Berlin: Akademie-Verlag, 1957.)

Loranger AW, Levine PM (1978): Age at onset of bipolar affective illness. Arch Gen Psychiatry 35:1345–1348.

Maj M, Magliano L, Pirozzi R, Marasco C, Guarneri M (1994): Validity of rapid cycling as a course specifier for bipolar disorder. Am J Psychiatry 151:1051–1019.

Marneros A (2001): Expanding the group of bipolar disorders. J Affect Disord 62: 39–44.

Mellor CS (1982): The present status of first-rank symptoms. Br J Psychiatry 140:423–424.

Morell V (1996): Manic-depression findings spark polarised debate. Science 272:31–32.

Mundo E, Walker M, Cate T, Macciardi F, Kennedy JL (2001); The role of serotonin transporter protein gene in antidepressant-induced mania in bipolar disorder: preliminary findings. Arch Gen Psychiatry 58:539–544.

Murphy FC, Rubinsztein JS, Michael A, Rogers RD, Robbins TW, Paykel ES, Sahakian BJ (2001): Decision-making cognition in mania and depression. Psychol Med 31:679–693.

Paykel E. S (1982): Life events and early environment. In Paykel ES (ed): "Handbook of Affective Disorders." New York: Churchill Livingstone, pp 146–161.

Perris C (1966): A study of bipolar (manic-depressive) and unipolar recurrent depressive psychoses: I. Genetic investigation. Acta Psychiatr Scand 42:15–44.

Potash JB, DePaulo JR (2000): Searching high and low: a review of the genetics of bipolar disorder. Bipolar Disord 2:8–26.

Roth M (1955): The natural history of mental disorder in old age. J Ment Sci 101:281–301.

Roth SM (2001): Unitary or binary nature of classification of depressive illness and its implications for the scope of manic depressive disorder. J Affect Disord 64:1–18.

Schwarz JE, Fennig S, Tanenberg-Karant M, Carlson G, Craig T, Galambos N, Lavelle J, Bromet EJ (2000): Congruence of diagnoses 2 years after first-admission diagnosis of psychosis. Arch Gen Psychiatry 57:593–600.

Spicer CC, Hare EH, Slater E (1973): Neurotic and psychotic forms of depressive illness: Evidence from age incidence in a national sample. Br J Psychiatry 123:535–541.

Strakowski SM, McElroy SL, Keck PE Jr, West SA (1996): The effects of antecedent substance abuse on the development of first-episode psychotic mania. J Psychiatric Res 30:59–68.

Tohen M, Greenfiend SF, Weiss RD, Zarate CA Jr, Vagge LM (1998): The effect of comorbid substance use disorders on the course of bipolar disorder: a review. Harvard Rev Psychiatry 6:133–141.

Van Os J, Takei N, Castle DJ, Wessely S, Der G, MacDonald AM, Murray RM (1996): The incidence of mania: Time trends in relation to gender and ethnicity. Soc Psychiatry and Psychiatr Epidemiol 31:129–136.

Veijola J, Rasanen P, Isohanni M, Tihonen J (1996): Low incidence of mania in northern Finland. Br J Psychiatry 168:520–521.

Verhulst FC, Van der Ende J, Ferdinand RF, Kasius MC (1997): The prevalence of DSM-III-R diagnoses in a national sample of Dutch adolescents. Arch Gen Psychiatry 54:329–336.

Weller RA, Weller EB, Tucker SG, Fristad MA (1986): Mania in prepubertal children: Has it been underdiagnosed? J Affect Disord 11:151–154.

Wertham FI (1929): A group of benign psychoses: Prolonged manic excitements: with a statistical study of age, duration and frequency in 2000 manic attacks. Am J Psychiatry 9:17–78.

Wing JK, Cooper JE, Sartorius N (1974): Measurement and classification of psychiatric symptoms. An instruction manual for the PSE and Catego Program. New York: Cambridge University Press.

Winoker G, Turvey C, Akiskal H, Coryell W, Solomon D, Leon A, Mueller T, Endicott J, Maser J, Keller M (1998): Alcoholism and drug abuse in three groups: Bipolar I, unipolars and their acquaintances. J Affect Disord 50:81–89

World Health Organization (1973): "The International Pilot Study of Schizophrenia." Vol. 1. Geneva: World Health Organization.

World Health Organization (1992): "International Classification of Disease." Chapter V. Mental and behavioural disorders. Geneva: World Health Organization.

CHAPTER 19

The Epidemiology of Alcohol Use, Abuse, and Dependence

NANCY L. DAY and GREGORY G. HOMISH

Western Psychiatric Institute and Clinic, University of Pittsburgh School of Medicine, 3811 O'Hara Street, Pittsburgh, PA 15213-2593

INTRODUCTION

Alcohol use and abuse occupy unique positions within our culture and history, influencing our attitudes toward drinking and our definitions of alcoholism. In colonial days, alcohol was a major part of life, serving as food, medicine, social facilitator, and a safe substitute for frequently nonpotable water (Levine, 1973). It provided, as well, a major source of revenue. Drinking was acceptable to the colonials who thought that people drank and got drunk by choice. Drunkenness was not proscribed; habitual drunkenness was considered an addiction, but an addiction to drunkenness, not to alcohol. It was conceptualized as a problem within the social and religious realms and punished with legal and religious sanctions.

Changes in social attitudes toward alcohol have created sweeping social movements throughout our history. The last of these resulted in the Eighteenth Amendment to the Constitution, Prohibition, which began in 1920 and was repealed in 1933. Some argue that there are signs that we may again be experiencing a return to prohibition sentiment (Room, 1991). What is less apparent but equally important is that, as a culture, we have maintained the earlier dual attitude toward alcohol, conceptualizing it as a positive benefit with restrained and appropriate use and a negative behavior when used to excess or harm. Similarly, we entertain at the same time the idea that alcoholism is a disease, or medical problem, and that alcoholism is a social problem related to excess consumption.

Two different research thrusts representing these differing approaches coexist within the field of alcohol studies. The sociological approach has documented the prevalence of drinking, drinking patterns, and problems within the population. This approach studies the continuum from abstinence to problem drinking and

Textbook in Psychiatric Epidemiology, Second Edition, Edited by Ming T. Tsuang and Mauricio Tohen. ISBN 0-471-40974-X

focuses on the social and environmental factors that affect position along this continuum. The medical approach has viewed alcoholism, or alcohol use disorder, as a disease, focusing on biological and genetic factors and clinical issues of diagnosis and treatment. Research covering both approaches will be presented in this chapter since both are needed to describe the range of alcohol effects, as well as the breadth of alcohol research within the United States.

DRINKING AND DRINKING PRACTICES

Population-based Estimates of Alcohol Use

On a population basis, there are several ways of estimating the amount of alcohol consumed. The most common is to estimate per capita alcohol consumption based on either alcohol production or sales. Apparent alcohol consumption, a measure derived by dividing the total quantity of alcohol sales by the total population in the United States aged 14 and older, was 2.21 gallons of absolute alcohol in 1994 (Stinson et al., 1997). This breaks down into 1.26 gallons of beer, 0.29 gallons of wine, and 0.66 gallons of spirits per capita. This is an underestimate of individual consumption, however, since abstainers were included in this calculation and illegal alcohol, home production, and duty free purchases were not included in this estimate. In the United States, the highest levels of per capita consumption occurred in the West (2.33 gallons per capita) and the lowest occurred in the Northeast (2.14 gallons). States with the highest per capita consumption included Nevada (4.15 gallons), New Hampshire (4.14 gallons) and Washington, DC (3.89 gallons) while states with the lowest per capita consumption included Utah (1.28 gallons), West Virginia (1.64 gallons), and Arkansas (1.68 gallons) (Stinson et al., 1997).

There has been a recent decrease in the consumption of alcoholic beverages, following a peak in the early 1980's (NIDA, 1991; Stinson et al., 1997). To examine this trend between 1984 and 1995, Caetano and Clark (1998) used data from two nationwide probability samples. The rate of abstention from alcohol increased in African-Americans and Hispanics but remained constant among Caucasians. Caucasian males decreased their levels of heavy drinking. There was no change among African-American and Hispanic men. Similarly, levels of heavy drinking decreased for Caucasian women but not for African-American or Hispanic women.

To evaluate this trend further, Greenfield et al. (2000) evaluated data from nationwide probability samples from 1984, 1990, and 1995. The overall trend of decreasing alcohol consumption appeared to stabilize around 1990. Just over 30% (30.6%) of the population abstained in 1984, 35% were abstainers in 1990, and 35.4% were abstainers in 1995.

These data, however, cannot give us individual patterns of use or the covariates of patterns of alcohol consumption. Individual interviews are necessary to collect specific levels and patterns of consumption.

Measurement of Drinking

Drinking is a behavior and, as such, can be described by the quantity, frequency, and type of beverage consumed. Quantity, the number of drinks per occasion, is a measure of drinking style while frequency, the number of occasions per unit time, is a measure of the role or the salience of alcohol in the individual's life-style. The type of beverage also is a marker of the style of drinking as well as of social status. Interestingly, although the percent of absolute alcohol differs among the different beverages, the amount of absolute alcohol per served drink is roughly equivalent. That is, a 12-oz. can of beer, a mixed drink containing 1.5-oz of spirits and a 5-oz. glass of wine all contain about the same amount of absolute alcohol.

The different variations of quantity, frequency, and beverage type can be combined to describe a drinking pattern. In fact, these patterns are used within our culture as markers of social status. Contrast, for example, the descriptors that come to mind when you compare the drinking patterns of two people: the first person drinks a six-pack after work every night and two to three six-packs on weekend nights, while a second person drinks wine every night with dinner, and on weekends, and either wine or a mixed drink before and with dinner. With high reliability, most readers will quickly be able to identify a gender, income, education, and occupational level for each of the individuals.

A number of scales have been developed that allow researchers to combine the various drinking parameters. The most common of these is average daily volume, an averaged estimate across all quantities, frequencies, and beverages. While this scale has the advantage that it is a continuous variable, it has the disadvantage that it ignores the diversity of drinking patterns. This diversity is important because, as noted above, drinking patterns correlate with other covariates of drinking, with consequences of drinking, and with alcohol abuse and dependence. Other ways of combining the data have also been developed, including measures of binge, or clustered drinking, or frequent heavy drinking, the frequency of consuming five or more drinks per occasion. Other researchers have constructed typologies of drinking to describe different patterns. These measures usually focus on only one dimension of drinking behavior and therefore can only be used to explore the effects of a specific pattern of use. At the top of the scale (the heaviest drinking levels) and the bottom (abstention and very light drinking) the concordance between scales is quite good. In the middle levels, there is considerable divergence, and in analyses that address more moderate levels of alcohol use, the type of scale that is selected becomes important.

The Prevalence of Alcohol Use

The National Household Survey on Drug Abuse is a nationwide probability sample of the prevalence of the use of alcohol and other drugs (Substance Abuse and Mental Health Services Administration 2000). Interviews included both individual households (for example, houses, apartments, military installations) and housing units with larger groups of people (for example, college dorms, homeless shelters but not institutions like hospitals or prisons). Enhanced sampling was used to increase the number of African-American and Hispanic subjects. Data from this study demonstrated that a majority of the population, 64.0%, drank at least once a year; specifically, 68.3% of the men and 60.0% of the women drank at least once a year. Just over 7% (7.2%) reported drinking 20 to 30 days of the month prior to interview. This was more common among men than women (10.5% compared to 4.1%). Men were also more likely to binge drink (five or more drinks on the same occasion on at least one day in the previous month) than were women (22.4% compared to 8.3%). Similarly, men were more likely than women to engage in heavy drinking (five or more drinks on five or more days in the past month); 9.3% of men reported heavy drinking compared to 2.3% of women.

Drinking and patterns of consumption changed with age (Substance Abuse and Mental Health Services Administration, 2000). Among men, the percentage who reported drinking in the past year did not vary greatly by age (79.3% for men aged 18–25; 77.7% for men aged 26–34; 70.2% for men over 35). However, younger men (18–25 years of age) were more likely to binge drink than were older men. Younger men (18–25 years of age) also had higher rates of frequent heavy drinking. One-fifth of the men aged 18–25 years reported drinking five or more drinks per occasion at least five or more times in the previous month, compared to 11.5% of the men 26–34 years of age, and 7.6% of the men aged 35 and over. Among women, similar patterns were found with respect to age although the levels of consumption were much lower.

There are two alternate interpretations to these age-related changes. They could result from aging, or they could be a cohort effect. In 1983, Stall (1986) followed up a group of men who had been interviewed in 1964. While stability was the mode, 25% of the men decreased their intake and 15% increased their drinking over the 20-year time period. The decrease was greatest among the heavy and moderate drinkers (80%) and the stability was determined mostly by men who had been light drinkers in the base period. Quantity was more likely to decrease than frequency. Findings from another study using both men and women corroborated the Stall report (Adams et al., 1990). These data demonstrate that the decrease over time is not a cohort effect, but a behavioral change associated with aging.

Caucasian men (61.2%) were more likely to have used alcohol in the past month than were Hispanic men (56.8%) or African-American men (49.0%) (Substance Abuse and Mental Health Services Administration, 2000). A similar pattern existed for women: more Caucasian women reported alcohol use in the past month (49.7%) than either Hispanic (33.6%) or African-American women (32.3%).

The prevalence of drinking increased with income (Stinson et al., 1998). Among those with incomes less than $10,000 per year, 53.3% of the men and 34.5% of the women drank 12 or more drinks in the past year, compared to 63.8% and 52.1%, respectively, among those whose incomes were over $25,000. However, when problematic alcohol use (as defined by DSM-IV diagnosis of alcohol dependence) is considered among those who drink, the pattern is reversed. Among men, 21.7% of those with incomes below $10,000 year had a dependence diagnosis compared to 6.9% of men with incomes greater than $25,000. Comparable figures for women were 12.3% and 4.1%, respectively.

Education level, like income level, was correlated with drinking patterns (Substance Abuse and Mental Health Services Administration, 2000). Among men and women, those with the most education were most likely to be drinkers. By contrast, those with less than a high school education were the most likely to report heavier drinking. For example, 7.5% of individuals with less than a high school education reported heavy drinking (five or more drinks on five or more occasions in the past 30 days) compared to 4% of college graduates.

Among men and women, those who were never married and those who were divorced or separated were the most likely to drink and had the highest rates of heavy drinking (Hilton, 1991a).

Religion also predicted drinking patterns, because of differing religious attitudes toward alcohol and because of the correlations between religion, ethnic identity, and socioeconomic status. Catholics and Jews were most likely to be drinkers (Midanik and Clark, 1994). Among Christians, Catholics were most likely to drink, followed by Liberal and then Conservative Protestants. Higher rates of heavier drinking (five or more drinks on at least one occasion per week) were found among those who reported their religious preference to be "other." People who were Jewish were least likely to be heavy drinkers.

Thus, drinking in the United States population followed patterns determined by individual, demographic, and socioeconomic factors. People who were older or of higher social status were more likely to be drinkers, but they were less likely to drink heavily or report drunkenness. Those of lower income and education were less likely to drink. Younger, unmarried men and women were more likely to drink and to drink heavily.

Measurement of drinking in a population sample is, at best, difficult. Because our cultural attitudes toward alcohol are still ambivalent, drinking is usually underreported. In fact, comparisons of alcohol production to reported use find that only about half of all alcohol produced is accounted for by surveys of drinking behavior (Embree and Whitehead, 1993; De Lint, 1981). Although researchers have assumed that the amount of underreporting is not correlated with the actual drinking practices of the individual (Popham and Schmidt, 1981), this has not been demonstrated and this inaccuracy could represent a significant bias.

DRINKING PROBLEMS

In addition to measuring the prevalence of drinking in the population, researchers have also focused on the consequences of alcohol use. These consequences are events such as accidents, family problems, and/or medical effects such as liver cirrhosis that may be attributed to drinking practices.

Definition of Drinking Problems

The measurement of drinking problems in survey research has a long history, extending back to the early national surveys on drinking and drinking problems (Clark, 1966; Keller, 1962), although considerable debate still exists regarding the list of eligible problems and/or the definition of such problems. There are also difficulties with the assessment of these consequences. The first of these is the issue of attribution. Although the definition of these items assumes that the outcome was the result of alcohol use and would not have occurred in the absence of alcohol consumption, none of the consequences is unique to alcohol exposure, and this assumption is difficult to prove. Moreover, as alcohol consumption increases, the tendency to blame problems on alcohol may also increase, confounding the relationship. In addition, negative labeling, as well as denial, both lead to a tendency to deny the role of alcohol in a given problem. The effect of these factors on the measurement of consequences is not known.

Hilton (1991b) divided drinking problems into three groups representing drinking patterns, consequences, and dependence. Consequences were variables such as fighting while intoxicated, problems with spouse, relatives, friends, job, or finances, resulting from drinking. Health problems and accidents due to drinking were also included in the listing (Hilton, 1991b). Dependence was defined by items such as loss of control and symptomatic behaviors such as tremors and blackouts. These symptoms parallel the diagnostic criteria for alcohol abuse and dependence, although the authors disavow this implication, arguing that they could reflect either a disease state or the immediate and short-term effects of too much drinking.

This reflects a still-current argument in alcohol research. While medical researchers and clinicians accept that the end product of alcohol use and the consequences of heavy alcohol use is a phenomenon defined as alcoholism, or alcohol abuse and dependence, social researchers argue that this construct is not applicable in the general population (Clark, 1991).

Prevalence and Correlates of Drinking Problems

In the National Household Study on Drug Abuse (Substance Abuse and Mental Health Services Administration, 2000), 22.8% of individuals reporting any alcohol use in the past year said that they experienced at least one of the components of dependence. These are comparable to the criteria listed earlier by Hilton and include physical health problems, psychological problems, increased tolerance, failed attempts to cut down, more use than intended, reduced involvement in other activities, and having a period of a month or more when a great deal of time was spent getting or using or recovering from the effects of alcohol.

More than 7% of those interviewed reported three or more of the components of dependence. Younger people reported more problematic use than older individuals. Among the heavier users (more than five drinks on more than five occasions in the past 30 days), 66.4% experienced at least one and 36.1% experienced three or more factors of dependence.

In an earlier national survey, 72% of all drinkers reported no drinking problems, 10% reported one problem, and 14% reported three or more problems (Hilton, 1991c). These drinking problems were more common among men than women and were found at higher rates among younger people (Hilton, 1991b). African-American men had higher rates of drinking problems than did Caucasian men. Ten percent of African-American men reported high levels of dependence symptoms (four or more) and 13.2% reported high levels of consequences (four or more, on a weighted scale) compared to 5.1% and 6.6% for Caucasian men, respectively. Caucasian women had more dependence problems than African-American women, with rates of 2.7% and 2.3%, respectively, but there was no difference in the rates of consequences. Among men, the rate of drinking problems was highest among divorced or separated men, 13.6% reported a high level of consequences, with widowed (12.5%) and never-married men (10.9%) next in order, compared to a low rate among married men (5.1%). Among women, the rates for never-married women were low (1.2% reported a high level of consequences) and the divorced or separated group had rates approximating the rates of the married women (2.5% and 2.7%, respectively). Rates of problems were highest among low-income groups and among those with the less education for males and females.

Jews, both male (0.8% for a high level of consequences) and female (0%) had the lowest rates of drinking problems. Within the Christian religion, Conservative Christians had the highest rates of drinking problems among current drinkers. Overall, the group that had no religion had the highest rates of drinking problems; 18.5% of the men and 3.9% of the women reported a high level of consequences.

In a survey completed in Iowa, Fitzgerald and Mulford (1993) found that 2.8% of the population reported a failure to fulfill responsibilities because of drinking. Most other consequences had prevalence rates of less than 1%. By contrast, in one of national surveys reported above, on the average, each item was endorsed positively by 2.8% of the subjects (Hilton, 1991c). The associations between problems were low, the average correlation coefficient between problems was 0.19 (SD = 0.10) for problems judged to be at a moderate level and 0.20 (SD = 0.09) for problems at a minimal level. There were higher correlations, on the level of 0.4, between loss of control, symptomatic behavior, and binge drinking and these three variables also correlated more highly with other problems.

The highest rates of drinking problems were found among men, those who were young, less educated, lower income, and single. The groups that had the highest rates of drinking problems also tended to be the groups that had the greatest proportion of abstainers, an indication that drinking problems are more prevalent among groups where drinking is less common and, perhaps, less approved. These predictors were, in general, the same factors that predicted heavy drinking. Hilton (1991d) assessed the predictability of these factors within a group of frequent heavy drinkers and found that after controlling for intake, few of the covariates remained significant.

Wechsler et al. (1995) found gender differences in the association between drinking and drinking problems, noting that women who drank four drinks during a drinking episode had approximately the same level of drinking problems as men who drank an average of five drinks on occasion. An analysis, using data from the National Household Survey on Drug Abuse, compared the rates of psychosocial consequences of alcohol and drug abuse between men and women (Robbins, 1989). This report found that while substance abuse was related more to intrapsychic problems among women and issues of social functioning among men, the majority of the gender differences were explained by the greater frequency of heavy drinking among men. Studies have also shown that women experience health consequences at lower levels of alcohol use than men (Mann et al., 1992; Hill, 1995).

In summary, studies in the general population demonstrate that the distribution of drinking is predicted by social and demographic factors, such as gender, age, education, and income. Those who are more advantaged drink more frequently. Heavier levels of drinking are more likely to occur within populations that are lower income, less educated, younger, and single. These latter factors also predict drinking problems, as does the rate of heavy drinking.

Relations Between the Sociological and Clinical Viewpoints

It is difficult to make a transition from drinking and drinking problems, a concept from the survey and sociological literature, to the diagnosis of alcoholism. These disparate approaches, as noted earlier, represent different conceptual models.

Those who support the sociological model contend that there is no unitary phenomenon, pointing to the fact that there is a wide distribution of drinking patterns, problems, and consequences and that the correlations between these variables are quite low in the general population (Clark, 1991; Tarter et al., 1991). Proponents of the disease concept of alcoholism point to the biological elements in the development of alcoholism, the development of tolerance and withdrawal, and the heritability of the disease. The diagnostic criteria for alcohol use disorder, in fact, incorporate the sociological approach. The diagnosis is the end of a continuum which is defined by a combination of drinking, consequences, and problems, and the point between having symptoms and having a diagnosable disease is arbitrary. Moreover, it is the number of symptoms rather than a specific progression or constellation of symptoms that defines the disorder.

ALCOHOLISM OR ALCOHOL ABUSE AND DEPENDENCE

Definition and Diagnosis

Benjamin Rush (1785) categorized drunkenness as a progressive disease and noted that the body progressively adapts to the use of alcohol until the person becomes habituated. It was the first definition of both the disease state and tolerance. He proposed strikingly nonmedical treatments, including terrors, whippings, and shaming, and advocated temperance; wine and beer were acceptable; the primary problem was spirits (liquor), particularly rum.

The use of the word "alcoholism" was proposed in Sweden in 1852 (Paredes, 1979) to remove the stigma of the term "drunkenness," and was defined as the biological and behavioral symptoms resulting from the damage caused by excessive ingestion, an irresistible urge to drink, and a functional disturbance of the central nervous system. Jellinek (1960) laid the groundwork for current diagnostic thinking. He proposed that there were two types of alcoholics, those who suffered physical and physiological changes resulting from prolonged use (chronic alcoholism), and others who had alcohol addiction, characterized by an urgent craving for alcohol.

There are as many different schemata for diagnosis as there are different names for the phenomenon. However, in general, the diagnoses include four concepts: tolerance to alcohol, withdrawal during abstinence, impaired control over alcohol consumption, and problems related to the use of alcohol (Beresford, 1991). These core factors that define the diagnosis, however, are only weakly correlated with each other (Cloninger, 1987).

Tolerance is defined as a physical dependence on alcohol, and reflects the amount of physical habituation that the body has developed (Beresford, 1991). As tolerance increases, the effect of a given amount of alcohol will decrease. Withdrawal constitutes a set of symptoms that occur when a person is abstinent. The resulting symptoms can range from anxiety, nausea, and tachycardia to seizures and delirium tremens. Thus, tolerance and withdrawal are markers of the biological effects of alcohol. Impaired control refers to the inability to control drinking once begun, to cut down or quit.

Social problems are problems that result directly from the use of alcohol. Driving or violence while intoxicated, neglect of responsibilities due to alcohol use, or failure to decrease alcohol use even in the face of physical problems caused by the exposure, such as cirrhosis, are all included in this category. This list parallels the list of consequences noted earlier and has been adapted from the studies of drinking problems. Accordingly, the same problems of attribution, labeling, and denial apply. Social consequences can be affected by a number of different drinking-related behaviors. They can result from the acute effects of intoxication, the effects of chronic drinking, or the prioritization of drinking over other roles and responsibilities.

These basic areas were combined into the diagnosis of alcohol abuse and dependence in the DSM-III (American Psychiatric Association, 1980). The diagnosis of alcohol dependence required either tolerance or withdrawal and either loss of control or social or physical problems because of alcohol use. A separate category, alcohol abuse, required the presence of impaired control or social consequences, in the absence of either tolerance or withdrawal. One weakness of the DSM-III system of classification for alcohol abuse and dependence was that there was no requirement that the symptoms occur together in time. Therefore, the estimates of lifetime prevalence may be considerably inflated as subjects experience symptoms over the course of their lifetime.

At the same time, Edwards (1986) developed a theoretical model, the Alcohol Dependence Syndrome (ADS). This model focused more on the salience of drinking and alcohol seeking behavior, and less on social consequences. It was defined by seven criteria: narrowing the drinking repertoire, salience of alcohol-seeking behavior, increased tolerance, repeated withdrawal episodes, drinking to relieve or avoid withdrawal, subjective awareness of a compulsion to drink, and reinstatement of established drinking patterns following a period of abstinence.

In 1987, the DSM criteria were revised, incorporating the theoretical model of the ADS into the conceptualization of the DSM-III-R (American Psychiatric Association, 1987). In the DSM-III-R, the diagnosis of alcohol dependence is made if three from a list of nine symptoms are present. Definitions of severity levels were also included in this revision, a recognition of the fact that alcohol dependence exists along a gradient. A diagnosis of alcohol abuse persists in the DSM-III-R and requires the presence of environmental problems due to alcohol use and recurrent use of alcohol when it is physically harmful.

A further revision, the DSM-IV, became official in 1994. The DSM-IV was also based on the ADS. To receive a diagnosis of alcohol dependence, a person must meet three of the following seven criteria: (1) tolerance, (2) withdrawal, (3) drinking in larger amounts or over a longer period than was intended, (4) a persistent desire to reduce consumption or unsuccessful efforts to cut down or control alcohol use, (5) spending a great deal of time obtaining, using, or recovering from the effects of alcohol, (6) giving up or reducing social, occupational, or recreational activities because of alcohol use, and (7) continued use even in the presence of physical or psychological problems caused or exacerbated by alcohol (American Psychiatric Association, 1994). In the DSM-IV, the symptoms must occur within the same twelve-month period although they need not occur at the same time. As a result of this addition, the prevalence of alcohol dependence is lower using the DSM-IV criteria, compared to the DSM-III. The DSM-IV also allows the clinician to specify whether or not alcohol dependence includes physiological dependence, either tolerance or withdrawal.

Alcohol abuse in the new system is diagnosed by the social effects of drinking, such as failure to fulfill major role obligations, use in situations in which drinking is physically hazardous, substance-related legal problems, and use despite problems caused by or exacerbated by drinking. In addition, dependence and abuse are now defined hierarchically, so that one cannot receive a diagnosis of abuse after meeting criteria for dependence. Using the DSM-III or DSM-III-R systems, it was possible to receive concurrent diagnoses of dependence and abuse. The hierarchical relationship in classification reduces the number of cases of alcohol abuse.

A parallel diagnostic system, the International Classification of Diseases (ICD) is used internationally. The tenth revision of this system is based on the ADS (WHO, 1990) and therefore is similar to recent versions of the DSM system. Two slight differences exist between the two systems (Bucholz, 1999). DSM-IVs alcohol abuse diagnosis is labeled "harmful use" in the ICD-10 criteria. Additionally, ICD-10 has incorporated a craving component into the diagnostic criteria, DSM-IV does not address craving in the diagnostic criteria.

Although differences still exist with regard to the specific criteria for diagnosing alcohol abuse and dependence and the definitions of the variables included in the diagnosis, the availability of standardized diagnostic criteria has been invaluable in the development of epidemiologic studies of these disorders. This standardization enables the field of alcohol research to achieve reliability across studies so findings can be compared. Further methodological advances have included the development of structured and semistructured instruments for interviewing, some of which are designed to be used by lay interviewers. These developments have made possible the general population surveys of psychiatric morbidity (for example, the Epidemiologic Catchment Area Study, National Comorbidity Study, etc. These will be discussed in greater depth in later sections).

Compared to other psychiatric diagnoses, two factors are unique in the diagnosis of alcohol abuse and dependence. First, substance abuse diagnoses require exposure to an outside agent as part of the causal sequence, and second, the diagnosis of alcoholism includes the effect of the disease on the environment as part of the diagnosis; a reflection of the unique history of alcohol.

Population Estimates

The Alcohol Epidemiologic Data System monitors data from the National Hospital Discharge Survey for discharges due to alcohol diagnoses (using the ICD-9-CM diagnostic criteria), including alcoholic psychoses, alcohol dependence syndrome, nondependent alcohol abuse, and alcoholic liver cirrhosis (Owings and Lawrence, 1997). These discharge data are a random sample drawn from nonfederal, short-stay hospitals. In 1997, there were 30,914,000 discharges, 1.8% had an "alcohol dependence syndrome" diagnosis listed as the primary diagnosis, an additional 0.5% had an alcohol abuse diagnosis listed as a primary diagnosis. Rates of alcohol diagnoses were higher for men than for women, and were highest within the age group 15–44.

Another means of assessing the prevalence of alcoholism uses the distribution of deaths from liver cirrhosis as a marker. Jellinek (WHO, 1951) developed a formula for estimating the rate of alcoholism based on the rate of liver cirrhosis, and the proportion of deaths from liver cirrhosis that can be attributed to alcoholism. In 1989, the age-adjusted mortality rate from cirrhosis of the liver was 9.1 per 100,000 persons in the United States (DeBakey et al., 1993), placing it as the ninth leading cause of death in the United States.

There are a number of problems with the use of cirrhosis mortality as a surrogate for alcoholism. Although historically, the rates of death from liver cirrhosis have responded quickly and dramatically to major changes in alcohol distribution, such as Prohibition or war (Terris, 1967), there was a 25% decrease in cirrhosis mortality between 1973 and 1983, in the absence of a comparable change in drinking practices (DeBakey et al., 1993). This reflects the relative success of treatment programs, for cirrhosis and for alcoholism, as well as changes in diagnostic practices and/or death certification. In addition, cirrhosis is more likely to occur with heavy daily drinking than with episodic or binge drinking (Smart and Mann, 1992), and with amounts above the range of 80 g of absolute alcohol per day (Savolainen et al., 1993), so many drinkers and drinking patterns are not represented by this measure. There are also biases in the determination and reporting of death from cirrhosis.

Prevalence of Alcohol Abuse and Dependence

Three large surveys provide data on the prevalence of alcohol dependence and abuse in the United States, the Epidemiologic Catchment Area (ECA) study, a study conducted collaboratively at five sites throughout the United States, the Alcohol Supplement to the National Household Interview Survey (NHIS), and the National Comorbidity Study (NCS).

The ECA study used standardized methods at all sites and diagnostic criteria from the DSM-III (Leaf et al., 1991). Data collection occurred between 1980 and 1984 across the separate sites. A structured diagnostic interview, the Diagnostic Interview Schedule (DIS), was developed and was administered by lay interviewers. Reliability studies of the diagnoses of alcohol abuse and dependence using this instrument are somewhat conflicting, however, the reliability seems to be moderate (Anthony et al., 1985; Helzer et al., 1985).

The ECA study found high prevalence rates for alcoholism (defined by the authors as either abuse or dependence); 13.8% of all subjects met criteria for a lifetime diagnosis and 6.3% met criteria in the year prior to interview (Robins et al., 1991). Alcohol disorders were second only to phobias in prevalence among psychiatric disorders. Alcohol disorders were more common in males, 23.8% of men and 4.6% of the women in the sample met criteria for a lifetime diagnosis of alcoholism (Helzer et al., 1991). The median age of onset was 21, and 90% of all subjects had experienced their first symptom before the age of 38 years.

Five percent of men and 0.9% of women met criteria for a diagnosis of alcoholism within the past month (Regier et al., 1993). Rates decreased across age categories, from 4.1% among those aged 18–24 to 0.9% among individuals over age 65. Rates were highest among Hispanics (3.6%), intermediate for African-

Americans (3.4%), and lowest for Caucasians (2.7%). People who were separated or divorced had the highest rate (5.9%) compared to rates of 2.0% for married and 4.2% for single people.

The ECA project also surveyed institutionalized individuals, sampling residents of mental hospitals, nursing, convalescent and rest homes, chronic hospitals, residential centers for alcohol and drug treatment, halfway houses, and correctional facilities (Leaf et al., 1991). Twelve percent of institutionalized individuals had alcoholism, compared to 6% of household residents. Most commonly, these people were in correctional facilities (78%), 11% were in psychiatric facilities, and 11% were in chronic care facilities (Robins et al., 1991).

While the rate of alcoholism in the institutionalized and treatment population is high, the proportion of people in the general population who meet criteria for a diagnosis of alcoholism who receive treatment is very small. Of the subjects with a lifetime diagnosis of alcoholism in the ECA Study, only 15% reported that they had ever mentioned their symptoms to a doctor. Only 10% of those who had a current diagnosis of alcohol abuse or dependence, in the absence of any comorbidity, received any mental health care; this was 9% of the men and 14% of the women (Robins et al., 1991).

In the ECA study, 49% of those who met criteria for a lifetime diagnosis of alcoholism reported a symptom within the recent year while 51% of those with a lifetime diagnosis did not (Helzer et al., 1991). These findings have been confirmed by other research as well. Skog and Duckert (1993), for example, studied a treatment sample and found that heavy drinkers and alcoholics were as likely to decrease as to increase their consumption. These findings parallel reports from the drinking practices literature that demonstrate significant changes in heavy drinking over time among subjects (Clark, 1966) and challenge the assumption that alcoholism is a chronic and unremitting disorder. Among remitted cases in the ECA study (symptom free for at least one year), 75% of the subjects reported no more than 11 years from first to last symptom (Helzer et al., 1991).

A second large national prevalence study was the Alcohol Supplement to the National Health Interview Survey. This project surveyed 22,418 and 43,809 individuals in 1984 and 1988, respectively (Williams and DeBakey, 1992). In 1984, using DSM-III criteria, 8.6% of the respondents met diagnostic criteria for alcohol abuse and dependence within the past year (Grant et al., 1991). A second wave of data collection was carried out in 1988. This wave used DSM-III-R criteria and found a prevalence rate of 9% for alcoholism (Grant et al., 1991). These rates compare to the rate of 6.3% for the ECA sample using DSM-III criteria (Helzer et al., 1991).

The National Comorbidity Study (NCS), the third nationwide survey to be considered here, sampled individuals 15 to 54 years old across the United States (Kessler et al., 1994). Only noninstitutionalized people were included in the survey. Between September 1990 and February 1992, 8,092 individuals participated in the survey. A modified version of the Composite International Diagnostic Interview was used to obtain DSM-III-R diagnoses. Lifetime prevalence rates for alcohol abuse and alcohol dependence were 9.4% and 14.1%, respectively. Yearly prevalence rates for abuse and dependence were 2.5% and 7.2%, respectively. Lifetime rates for abuse and dependence were greater in men (abuse: 12.5%; dependence: 20.1%) compared to women (abuse: 6.4%; dependence: 8.2%). More men, compared to women, met criteria for a diagnosis of abuse or dependence in the past year.

Correlates of Alcohol Abuse and Dependence

There were differing patterns in the prevalence of alcoholism by age, sex and race in the ECA study (Helzer et al., 1991). The lifetime prevalence rate for alcoholism in Caucasian males decreased from 28.3% to 27.0% between age groups 18–29 and 30–44, respectively, and the rate in Caucasian females decreased across the same ages from 7.5% to 5.5%. Thereafter, in both genders, the rates decreased with age. The decrease was greater for females and the male to female ratio increased from 3.8 to 1 in the youngest age group to 8.6 to 1 in the oldest.

With respect to age, the pattern of alcoholism among Hispanics had a pattern similar to that of Caucasian men and women although the prevalence rates were higher for Hispanic males (35.9% at ages 30–44) and lower for Hispanic females (3.7% at ages 30–44). The pattern by age was different among African-Americans. For both males and females, the highest prevalence rates were found in the middle age groups, between ages 45 and 64, 32.9% for males and 7.3% for females. Thus, although there was little difference in the overall rate of alcoholism between African-Americans and Caucasians, there were quite different patterns in the distribution of prevalence rates by age.

There was an inverse relationship between alcoholism and educational level and few of the identified alcoholics (9%) had a stable marriage (Helzer et al., 1991). Concordant with the findings on education, there was an inverse relationship between occupational level, income, and the prevalence of alcoholism. It is notable that these covariates are quite different from those that predict drinking and heavy drinking in the general population. They are similar, however, to those that predict drunkenness.

For the NHIS, the rate of alcoholism was 13.3% among males and 4.4% among females. Caucasians had a higher prevalence than African-Americans, 9.1% compared to 5.6%, respectively. The 1988 NHIS survey also found that at younger ages, more Caucasians met criteria for alcohol abuse and dependence, while at older ages the ratio was tipped toward African-American respondents. In the ECA project, the rates of diagnosis for males and females were most similar among the younger-aged cohorts and diverged sharply among the older subjects.

The rates found in the two NHIS surveys using DSM-III (8.6%) and DSM-III-R (9%) criteria were comparable. Both of these rates were higher than the rate reported by the ECA project using DSM-III criteria (6.3%). The discrepancies in the data are mostly in the younger aged groups where the prevalence rates are much higher in the NHIS study, particularly among Caucasians, compared to the ECA study. Prevalence rates for the NCS were midrange between the ECA and NHIS findings (7.2% for alcohol dependence).

Alternative Models of Alcoholism

There are other formulations of the diagnostic spectrum of alcohol abuse and dependence, although few epidemiologic data exist for these proposed models.

Cloninger (1987) has proposed a neurobiological learning model of alcoholism, based on personality dimensions, that has two subtypes. Type I or milieu-limited alcoholics have a later onset, psychological rather than physiological dependence, and they experience guilt over their use. Type II or male-limited alcoholics have problems at an earlier age, exhibit spontaneous alcohol-seeking behavior and are socially disruptive when drinking. Johnson and colleagues (2000) suggested that subtypes of alcoholics could be differentiated by age of onset. In contrast to the early onset–late onset subtyping, they considered age of onset in three categories: under 20 years old, 20–25 years old, and over 25 years old. Zucker (1987), on the basis of developmental studies, has proposed a four-group subtype of alcoholism. Babor et al. (1992), using empirical clustering, have proposed two types of alcoholics based on premorbid risk factors, pathological use of alcohol and other substances, and the chronicity and consequences of drinking. Other reviewers have questioned the validity of the conceptualization and have recommended a rethinking and reformulation of our ideas about alcoholism (Tarter et al., 1991).

All of these typologies have in common an attempt to combine the various effects of drinking, drinking patterns, social problems, predictors, including genetic background and environmental factors, and psychosocial variables into a pattern. Many were developed using clinical populations and thus reflect the biases inherent in such samples, including the preselection of subjects to a treatment facility for alcohol abuse and dependence.

Genetic Factors in Alcohol Abuse and Dependence

Family studies have demonstrated that the risk of alcoholism was much higher among first-degree family members of an alcoholic; on average, the risk was increased seven times (Merikangas, 1990). More recent work has also found a higher rates of alcohol dependence in adult siblings of an alcoholic (Bierut et al., 1998). In a sample of individuals diagnosed with DSM-III-R alcohol dependence, 49.7% of their brothers and 23.8% of their sisters also had a diagnosis of alcohol dependence. This compared to 19.8% of brothers and 6.0% of sisters of a nonalcohol dependent control group. Studies of twin pairs also demonstrated a genetic influence, although the effect was moderated by gender and diagnosis. Concordance rates were higher for men than for women and for alcohol dependence compared to alcohol abuse (Pickens, 1991).

Comorbidity

Alcohol abuse and alcohol dependence are commonly associated with other disorders. In the ECA study (Helzer et al., 1991), the comorbidity rate was 32%. Among those with a diagnosis of alcohol abuse and dependence, 47% had a comorbid diagnosis. The most common second diagnosis among alcoholics was drug abuse and dependence, but other diagnoses, including antisocial personality, mania, and schizophrenia were also highly associated with alcoholism. Although in clinical samples depression is the disorder most commonly associated with alcoholism, this phenomenon was not particularly notable among the general population study. Female alcoholics had the highest rates of comorbidity, 65%, compared to 44% for the male alcoholics (Helzer et al., 1991).

High rates of comorbidity were also found in the National Comorbidity Study (Kessler et al., 1997). The NCS compared rates of comorbidity for men and women with a lifetime diagnosis of alcohol abuse and alcohol dependence. For most comorbid disorders, there was a greater association between alcohol dependence than there was for alcohol abuse. For men with a lifetime diagnosis of alcohol abuse or dependence, the most common second lifetime diagnosis was drug abuse or dependence (29.7% vs. 40.6%, respectively). Among women, a lifetime history of anxiety disorders was the most common second diagnosis for those with a lifetime diagnosis of alcohol abuse (48.8%) or alcohol dependence (60.7%).

Alcohol use and particularly drunkenness also contribute to morbidity and mortality rates for accidents, violence, cardiovascular disease, liver cirrhosis and certain types of cancer (National Institute on Alcohol Abuse and Alcoholism, 1993). Further, alcohol use affects reproductive functioning among women (National Institute on Alcohol Abuse and Alcoholism, 1993), and use during pregnancy causes growth, morphologic and neurological deficits in the offspring (Day, 1992).

SUMMARY

Drinking is the modal behavior in the United States. Overall, 70% of the population drinks at least once a year. Drinking behavior correlates with social and demographic status and is more prevalent among those who have higher levels of education and income. Heavy drinking and drunkenness are also frequent. Approximately 6% of the population reports drinking eight or more drinks in a day at least once a week and 3% of respondents report being drunk as often as once a week. In contrast to drinking and heavy drinking, drunkenness is correlated with younger age, less education, and lower income.

Epidemiologic research in the area of drinking practices can make substantial contributions to the field in several areas. The first is in the measurement of drinking and drinking patterns. As noted above, general population estimates of drinking only account for a portion of the actual alcohol that is produced. It is necessary to explore new means of measuring alcohol use and to develop new techniques of interviewing that may diffuse some of the social stigma associated with drinking. This will allow researchers to estimate more accurately the level of alcohol use, the pattern of use by demographic and social predictors, and to identify the segments of the population that do not report their use accurately.

In addition, although we have identified the correlates of drinking, drinking problems, and alcohol dependence and abuse, we do not know what factors may predict the transition from one level of drinking to another. For example, although drinking is more prevalent among those who are better educated and have higher incomes, drunkenness is found among those who are less educated and have lower incomes. We do not know what factors may trigger the transition from alcohol use to abuse and/or what it is about education and income (for example) that may affect this transition.

Six percent of the adult population reports current drinking problems at a high level, and 6 to 9% of the general population of adults meet criteria for alcohol abuse and dependence within the year prior to interview. These rates are mirrored by the proportion of all hospitalized patients with alcohol diagnoses, 5%. The prevalence rates and the covariates are remarkably similar for heavy drinking, drinking problems, and alcohol abuse and dependence. We can conclude from this that while these approaches come from different conceptual models, they are evaluating the same symptoms and identifying equivalent proportions of the population.

To understand the relations between drinking, drinking problems, and alcoholism will require the collection of these data on both clinical and general population samples. A clearer view of the relations between drinking problems and alcoholism will also allow more definitive studies of the essential diagnostic elements of the disorder and allow better separation of the disease process from the consequences of alcohol misuse.

Future directions of epidemiological research on alcohol disorders should include further refinement of measurement techniques and exploration of the relationship between the social aspects of alcohol use, misuse, and alcoholism. This should allow more insight into the diagnosis of alcohol disorders, which in turn would allow us to develop a better understanding of the factors that affect the transition from drinking to alcoholism.

REFERENCES

Adams WL, Garry PJ, Rhyne R, Hunt WC, Goodwin JS (1990): Alcohol intake in the healthy elderly. Changes with age in a cross-sectional and longitudinal study. Am Geriatr Soc 38:211–216.

American Psychiatric Association (1980): "Diagnostic and Statistical Manual of Mental Disorders," 3rd ed. Washington, DC: American Psychiatric Association.

American Psychiatric Association (1987): "Diagnostic and Statistical Manual of Mental Disorder," 3rd ed. revised. Washington, DC: American Psychiatric Association.

American Psychiatric Association (1994): "Diagnostic and Statistical Manual of Mental Disorders," 4th ed. Washington, DC: American Psychiatric Association.

Anthony JC, Folstein M, Romanoski AJ, Von Korff MR, Nestadt GR, Chahal R, Merchant A, Brown CH, Shapiro S, Kramer M, Gruenberg EM (1985): Comparison of the lay Diagnostic Interview Schedule and a standardized psychiatric diagnosis: Experience in eastern Baltimore. Arch Gen Psych 42:667–675.

Babor TF, Hofmann M, DelBoca FK, Hesselbrock V, Meer RE, Dolinsky ZS, Rounsaville B (1992): Types of alcoholics, I: Evidence for an empirically derived typology based on indicators of vulnerability and severity. Arch Gen Psych 49:599–608.

Beresford TP (1991): The nosology of alcoholism research. Alcohol Health Res World 15:260–265.

Bierut LJ, Dinwiddie SH, Begleiter H, Crowe RR, Hesselbrock V, Nurnberger JI Jr, Porjesz B, Schuckit MA, Reich T (1998): Familial transmission of substance dependence: alcohol, marijuana, cocaine, and habitual smoking. A report from the collaborative study on the genetics of alcoholism. Arch Gen Psych 55:982–688.

Bucholz KK (1999): Nosology and epidemiology of addictive disorders and their comorbidity. Psychiatric Clinics of North America 22:221–240.

Caetano R, Clark WB (1998): Trends in alcohol consumption patterns among whites, blacks and hispanics: 1984 and 1995. J Stud Alcohol 59: 659–668.

Caetano R, Kaskutas LA (1996): Changes in drinking problems among whites, blacks, and Hispanics: 1984–1992. Subst Use Misuse 31:1547–1571.

Clark WB (1966): Operational definitions of drinking problems and associated prevalence rates. Quart J Stud Alcohol 27:648–668.

Clark WB (1991): Conceptions of alcohol problems. In Clark WB, Hilton ME (eds): "Alcohol in America." Albany, NY: State University of New York Press, pp 165–172.

Cloninger CR (1987): Neurogenetic adaptive mechanisms in alcoholism. Science 236:410–416.

Day N (1992): The effect of alcohol use during pregnancy. In Zagon I, Slotkin T (eds): "Maternal Substance Abuse and the Developing Nervous System." Orlando: Academic Press, pp 27–44.

DeBakey SF, Stinson FS, Dufour MC (1993): "Liver Cirrhosis Mortality in the United States, 1970–1989" (Surveillance Report No. 25). Washington, DC: U.S. Dept of Health and Human Services, National Institute on Alcohol Abuse and Alcoholism.

De Lint J (1981): "Words and deeds": Responses to Popham and Schmidt. J Stud Alcohol 42:359–361.

Edwards G (1986): The alcohol dependence syndrome: A concept as stimulus to enquiry. Brit J Addict 81:171–183.

Embree BG, Whitehead PC (1993): Validity and reliability of self-reported drinking behavior: Dealing with the problem of response bias. J Stud Alcohol 54:334–344.

Fitzgerald JL, Mulford HA (1993): Alcohol availability, drinking contexts and drinking problems: The Iowa experience. J Stud Alcohol 54:320–325.

Grant BF, Harford TC, Chou P, Pickering R, Dawson DA, Stinson FS, Noble J (1991): Prevalence of DSM-III-R alcohol abuse and dependence, United States, 1988. Alcohol Health Res World 15:91–96.

Greenfield TK, Midanik LT, Rogers JD (2000): A 10-year national trend study of alcohol consumption, 1984–1995: Is the period of declining drinking over? Am J Public Health 90:47–52.

Helzer JE, Robins LN, McEvoy LT, Spitznagel EL Stoltzman RK, Farmer A, Brockington IF (1985): A comparison of clinical and Diagnostic Interview Schedule diagnoses. Arch Gen Psychiat 42:657–666.

Helzer JE, Burnam A, McEvoy LT (1991): Alcohol abuse and dependence. In Robins LN, Regier DA (eds): "Psychiatric Disorders in America. The Epidemiologic Catchment Area Study." New York: The Free Press, pp 81–115.

Hill SY (1995): Mental and physical health consequences of alcohol use in women. Recent Dev Alcohol 12:181–197.

Hilton ME (1991a): The demographic distribution of drinking patterns in 1984. In Clark WB, Hilton ME (eds): "Alcohol in America." Albany, NY: State University of New York Press, pp 73–86.

Hilton ME (1991b): The demographic distribution of drinking problems in 1984. In Clark WB, Hilton ME (eds): "Alcohol in America." Albany, NY: State University of New York Press, pp 87–104.

Hilton ME (1991c): A note on measuring drinking problems in the 1984 national alcohol survey. In Clark WB, Hilton ME (eds): "Alcohol in America." Albany, NY: State University of New York Press, pp 51–72.

Hilton ME (1991d): Demographic characteristics and the frequency of heavy drinking as predictors of self-reported drinking problems. In Clark WB, Hilton ME (eds): "Alcohol in America." Albany, NY: State University of New York Press, pp 194–212.

Jellinek EM (1960): "The Disease Concept of Alcoholism." Highland Park, NJ: Hillhouse Press.

Johnson BA, Cloninger CR, Roache JD, Bordnick PS, Ruiz P (2000): Age of onset as a discriminator between alcoholic subtypes in a treatment-seeking outpatient population. Am J Addict 9:17–27.

Keller M (1962): The definition of alcoholism and the estimation of its prevalence. In Pittman D, Snyder C (eds): "Society, Culture and Drinking Patterns." New York: Wiley, pp 310–329.

Kessler RC, Crum RM, Warner LA, Nelson CB, Schulenberg J, Anthony JC (1997): Lifetime co-occurrence of DSM-III-R alcohol abuse and dependence with other psychiatric disorders in the National Comorbidity Survey. Arch Gen Psych 54:313–321.

Kessler RC, McGonagle KA, Zhao S, Nelson CB, Hughes M, Eshleman S, Wittchen HU, Kendler KS (1994): Lifetime and 12-month prevalence of DSM-III-R psychiatric disorders in the United States. Results from the National Comorbidity Survey. Arch Gen Psych 51:8–19.

Leaf PJ, Myers JK, McEvoy LT (1991): Procedures used in the epidemiologic catchment area study. In Robins LN, Regier DA (eds): "Psychiatric Disorders in America. The Epidemiologic Catchment Area Study." New York: The Free Press, pp 1–32.

Levine HG (1973): The discovery of addition: changing conceptions of habitual drunkenness in America. J Stud Alcohol 39:143–174.

Mann K, Batra A, Gunthner A, Schroth G (1992): Do women develop alcoholic brain damage more readily than men? Alcohol Clin Exp Res 16:1052–1056.

Merikangas KR (1990): The genetic epidemiology of alcoholism. Psychol Med 20;11–22.

Midanik LT, Clark WB (1994): The demographic distribution of US drinking patterns in 1990: Description and trends from 1984. Am J Public Health 84:1218–1222.

National Institute on Drug Abuse (1991): "National Household Survey on Drug Abuse, Highlights 1990." Washington, DC: U.S. Department of Health and Human Services Publication Number (ADM) 1789-91.

National Institute on Alcohol Abuse and Alcoholism (1993): "Eighth Special Report to the U.S. Congress on Alcohol and Health." Washington, DC: U.S. Department of Health and Human Services.

Owings MF, Lawrence L (1997): "Detailed Diagnoses and Procedures. National Hospital Discharge Survey." Vital Health Stat Series 13(145). (DHHS Pub No. 2000-1716). Hyattsville, MD: National Center for Health Statistics.

Paredes A (1979): The history of the concept of alcoholism. In Tarter R, Sugarman A (eds): "Alcoholism—Interdisciplinary Approaches to an Enduring Problem." Reading MA: Addison-Wesley, pp 9–52.

Pickens RW, Svikis DS, McGue M, Lykken DT, Heston LL, Clayton PJ (1991): Heterogeneity in the inheritance of alcoholism. Arch Gen Psychiat 48:19–28.

Popham RE, Schmidt W (1981): Words and deeds: The validity of self-report data on alcohol consumption. J Stud Alcohol 42:355–358.

Regier DA, Farmer ME, Rae DS, Myers JK, Kramer M, Robins LN, George LK, Karno M, Locke BZ (1993): One-month prevalence of mental disorders in the United States and sociodemographic characteristics: The Epidemiologic Catchment Area study. Acta Psychiat Scand 88:35–47.

Robbins C (1989): Sex differences in psychosocial consequences of alcohol and drug abuse. J Health Soc Behav 30:117–130.

Robins LN, Locke BZ, Regier DA (1991): An overview of psychiatric disorders in America. In Robins LN, Regier DA (eds): "Psychiatric Disorders in America. The Epidemiologic Catchment Area Study." New York: The Free Press, pp 53–81.

Room R (1991): Cultural changes in drinking and trends in alcohol problems indicators: Recent U.S. experience. In Clark WB, Hilton ME (eds): "Alcohol in America." Albany, NY: State University of New York Press, pp 149–164.

Rush B (1785): "An Inquiry Into the Effects of Ardent Spirits Upon the Human Body and Mind, with an Account of the Means of Preventing and of the Remedies for Curing Them" (8th ed. 1814). Reprinted in Keller M, "Classics of the Alcohol Literature" Quart J Stud Alcohol 4:321–341 (1943).

Savolainen VT, Liesto K, Mnnikk A, Penttil L, Karhunaen PJ (1993): Alcohol consumption and alcoholic liver disease: Evidence of a threshold level for effects of ethanol. Alcohol Clin Exp Res 17:1112–1117.

Skog O, Duckert F (1993): The development of alcoholics' and heavy drinkers' consumption: A longitudinal study. J Stud Alcohol 54:178–188.

Smart RG, Mann RD (1992): Alcohol and the epidemiology of liver cirrhosis. Alcohol Health Res World 16:217–222.

Stall R (1986): Change and stability in quantity and frequency of alcohol use among aging males: A 19-year follow-up study. Brit J Alcohol 81:537–544.

Stinson FS, Lane JD, Williams GD, Dufour MC (1997): "US Apparent Consumption of Alcoholic Beverages. Based on State Sales, Taxation, or Receipt Data" (US Alcohol Epidemiologic Data Reference Manual, Vol 1, 3rd ed. NIH Pub No 97-4263) Bethesda, MD: National Institute of Alcohol Abuse and Alcoholism, US Department of Health and Human Services.

Stinson FS, Yi H, Grant BF, Chou P, Dawson DA, Pickering R (1998): "Drinking in the United States: Main findings from the 1992 National Longitudinal Alcohol Epidemiologic Survey (NLAES)." (US Alcohol Epidemiologic Data Reference Manual, Vol 6, 1st ed. NIH Pub No 99-3519). Bethesda, MD: National Institute of Alcohol Abuse and Alcoholism, US Department of Health and Human Services.

Substance Abuse and Mental Health Services Administration (2000): "National Household Survey on Drug Abuse: Main Findings 1998." Rockville, MD: U.S. Department of Health and Human Services.

Tarter RE, Moss HB, Arria A, Mezzich AC, Vanyuko MM (1991): The psychiatric diagnosis of alcoholism: Critique and proposed reformulation. Alc Clin Exp Res 16:106–116.

Terris M (1967): Epidemiology of cirrhosis of the liver: National mortality data. Am J Public Health 57:2076–2089.

Wechsler H, Dowdall G, Davenport A, Rimm E (1995): A gender-specific measure of binge drinking among college students. Am J Public Health 85:982–985.

Williams GD, DeBakey SF (1992): Changes in levels of alcohol consumption: United States, 1983–1988. Brit J Addict 87:643–648.

World Health Organization Expert Committee on Mental Health (1951): Report on the First Session of the Alcoholism Subcommittee. Geneva: World Health Organization, Technical Report Series No. 42.

World Health Organization (1990): "Proposed 10th Revision of the International Classification of Diseases (ICD-10). Clinical Descriptions and Diagnostic Guidelines." Geneva: World Health Organization.

Zucker RA (1987): The four alcoholisms: A developmental account of the etiological process. In Rivers PC (ed): "Alcohol and Addictive Behavior." Lincoln NB: University of Nebraska Press, pp 27–83.

CHAPTER 20

Epidemiology of Drug Dependence

JAMES C. ANTHONY, with JOHN E. HELZER

Department of Mental Hygiene, Bloomberg School of Public Health, The Johns Hopkins University, Baltimore, MD 21205 (J.C.A.); Department of Psychiatry, School of Medicine, University of Vermont, Burlington, VT 05401 (J.E.H.)[1].

INTRODUCTION

This is a chapter on the epidemiology of drug dependence and related psychiatric disturbances such as drug abuse—all of which are conditions that recently have been recognized as major sources of the global burden of health problems (Murray and Lopez, 1998). The chapter introduces the main clinical features of drug dependence and a set of contemporary case definitions now being used in clinical and epidemiologic research. It also provides an overview of recent basic epidemiologic evidence on drug dependence, with and without the related condition of drug abuse, including some coverage of adolescent drug use. The chapter offers several recommendations for future epidemiologic studies of drug dependence.

In this chapter, the term "drug" is used to encompass a set of internationally regulated substances such as marijuana and heroin, which generally are not available by medical prescription. This set of drugs also includes medicines more often available through legal channels, as well as illegal channels, of supply and distribution: cocaine and prescribed amphetamines; oxycodone (e.g., OxyContin) and other analgesic drugs; diazepam (e.g., Valium) and other anxiolytic drugs; and flurazepam, secobarbital, and other sedative-hypnotic drugs. Tobacco (nicotine), coffee (caffeine), and alcohol (ethanol) also are drugs, although they are not subject to international controlled substances law. Tobacco dependence and caffeine dependence are discussed in this chapter, briefly. The epidemiology of alcohol dependence is the topic of a separate chapter.

There are many reasons to study drug-related problems by considering each drug compound or drug category, one at a time. Doing so, it is possible to take into account the individual pharmacologic and pharmacokinetic profile of each drug, which help to shape the biologic response to drug exposure, including the function of each drug as a reinforcer of human behavior. In turn, the biologic response to drug exposure and each drug's efficacy as a reinforcer help to determine, in part,

[1]Dr. Helzer joined Dr. Anthony as coauthor for this chapter in the first edition of the textbook.

Textbook in Psychiatric Epidemiology, Second Edition, Edited by Ming T. Tsuang and Mauricio Tohen.
ISBN 0-471-40974-X

whether drug dependence or other drug problems will occur within populations of drug users. As we shall see, responses to drug exposure or self-administration include a profile of effects on presynaptic and postsynaptic signaling mechanisms, many of them involving dopamine and serotonin. These responses create an important articulation for recent and future epidemiological research on initiation of drug use and the risk of drug dependence syndromes.

Studying drug dependence epidemiology, investigators often have devised groups of drugs, or have designated a set of specific drug-related behaviors for special investigation. For example, much of the evidence presented in this chapter concerns a set of behaviors we have called "extra-medical drug use" (Anthony et al., 1994). As the name implies, this set includes drug-taking that occurs outside the boundaries of generally accepted medical practice. As a concept, "extra-medical drug use" encompasses the use of so-called illegal drugs such as heroin, marijuana (cannabis, hashish), and LSD, which are assigned by international agreement to Schedule I, the highest level of regulatory control reserved for drugs designated via international treaties and conventions as having no acceptable use in the practice of medicine. The concept of extramedical drug use also encompasses the illegal use of cocaine, morphine, and methadone, as well as other marketed pharmaceutical products such as OxyContin, all of which have been assigned to lower levels of regulatory control (Schedules II through V), because they are regarded as having acceptable use in medical practice. As measured, "extra-medical drug use" also encompasses the use of these pharmaceutical products for reasons or in a manner that goes beyond the bounds set by the prescriber's instructions, or beyond the limits of the package insert directions on proper use of nonprescription drugs in Schedule V, which may be purchased over-the-counter (OTC) and without a prescription.

In order to be clear about this broad set of drug-taking behaviors in epidemiological studies, the assessment of extra medical drug use generally includes specific questions on using prescription drugs "to get high," or "taking more than the doctor prescribed." In consequence, when the epidemiological research implements this concept of extra-medical drug use, it should be understood as more than "illegal drug use" because some of these behaviors are not actually violations of law. In addition, the concept does not encompass all use of prescription or OTC drugs listed in Schedules II through V. There are few epidemiological studies on the risk of becoming drug dependent when individual pharmaceutical products are used exactly as specified by a prescribing doctor. For reasons to be described in this chapter's section on assessment methods, there are special difficulties to be faced when standard epidemiological procedures are used to assess the risk of dependence after doctors have prescribed these drugs as medicines, and there are extraordinary difficulties when the context is that of forensic psychiatry.

Notwithstanding difficulties of this type, there is good reason to develop an epidemiology of drug dependence as it pertains to individual pharmaceutical products and to individual drugs such as marijuana, cocaine, methamphetamine and methylenedioxymethamphetamine. At the time of writing this chapter, there is intense public interest in the risks associated with using OxyContin, which is the analgesic drug oxycodone in a sustained release dosage formulation. American media reports on this drug describe an atypical epidemiological pattern of distribution, with outbreaks mainly east of the Mississippi River in small communities and rural areas often characterized as impoverished or with high levels of unemployment; this drug has not been as prominent in similarly disadvantaged urban or inner city areas, notwithstanding recent mentions of oxycodone in the National Institute on Drug Abuse (NIDA) Community Epidemiology Work Group findings (United States Department of Health and Human Services, 2001).

A different epidemiological pattern has been observed with respect to "ice" (the psychostimulant methamphetamine formulated for ease of heating, so that fumes may be inhaled by mouth or "smoked"). Supplied primarily by Asian drug traffickers, ice smoking outbreaks reached a peak on Guam and other Pacific Islands between 1986 and 1994. During the 1990s a combination of Asian and Latin American suppliers fueled outbreaks in southern California and the American Southwest until ice displaced cocaine as the primary drug of abuse for patients being admitted to drug treatment agencies in those areas of the United States. Subsequently, the manufacture of ice and the practice of ice smoking spread into the less metropolitan and rural communities of the American Midwest; outbreaks have been much less common east of the Mississippi. There is a completely separate epidemiology for methylenedioxymethamphetamine (MDMA), despite a chemical relationship to methamphetamine. A stimulant-hallucinogen, MDMA has appeared in epidemiological reports on youthful drug-taking on and off since the late 1960s, when it became known as a "love drug" or "Ecstasy" (e.g., see Anthony and Trinkoff, 1989). Recently, MDMA has resurfaced, often in connection with youth "raves," dance parties, and hip-hop clubs of urban communities, but with a more widespread distribution throughout North America and in both hemispheres —sometimes with focal points in isolated or rural areas selected and marketed as international tourist destinations (Schutz and Tancer, 2001).

Drug-specific variation of this type can make drug dependence epidemiology an especially fascinating branch of the biomedical sciences. This variation highlights a special role for anthropology, ethnography, and the other social sciences in drug dependence epidemiology, as compared to most other branches of psychiatric epidemiology and epidemiology when applied to health conditions of multifactorial origin (Trostle and Sommerfeld, 1996). Serious ethnographic studies can return data and information to communities to guide more formal surveillance operations and interventions in the early stages of these drug-taking outbreaks, before the public imagination is captured and misled by less rigorous eyewitness and journalistic accounts (Trostle and Sommerfeld, 1996; Agar, 1995). To the extent that the epidemiology of drug-taking is governed by drug product market structure and by pricing variations, contributions from the disciplines of economics and pharmacoeconomics are required (Manski et al., 2001). The person-to-person spread of new drug formulations (e.g., ice, OxyContin) or reintroduced drugs (e.g., Ecstasy) resembles more general social phenomena such as the diffusion of behavioral innovations, or "social contagion." For this reason, progress in drug dependence epidemiology requires a borrowing of principles, concepts, and methods developed in social psychology and the behaviorally oriented social sciences (e.g., Valente, 1999), as well as the tools of infectious disease epidemiology (e.g., see de Alarcon, 1985). As we shall see later in the chapter, there also has been useful borrowing from the domains of developmental science and educational research, from which longitudinal growth curve methodologies and multilevel methods have emerged. These methods have helped in epidemiological research on the developmental trajectories of youthful drug-taking (e.g., see Brook et al., 2000), and in multilevel research where the hypotheses cut across levels of organization from the neighborhood context down to the individual-level characteristics (e.g., see Petronis and Anthony, 2000).

Drug dependence epidemiology also has become more fascinating due to recent progress in bench science research, genetics, and clinical therapeutics. In epidemiological research on drug dependence problems completed almost 20 years ago, it was possible to estimate that approximately one in five extramedical drug users developed problems of clinical significance (Anthony and Helzer, 1991). Advances in neuroscience, molecular biology, pharmacology, and clinical therapeutics have clarified some of the differentiating neuroadaptational mechanisms that might help us to explain why some drug users make the transition from nondependent drug-taking and become drug dependent, and why there might be drug-to-drug variations in the transition probabilities (e.g., as summarized by Koob and LeMoal, 2001). This progress has necessitated close inspection of individual drug compounds and drug classes in epidemiological studies. It now is possible to offer drug-specific epidemiological estimates on transition probabilities from drug use to drug dependence. For example, in the United States, an estimated one in three tobacco smokers has developed tobacco dependence; an estimated one in six cocaine users has developed cocaine dependence; an estimated one in eleven marijuana users has developed marijuana dependence (Anthony et al., 1994).

Concurrently, research advances in behavior genetics and genetic epidemiology challenge us to consider a possibility that human genetic susceptibility to develop drug dependence is largely generic, cutting across essentially all drugs that function as reinforcers of human behavior, with drug-specific susceptibilities of lesser importance. To be sure, some findings from the genetics research are consistent with prior conceptualization of pharmacological classes (e.g., opioids, psychostimulants, sedative-hypnotics) or individual drugs (e.g., alcohol, tobacco, marijuana, cocaine). In addition, there are association and linkage studies, twin studies, adoptee studies, and research on familial aggregation that are focused upon individual drugs or drug groups (e.g., Uhl et al., 1992; Kendler and Prescott, 1998a, b; Newlin et al., 2000; Luthar et al., 1992a; Merikangas et al., 1998). Nonetheless, as will be discussed later in this chapter, there also are findings to suggest that alcohol, tobacco, marijuana, and cocaine dependence are manifestations of a common genetic susceptibility, with convergent epidemiological estimates of a substantial intercorrelation between these traits.

It now should be clear that mastery of drug dependence epidemiology poses some special challenges for students of psychiatric epidemiology specifically and for epidemiology in general, and often necessitates an appeal to advanced biostatistics and other branches of statistical methods. At the same time, drug dependence epidemiology is fascinating because of its reach from pharmacology, molecular genetics, and other sciences "of the bench" to ethnography, human genetics, and the other sciences "of the field." If it is successful, this chapter will provide an introduction to many of these challenges and will open many doors to this fascinating domain of epidemiological research.

A note about terminology may be in order. In the current edition of the textbook, this chapter has been rewritten to eliminate the use of the term "risk factor," always an element of epidemiological jargon, now a source of confusion when epidemiologists seek to communicate with scientists trained in other disciplines. Since we typically mean "suspected cause" when we speak of "risk factors," we should say what we mean. Hence, in the place of the term "risk factor," the reader will find alternative terms such as "causal influence," "suspected cause," and "suspected determinant of risk." When there is no reach toward causal inference, or when the exact nature of a possible causal relationship is uncertain, the terms "risk indicator" or "predictor" serve well.

The term "protective factor" has been dropped for similar reasons. The concept of protective factor sometimes has been specified as if it were simply an inverse risk factor (i.e., inversely associated with risk of disease). However, not too long ago, Sir Michael Rutter suggested a criterion for use of the term "protective factor"—namely, use of this term should be limited to contexts in which one condition or process is buffering the insalubrious effects of some other condition or process (e.g., see Rutter, 1991). This redefinition of protective factor creates its own problems, illustrated when we think about iodinized salt as protection against mental retardation (MR). What exactly is the risk-buffering interaction we would have to detect in order to evaluate the efficacy or effectiveness of iodinized salt in a trial to prevent MR? In theory, as a human species, we all suffer an iodine deficiency disease trait of genetic origin, expressed as MR when dietary iodine is below a threshold level, but we are not yet able to specify and measure the sites of genetic influence. Hence, the evidence from research to study iodine as a protective factor would not meet Sir Michael's criterion.

In the context of drug dependence epidemiology, one might think of Schedule II regulatory restrictions on methaqualone, a sedative-hypnotic medicine, as having had a protective influence with respect to the risk of methaqualone overdose; there is some evidence that overdose rates dropped not too long after methaqualone was assigned to Schedule II (Anthony, 1982). Thereafter, faced with declining sales, the licensed manufacturers of methaqualone decided to stop manufacturing and marketing the drug, partly due to burdens associated with Schedule II restrictions, and apparently also due to introduction and widespread marketing and sales of newer and less toxic sedative–hypnotic medicines such as flurazepam.

Similarly, there is a reduced risk of early onset drug use observed in relation to elevated levels of parental supervision and monitoring of 8–10 year old children (e.g., see Chilcoat and Anthony, 1996). Research to assess the possibly salubrious, protective effects of parental supervision and monitoring of children would not seem to require any interaction analysis.

DISTRIBUTION OF DRUG-RELATED PROBLEMS IN SPACE AND TIME

As was just mentioned in this chapter's Introduction, the epidemiologic study of individual drugs and drug classes reveals noteworthy variations in the global distribution of drug-related problems. Some relatively crude generalizations can be made on the basis of systematic reports to the World Health Organization and the United Nations, although recent estimates are not available for many parts of

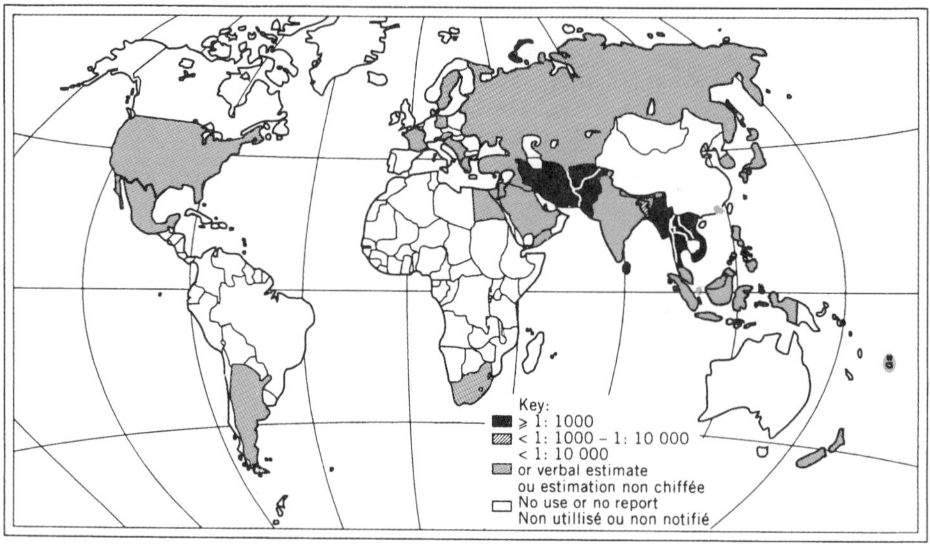

Map 1. Opium. (From Hughes et al., 1983.) *NOTE:* For Maps 1 to 7, the key shows countries in which the prevalence of active cases is estimated to be greater than or equal to 1 per 1,000 persons, less than 1 per 10,000 persons, or intermediate.

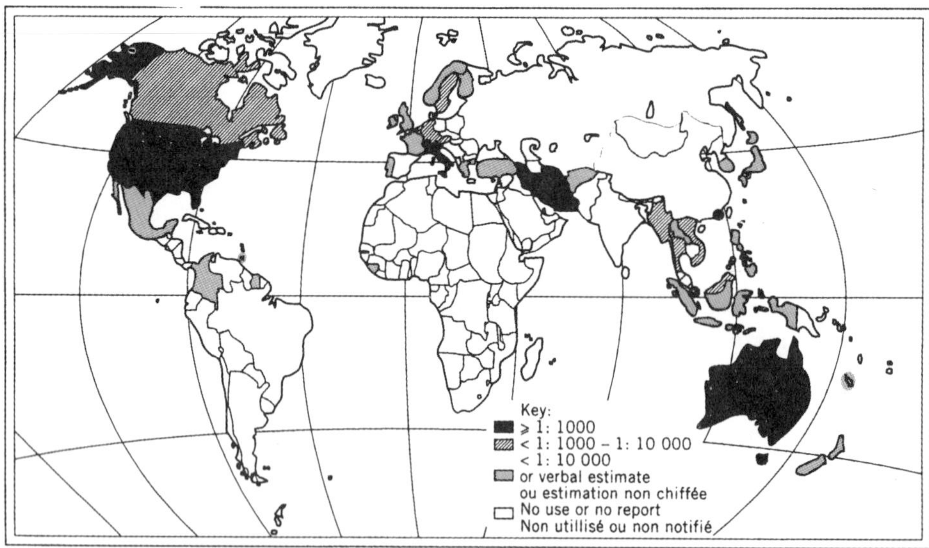

Map 2. Heroin. (from Hughes et al., 1983.)

the world, and there is no good compendium of statistics of the type compiled for alcoholic beverages (e.g., World Health Organization, 2000). Nonetheless, it has been observed that problems associated with use of opium traditionally have been observed more often in South and Southeast Asia, where opium poppy cultivation is widespread (see Map 1). Heroin is derived from the opium poppy, but heroin problems have had a substantially different global distribution (Map 2),

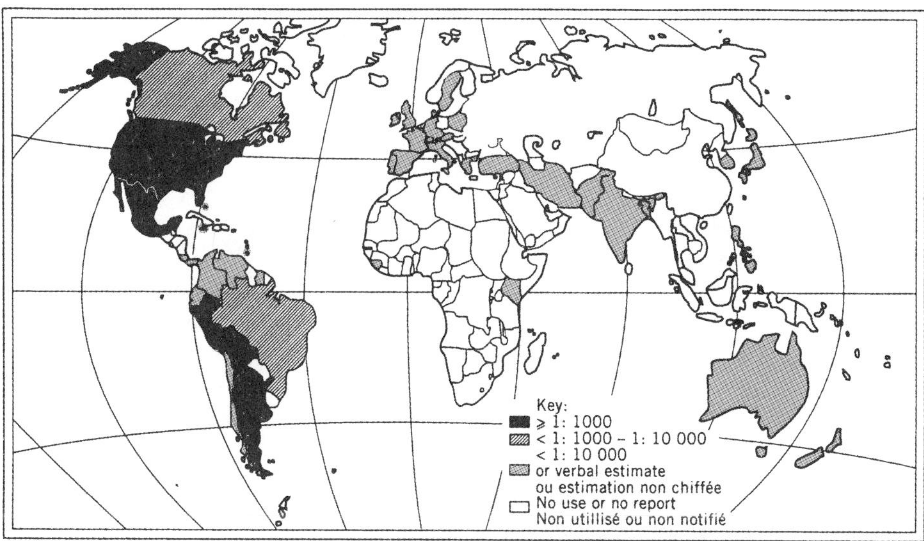

Map 3. Cocaine and other cocoa derivatives. (From Hughes et al., 1983.)

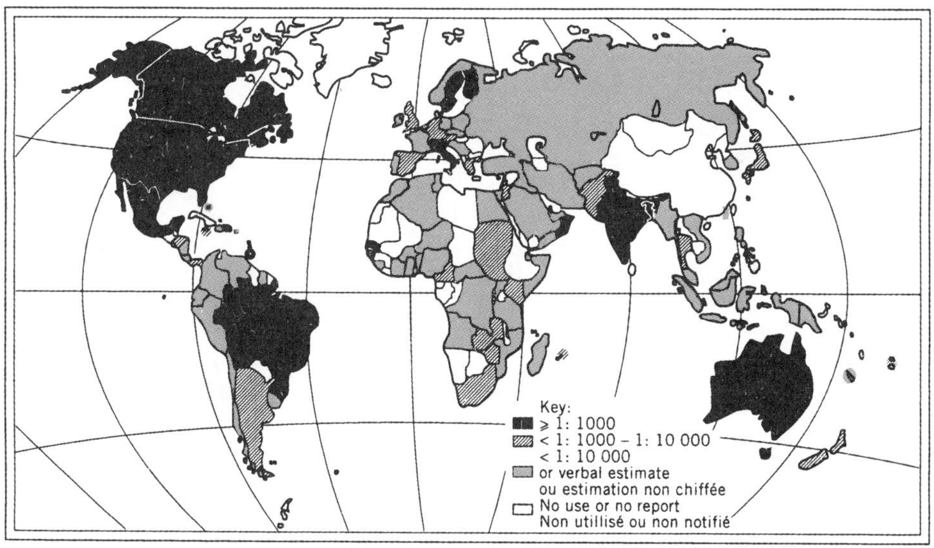

Map 4. Cannabis. (From Hughes et al., 1983.)

related more to sites where heroin is refined from opium or morphine and to lines of supply and distribution from the clandestine heroin laboratories (Hughes et al., 1983).

By studying global maps of human drug experience such as these (Maps 1–7), the scholar interested in drug dependence will be led toward fascinating accounts of historical epidemiology, which add to our understanding of how drug-related

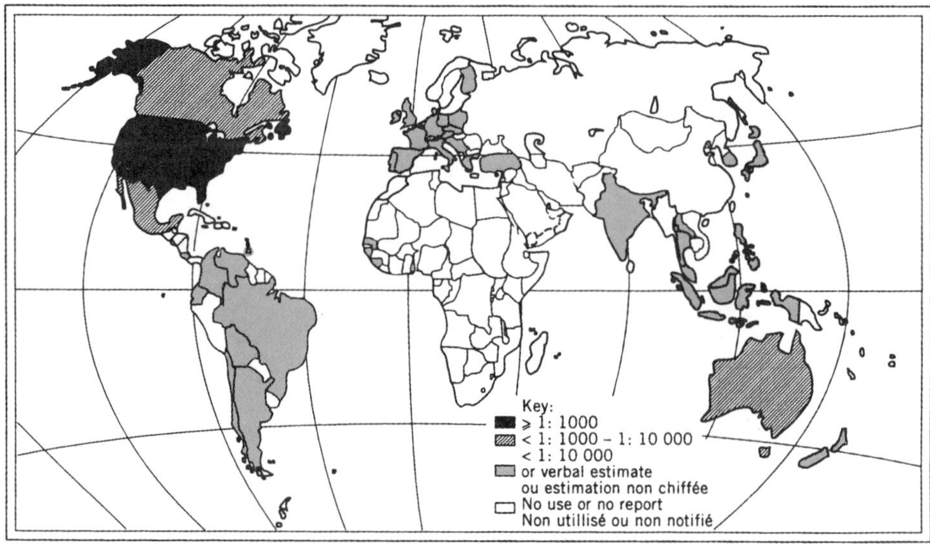

Map 5. Hallucinogens. (From Hughes et al., 1983.)

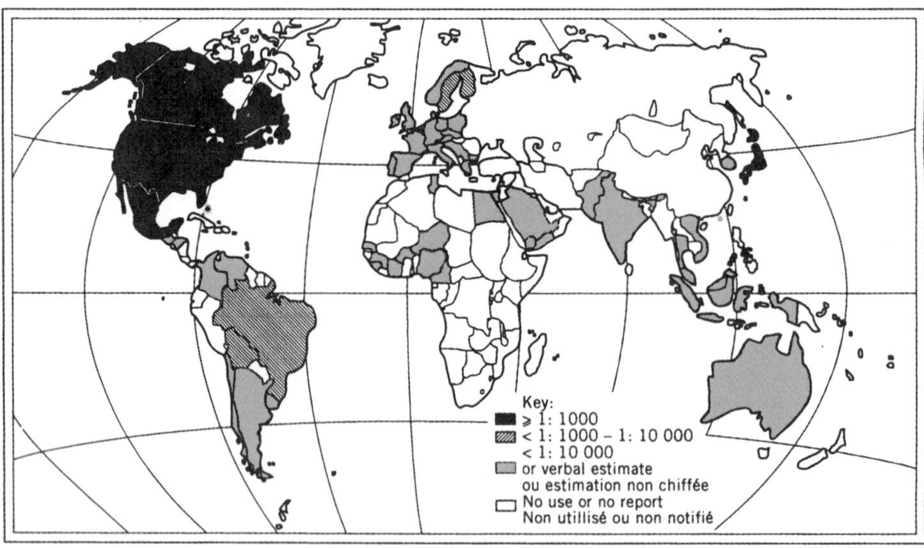

Map 6. Amphetamines. (From Hughes et al., 1983.)

problems are distributed in time as well as space (e.g., see Musto, 1987; Courtwright, 2001). For example, since the middle of the twentieth century, the people of Japan and the western Pacific seem to have been more affected by dependence on the psychostimulant amphetamine drugs than by other drugs, although in recent years problems associated with marijuana and other cannabis products (e.g., hashish) have become more prominent in Japan and elsewhere around the globe (Hughes

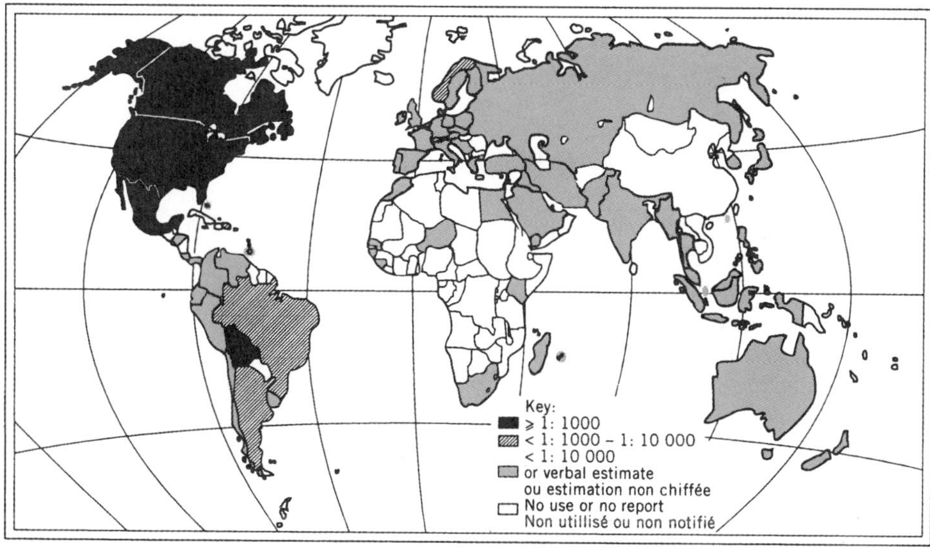

Map 7. Babituratures or other sedatives, and tranquilizers. (From Hughes et al., 1983)

TABLE 1. One-Year Interval Prevalence Estimates From the NIDA National Household Survey on Drug Abuse, Depicting the Recent Epidemic of Cocaine Use in the United States[a]

Year of Survey	Estimate for Persons Aged 12–17 Years	Estimate for Persons Aged 18–25 Years	Estimate for Persons Aged 26 Years and Older
1972	1.5	NA	NA
1974	2.7	8.1	< 0.5
1976	2.3	7.0	0.6
1977	2.6	10.2	0.9
1979	4.2	19.6	2.0
1982	4.1	18.8	3.8
1985	4.0	16.3	4.2
1988	2.9	12.1	2.7
1990	2.2	7.5	2.4
1991	1.5	7.7	NA
1992	1.1	6.3	NA

[a]Estimated prevalence of cocaine use in the past year (in percent) by year and age group at the time of the survey. Data are from the National Institute on Drug Abuse National Household Survey on Drug Abuse, 1972–1992.

et al., 1983). In the Americas, coca leaf chewing has been practiced for centuries, apparently with minimal health effects (Buck et al., 1968; Carroll, 1977). Nonetheless, after cocaine was extracted from the coca leaf in the 19th century, the U.S. population has experienced two epidemics of cocaine use and associated problems. The first American cocaine epidemic extended from the late nineteenth century into the early years of this century, and the second started in the mid-1970s, with a peak in the early 1980s, and a subsequent decline since then (Petersen, 1977;

Musto, 1990, 1991; Harrison, 1992; United States Substance Abuse and Mental Health Services, 1993, 2000). Table 1 illustrates the rise and fall of the second of these epidemics, 1972–1992.

PRESENTING CLINICAL FEATURES AND CASE DEFINITIONS

By comparison with typically more short-lived or acute problems such as drug intoxication, dependence on one of the internationally controlled drugs can be a chronic and debilitating mental and behavioral disorder (e.g., see Hser et al., 2001). Dependence almost always develops insidiously over a time course of months or years, part and parcel with repeated bouts of drug intoxication. In the largest available epidemiologic sample of cases with a history of drug dependence and/or drug abuse, the estimated median time from initial drug use to the initially recognized symptom was 23 years (Anthony and Helzer, 1991).

Our most recent epidemiological studies have suggested a substantial drug-specific variation in estimates of this type, as well as possible differences associated with studying the experience of different birth cohorts and different periods of time. As shown in Figure 1, with evidence from a nationally representative survey of 15–54 year old household residents in the United States, the estimated elapsed time from first extra-medical use until occurrence of dependence is substantially shorter for users of cocaine than for users of either alcohol or marijuana. Depicted in the inset figure for Figure 1, "instantaneous" risk of cocaine dependence peaked within 1–3 years after first cocaine use, whereas the peaks for alcohol and marijuana were later (Wagner and Anthony, in 2002a).

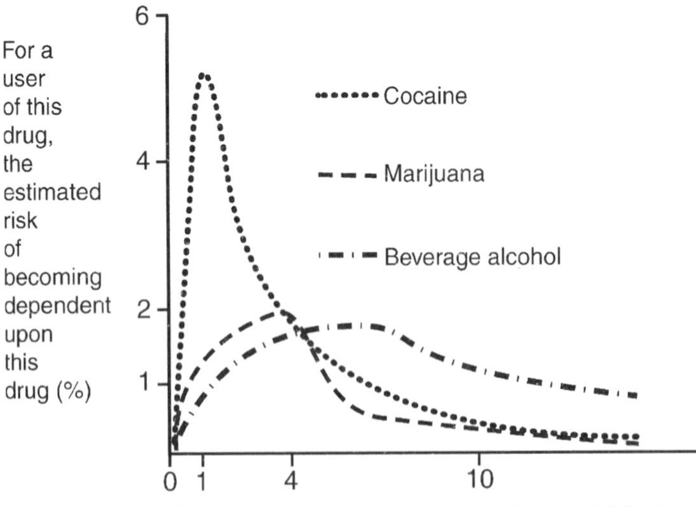

Figure 1. Estimated risk of developing DSM-III-R dependence upon cocaine, marijuana, and beverage alcohol, plotted in relation to the number of elapsed years since the age at first use of the drug. From data reported by Wagner and Anthony (2002a), based upon estimates from the National Comorbidity Survey, USA, 1990–92. (Reproduced with permission of copyright holder James C. Anthony, 2002).

Contemporary case definitions used in clinical practice and in this type of epidemiological research on drug dependence are based primarily on neuropsychopharmacologic criteria (e.g., tolerance and withdrawal) and on behavioral criteria (e.g., drug seeking and drug taking). In some instances, the case definitions also refer to social maladaptation secondary to drug use; some stress a subjectively felt compulsion to take the drug, a craving, or some other similar disturbance in the mental life that can be linked to drug use. When attempts have been made to distinguish drug dependence from drug abuse and harmful drug use this typically has been accomplished by restricting the latter to socially maladaptive or harm-causing drug use without the complications implied by neuropsychopharmacologic criteria or by subjectively felt compulsions and craving (World Health Organization, 1992; Babor, 1992).

The neuropsychopharmacologic criteria of central importance to the diagnosis of drug dependence involve neuroadaptation that occurs secondary to drug exposure. Some aspects of neuroadaptation can be documented very early in the drug dependence process; for example, a pharmacologic tolerance is manifest by change in the slopes or intercepts of dose response curves upon repeated drug exposures. Other signs of neuroadaptation, such as the appearance of a drug withdrawal syndrome, are not readily apparent as clinical phenomena unless the drug dependence process is challenged by (1) administration of antagonists, such as the opioid antagonist naloxone in the case of dependence on heroin or other opioids, or (2) an abrupt reduction in dosage or a complete cessation of drug use after drug taking has been sustained for days or weeks.

In some cases, withdrawal symptoms appear several times daily and serve as a forerunner for subsequent drug-seeking and drug-taking behavior that can relieve the withdrawal symptoms for a time. In other cases, withdrawal symptoms are mild and infrequent and may escape clinical detection unless the drug-dependent patient is challenged under restrictive conditions.

Going beyond neuroadaptation, drug seeking and drug taking are represented among the criteria of drug dependence that tap its behavioral dimensions. Consistent with a description of the alcohol dependence syndrome first stated by Edwards and Gross (1976), these behavioral manifestations of drug dependence can be grouped under headings such as "salience" and "withdrawal avoidance." Salience of drug seeking or drug taking occurs together with the increasing time demands associated with drug use, concurrent with reduced commitment to social, occupational, and recreational activities and sometimes to a general narrowing in the behavioral repertoire unconnected to drug taking. Withdrawal avoidance implies drug taking in order to prevent or reduce the severity of drug withdrawal symptoms.

There is not yet a universal consensus that a subjectively felt compulsion to take a drug should be included as a *sine qua non* criterion in drug dependence case definitions. Nonetheless, this disturbance of the mental life has become prominent in some of the newer case definitions and diagnostic criteria for drug dependence. Neither compulsions to take drugs nor drug cravings were represented in dependence criteria written for the 1980 *Diagnostic and Statistical Manual of Mental Disorders*, 3rd ed (DSM-III; American Psychiatric Association, 1980). As shown in Table 2, drug-related desires and/or compulsions appeared in diagnostic guidelines written for the *International Classification of Disease*, 10th rev (ICD-10; World

TABLE 2. DSM-III-R and ICD-10 Case Definitions

DSM-III-R

Diagnostic criteria for psychoactive substance dependence

A. At least three of the following:
1. Substance often taken in larger amounts or over a longer period than the person intended.
2. Persistent desire or one or more unsuccessful efforts to cut down or control substance use.
3. A great deal of time spent in activities necessary to get the substance (e.g., theft), taking the substance (e.g., chain smoking), or recovering from its effects.
4. Frequent intoxication or withdrawal symptoms when expected to fulfill major role obligations at work, school, or home [e.g., does not go to work because hung over, goes to school or work "high," intoxicated while taking care of his or her children or when substance use is physically hazardous (e.g., drives when intoxicated].
5. Important social, occupational, or recreational activities given up or reduced because of substance use.
6. Continued substance use despite knowledge of having a persistent or recurrent social, psychological, or physical problem that is caused or exacerbated by the use of the substance (e.g., keeps using heroin despite family arguments about it, cocaine-induced depression, or having an ulcer made worse by drinking).
7. Marked tolerance: need for markedly increased amounts of the substance (i.e., at least 50% increase) in order to achieve intoxication or desired effort, or markedly diminished effect with continued use of the same amount.

Note: The following items may not apply to cannabis, hallucinogens, or phencyclidine (PCP):

8. Characteristic withdrawal symptoms (see specific withdrawal syndromes under Psychoactive Substance-Induced Organic Mental Disorders).
9. Substance often taken to relieve or avoid withdrawal symptoms.

B. Some symptoms of the disturbance have persisted for at least 1 month or have occurred repeatedly over a longer period of time.

Diagnostic criteria for psychoactive substance abuse

A. A maladaptive pattern of psychoactive substance use indicated by at least one of the following:
1. Continued use despite knowledge of having a persistent or recurrent social, occupational, psychological, or physical problem that is caused or exacerbated by use of the psychoactive substance
2. Recurrent use in situations in which use is physically hazardous (e.g., driving while intoxicated).

B. Some symptoms of the disturbance have persisted for at least 1 month or have occurred over a longer period of time.

C. Never met the criteria for Psychoactive Substance Dependence for this substance.

ICD-10

Diagnostic guidlines for the dependence syndrome due to psychoactive drug use

A definite diagnosis of dependence should usually be made only if three or more of the following have been experienced or exhibited at some time during the period year:

A. A strong desire or sense of compulsion to take the substance.

TABLE 2. (*Continued*)

ICD-I0

Diagnostic guidlines for the dependence syndrome due to psychoactive drug use

B. Difficulties in controlling substance-taking behavior in terms of its onset, termination, or levels of use.
C. A physiological withdrawal state when substance use has ceased or been reduced, as evidenced by the characteristic withdrawal syndrome for the substance or use of the same (or a closely related) substance with the intention of relieving or avoiding withdrawal symptoms.
D. Evidence of tolerance, such that increased doses of the psychoactive substance are required in order to achieve effects originally produced by lower doses.
E. Progressive neglect of alternative pleasures or interests because of psychoactive substance use; increased amount of time necessary to obtain or take the substance or to recover from its effects.
F. Persisting with substance use despite clear evidence of overtly harmful consequences, such as harm to the liver through excessive drinking, depressive mood states consequent to periods of heavy substance use, or drug-related impairment of cognitive functioning: efforts should be made to determine that the user was actually, or could be expected to be, aware of the nature and extent of the harm.

Source: American Psychiatric Association, 1987; World Health Organization, 1992.

Health Organization, 1992), in the revised DSM-III known as DSM-III-R (American Psychiatric Association, 1987), and in the DSM-IV (American Psychiatric Association, 1990).

Careful study of the diagnostic guidelines and criteria in Table 2, with comparison to DSM-III and earlier criteria, will be repaid by a greater appreciation for how drug dependence case definitions are changing. The observable variations in these several diagnostic systems emerged over a span of less than 20 years.

The history of the concept of opioid dependence suggests that we should expect continual refinement of the drug dependence diagnostic criteria for many years to come and possibly some radical changes coincident with new findings from laboratory, clinical, or epidemiologic studies. Emerging originally from primitive concepts of customs, habit, and addiction as a moral enslavement or a defect of human will, these contemporary case definitions now are among the accumulated results of more than 40 years of work by the World Health Organization's Expert Committee on Drug Dependence, by task panels organized for DSM-III, DSM-III-R, and DSM-IV, and by others. Until strengthened by a more confirmatory body of empirical evidence, the criteria most likely will continue to be changed every half-decade or so (e.g., see Sonnedecker, 1962; Eddy et al., 1965; Musto, 1987; Kosten and Kosten, 1991; Woody et al., 1993).

Of course, continual change in the drug dependence case definitions tends to complicate research progress in this field. For example, in the United States, the first of our largest and most definitive epidemiologic studies of drug dependence was the National Institute of Mental Health Epidemiologic Catchment Area (ECA) surveys, with fieldwork conducted between 1980 and 1985, followed by the

National Comorbidity Survey and the National Longitudinal Alcohol Epidemiology Study (NLAES), conducted in the early 1990s. The ECA Program was a multisite collaborative study, with an aggregate sample that included almost 20,000 interviewed respondents aged 18–96 years, selected by probability sampling from households, prisons, mental hospitals, and other institutions and group quarters. The ECA Program was the first to provide epidemiologic findings based on the DSM criteria for drug dependence as implemented by the Diagnostic Interview Schedule (DIS) method, which combined assessments by standardized interview with computer-assisted diagnostic procedures (Robins et al., 1985; Anthony and Helzer, 1991).

In contrast, the National Comorbidity Survey (NCS) and the NLAES involved large national probability samples. To illustrate the scale of the research, the NCS sample included 8,098 respondents 15–54 years of age, selected by probability sampling of household residents. The NCS assessment plan made use of a DIS-like method known as the Composite International Diagnostic Interview (CIDI), with standardized interview items and a computer program based on diagnostic criteria from DSM-III-R (Kessler et al., 1994). The NLAES also drew participants by probability sampling and used a related field survey diagnostic method (e.g., see Grant, 1996).

According to results from population surveys in the five ECA sites, cocaine dependence was nonexistent among American adults in the early 1980s. By comparison, findings from the NCS showed that an estimated 2.7% of Americans aged 15–54 years qualified as currently active or former cases of cocaine dependence. While it is plausible that the prevalence of cocaine dependence actually increased between 1985 and 1990, concurrent with declines in the recent American epidemic of cocaine experimentation, this difference in findings from the two surveys is attributable entirely to a change in the drug dependence case definitions. The DSM-III did not include a category of cocaine dependence, and this by itself explains why no cases were detected or reported in the ECA survey.

However, the DSM-III-R had adopted a diagnostic category for cocaine dependence. When the NCS applied this case definition, some cocaine users were found to have become affected by this newly recognized form of drug dependence. This recent experience serves to illustrate that between-study comparisons depend heavily on constancy or at least rough similarity in case definitions and in the manner of making case definitions operational in each study's assessment plan (Anthony et al., 1994).

CASE ASCERTAINMENT METHODS

There are many possible approaches to the clinical assessment of drug problems among adolescents and adults (e.g., see U.S. Department of Health and Human Services, 1994), but the ECA and NCS initiatives offer a good example of contemporary practice in epidemiologic studies of drug dependence. These studies now rely for the most part on interview-administered standardized questions on the manifestations of drug dependence. Sometimes computer-assisted interviewing takes place after an field staff member has introduced the study, developed some trust and rapport with the individual respondent, and provided instructions to get the respondent started with the computer (U.S. Substance Abuse and Mental Health Services, 2000). In general, the standardized questions in these field survey diagnostic assessments are directed toward the individual respondent, with no attempt to augment the information base by gathering data from collateral informants (e.g., spouses, supervisors, coworkers) or by drawing biologic specimens to test for recent drug exposure.

For clinicians familiar with denial of drug-related problems and other complicating features of drug dependence, this method of assessment may seem to leave something to be desired, and the problem of false-negative assessments of drug dependence has been a preoccupation in epidemiological circles for many years (e.g., see Anthony et al., 2000). Nonetheless, it is important to recognize that denial can be a fluctuating clinical characteristic of drug dependence, perhaps most readily apparent in clinical or judicial proceedings that provide the suspected case with no shelter from self-incrimination. In contemporary epidemiologic studies such as the ECA surveys, the NCS, and the NLAES, the investigators made special efforts to develop a respondent's trust and rapport *before* broaching sensitive topics of illicit behavior, and they provided special assurances of confidentiality so that the respondents would be protected from harm that otherwise might come from self-disclosure of drug dependence (e.g., see Robins, 1983; Eaton et al., 1984; Johnston, 1985; Anthony et al., 1994, 2000).

The actual translation of diagnostic criteria for drug dependence into standardized interview questions for case ascertainment and diagnosis is a topic of several papers (Boyd et al., 1985; Anthony and Helzer, 1991). The underlying concept is a simple one that can be illustrated without difficulty by considering the example of pharmacologic tolerance.

When the DIS and DSM criteria ask for evidence that pharmacologic tolerance has developed, the DIS and CIDI seek the respondents' answers to standardized questions such as the following:

DIS: Did you find you needed larger amounts of these drugs to get an effect or that you could no longer get high on the amount you used to use?

CIDI: Did you ever find that you had to use more drug than usual to get the same effect or that the same amount had less effect on you than before?

Once the answers to questions of this type have been entered into an electronic database, the diagnostic computer program checks the respondent's data record and counts an affirmative answer toward the tolerance criterion of the dependence diagnosis. A corresponding process is followed for each of the diagnostic criteria for drug dependence; respondents who meet the required criteria are designated as cases, and all others are designated as noncases.

There is universal agreement that we need more studies on the reliability and validity of this form of standardized drug dependence diagnosis. Nevertheless, to date, the result of this approach to assessment in epidemiologic field studies has been a set of alcohol and drug dependence diagnoses with levels of reliability and validity that are appreciably better than corresponding diagnoses for other categories of mental disorders (e.g., see Anthony et al., 1985; Helzer, 1985; Wittchen, 1996; Prusoff et al., 1988; Lagenbucher et al., 1994; Shillington et al., 1995; Wittchen et al., 1989, 1998; Wittchen et al., 1999; Shillington and Clapp, 2000).

In relation to the issue of diagnostic validity, it is important to remember that individuals can be drug dependent even when bioassays show no recent drug exposure, to the extent that symptoms such as compulsion to take a drug remain present for some time after drug use. It also is important to remember that many individuals who test positive for recent drug use would not qualify as cases of drug dependence: many drug users are not drug dependent (Anthony et al., 1994). For these reasons, drug dependence is evaluated on clinical grounds, and the validity of drug dependence diagnoses does not depend on agreement between a bioassay for recent drug use versus a clinical diagnosis of drug dependence.

There are some conditions under which the validity of diagnostic assessments for drug dependence might be compromised, and three examples of these conditions will be mentioned here. First, in the context of forensic psychiatry or in criminal justice research, there are special problems. On one side, we may have a defendant about to be found guilty or sentenced to a prison for a crime. In this context, we may expect some failure of our standard clinical and epidemiological survey diagnostic procedures for drug dependence. Many prisoners believe, perhaps correctly, that the drug dependence diagnosis is a mitigating circumstance. If they report experiencing the clinical features of drug dependence, the judicial consequences might be more to their liking—such as a judge's decision of 'probation before judgment' rather than a felony conviction, or referral to a residential drug treatment program as opposed to sentencing to prison time. On another side, we may have a patient as plaintiff, making a claim of medical malpractice or negligence, with either a prescribing doctor as defendant, the pharmaceutical manufacturing company as defendant, or both. This is another context in which our standard clinical and epidemiological survey diagnostic procedures can fail, with the plaintiff claiming to have experienced clinical features of drug dependence when the condition of drug dependence never has existed in actual fact.

In the context of forensic psychiatry and criminal justice research, there is good reason to be suspicious about the validity of standard diagnostic procedures that are used routinely in clinical and epidemiological studies. Some degree of cross-examination and ancillary investigation by a well-trained, broadly experienced, and highly qualified diagnostician is required. Anthony et al. (1985) introduced the logic for a cross-examination strategy that can be used to strengthen standard procedures, and provided examples of information obtained when a well-trained diagnostician is allowed to cross examine during the course of diagnostic assessments. However, even with detailed cross-examination and ancillary investigations, it may be difficult or impossible to identify an individual who falsely claims to have become drug dependent. Some of the above-mentioned advances in neuroscience have included neuroimaging findings that correlate with subjectively experienced craving for drug use (e.g., see Childress et al., 2000) and separate correlations when research subjects are engaged in deception (Langleben et al., 2000). Nonetheless, these neuroimaging procedures have uncertain sensitivity and specificity as diagnostic assessments for drug dependence. In the final analysis, if prisoners or patients feel that something is to be gained by an exaggeration of their cravings or other subjectively felt clinical features of drug dependence, we have no certain diagnostic procedure that will identify this source of a falsely positive diagnosis. In many branches of medicine, there are more definitive procedures with essentially no reliance upon self-reporting of the clinical features (e.g., glucose tolerance assays for diabetes). Drug dependence is more akin to other psychiatric disturbances for which there is no such procedure (e.g., post-traumatic stress disorder), and we must rely heavily upon self-report (Anthony et al., 2000).

Another context provides an additional example of possible invalidity of standard diagnostic assessments of drug dependence under field survey conditions, and draws upon the perspectives of developmental psychopathology. The context is that of comparative epidemiological research in which the goal is to compare and contrast age-specific or development-specific estimates of the prevalence or risk of becoming drug dependent. For example, in several studies during the 1990s, we found some evidence that adolescents are at increased risk of being or becoming dependent upon marijuana, once marijuana use starts, as compared to marijuana users who are young adults or middle age (e.g., see Anthony et al., 1994; Kandel et al., 1997; United States, 1999). This comparison rests upon two important assumptions: (1) the phenomenological form and content of marijuana dependence is the same for adolescents and adults, with no complications of 'age-appropriateness' or 'symptom equivalence' in diagnosis, of a type seen in relation to the mood disorders (e.g., see Angold and Costello, 1995); and (2) there is no special overreporting or underreporting of clinical features of marijuana dependence for adolescents versus the other adult marijuana users. However, there now is evidence of possible overreporting of the clinical features of marijuana dependence by adolescent recent-onset marijuana users versus adult recent-onset marijuana users, when an abbreviated DIS-like diagnostic assessment was used in our most recent nationally representative epidemiological surveys of drug dependence, conducted between 1995 and 1998. That is, in this comparison of adolescents and adults who had recently started to use marijuana during the mid-to-late 1990s, with multivariate response models used to hold constant the levels of marijuana dependence and the cumulative number of occasions of marijuana use, the adolescent users were more likely to report clinical features of marijuana dependence such as self-reported pharmacological tolerance and an inability to cut down on marijuana use when reductions in use had been attempted. Even with a constraint on the possible occurrence of marijuana-related toxicity (i.e., by restricting these analyses to adolescents and adults who had used marijuana just one or two times), adolescent users were more likely to report clinical features of marijuana dependence during this epidemiological field survey's diagnostic assessment (Chen and Anthony, in press for 2002).

Methodological research of this type demonstrates some of the special challenges faced when epidemiologists must rely upon diagnostic assessments that can differ in validity across subgroups under study. The contexts of forensic psychiatry and criminal justice research also pose special challenges. These challenges do not constitute a complete invalidation of inferences to be drawn when we use field survey diagnostic procedures. Indeed, in the methodological study of marijuana dependence, the multivariate response model provided evidence that adolescent marijuana users had higher levels of marijuana dependence than adult marijuana users, even when possible adolescent overreporting of clinical features was taken into account (Chen and Anthony, in press for 2002). Nevertheless, there is need for additional methodological research on these diagnostic procedures, with an expectation of refinements over time, perhaps with improvements based upon some of the newer experience sampling methods and computerized adaptive testing (Anthony et al., 2000).

Some epidemiology readers may be surprised at this field's emphasis upon epidemiological field surveys, and might ask why the chapter gives short shrift to studies based upon hospital records or cases seeking treatment. The answer is that there actually are useful epidemiological studies based on hospital records and registries of cases seeking treatment or who have been apprehended by the police authorities. For example, Robertson and Bucknall (1985) have described characteristics of the heroin users brought to the attention of the United Kingdom's registry; Vaillant (1966) described the clinical course and medical problems experienced by recognized cases; Hser et al. (2001) recently described the experiences of heroin users who first were identified during the course of treatment or rehabilitation for opioid problems. Shapiro et al. (1975) estimated the risks of developing drug dependence problems after hospitalized patients received controlled opioid drugs. However, there is good reason to believe that the officially recognized cases are just the tip of the iceberg, so to speak; many cases of drug dependence never have become officially recognized in health or criminal justice agency statistics (e.g., see Anthony and Helzer, 1991). Plus, there is good reason to suspect that there are important transition biases that influence which drug users or drug dependence cases come to the attention of the medical or criminal justice authorities. This problem will be discussed later in this chapter under the heading of "Race as a Possible Causal Determinant of Drug Dependence."

PATHOGENESIS, NATURAL HISTORY, AND CLINICAL COURSE OF DRUG DEPENDENCE

There now are several competing conceptual models for the pathogenesis of drug dependence and its natural history, as well as for the clinical course of drug dependence, which is natural history modified by one or more clinical interventions intended to be more than palliative in character. The "Jellinek curve" with its notion of "bottoming out" was among the first of these conceptions—a concept applied originally to alcohol, with later extension to other drugs (e.g., in Narcotics Anonymous self-help groups). Many investigators have ignored drug dependence or studied it as if the dependence phenomenon were more or less an extension of the initial levels of drug involvement, for example, by counting up the numbers of occasions of illegal drug use: the more the number of occasions, the greater the level of drug involvement, with no incorporation of clinical features of drug dependence such as salience, tolerance, or withdrawal states as described above (e.g., see Brook et al., 2000a, b).

Many clinically oriented investigators have become dissatisfied with this conception, and first offered an alternative model that emphasized transitions, such as the transition from nonuse to first use, the transition from first use to first problem, and the transition from first use to a formal diagnosis of drug dependence (e.g., see Helzer, 1985; Anthony and Helzer, 1991). One advantage of this initial "transitions" model is that it is true to the discrete character of the different stages of drug-related experiences: either a person has had a chance to try a drug, or has not; either a person has tried a drug or has not, has developed a drug problem or has not, and so on. One disadvantage of the initial transitions model was that it ignored the dimensional character of progressions within each stage. For example, for many individuals, the initial drug-taking experience is followed by an increasing number of drug-taking occasions before the threshold of formal clinical diagnosis is crossed. Once the clinical threshold is crossed, the drug dependent individual may or may not progress toward more serious drug involvement.

Dissatisfaction with the initial transitions–progression model produced a hybrid transitions–progressions model described by Anthony (1999): "At a very simplistic level, we can decompose the process or causal mechanisms for becoming drug dependent into a linked sequence of stages or transitions, with intermediate dimensional progression within these stages." Leshner (2001) has characterized this type of conceptualization as a "canal lock" model, with each stage-transition in correspondence with a new lock, and with progression within each stage or lock of the canal. A "downward spiral" model offered by Koob and Le Moal (2001) resonates with the "bottoming out" facet of Jellinek's curve, is limited because the model fails to acknowledge that many individuals have opportunities to try drugs but never do so, but is attractive because it seeks to integrate a large body of evidence from laboratory, clinical, and epidemiological studies on changes in cognitive preoccupations, frequency of binge intoxication, reward processes, mood dysregulation, and neuroadaptation in accompaniment with the start of drug taking and later experience of clinical features of withdrawal states.

No matter which conceptual model is chosen, drug dependence will not occur, and the full syndrome of drug dependence cannot persist, in the complete absence of a drug. For this reason, it makes sense to think of each drug as an important etiologic agent in relation to the occurrence of dependence on that drug. Analogous to an agent of infectious disease that must be conveyed from its reservoir of origin toward effective contact with a human host, a drug must be conveyed to its users from the point or points of origin, which might include agricultural fields (e.g., for marijuana, opium poppy, or coca leaf) as well as chemistry laboratories (e.g., for a barbiturate sedative–hypnotic or for methamphetamine). Humans are the vectors that bring drugs out of their reservoirs and into contact with drug users (e.g., see Anthony, 1983); once drug taking begins, there is person-to-person diffusion of drug-taking behavior and drug dependence (e.g., see de Alarcon, 1969; Hanzi, 1976).

Working from the reservoir of drug supply toward the clinical case of drug dependence, it is possible to identify moments or intervals of exposure opportunity before which there is no chance of drug dependence. Here, the "exposure opportunity" for drug involvement is analogous to the same concept Wade Hampton Frost described in relation to his theory of infectious disease epidemiology (Frost, 1927). For many individuals, drug exposure opportunities are presented by members of their peer groups, and in theory, exposure opportunity may be determined in part by an individual's sex or gender (Van Etten et al., 1997), race, region of residence, urban–rural residence (Van Etten and Anthony, 2001), social class, level of paternal alcohol consumption, history of childhood misbehavior (e.g., truancy) or aggressiveness (Rosenberg and Anthony, 2001a), low emotional control, and patterns of social interactions with peers and others. It follows that effective prevention and control of drug dependence depend in part on regulation of exposure opportunities and by attention to the determinants of these exposure opportunities (e.g., see Hawkins et al., 1992; Stenbacka et al., 1993; Crum et al., 1994; Van Etten et al., 1997; Wagner and Anthony, 2002b).

Observations about "steppingstone" and "gateway" associations in adolescent drug involvement (e.g., Kandel et al., 1992) also can be linked to the concept of drug exposure opportunity. O'Donnell speculated about the contribution of tobacco, alcohol, and marijuana use to later use of cocaine, heroin, and other drugs, as follows:

> Cigarette and alcohol use, *by mechanisms not considered*, contribute to marijuana use. Marijuana use, in turn, is one of the causes of further nonmedical drug use.... One of the mechanisms by which this probably occurs is that continued use of marijuana, especially heavy use, makes more probable contact with drug sellers and the drug subculture to assure a continuous supply. This contact in some cases leads to friendship with users of other drugs, which, in turn, increases the probability of using other drugs. (O'Donnell, 1985)

Seeking to understand the development of increasing drug involvement, Wagner and Anthony (2002b) have tried to address mechanisms not considered by O'Donnell. As explained in their study of the "gateway" phenomenon,

> Simply put, the idea is that young people using alcohol or tobacco are more likely to be offered a chance to try marijuana, or to face some other form of "marijuana exposure opportunity" at home or within a peer group setting. In addition, as an elaboration of the trajectory, marijuana smokers might be more likely to have chances to try cocaine in similar settings, as compared to youths who do not smoke marijuana.
>
> A separate idea about mechanisms takes exposure opportunity as a given: once the "marijuana exposure opportunity" has occurred, alcohol or tobacco users are more likely to actually use marijuana, as compared to youths who have not started to smoke tobacco or use alcohol. Next in sequence, once the "cocaine exposure opportunity" has occurred, a marijuana-smoking young person is more likely to actually use cocaine (Wagner and Anthony, 2002b).

These recent observations are consistent with the idea that once an exposure opportunity has occurred, drug dependence cannot develop unless there is an effective contact manifest in some form of biologic response—for example, a drug intoxication state. As in the case of infective agents, effective contact with a drug also can be measured in the form of immune response to antigen. Current molecular biologic research supported by the National Institute on Drug Abuse and others holds promise for future development of improved immunoassays for drug exposure as well as possible immunizing agents that might modulate biologic responsivity once drug exposure occurs (e.g., see Landry et al., 1993; Kosten et al. 2000).

A single effective contact is not sufficient for the development of drug dependence, and many drug users do not become drug dependent, as illustrated in Figure 1 of this chapter. Typically, drug dependence does not develop unless there are repeated bouts of drug intoxication over a span of days or weeks, signifying multiple effective contacts. The reinforcing function of drug taking may become apparent as early as the second occurrence of effective contact; multiple bouts of drug intoxication may serve as an indicator of the reinforcing efficacy of drug use.

However, differences in availability of individual drugs can determine the frequency and duration of their use, notwithstanding a broad contrast in the laboratory evidence on relative reinforcement potential of these drugs. For example, in laboratory research it has been difficult to show that marijuana smoking is a powerful reinforcer; not so for cocaine (e.g., see Pickens et al., 1973). Nonetheless, in the United States, persistent marijuana users have outnumbered persistent cocaine users for more than two decades, most likely due to generally greater availability of marijuana (e.g., see Kandel, 1991, Kandel et al., 1992; Harrison, 1992, United States Substance Abuse and Mental Health Services, 2000).

Neuroadaptation and the clinical features of drug dependence develop during the course of repeated bouts of drug intoxication. Whereas the diagnostic criteria and case definitions often imply a clear transition point before and after drug dependence, the more general experience is consistent with an insidious onset and there is no clear first episode of drug dependence, as is true for many other medical conditions (Beiser et al., 1993). For this reason, an incident case of drug dependence is one who is found upon assessment to meet the diagnostic criteria, against a background history of one or more prior assessments when full criteria have not been met (Eaton et al., 1989; Wagner and Anthony, 2002a).

In general, retrospective data cannot give a clear or distinct impression of when criteria were met for the first time, and prospective data on the timing of a first episode are no more fine-grained than the interval from one observation to the next. In this respect, drug dependence is no different from many other diseases with insidious onset that are studied routinely by epidemiologists. Research progress must be made by specifying sometimes arbitrary rules about when to date the age or time of initial onset, and age at first diagnosis sometimes is the only possibility, as discussed by Wagner and Anthony (2002a).

Notwithstanding some notable exceptions (e.g., Chen and Kandel, 1995), most of the scientific and clinical literature on the natural history of drug dependence actually concerns its clinical course in that the literature draws heavily on the experience of cases who have been treated or incarcerated with an intent to change the nature of the individual's drug dependence status rather than merely to provide temporary palliative relief (e.g., see Vaillant, 1966; Sells, 1977; McGlothlin, 1985; Anglin et al., 1986; Nurco et al., 1989; Hser et al., 2001). The result can be a distorted view of what happens in nature when drug dependence is left without intervention, as often has been the case (e.g., see Smart, 1977; Anthony and Helzer, 1991; Robins, 1993).

The clinical course of drug dependence is its natural history modified by one or more experiences of clinical intervention, where the goal is more than palliative care. Under these circumstances, the course generally is portrayed as chronic and with few lasting remissions: relapse is said to be the rule rather than the exception. Often, the course is complicated by legal problems connected to drug seeking or drug taking, as well as intervals of incarceration within the criminal justice system (e.g., see Haastrup, 1973; Nurco et al., 1989; Hser et al., 2001).

Mortality rates for drug-dependent cases have been observed to exceed those of age-matched controls, even when differences in gender and social class are taken into account. Although drug dependence is allowable as a recognized cause of death, many drug-dependent individuals die prematurely from other proximal causes, such as homicide, suicide, opportunistic infections secondary to drug injection practices, and drug overdosage (e.g., see Sapira et al., 1970; Sells, 1977;

Neumark et al., 2000; Rosenberg and Anthony, 2001a, b). Of course, many of these premature deaths might be prevented if drug dependence were to be recognized, kept under medical surveillance, and treated as a chronic medical condition.

Given the overwhelming impression of a serious and chronic condition that does not respond well to treatment or to changes in environmental conditions, the experience of Vietnam veterans returning to the United States is noteworthy and deserves careful scrutiny (e.g., see Robins, 1977; 1993; Helzer, 1985). Consistent with evidence from recent epidemiologic surveys in the United States (e.g., see Anthony and Helzer, 1991; Anthony et al., 1994), the experience of these soldiers seems to suggest that it was relatively common to become drug dependent and then to return to nondependent periods of abstinence, without treatment. One of the pressing items on the research agenda for drug dependence is to clarify this difference between findings on the clinical course of drug dependence based on studies of treated or incarcerated cases versus findings on its natural history based on both treated and untreated cases.

THE OCCURRENCE AND FREQUENCY OF DRUG DEPENDENCE

In common with most mental disorders, drug dependence takes its toll during life and leaves very little trace after death. For this reason, mortality rates based on deaths attributed to drug dependence are an unstable foundation for epidemiologic inferences, and with no more than a few exceptions epidemiologists generally have turned to the field survey method in order to study the occurrence (incidence) and frequency (prevalence) of this condition in human populations.

In the context of this general endorsement of epidemiological field survey methods, some readers may be interested in whether occurrence of drug dependence can be measured surveillance of the routine administrative statistics of hospital or managed care organizations. Any evaluation of this type of surveillance brings an epidemiologist face to face with some of the traditional concerns of psychiatric epidemiology, such as the influence of "nosocomial" and "threshold" effects (e.g., see Anthony and Van Etten, 1995). The results of these effects include a familiar iceberg phenomenon: cases identified in the administrative statistics may be no more than a small fraction of the total number of cases in a population (e.g., see Anthony, 1999, for an illustration of the "iceberg" phenomenon). With respect to the occurrence of dependence on prescribed Schedule II-III analgesic drugs such as morphine and oxycodone, it is difficult to inspect published evidence of the Boston Collaborative Drug Surveillance Project (BCDSP) without giving serious consideration to a kind of "iceberg" phenomenon (Shapiro et al., 1978); the BCDSP estimates for risk of developing dependence upon these analgesic drugs are extremely small (under 1 case of dependence per 1000 patients treated)—perhaps too small to be credible or convincing.

The Occurrence (Incidence) of Drug Dependence

Incidence values are rates that deserve special attention because they help to convey the probability of becoming a case of drug dependence for the first time, among members of a defined population. An incidence estimate is one way to express the risk of developing drug dependence during some span of time. By comparing incidence or risk estimates for different subgroups of a population, it is possible to discriminate conditions of heightened risk and suspected determinants of risk, as distinct from prevalence correlates that do not determine risk of drug dependence (e.g., see Anthony et al., 1994).

It is important to recognize that drug taking can be conceptualized and measured in relation to an underlying dimension that runs from no drug use upward through increasing levels of drug involvement, as discussed in relation to the pathogenesis of drug dependence. Many strengths and benefits accrue by studying drug taking in this fashion (e.g., see Pandina et al., 1981; Brook et al., 2000b). Nonetheless, when investigators specify dimensional drug taking as an outcome in their studies, they have abandoned the statistical concept of risk, and in a formal sense they no longer can gain a direct view of the determinants of risk for drug taking or drug dependence. Indeed, there is no compelling reason to think that a profile of causes for the transition from no use to initial drug use should be identical to the profile of causes for the transition from drug experimentation to fully developed drug dependence (e.g., see Robins, 1977; Anthony, 1991a; Glantz, 1992; Smart, 1992; Anthony et al., 1994). As will be noted later in this chapter, some of the twin studies of drug dependence have derived considerably different models of causal influence on the liability to initiate drug use versus the liability to become dependent or a persistent user, once use has started (e.g., see True et al., 1997).

To our knowledge, the ECA program was the first epidemiologic study that sought to estimate prospectively the incidence of drug dependence for a general population, using standardized diagnostic assessments in the context of an epidemiologic field survey. By means of a prospective study design and taking advantage of repeatedly administered DIS assessments, ECA surveys conducted in four American communities have provided evidence on the occurrence of drug dependence in adulthood, measured as a cumulative annual incidence estimate of 1.09% for the diagnostic category of drug dependence combined with drug abuse (Eaton et al., 1989). Approximately 40% of identified cases in the ECA surveys have been found to qualify for a diagnosis of drug abuse without drug dependence; the remaining 60% qualified for drug dependence with or without drug abuse (Anthony and Helzer, 1991). Thus, assuming generalizability of these estimates from the ECA sites to the nation as a whole, for adults living in the United States during the early 1980s, an estimated 0.6%, or 6 per 1,000, were found to become incident cases of drug dependence during a 1-year interval of observation.

By comparison with this approximate annual incidence value of 6 cases of drug dependence per 1,000 adults in the population, an estimated 6 per 1,000 American adults become incident cases of panic disorder each year, and an estimated 7 per 1,000 develop obsessive-compulsive disorder. For major depression and alcohol abuse and dependence syndromes, the estimated risk is slightly more than 15 incident cases per 1,000 per year. Phobic disorders among adults developed at an annual rate of 40 cases per 1,000 per year, and the other mental disorders were observed to occur too infrequently for suitable estimates, despite the unprecedented large size of the ECA sample within the field of psychiatric epidemiology (Eaton et al., 1989).

The Frequency (Prevalence) of Drug Dependence

Lifetime Prevalence. In contrast with incidence, prevalence values are proportions that communicate the probability of being affected by drug dependence within a defined population. Among persons who have survived to some specific time, the lifetime prevalence expresses the probability of being a currently active or a former case of drug dependence. That is, among these survivors, lifetime prevalence is the probability of having become a case during the span of life prior to assessment (Kramer et al., 1980).

When studying drug dependence, it is especially important to link the concept of survivorship with the concept of lifetime prevalence. To the extent that drug dependence accounts for excess mortality, a lifetime prevalence value can understate the cumulative probability of developing drug dependence. Furthermore, lifetime prevalence comparisons can give a distorted view of high-risk groups. That is, if two groups have equal risk of developing drug dependence, but different risks of dying from drug-related causes, then lifetime prevalence comparisons will suggest falsely that the group with long-surviving cases is at greater risk of drug dependence than the group whose cases die sooner (Kramer et al., 1980).

Because lifetime prevalence confounds the forces of becoming drug dependent together with the forces of mortality, our analyses of lifetime prevalence data generally cannot provide the definitive epidemiologic evidence required to discriminate determinants of risk or conditions of heightened risk from other correlates of prevalence. Nonetheless, lifetime prevalence estimates can help us to understand how commonly drug dependence has affected a population and may serve as a guide toward more definitive epidemiologic research on the determinants of risk (Anthony et al., 1994).

An increasing number of epidemiological field surveys are producing estimates for lifetime prevalence of drug dependence, separated from the condition of drug abuse. For example, when a DIS-like method and DSM-III criteria were used in a survey of adults in Taiwan, an estimated 0.8% of metropolitan Taipei residents were found to have become drug dependent as compared with a prevalence estimate of 2.0% for residents of small towns. In the rural villages of Taiwan, no cases of drug dependence were found (Hwu et al., 1989).

In the United States between 1980 and 1985, the ECA surveys of adults aged 18 years and older found lifetime prevalence of drug dependence to be close to 3.0%, according to the DIS/DSM-III method. In 1990–1992, the NCS survey of 15–54-year-old American household residents applied the CIDI/DSM-III-R method and produced a lifetime prevalence estimate of 7.5%; Grant (1996) reported a generally congruent estimate from her separate National Longitudinal Alcohol Epidemiology Study (NLAES), which applied a method similar to that of the CIDI, but with a slightly different diagnostic algorithm, and which was based on DSM-IV diagnostic criteria. The larger NCS value appears to be due primarily to changes in the diagnostic criteria for drug dependence from DSM-III to DSM-III-R, including the addition of a DSM-III-R cocaine dependence category. Another potential source of variation in survey estimates was a slightly different way of grouping the controlled substances for the NCS, and inclusion of a new category for dependence on inhalants such as glue and other volatile intoxicants (Anthony et al., 1994). In a later section of this chapter, there is a discussion of how different age compositions of the samples might have led to larger overall NCS prevalence values.

Grouping drug dependence with the problems associated with drug abuse, and applying the DIS/DSM-III method or similar methods, epidemiologists studying adults in different geographic locations have produced lifetime prevalence estimates with a range from under 1% (Taiwan, Korea, and Puerto Rico) to 6.9% (Edmonton, Canada), 7.6% (Los Angeles, CA), and 13.3% (Fresno, California)—some of this variation may be due to differences in the case definitions or measurement strategies. In Christchurch (New Zealand), and in ECA surveys of Baltimore, New Haven, and St. Louis, the lifetime prevalence estimates have been within the range from 5.6% to 5.9%. A lower value of 3.8% was found in the Durham-Piedmont ECA site, and in Munich (Germany) a modified DIS-like method was used for follow-up assessments of an adult population sample, yielding a lifetime prevalence value of 1.8%. Differences in sampling plans and samples (e.g., age composition) account for some unknown part of the variation in these estimates (Bland et al., 1988a; Hwu et al., 1989; Wells et al., 1989; Lee et al., 1990a,b; Anthony and Helzer, 1991; Wittchen et al., 1992; Canino et al., 1993; Merikangas et al., 1998a, b).

The lifetime prevalence of alcohol dependence and/or abuse generally has been found to be roughly two to three times greater than the lifetime prevalence of the drug abuse/dependence syndromes. For example, lifetime prevalence estimates from the NCS in the USA are 14% for alcohol dependence and 7.5% for dependence on controlled substances (Anthony et al., 1994); similar NLAES estimates have been reported (e.g., see Grant, 1996). Corresponding values from epidemiological samples in Germany are 6% and 2%, in Mexico 7% and 2%, in the Netherlands 6% and 2%, and in Ontario, Canada, 9% and 8.5% (Merikangas et al., 1998). However, to date, no ECA-like or NCS-like surveys have been conducted in a Muslim country, where the relative prevalence of these conditions might be reversed due to religious proscription of alcohol use.

By grouping alcohol abuse/dependence syndromes together with abuse/dependence syndromes involving internationally controlled substances, it is possible to gain a better appreciation for the magnitude of psychiatric disorders directly connected with the use of these psychoactive substances. By this standard, in the United States an estimated 17% of adults 18 years of age or older have become cases as identified by the DIS/DSM-III method (Anthony and Helzer, 1991). Using the CIDI/DSM-III-R method to study younger Americans aged 15–54 years, and combining the alcohol and other drug use disorders in a similar fashion, Kessler et al. (1994) reported that 26.6% had become cases of abuse and/or dependence. The corresponding estimate for Christchurch (New Zealand) and Edmonton (Canada) was 21%, while it was 13.5% according to the modified DIS-like method used in the Munich Follow-Up Study (Bland et al., 1988a; Wells et al., 1989; Helzer et al., 1990; Wittchen et al., 1992).

The ECA and NCS initiatives have provided a useful glimpse of drug-specific lifetime prevalence values, as depicted in Table 3. The lifetime prevalence of alcohol dependence was 14.1% in the NCS data, mentioned above. According to ECA estimates, some 13% had become cases of alcohol dependence and/or abuse (Helzer et al., 1991). Given that some 80%–90% of adult Americans have con-

TABLE 3. A Comparison of Lifetime Prevalence Estimates for Drug Dependence Syndromes, Based on the National Comorbidity Survey (NCS) and the Epidemiologic Catchment Area (ECA) Surveys, Specific for Individual Drug Groups[a]

Drug Group	NCS Estimate (%)	ECA Estimate (%)
Alcohol	14.1	13.0
Cannabis	4.2	4.4
Cocaine	2.7	NA
Heroin	0.4	< 0.7
Stimulant[b]	1.7	1.7
ASH drug[c]	1.2	1.2
Hallucinogens	0.5	0.4
Inhalants	0.3	NA

[a]The NCS surveyed U.S. household residents 15–54 years of age from 1990–1992, with CIDI/DSM-III-R assessment of the drug dependence syndromes. The ECA surveys were conducted between 1980 and 1984, encompassed both household and nonhousehold residents 18 years of age and older, and used Diagnostic Interview Schedule assessments of drug dependenve and drug abuse, defined in terms of the DSM-III criteria.
[b]Here, the stimulant group includes methamphetamine and other amphetamines as well as methylphenidate and other psychostimulants, but does not include cocaine products.
[c]The ASH drugs are anxiolytic (tranquilizer), sedative, and hypnotic drugs, such as diazepam and other benzodiazepines marketed at the time of each survey, and the barbiturates.
Sources: Anthony and Heizer, 1991; Anthony et al., 1994.

sumed alcohol, roughly 15%–20% of alcohol users had become cases (Anthony et al., 1994).

About 4% of the 15–54-year-old household population of the USA had become cases of cannabis dependence by NCS estimates. A corresponding value of 4.4% was obtained from the ECA surveys of all adults, which combined cannabis dependence with cannabis abuse. Among cannabis users, approximately 9%–20% had become cases (Anthony and Helzer, 1991; Anthony et al., 1994). By comparison, reporting on their valuable longitudinal sample of young men and women in New York State, Kandel and Davies (1992) have estimated that almost one-half of the young male marijuana users had started near-daily marijuana use by ages 28 or 29, and about 37% of the young female marijuana users had done so.

Some recent data from Australia raise some interesting questions about the epidemiology of cannabis use and dependence. Drawing upon estimates from an NCS-like national sample survey of Australians, Swift et al. (2001) reported that an estimated 1.5% met DSM criteria for recently active cannabis dependence and 0.7% met criteria for recently active cannabis abuse. Whereas some 9%–20% of cannabis users in the United States had become dependent upon cannabis, the corresponding estimate from the Australian survey is somewhat larger (Marie Teesson and Michael Lynskey, personal communication to the author). This greater occurrence of the problems associated with cannabis dependence in an Australian sample as compared to a U.S. sample merits scrutiny in new cross-national research.

Close to 3% of adults had become cases of cocaine dependence by NCS estimates, and 0.2% qualified for cocaine abuse by ECA estimates; cocaine dependence was not assessed in the ECA study. Among cocaine users, slightly more than 15% had become cocaine dependent, and about 3% had qualified for the DSM-III cocaine abuse diagnosis (Anthony and Helzer, 1991; Anthony et al., 1994).

It would appear that, globally, prevalence of cocaine dependence achieved peak values some time during the last two decades in the United States (i.e., between 1980 and 1995). To date, no epidemiological surveys have produced lifetime prevalence estimates larger than the three percent value obtained in the NCS initiative. Nonetheless, it is possible that the prevalence of cocaine dependence is greater in selected regions of the Andes or elsewhere in South America, where smoking of coca paste ("basuco" and "pastabas") has become surprisingly common, even among school-attending youths (e.g., see Caris and Anthony, 2000).

With respect to controlled substances other than cannabis and cocaine, NCS estimates for the dependence syndrome did not differ appreciably from the ECA estimates for the dependence syndromes combined with the category of drug abuse. Among heroin users, more than 20% had developed heroin dependence and/or abuse. Among users of stimulants (other than cocaine), more than 10% had become cases of stimulant dependence or abuse. Among users of sedative, hypnotic, or anxiolytic drugs, an estimated 10%–25% had developed dependence or abuse involving these drugs. For hallucinogens, the corresponding value was under 10% (Anthony and Helzer, 1991; Anthony et al., 1994). Corresponding estimates for these drugs from other countries are not yet available, due to small numbers of users and imprecise estimates from the other surveys.

It may be instructive to make a comparison to lifetime prevalence values for tobacco dependence, now available only for several locales. Using a DIS-like method and DSM-III criteria to study adults (aged 18–64) in urban and rural Korea, epidemiologists found that 20% of urban residents and 21% of rural residents had become tobacco dependent (Lee et al., 1990b). When the same methods were used in Taiwan, the lifetime prevalence of tobacco dependence was found to be 7.8% in metropolitan Taipei, 12.2% in small towns of Taiwan, and 13.6% in the rural villages of Taiwan (Hwu et al., 1989). The NCS estimate for lifetime prevalence of tobacco dependence, based on the CIDI/DSM-III-R method, was 24.1%. Among those who had used tobacco, roughly 32% had developed tobacco dependence, a value not too distant from a corresponding estimate of 27% based on a population sample of young adults living in the Detroit, Michigan area (Breslau et al., 1993).

This overview of lifetime prevalence estimates helps to substantiate a growing awareness in psychiatry and public health that many persons are affected by dependence on the internationally regulated drugs such as marijuana, cocaine, and heroin, particularly in nations of the Western world, where a general finding is that well over 1% of the adult population has become drug dependent. Moreover, there are some areas where an estimated 7%–8% of adults can be discovered to have a history of drug dependence, not counting alcohol dependence (e.g., see Bland et al., 1988b; Wells et al., 1989; Anthony et al., 1994; Merikangas et al., 1998a, b).

These forms of drug dependence occur against a background of somewhat higher lifetime prevalence values for alcohol and tobacco. To the extent that drug dependence is sustained by some of the same forces that give rise to high frequency of alcohol dependence and tobacco dependence, effective control of drug dependence may require coordinated action in relation to alcohol and tobacco as well.

Research to be conducted over the next decade quite likely will show that dependence on coffee and other caffeine-containing products is a widely prevalent condition in many countries of the world, given that caffeine is one of the most widely used psychoactive drugs. For example, in the United States, an estimated 15%–20% of the population drinks at least five cups of coffee per day, and this estimate does not encompass the use of xanthine-containing beverages such as tea and the colas (Anthony and Arria, 1999). If caffeine supplies were disrupted, symptoms of headache and other manifestations of caffeine withdrawal would affect many individuals. Nonetheless, it is not at all clear that caffeine dependence merits inclusion within diagnostic classifications for mental disorders; caffeine-associated disruptions in the normative behavioral repertoire appear to be minimal, and this disruption may be a *sine qua non* with respect to societal concern about the drug dependence syndromes.

Dependence syndromes associated with the use of betel nut, kava or sakau (Piper methysticum), kola, ayahuasca, yohimbine, and other psychoactive products consumed in the emerging market economies of the world has not been studied to any great extent. These are generally unexplored territories with respect to the epidemiology of drug dependence. Insights from anthropological and ethnographic studies exist, but there are no systematic epidemiological studies to support firm inferences about risk of dependence upon these drugs.

Point Prevalence and Interval Prevalence. Complementing the information from lifetime prevalence estimates, interval prevalence estimates can be used to express the probability of being a recently active case of drug dependence. For example, a 1-year prevalence value conveys the probability of being active within a 1-year interval prior to the assessment session (e.g., see Kessler et al., 1994).

The published literature includes 1 month and 6 month prevalence estimates, as well as 1-year prevalence estimates for drug dependence (e.g., see Myers et al., 1984; Regier et al., 1988; Kessler et al., 1994; Warner et al., 1995; Grant, 1996). To our knowledge, no one has published estimates for point prevalence, that is, the proportion affected by drug dependence at some specific defined point in time.

In common with lifetime prevalence, interval prevalence is affected by survivorship of cases relative to noncases and does not give a clear view of the risk to become a case. In addition, interval prevalence is affected more generally by the duration of drug dependence, where duration can be influenced by factors such as availability and access to early intervention or treatment. That is, even when two groups have equal risk of developing drug dependence and equal risk of dying from drug-related causes, the probability of being an active case can be shown to depend on the duration of being an active case. For example, if the advantage of earlier or more effective intervention leads one group to have mainly short-duration cases relative to the longer-duration and more chronic cases in another less-advantaged group, then the two groups will differ in their 1-year prevalence values: Earlier and more effective intervention will lead to lower interval prevalence values (see Anthony et al., 1992, for a detailed discussion of this issue in relation to causal research on drug dependence syndromes).

Despite these complications, interval prevalence estimates are useful because they serve to tell us how many persons have recently been affected by drug dependence. As distinct from the former cases, these recently active cases represent the potential burden and caseload for current early intervention and treatment programs.

According to ECA 1-year prevalence values for the adult population of the United States, an estimated 2.7% (±0.2%) were recently active cases of drug dependence and/or drug abuse with at least one symptom or drug-related problem occurring in the 1 year prior to assessment (Anthony and Helzer, 1991); values not appreciably different from the NCS estimates have been obtained from the NCS and NIAAA surveys in the United States (Warner et al. 1995; Grant, 1996). In the small towns of Taiwan, the 1-year prevalence of drug dependence/abuse was 1.3%, but in metropolitan Taipei and in rural villages the survey found essentially no recently active cases (Hwu et al., 1989). For Christchurch (New Zealand), a comparable 6-month prevalence estimate was 1.5%, as reported by Oakley-Browne and colleagues (1989); in the Munich Follow-Up Study (Wittchen et al., 1992), it was 0.6%.

In more recent surveys of interval prevalence, Metzler et al. (1994) have reported that an estimated 2.2% of the United Kingdom's population is affected by drug dependence syndromes. However, this estimate may be an underestimate relative to the values obtained in the ECA and NCS surveys in the United States, due to the use of a different method of case ascertainment in the U.K. survey (Furr-Holden and Anthony, in press).

For many purposes, it can be useful to say that a case of drug dependence remains active until drug use stops: Among cases of drug dependence, continuing drug use may be taken as an indicator that the dependence process has not been interrupted. In some instances, this approach to dating the recency of drug dependence produces an increase in the number of active cases and in the 1-year prevalence estimate. For example, the 1-year prevalence of active drug dependence and/or abuse in the Baltimore ECA was 2.9% (±0.3%) when cases were defined as active if they had experienced at least one dependence symptom or drug-related problem within the year prior to assessment; the estimate was 4.0% (±0.4%) when cases were defined as active if they reported drug use within the year prior to assessment. In the Los Angeles ECA, the increase was from 2.9% (±0.3%) to 4.6% (±0.4%). Of course, this approach to prevalence estimation is available only when investigators assess recency of drug use in addition to recency of drug problems (Anthony and Helzer, 1991).

By the same token, an extremely conservative approach can be taken by requiring a case to meet all of the criteria for drug dependence in the recent past. Working along these lines, and focusing specifically on cases of DSM-III-R drug dependence who met the full criteria for dependence during the 1 year prior to assessment, the NCS has estimated that 1.8% of 15–54-year-old Americans (±0.2%) qualify as recently active drug dependence cases (Kessler et al., 1994). The group of recently active cases primarily was affected by marijuana dependence, cocaine dependence, and/or dependence on other psychostimulant drugs such as the amphetamines. The corresponding 1-year prevalence estimate for alcohol dependence, from the same source, was 4.4% (±0.4%).

Summary Overview

Currently available prospective data indicate that the risk of developing drug dependence is just under 1% per year for adults in the United States. Studies are under way to produce incidence estimates for teenagers and for other countries of the world.

Recent estimates for the lifetime prevalence of drug dependence indicate a broad range from under 1% in some countries (e.g., Korea, Puerto Rico) to above 3% in other locales (e.g., Christchurch, New Zealand; Edmonton, Canada; Los Angeles, CA). The proportion of drug users who develop drug dependence seems to vary considerably from one drug category to another and most likely is determined by factors such as drug availability as much as by the reinforcing functions served by these drugs. For example, among alcohol users, the proportion who had become cases of alcohol dependence and/or abuse has been estimated to be 15%–20%, not too distant from that observed for users of cocaine but slightly greater than the proportion observed for cannabis users. For users of tobacco and users of heroin, the proportion appears to be higher, sometimes approaching or exceeding 30% (e.g., see Anthony et al., 1994).

In the United States, the 1-year prevalence of drug dependence is between 1.4 and 2.2 active cases per 100 persons aged 15–54 years. In other countries where comparable surveys have been taken, the 1-year prevalence of drug dependence is lower than this. However, there is reason to look closely at recent evidence from Australia with respect to cannabis. The apparent excess occurrence of cannabis dependence among cannabis users in Australia remains a neglected issue that epidemiologists must resolve.

Based on the reported estimates for adults living in the United States, the one-year prevalence of drug dependence is some two to four times the cumulative annual incidence of drug dependence. This relationship between one-year prevalence and cumulative annual incidence is consistent with the concept of drug dependence as a persistent psychiatric disturbance with a duration of more than one year. For every newly developed incident case of drug dependence in the adult population at present, there are several other adults whose drug dependence started some years back and who continue to be burdened by its complications in their present lives.

SUSPECTED DETERMINANTS OF DRUG DEPENDENCE PREVALENCE

An important goal for epidemiologic research on drug dependence, beyond quantifying occurrence and frequency, is to identify the determinants of drug dependence in human populations and to translate these research findings into practical strategies for public health work and preventive psychiatry. As discussed in the prior section of this chapter, prevalence is influenced not only by the conditions and processes out of which drug dependence develops but also by forces that extend or shorten the duration of drug dependence, including mortality rates.

In this context, mortality rates are important for two reasons. First, excess mortality associated with drug dependence will reduce the duration of drug dependence and the survivorship of cases, with a resulting downward impact on prevalence values. Second, mortality rates together with birth rates can affect the broad age structure of human populations, and certain changes in age structure can yield either dramatic increases or dramatic declines in the number of cases of drug dependence over spans of 10–20 years, even when there is no change in other factors that influence risk or duration of drug dependence. For example, as discussed in the following section on age-specific risk and prevalence of drug dependence, the number of cases of drug dependence in many countries will increase dramatically between 1990 and 2010 solely as a result of demographic shifts in the population of these countries, due largely to high birth rates and declining mortality rates. These increases will occur unless there are compensatory changes in the other determinants of prevalence, including such factors as more effective prevention or treatment initiatives (Anthony, 1992).

As in all of epidemiology, our capacity to translate drug dependence research findings into practical strategies rests in part on our discrimination of risk-modifying conditions and processes from duration-modifying conditions and processes. This capacity is impaired to the extent that our epidemiologic research on drug dependence has produced no more than prevalence estimates and has failed to shed light on incidence, risk, and suspected causal influences on risk (e.g., see Anthony, 1993). What follows is a summary overview of promising leads in relation to what might influence prevalence of drug dependence either by reducing risk or by shortening its duration. In many instances, our knowledge is constrained because we have many studies based on prevalent cases found in cross-sectional surveys but few estimates from good epidemiologic studies of incident cases of drug dependence. Our knowledge has been enhanced in relation to some important prevention research studies that have helped shed light on the determinants of risk of initiating drug use and making the transition to more serious drug involvement.

The breadth of suspected determinants of prevalence has a range from the microscopic to the macroscopic, from maps of our human genome to maps of human social environments and group characteristics such as shared social values and customs. The current program of genome mapping will help to clarify possible genetic vulnerability to drug dependence by identifying specific candidate genes for drug dependence. New research on families headed by drug-dependent parents will shed light on impaired parenting practices, supportive community and school programs, and other suspected environmental determinants of drug dependence.

The search for these determinants is made more exciting and challenging by the prospect of interactions between various determinants—for example, the discovery of protective environmental factors that might modify what otherwise should be moderate or high risks linked to heredity or other family factors. Our plans for these discoveries can build from what has been observed about drug dependence in relation to demographic factors associated with sex and age, for which we have some risk estimates as well as prevalence estimates. Ultimately, it should be possible to develop more effective prevention and control strategies for public health work by drawing on new knowledge about the separate and interrelated contributions of social, psychological, and other biologic conditions that foster and sustain drug dependence in human populations.

Demographic Risk Indicators: Sex and Age

Sex, Gender Roles, and Drug Dependence. Modern awareness of drug dependence emerged from a nineteenth century view of morphine addiction as a soldier's disease, mainly affecting American Civil War veterans, men who had received morphine by injection for relief of pain due to wounds of battle and associated trauma. By the early twentieth century, clinical attention shifted somewhat, more in the direction of problems experienced by women who were taking large daily doses of nonprescription patent medicines and other products containing alcohol, tincture of opium, or morphine, or perhaps the newer products of a growing pharmaceutical industry: heroin derived from the opium poppy; cocaine extracted from coca leaf; chloral hydrate or other drugs used to calm, sedate, or bring sleep. Some attention also was given to opium smoking, apparently practiced by Chinese of both sexes, but made notorious in the United States by popular stories of Chinese immigrant-laborers whose opium dens lured not only men but also women later entrapped into prostitution and slavery (Musto, 1987).

With enforcement of laws to regulate supply, distribution, and use of these drugs, including early twentieth-century international treaties, the bulk of clinical and scientific attention shifted back to drug dependence among individuals, mainly men, who would break the law to sustain their drug taking. In part, this emphasis on men may have been due to creation in the late 1920s of a United States Public Health Service research program on drug addiction, which until the 1970s drew study subjects primarily from men incarcerated for drug-related federal offenses. However, from the late nineteenth century onward, there has been a continuing stream of clinical case reports and occasional sociologic or ethnographic studies featuring narrative descriptions of women who suffered from drug dependence. This early research set the stage for more contemporary epidemiologic studies of drug taking and drug dependence in various countries, which now generally show that both sexes are affected, men somewhat more than women (e.g., see Rae and Braude, 1989; Kandel, 1991).

ECA estimates for annual incidence of drug dependence and/or drug abuse corroborate a general pattern of male preponderance among drug-dependent individuals. Based on ECA estimates for adult men, the risk of developing a drug dependence or drug abuse syndrome has been observed to be close to 1.7% per year; the corresponding value for adult women is lower, at about 0.7% per year (Eaton et al., 1989). Lifetime prevalence values for men have exceeded those for women in epidemiologic surveys conducted in New Zealand, Canada, the five ECA populations, and the United States household population surveyed for the NCS. Surveys conducted in Taiwan and Korea suggest a greater balance in prevalence for men and women, but the number of detected cases in these surveys was small and the statistical power to detect male–female differences was not optimal (Bland et al., 1988a; Hwu et al., 1989; Wells et al., 1989; Lee et al., 1990a,b; Anthony and Helzer, 1991; Wittchen et al., 1992; Canino et al., 1993).

Considering our general model for pathogenesis of drug dependence, it is helpful to ask whether the observed differences are due entirely to more prevalent use of controlled substances by men or whether men who take these drugs might be more likely to become drug dependent than female drug users. According to available epidemiologic data for most of the psychoactive drugs we have studied, males generally are more likely to be exposed to opportunities to try drugs and are more likely to take controlled substances. In addition, once drug use begins, they are more likely to become daily users and to develop drug dependence and/or drug abuse (e.g., see Kandel and Davies, 1992; Anthony et al., 1994; Van Etten et al., 1997; Van Etten and Anthony, 2001). However, once an opportunity to try a drug has occurred, females seem no less likely than men to try illegal drugs (Van Etten and Anthony, 2001). This evidence summarizes what is known about recent experiences in the United States. We have only started to examine whether this evidence holds for other countries of the world and for subgroups within the United States (e.g., see Delva et al., 1999).

Hence, it is possible that observed male–female differences in occurrence or frequency of drug dependence may be traced back to greater exposure opportunities for men versus women. If a male/female difference in exposure opportunity exists, this would point more directly toward a possible variation based on gender identities and social roles linked with sex, perhaps separate from any hypothesized sex-linked biologic differences (e.g., see Van Etten and Anthony, 2001). At present, no studies speak clearly and definitively to the issue of sex versus gender identity and gender roles in relation to the prevalence of drug dependence syndromes.

Finally, there is some evidence of male–female differences in the probability of stopping drug use once it begins (e.g., Kandel and Raveis, 1989; Anthony and Helzer, 1991). That is, for women, drug use appears to be more short-lived than for men.

In conclusion, it appears that male–female differences in prevalence of drug dependence may be determined in part by differences in risk of experiencing opportunities to try drugs. Other plausible sources of variation, not yet contradicted by evidence, include sex-linked differences in risk of becoming drug dependent (e.g., with respect to drugs such as marijuana and cocaine), and by differences in duration of drug dependence.

Age and Drug Dependence. From 1870 through the 1970s, cases of virtually all ages have been described in the world literature on clinical and other scientific studies of drug dependence, with some reports on cases occurring among very mature adults in late life. The drug problems of adolescents and young adults began to receive considerably increased attention after passage of drug regulations in the early twentieth century, although in the 1950s there was some shift in focus of concern toward problems linked to adult use of legally available pharmaceutical products: for example, truck drivers and homemakers taking stimulant, sedative, and hypnotic (sleep-promoting) drugs for nonmedical reasons (e.g., see Musto, 1987).

Between 1960 and the present, a societal concern about youthful drug taking has stimulated organization of surveys of adolescent drug use in many countries of the world, as well as cross-sectional household surveys in some countries. In the United States, repeated cross-sectional surveys of students and household residents now provide epidemiologic trend data on drug taking in the population, but until recently these surveys have not attempted to assess clinical conditions such as drug dependence. Nonetheless, it is important to note that the most recent epidemiologic surveys show some evidence of increased prevalence of drug taking among adults aged 35 years and older, perhaps as a sign that drug-taking patterns acquired in adolescence and young adulthood are being carried over into middle-age (e.g., see United States Substance Abuse and Mental Health Services, 1993, 2000). Johnson and Gerstein (1998) have drawn attention to some impressive differences that can be seen in the illegal drug experiences of different cohorts within the United States since World War II; Golub and Johnson (2001) have stressed more recent birth cohort experiences, and also draw attention to subgroup variation in birth cohort drug experiences within the United States, with a specific focus on the "gateway" progressions from alcohol and tobacco to marijuana and other illegal drug use.

Within the United States, trend data from cross-sectional surveys of drug taking were strengthened with the addition of drug dependence assessments for the ECA Program in the early 1980s. According to both cross-sectional and prospective data from the ECA surveys, the risk of developing a syndrome of drug dependence or drug abuse now varies considerably from one age stratum to the next. For example, according to the prospective study conducted by Eaton et al. (1989), the estimated risk of developing drug dependence or drug abuse was observed to be 2.8% per year for persons 18–29 years old in the early 1980s (±0.5%); 0.7% per year for 30–44 year olds (±0.2%); and less than 0.1% per year for older adults. The estimated annual incidence for males 18–29 years old was 4.4% per year (±1.1%); for females 18–29 years old, it was 1.6% per year (±0.45%).

Figure 2 gives predicted annual incidence rates for males and females aged 18 or older, derived from a logistic regression analysis of prospective data from the ECA surveys. The shape of these age-specific curves is noteworthy, with peak values at 18 years for men (almost 8% per year) and for women (2.8% per year). By implication, risk of developing drug dependence or drug abuse also must be at fairly high levels among slightly younger teenagers (aged 15–17). Retrospective data from the ECA Program, subject to limitations discussed in an earlier section of this chapter, provide some evidence on this point: The risks of developing drug dependence and drug abuse are observed to rise in early adolescence, reaching peak values between the ages of 15 and 25, and with lower values for later age strata (Burke et al., 1990). To some extent, these age-specific patterns reflect age-specific risk of initiating drug use, taking into account a possible induction period of 13 years from the time of initial drug use to the time of meeting full criteria for drug dependence. Wagner and Anthony (2002a) have suggested that the induction period for cocaine is substantially shorter than the corresponding induction period of alcohol or marijuana, as depicted in Figure 1 of this chapter.

Age-specific prevalence values for drug dependence correspond with age-specific incidence values and the observed chronic course of drug dependence. The ECA lifetime prevalence estimates are highest among younger American adults: considering 18–29 year olds, an estimated 9% of men and 5.5% of women have developed drug dependence. Corresponding values for 30–44 year olds are 5.1% (men) and 3.0% (women), and for older men and women the values are under 1% (Anthony and Helzer, 1991).

The generally strong relationship between age and drug dependence draws attention to the potential importance of age composition of epidemiologic samples, as well as the impact of demographic forces on the number of drug-dependence cases in the population. For example, the youngest subjects in the ECA samples

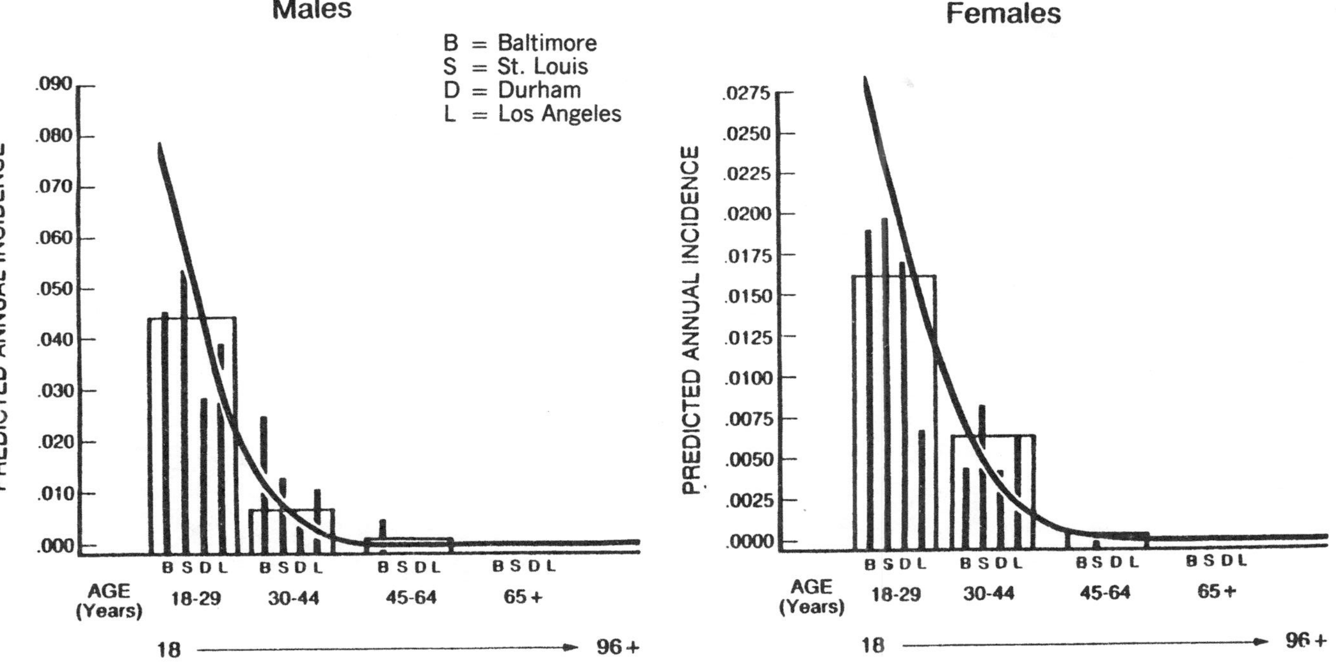

Figure 2. Annual incidence of DIS/DSM-III drug abuse/dependence syndromes. The smoothed curve presents annual incidence estimates for each age of adulthood, separately for males and females. The broad histogram bars give summary estimates of annual incidence for each of the following age strata: 18–29 years, 30–44 years, 45–64 years, and 65 years and older. The narrow histogram bars show variation from site to site within each given age stratum. Lack of a histogram bar for persons age 65 + years indicates an annual incidence estimate of zero, corresponding to no observed incidence cases in this age group, despite large numbers of elderly study participants in the Epidemiologic Catchment Area surveys. (Reproduced with permission from Eaton et al., 1989.)

were 18 years and the oldest was 96 years; many ECA subjects were 65 years or older. By comparison, the age range of subjects in the NCS was 15–54 years. In view of the association between age and drug dependence, and the exceptionally low prevalence values for adults 55 years or older, it follows that NCS prevalence estimates for drug dependence should be greater than ECA prevalence estimates, and would have been even larger if identical survey methods had been used in these two research programs. When considering lifetime prevalence values from DIS/DSM-III surveys in New Zealand, Munich, Korea, and Puerto Rico, it is important to consider that population coverage of these surveys was extended from ages 18 through 64 and did not include elderly residents of these countries.

Forecasting methods advocated within psychiatric epidemiology by Professor Morton Kramer make use of age-specific prevalence estimates and global projections for a changing age structure of human populations to disclose which countries should expect to maintain a stable number of mental disorder cases, which should experience increased caseloads, and which should experience decreased caseloads, all else being held constant. By applying these methods, Kramer and others have been especially effective in drawing worldwide attention to an increasing prevalence of cognitive disorders such as dementia, which differentially affect the very rapidly growing elderly segments in every country's population (e.g., see Kramer, 1989).

It is less widely appreciated that the same projection methods can be applied to drug dependence and other mental disorders with a different pattern of age relationships (Kramer, 1992a). In an initial effort, Kramer has used these methods to project a stable number of white Americans with drug dependence in the United States and concurrent increases in the number of African-Americans and Hispanic-Americans affected by drug dependence (Kramer, 1992b; also discussed by Anthony, 1992).

M. Piazza applied the NCS age-specific prevalence estimates for drug dependence in order to study demographic trends in various regions and countries of the world and to forecast where health planners and policy makers in each country should be preparing for an increased drug dependence caseload. Table 4 illustrates this work as applied to Brazil, where the projection method forecasts dramatic increases in the number of drug-dependent cases between 1990 and 2010. These increases are due to Brazil's recent twentieth-century experience of high birth rates and declining infant mortality rates: more inhabitants of Brazil are surviving to ages when drug dependence develops. As noted elsewhere, many countries and regions are slated for increases in the number of drug-dependent persons over the decades from 1990 to 2010, although in North America and Western Europe the projection method shows considerable stability because the population age structure in these areas already has changed. In these regions, population growth primarily is in the very old age groups, where prevalence of drug dependence is not so high (M. Piazza, unpublished manuscript, 1993).

Values obtained from this projection method now are based on a very consistent age-specific pattern of low prevalence rates for drug dependence among the very young (under 15 years of age) and among mature adults (over 45 years of age), with higher prevalence rates among 15–44 years olds. This age-specific pattern, with the burden of drug dependence concentrated among 15–44 year olds, now generally seems to hold wherever drug-dependence surveys have been conducted and also

TABLE 4. Projected Increase in Brazil's Caseload for Treatment of Drug Dependence, for the Years 1990–2010

Age Groups	Population Size in 1990	NCS Age-Specific Rate[a]	Projected Number of Active Cases in 1990	Projected Population Size in 2010	NCS Age-Specific Rate[a]	Projected Number of Active Cases in 2010	Projected Increase in Treatment Caseload from 1990 to 2010
All ages							
0–4							
5–9							
10–14	52,978,000	0.001	52,978	58,467,000	0.001	58,467	5,489
15–19							
20–24	28,670,000	0.033	946,110	37,256,000	0.033	1,229,448	283,338
25–29							
30–34	24,981,000	0.016	399,696	33,147,000	0.016	530,352	130,656
35–39							
40–44	17,478,000	0.013	227,214	27,380.000	0.013	355,940	128,726
45–49							
50–54	11,352,000	0.007	79,464	23,053,000	0.007	151,441	81,977
55 +	14,909,000	0.001	14,909	28,141,000	0.001	28,141	13,232
Total number of projected cases			1,720,371			2,363,789	643,418

[a]These are estimates from the U.S. National Comorbidity Survey, indicating the proportion of each age group found to qualify as a current or recently active case of DSM-IIIR drug dependence (with symptoms within one year of assessment. Even if these particular estimates do not apply to Brazil, there will be an increase in the number of age-specific relationships is roughly comparable to what has been observed in the United States and elsewhere, unless there are new changes in compensating conditions that determine prevalence levels.

where health statistics have been gathered on occurrence of deaths associated with drug dependence. Thus, even if the absolute number of projected cases is in error for an individual country, the overall impression of change or stability in drug dependence caseload should be correct, provided the relative differences in prevalence across age groups follow this generally observed pattern (Anthony, 1995).

In summary, recent epidemiologic surveys have revealed a general pattern for the age-specific occurrence and frequency of drug dependence: Until age 15 and after age 45, the occurrence and frequency of drug dependence are low; between 15 and 44, higher values are observed, with peak values typically between 15 and 25. There certainly may be exceptions to these general observations (e.g., when elderly patients become dependent upon prescription drugs). Countries and regions that project new population increases for 15–44 year olds may be expected to experience increased caseloads of drug dependence, unless there are compensating conditions such as increased application of effective prevention and control strategies.

Race as a Determinant of Risk for Drug Dependence

One of the most common preconceptions about race and drug dependence, sometimes appearing in the drug-dependence literature, is that there is something about African-Americans to make them more vulnerable. This preconception is buttressed by studies of public treatment for drug dependence and by criminal justice research, which show disproportionate representation of African-Americans among drug-dependent patients and among persons arrested and convicted for drug-related crimes (e.g., see Kandel, 1991).

Science ethics, by itself, dictates that no epidemiologist should make superficial or casual statements about race and drug dependence, given the long tradition of research tinged with racism or used to bolster white supremacist or racist arguments. More than most observers, epidemiologists are well equipped to understand that race is strongly confounded with social disadvantage in the Western world, where most drug dependence studies have been conducted, and elsewhere. More than most scientists, epidemiologists can design and interpret population studies that seek to disentangle the effects of social disadvantage and other high-risk environmental conditions from the effects of race as a biologic and inherited characteristic. These studies must be conducted before conclusive statements about race and drug dependence can be made (e.g., see Jones et al., 1991). In this regard, Kaufman and Cooper (2001a, b) have contributed some useful insights about epidemiological research on race as a potentially risk-associated predisposing characteristic versus racism as a manifestation of social processes, with additional useful commentary by Camara Phyllis Jones (2001).

Against this background, it is important to draw attention to recent epidemiologic studies in which social disadvantage and neighborhood environment have been taken into account. In these studies, African-Americans have *not* been found to be at increased risk of developing drug dependence or drug abuse, relative to white Americans (Anthony, 1991a). Nor have they been found to have higher rates of taking cocaine or smoking crack (Lillie-Blanton et al., 1993; Flewelling et al., 1993). Indeed, some studies show that African-American youths are less likely to start taking drugs and alcohol than their white American adolescent peers (United States Substance Abuse and Mental Health Services, 1993).

In a most interesting study of social causation versus social selection in relation to ethnicity and the occurrence of drug dependence, Dohrenwend et al. (1992) assembled an epidemiological sample of both Sephardic and Ashkenazi Jews living in Israel. Studying the risk of having developed drug dependence across strata defined by achieved levels of education, the research team found more substantial evidence favoring a social causation model in relation to the risk of drug problems. It is important to say that the evidence favored a social selection model in relation to the risk of having developed schizophrenia (Dohrenwend et al., 1992).

Within the United States, it may be premature to draw firm conclusions about social causation and social selection hypotheses in relation to race and ethnicity. The excess frequency of African-Americans among patients receiving publicly funded treatment for drug problems and among those arrested or incarcerated for drug-related crimes most likely exemplifies one or more biases in a sequence of transitions leading from the total population of cases and noncases, a transition that occurs to differentiate a more selected subpopulation admitted to public treatment and criminal justice facilities. Like the fallacy of medical statistics identified by Berkson (1946), these transition biases can lead to erroneous inferences about the causes of drug dependence. We are aware of no careful epidemiologic study showing race per se to be an important causal factor for dependence on drugs such as cocaine or heroin, once race-related differences in social status and disadvantage have been taken into account.

Having said this, one must note that the absence of evidence does not imply the absence of association. For example, in many studies, we now allow participants to characterize their racial heritage in relation to multiple categories of family background: African heritage, Hispanic heritage, Asian heritage, Pacific Islander heritage, and so on. This approach can be devised with an appreciation of the possibility that "race" does not necessarily reflect a "fixed biologic characteristic *internal* to the study subject" as opposed to a "complex and historically contingent set of social relations that exist external to the study subject" (Kaufman and Cooper, 2001b; Jones 2001). If we will allow participants to characterize themselves in this fashion, we may find that the size of the human genome creates opportunities for variation in risk of drug dependence in relation to subgroups self-designated in relation to their own perceptions of racial heritage, notwithstanding the vast similarity of individual genomes across subgroups within the human species, and with statistical control over differences associated with social disadvantage and status.

Examples from alcohol and tobacco research suggest that it is only a matter of time before pharmacogenetic studies will identify robust differences in some of the inherited substrates of dependence upon cocaine and heroin, differences that will appear in contrasts between individuals who self-designate themselves as being of African heritage, Asian heritage, or Caucasian heritage. Asian-African-Caucasian contrasts already have identified important pharmacogenetic variation with respect to phenotypic response to ethanol exposure (e.g., postethanol "flushing" response) and substrates in genetic polymorphisms regulating alcohol dehydrogenase (ADH) isoenzymes and aldehyde dehydrogenase (ALDH) isoenzymes, found on chromosomes 4 and 12. Considerable pharmacogenetic variation within subgroups also has been found, and not just within Asian subgroups. For example, studying an epidemiological sample restricted to Jewish males in Israel, Neumark et al. (1998) recently reported findings suggesting that alleles at one of the ADH loci (ADH2*2) might be protective against heavy ethanol consumption among Jews. With respect to tobacco, Sellers et al. (2000) recently reported race-related variation in the frequency of the CYP2A6 mutant allele that has been implicated as a source of variation in degree of tobacco involvement among smokers. Findings such as these substantiate a base of evidence to help us understand observed race-related differences in response among drug users.

It also may be important to note that the profiles of risk-influencing conditions and processes may not be the same, once self-designated race has been used to form population subgroups. A simplifying assumption might be that all subgroups will benefit equally from preventive interventions directed toward the same conditions and processes. Ellickson and Morton (1999) recently offered prospectively gathered evidence that this assumption might not hold. With respect to the use of drugs such as cocaine and heroin, the profile of risk-influencing conditions observed for self-designated white and non-Hispanic subgroups in the longitudinal study sample was not entirely the same as the profile observed for other subgroups (Black, Asian, Hispanic). Indeed, they found that low parental educational attainment was associated with increased risk of drug involvement for white non-Hispanic youths, but was associated with reduced risk of drug involvement for Hispanic and black youths. Consistent with speculations about population heterogeneity offered by Golub and Johnson (2001), among blacks, earlier marijuana and tobacco use were not associated with later risk of starting to try drugs like heroin and cocaine.

Other Suspected Determinants of Drug Dependence

The moderate-to-strong associations between sex, age, and drug dependence pose a challenge in epidemiologic research on other suspected determinants of drug dependence, which also might be related to sex and age. To protect against confounding by these factors, investigators interested in drug dependence can turn to epidemiologic strategies such as matching, stratification, or statistical modeling. More often, however, they have restricted the sex or age composition of their study samples. For example, there are more epidemiologic studies of drug dependence among males than among females, and there is essentially no strong evidence on causes of drug dependence syndromes that occur past age 40. Study of individual cases shows that syndromes of drug dependence do occur in the middle and later years of adulthood; however, after ages 45–55 years, the risk of developing these syndromes for the first time in ones life is quite small (e.g., see Eaton et al., 1989).

Heredity and Genetics Research. The search for determinants of drug dependence can be conceptualized in relation to a human developmental sequence that runs from conception through childhood and adolescence to adulthood. Early clinical observations about familial aggregation of alcohol and other drug dependence and notes on possible concordance of monozygotic twins sparked considerable interest in research on hereditary factors in relation to these syndromes. Vanyukov and Tarter (2000) provide a useful introduction and overview to the several lines of genetic research on the drug dependence syndromes. They use

Falconer's concept of liability as an organizing principle, and describe a dynamic developmental model of liability to drug dependence in terms of vectors of influence that determine an "ontogenetic trajectory" leading toward or away from expression of the drug dependence liability. As defined by Falconer (1965), liability for disease traits not inherited in a Mendelian fashion may appear as a nonrandom familial distribution of disease, expressed "...not only the individual innate tendency to develop or contract the disease, i.e., his susceptibility in the usual sense, but also the whole combination of external circumstances that make him more or less likely to develop the disease." This liability concept and the Tarter–Vanuykov ontogenetic trajectory model are generally consistent with a conception of behavior genetics research in terms of studies of the sources of variation in behavior, whether these sources of variation can be traced back to familial inheritance or to environmental conditions and processes. In relation to drug dependence, the profile of these studies now includes association and linkage studies, twin studies, adoption studies, and studies of familial aggregation.

Discovery of polymorphisms for the D2 dopamine receptor in the q22q23 region of chromosome 11 contributed new enthusiasm for a new line of association and linkage studies about drug dependence, in part because dopamine neurotransmission is central in brain reward and learning circuitry, and in relation to reinforcing functions of drug self-administration. Later, this line of research was broadened to encompass the entire family of dopamine receptor genes, as well as genes regulating isoenzymes that are active in biotransformation or metabolism of drugs. Against a backdrop of concern about false-positive findings (e.g., see Gerlernter et al., 1993; Vanyukov, 1999) and inconsistent or subtle findings (e.g., see Wong et al., 2000), there now is an ever-increasing number of studies in the hunt for drug dependence genes, using strategies of genetic epidemiology as well as those of molecular genetics (e.g., see Crabbe et al., 1994; Suarez et al., 1994; Reich et al., 1998; Nestler and Landsman, 2001).

Laboratory studies have demonstrated that dopamine is a neurotransmitter of central importance in relation to repetitive drug taking and the reinforcing functions of drug use, not only for cocaine, but also for alcohol, opioids, and other drugs. Other neurotransmitters and aminergic pathways also have been implicated (e.g., serotonin), but not as strongly nor consistently as dopamine. Studies of dopamine activity sites within the mammalian nervous system initially identified two receptors, D_1 and D_2, with later discovery of D_3, D_4, and D_5 receptors. In initial research to clone and express complementary DNA of the D_2 dopamine receptor, it was possible to map a D_2 receptor gene in the q22q23 region of human chromosome 11. Subsequently, restriction fragment length polymorphisms of this gene (TaqI A and B RFLPs) were examined in case–control studies of both alcoholism and drug dependence. In some (but not all) studies, cases of alcoholism that have been observed to have an excess frequency of the TaqI A1 RFLP relative to control subjects; the case–control findings generally have not been supported in family or linkage studies (e.g., see Blum et al., 1990; Conneally, 1991; Turner et al., 1992; Smith et al., 1992; Goldman, 1993; Pato et al., 1993; Comings, 1998; Gerlernter and Kranzler, 1999; Wong et al., 2000). Heavy drug use or drug abuse was initially associated with the TaqI B1 RFLP located near the first coding exon of the D_2 dopamine receptor gene, and less strongly with the TaqI A1 RFLP previously found in association with severe alcoholism (Uhl et al., 1992); there also are observed associations between the D_2 dopamine receptor gene and tobacco smoking (e.g., Comings et al., 1996). However, there is much inconsistency of findings and non-replication in both Caucasian samples (e.g., Gerlernter et al., 1999) and African-American samples (e.g., Berrettini and Persico, 1996). The same general pattern of inconsistency characterizes a growing body of research on the other dopamine receptor genes (e.g., see Wong et al., 2000).

A central role for dopamine in the actions of many different psychoactive drugs enhances the biological plausibility of its link to inheritance of drug dependence syndromes. In addition, there also are distinctive neuroanatomical distributions of dopamine receptors in brain regions associated with reward, learning, emotions, and cognitions—all associated with drug dependence. However, the hunt for drug dependence genes has not been restricted to the family of dopamine receptor genes, and there is good reason to look elsewhere for candidate genes and for protein expression involved in neuronal response to psychoactive drugs (Crabbe et al., 1994; Radel and Goldman, 2001; Nestler and Landsman, 2001). For example, Vandenbergh et al. (1997) reasoned that there might be an important modification of association between dopamine and drug dependence, and tested for an interaction with alleles for catechol-o-methyltransferase (COMT), which is a dopamine degrading enzyme. This research team found that volunteer subjects with higher levels of illegal drug involvement were more likely to have an allele that encodes a high activity form of COMT. The association with COMT appears to be independent of a separate association involving the D_4 dopamine receptor gene (Vandenbergh et al., 2000). The genetic epidemiology of COMT and its relationship to drug dependence remains to be exploited.

Also with an interest in the enzymes that degrade centrally active neurotransmitters, Vanyukov et al. (1995) inaugurated a line of research on a dinucleotide repeat length polymorphism at the monoamine oxidase A gene in the p11.23—11.24 region of the human X chromosome (MAOCA-1). (Monoamine oxidase A is an enzyme that degrades serotonin and norepinephrine.) The research team found evidence that longer repeat lengths of MAOCA-1 (above 115 base pairs) have a relatively modest association with risk of early-onset psychoactive substance use disorder for males but not for females. This association is intriguing when considered against a backdrop of findings on behavioral and brain chemistry disturbances secondary to cocaine dependence, including effects on serotonin pathways and aggression against self and others (Petronis et al., 1996). For example, a small and suggestive but not yet replicated family-genetic study has described a syndrome of aggressive behavioral disturbances affecting men with a point mutation in the gene encoding MAOA and abolishing MAOA catalytic activity (Brunner et al., 1992). Laboratory studies of transgenic mice have added new evidence of importance. These mice, generated to have a deletion of the gene encoding MAOA, show (1) altered levels of brain serotonin and norepinephrine, and (2) excess aggressive behavior, especially among males (Cases et al., 1995). Finally, tapping a capacity to conduct Harlow-style rearing experiments in their primate colony, an NIH intramural research team has found important new evidence of gene-environment interaction in relation to aggression and heavy ethanol consumption, with a maternal rearing environment found to dampen aggression and drinking associated with one of the serotonin transporter genes. Hence, there is good reason to pursue a line of genetic epidemiological research on MAOCA-1, serotonin, and their relationship to drug dependence.

Many initial signals of associations with genes that regulate neurotransmitter receptor sites or enzymes that degrade these neurotransmitters in the brain may well prove to be falsely positive in the long run, especially in the context of genome-wide scans (e.g., see Gerlernter et al., 1993; Reich et al., 1998). However, as noted by Comings (1998), it may be too much to expect strong and consistent findings at this stage of genomic research on drug dependence and related polygenic conditions.

An interesting pattern of evidence has emerged in relation to the allelic variants associated with drug metabolizing enzymes that function outside the central nervous system, such as the cytochrome P450 monooxygenases as well as certain non-P450 monooxygenases. In the first group are CYP2D6 and CYP2A6, which catalyze metabolism of tobacco, opioids, and many other drugs, despite relatively low abundance outside the liver (e.g., see Tanaka, 1999). For example, CYP2A6 activates some tobacco procarcinogens and inactivates nicotine to form cotinine; smokers with CYP2A6 mutant alleles smoke less tobacco (Pianezza et al., 1998). Boustead et al. (1997) have reported that smokers with two mutant CYP2D6 alleles are more committed to their first cigarette in the morning than any other, but this observation requires replication: it was derived from a *post-hoc* analysis after the investigators failed to find allele-related differences in the total score from the Fagerstrom Tolerance Questionnaire.

One of the more intriguing lines of research on genetics of drug dependence in recent years seeks to link personality traits and drug dependence back to specific genes, and there are some fascinating conceptual models of these linkages (e.g., see Cloninger et al. 1996). On occasion, this research has been oriented toward a facet of personality termed "harm avoidance," but most of the empirical studies have been designed in relation to the three-factor personality model advanced by Costa and McCrae (McCrae and Costa, 1990), with emphasis upon the factor called "openness to experience" (or closely related facets of personality known by the names of "sensation seeking" or "risk taking"). Empirical links between risk of illegal drug use and openness, sensation seeking, and risk-taking are well known (e.g., see Miles et al., 2001), but less well known is a pattern of findings that link dopamine receptor genes to this aspect of personality (e.g., see Ebstein et al., 1996; Benjamin et al., 1996). Hence, there is intriguing evidence of a causal mechanism to link the dopamine receptor genes to risk of drug dependence via a possible intermediate role of personality. Of course, the pattern of empirical evidence is not entirely consistent and (as might be expected) Gerlernter's research team has not been able to replicate a relationship between the implicated DRD4 polymorphism and novelty seeking in their sample (Gerlernter et al., 1997). We must wait for more definitive evidence on this eminently plausible linkage.

In sum, new lines of genetic epidemiological research on drug dependence have produced intriguing leads about a profile of hereditary influences on drug dependence, which now deserve additional study and systematic replication using more definitive epidemiologic research strategies in multiple sites, coupled with the methods of molecular genetics. The desirability of conducting these studies is supported by a concurrent trend of new findings now emerging from recent family and twin studies of drug dependence, despite methodologic problems due to sampling and ascertainment biases, as well as other limitations widely known to practitioners in the rapidly evolving fields of behavior genetics and genetic epidemiology. With the possible exception of the family of dopamine receptor genes, there is not yet sufficient evidence to warrant a Human Genome Epidemiology (HuGE) review of the type recently completed for the ALAD gene and lead toxicity (Kelada et al., 2001), but this is one of the target goals for genetic epidemiologists interested in drug dependence.

Twin research. Twin studies of drug use and drug dependence blossomed in the last decade of the twentieth century. Virtually all of these studies provided evidence of (1) substantial heritability of drug dependence at the 20%–25% level and sometimes as large as 60%–80%, (2) generally more modest heritability for initiation of drug use, and (3) substantial influence of environmental conditions, often characterized in relation to shared environment as opposed to nonshared environment (Kendler et al., 2000). For example, one of the first studies showed an excess of monozygotic (MZ) male twin concordance for drug dependence and/or abuse (63%) relative to dizygotic (DZ) male twin concordance (43%) and a generally consistent but less pronounced difference for female twin pairs. Although constrained somewhat by a possibility that MZ twins share environments more closely than DZ twins, the data from this study also provided preliminary estimates for the genetic components of liability for drug dependence and/or abuse: an estimated 31% for male twins (6–18%); an estimated 22% for females (6–45%). That is, even granting an inherited component, the evidence favors a large contribution from environmental conditions, larger than that observed for alcoholism and perhaps attributable to shared exposure opportunities for illicit drug use, even within MZ twin pairs (Pickens et al., 1991; Labuda et al., 1993). Kendler and Prescott (1998a) deserve credit for the largest reported heritability estimates from a twin study of cocaine use and problems of cocaine dependence. In their female twin sample, they found heritability of 39% for cocaine use, 79% for DSM-IV cocaine abuse, and 65% for DSM-IV cocaine dependence. By comparison, their estimates for cannabis are as follows: cannabis use, 35%–40%; DSM-IV cannabis abuse, 72%; DSM-IV cannabis dependence, 43%–62%, depending upon the model chosen.

Each of the recent twin studies merits close inspection, with differentiation of findings from studies of adult twins versus adolescent twins. Each research team is starting to add new evidence on the relative contributions of genes, shared or "common" environments, and nonshared or "unique" environments, notwithstanding an initial focus on estimation of heritability as a summary measure of the relative importance of genetic factors for a specific population at a specific time, given the genetic composition and range of environments available in that population (Kendler and Prescott, 1998a). In addition, each team has selected different facets of drug dependence epidemiology to explore in detail. Several examples will be presented.

Both McGue et al. (2000) and Maes et al. (1999) studied adolescent twin pairs in the United States, and found stronger estimates of heritability for tobacco use than for marijuana use and other illegal drug use. McGue et al. (2000) characterized the published heritability estimates of 22% and 18% for adolescent marijuana use as modest, although these values are sufficiently ample to motivate a search for underlying genetic substrates. Both McGue et al. (2000) and Maes et al. (1999) reported more substantial heritability estimates for tobacco use (55%–85%) and nicotine dependence (44%), consistent with the review prepared by Heath and Madden (1995).

An attempt by McGue's research team to investigate the relative balance of sources of variation in relation to shared and nonshared ("unique") environmental factors generally favored the shared environment, except with respect to the use of psychostimulant amphetamine drugs, for which the influence of nonshared environments was prominent (McGue et al., 2000). Whereas the use of multivariate models to partition sources of variation has become commonplace in these studies (e.g., via ACE models: Additive genetic, Common environment, Unique environment), estimates from these models generally rest upon an assumption of no gene-environment interactions, which on the surface would seem to be questionable in research on illegal drug taking and other behavioral disturbances such as conduct problems and drinking problems (e.g., see Cutronia et al., 1994; Cadoret et al. 1995a, b). There is an added complexity that might promote familiality in twin studies of illegal drugs, in that one twin (whether MZ or DZ) may be the vector introducing the other twin to the illegal drug use, and sustaining the twins' drug-taking once it begins. This kind of diffusion of an innovation from one twin to the other, and the sustained social reinforcement of the behavior, are processes that deserve greater scrutiny in twin research (e.g., see Kendler and Gardner, 1998). These are processes that also may be operational in relation to conditions such as bulimia and possibly childhood conduct disorder or adult antisocial personality disorder, but they are likely to be less prominent in twin studies of conditions such as Alzheimer's disease or post-traumatic stress disorder. The prominence of diffusion processes in relation to illegal drug use and drug dependence may help account for the size of the "shared environment" component of familiality estimates in the recent twin studies on these conditions, which tend to be larger than one sees in twin research on other behavioral traits (Plomin and Daniels, 1987), as noted by McGue et al.

The study by McGue and colleagues also is noteworthy for its failure to discover male–female differences in heritability estimates, which have been prominent in other studies that have included both male and female twin pairs (e.g., see Pickens et al., 1991). They have suggested that low statistical power might be an explanation for this lack of male–female differences. However, there is another possible explanation, related to a differentiation of adult twin studies and adolescent twin studies. McGue and colleagues are studying a sample of 17-year-old twin pairs. It is possible that the male–female differences emerge later in life. As they note, the prominence of shared familial influence during adolescence includes conditions such as family attendance at religious services or involvement in church-related activities, found elsewhere to have an inverse association with adolescent drug involvement (e.g., see Johanson et al., 1996; Maes et al., 1999).

In a recent adolescent twin study of more modest size and statistical power, but with the advantages gained by identifying adolescent twins from within a nationally representative survey sample, Miles et al. (2001) offer interesting evidence that to some extent contradicts the above-mentioned hypothesis linking genetic polymorphisms, illegal drug involvement, and sensation seeking or risk taking. Miles and colleagues found correlations between marijuana use and many of the manifestations of risk taking (e.g., not wearing a seat belt), but their models indicated that this covariation was due largely to influence of twin similarity in environmental experiences or conditions and not to genetic factors. One suspects that this difference in findings might be attributable to differences in the phenotype under study (e.g., dependence syndromes versus less involved adolescent use of marijuana as observed in a sample of school-attending youth).

Twin studies based on the Virginia Twin Registry, until recently mainly studies of adult female twins, have illuminated a variety of facets of the genetics of drug dependence, and are especially noteworthy because of a very fastidious approach to possible sources of bias in estimation, such as error due to unreliability in reporting on drug use and problems of drug dependence, noncooperation bias, and "social zygosity"—whether MZ twins are more likely to socialize together (Kendler and Prescott, 1998b, Kendler et al., 2000). To illustrate, Kendler and Gardner (1998) have provided some important new evidence on the "equal environment" assumption: that MZ and DZ twins are equivalent with respect to exposure to environmental influences. As these authors have noted, if the equal environment assumption is incorrect, then it is not just genetic similarity that accounts for greater concordance of drug dependence observed among MZ twins relative to DZ twins; at least some of the greater MZ concordance is attributable to environmental influences. By probing the EEA assumption via statistical modeling of data from Caucasian female same-sex twins recruited for the Virginia Twin Registry, they found evidence of an upward bias in the estimates of heritability for initiation of drug use, but not in heritability estimates for drug dependence. However, their models suggested that the magnitude of upward bias in the heritability estimate was no more than modest in their sample (Kendler and Gardner, 1998).

Tsuang et al. (1998), studying a sample of adult male twins from the Vietnam era twin registry, and Karkowski et al. (2000), studying a sample of adult female twins, have both arrived at a conclusion that there is substantial commonality in the vulnerability to drug dependence. Tsuang and colleagues found their strongest evidence favoring drug-specific vulnerability for heroin, and to a lesser extent, marijuana, but concluded that much of the vulnerability is common across drugs. Karkowski and colleagues summarize a similar result: "... just one general genetic factor and one general familial environmental factor in additional to nonfamilial environmental factors that influence drug use, regardless of type of substance" (Karkowski et al., 2000, p. 668).

Lyons et al. (1997) extended the line of twin research about marijuana by looking into possible genetic variation in response to marijuana use, in the form of subjectively experienced positive and negative effects, also drawing upon the Vietnam era twin registry samples. A very interesting result was that these marijuana effects, whether positive or negative, appear to be influenced mainly by nonshared or unique environmental conditions, with essentially no contribution from the common environment. The study produced a heritability estimate of 27% for experiencing negative effects of marijuana use, as reflected in a latent factor tapped by questions about experiences such as whether the twin ever felt paranoid shortly after using marijuana, and a heritability estimate of 29% for experiencing positive effects, as reflected in a separate latent factor tapped by questions about experiences such as whether the twin ever felt energetic or creative shortly after using marijuana. Of course, here again the ACE multivariate model's assumptions may be violated. For example, it seems likely that the experience of subjectively felt positive or negative reactions to marijuana depends upon gene-environment interactions.

True et al. (1997) also turned to the Vietnam era twin registry sample to investigate the possibility that liability to tobacco smoking initiation and smoking persistence are determined by the same or different factors. They considered a single liability dimension (SLD) model, an independent liability dimension (ILD) model, and a combined liability dimension (CLD) model, and found that twin-pair resemblance of smoking experiences were best explained by a combined liability dimension model with two component processes. The first process is expression of liability for initiation of tobacco smoking behavior, with substantial influences from genetic susceptibility and shared environmental factors. The second process is an expression of liability for persistence of tobacco smoking, with a strong genetic contribution and relatively little influence of shared or unique environmental factors. As with the other contributions from the Vietnam twin research team, this paper was a model of careful exposition for complex multivariate models, demonstrating how alternative conceptual models for stages of drug dependence can be compared and contrasted usefully.

The current evidence from twin studies of drug dependence also includes a finding that risk of drug abuse is greater for twins adopted away from biologic families with a history of alcohol problems (e.g., see Cadoret et al., 1980, 1986; Cadoret, 1992). The observed occurrence of drug abuse also was greater for twins adopted into families characterized by divorce or a history of psychiatric disturbances, even when there was no biologic family history of drug abuse.

Elaborating this line of research, Cadoret et al. (1995a, b, 1996) found evidence in support of two independently operating genetic pathways toward drug dependence for males, but a somewhat different result for females. One pathway leads from alcohol dependence problems in a biological parent for males but not females; the other pathway leads from the biological parent's antisocial behavior and personality traits, via intermediate adoptee aggression and the adoptee's own antisocial behavior and personality traits. Although it leaves open the possibility of drug-specific susceptibilities to drug dependence for females (as well as males), this adoption study adds strength to the inference that some of the risk of dependence on illegal drugs comes from genetic susceptibility to alcohol dependence, a "common factor" model in which the alcohol dependence of a biological parent confers increased risk of both alcohol dependence and dependence on other drugs, perhaps more readily detected in males than in females because of the above-mentioned male excess in occurrence of alcohol dependence.

Clearly the best approach to clarify the inherited vulnerabilities to drug dependence will be multifaceted. One facet will involve molecular genetics and a search for candidate genes and their expressed proteins, but this research will not stop when candidate genes for drug dependence are identified. The second facet will involve a discovery process to find or to design mutable environmental conditions or other interventions capable of modifying genes or gene products that predispose toward drug dependence. The earliest indication of these conditions may come from studies of siblings, including MZ and DZ twin pairs, who are discordant for drug dependence and whose history of experience from the chorionic sac onward can be traced with reasonable accuracy and precision. While the MZ-DZ concordance ratios signal important genetic vulnerabilities to drug dependence, the existence of many discordant MZ twins now constitutes our strongest evidence that environmental conditions are major causal influences with respect to drug dependence.

Family-Genetic Studies and Drug Dependence. Even before the human genome mapping project, the discovery of RFLPs linking the D_2 dopamine receptor gene with drug dependence, and recent twin study evidence on concordance of drug dependence, there was considerable research activity in relation to a possible familial aggregation of drug dependence. By 1985, Croughan was able to review nine studies concerning the occurrence of alcohol or drug dependence in families of patients admitted to drug treatment facilities. Compared with historical controls rather than internal controls for each study, the overall observed occurrence of drug dependence in parents and siblings seemed to be higher than expected values, especially among males, consistent with patterns of hypothesized familial aggregation (Croughan, 1985). Since then, many different research groups have contributed evidence on this topic, mainly consistent with patterns of hypothesized familial aggregation among parents and siblings (Mirin et al., 1991; Rounsaville et al., 1991; Merikangas et al., 1992; Luthar et al., 1992a, b, 1993).

Four important advances were made in the early work led by Rounsaville and Merikangas. First, many of the siblings of opioid-dependent subjects had not experimented with illicit drug use, although more than a majority had done so. In this respect, they were no different from most adolescents and young adults growing up in the United States. However, in contrast with available epidemiologic evidence on the transition from drug use to drug dependence, virtually all of the drug-using siblings later developed drug dependence and/or drug abuse. Second, in this research statistical models were used to hold constant alternative suspected determinants of risk (e.g., sex and age) as well as methodologic conditions (e.g., method of case ascertainment). Even under these more rigorous circumstances the investigators found evidence that parental drug disorders signaled an increased risk for drug dependence or abuse among siblings of opioid-dependent patients. Third, drug dependence and/or abuse was more likely to occur when both parents were affected by drug disorders compared with the experience of siblings with only one parent or neither parent affected. Finally, a very large majority of the spouses of opioid-dependent patients were found to have developed drug dependence and/or drug abuse themselves, with implications not only for future studies of assortative mating in relation to drug disorders but also for studies that seek to understand how children might be influenced by drug dependence within the family. One important implication of these findings is that the offspring of drug-dependent parents are not universally disadvantaged by drug dependence or related problems: Unlike many of their contemporaries and as distinct from their opioid-dependent siblings, a large number had not experimented with illicit drug use. Similar findings have emerged from other recent investigations into the offspring of alcohol- and drug-dependent parents based on yoking together small clinical and community samples.

As was observed for twin research on drug dependence, there now is an accumulating number of studies on familial aggregation of various forms of drug dependence, some with ascertainment via clinical samples, some with more general epidemiological field survey sampling. One of the important observations from these studies involves a question raised in the introduction to this chapter and in relation to the twin and adoption studies. Namely, should we think of a single diathesis or genetic susceptibility for alcohol, tobacco, and other drug dependence, such as a common tendency to become dependent? Another possibility is that there is some degree of drug-specificity in this tendency, with some individuals predisposed toward dependence on alcohol, and a different inherited predisposition for dependence on cocaine or marijuana or tobacco. The accumulated evidence on this research question is not yet definitive, but there are some recent studies suggesting existence of a source of familial aggregation that is generic across drugs (alcohol, tobacco, marijuana, cocaine), not entirely explained by similarity in drug exposure opportunities, as well as existence of drug-specific predispositions toward dependence upon cocaine or marijuana (e.g., see Merikangas et al., 1998a, b; Beirut et al., 1998).

Several research groups have offered recent extensions of the family-genetic research design by studying adoptees who have been recruited after contacts with adoption agencies or as members of large epidemiological survey samples. Newlin et al. (2000) studied adoptees recruited from within the NLAES study sample, and found that the adoptive father's alcohol dependence problems might have influenced risk of dependence on illegal drugs as well as risk of alcohol dependence. This evidence in support of a common factor model was not observed when the adoptive mother had drinking problems. McGue et al. (1996) investigated parental and sibling influences on drinking by studying an adoption sample recruited from agencies, but focused their attention on siblings within the family. Their sample included adoptees as well as the birth offspring of the adoptive parents. Within the sample of birth offspring, there was evidence to link the father's problem drinking with the adolescent son's alcohol involvement, and to link the mothers problem drinking with the adolescent daughters alcohol involvement, but evidence did not link the opposite-sex pairs of parents and offspring. Moreover, if the observed relationships were a manifestation of social learning and offspring imitation of the same-sex parent's behavior, then there ought to be similar links in the data on the adopted children. Surprisingly, there was no association between father's or mother's problem drinking and the adolescent alcohol involvement of the adopted children. However, there were sib–sib associations in alcohol involvement, leading the investigators to conclude that perhaps there is a substantial environmental effect of sibling drinking that has been neglected in research on children of alcoholic parents. Whether these findings can be replicated by others, and whether they apply to drug dependence problems are open questions for future research.

In summary, each line of research on genetic susceptibilities for drug dependence has produced evidence to challenge a belief that occurrence of drug dependence can be explained entirely by sociologic or psychological factors. To be sure, more definitive research is needed before we can identify and control the mechanisms that account for observed familial aggregation of drug dependence. The present state of knowledge indicates that some of these mechanisms will involve inherited predispositions, while others surely will involve congenital, perinatal, or postnatal experiences leading toward and past the initial experience of drug exposure (Turner et al., 1993).

Kendler and colleagues recently outlined four questions that will assume increasing importance in the next stage of genetics research on the drug dependence syndromes.

1. What are the pathways from genes to substance misuse and to what extent do they involve personality, psychopathologic processes, variations in metabolism, target receptors, and/or postreceptor mechanisms (such as the signaling pathways studied by Maldonado et al., 1996; Blendy and Maldonado, 1998)?
2. What is the relationship between the genetic and environmental factors that influence initiation versus subsequent misuse?
3. How specific are genetic risks for the use and misuse of individual psychoactive substances?
4. What are the chromosomal locations of susceptibility genes for the [psychoactive substance use disorders]?

These four questions lay out points on a map for the future of a genetic epidemiological perspective as applied to the study of drug dependence. To this list may be added some new questions that elaborate the above. Namely, how do genetic susceptibilities combine to influence the selection of environmental conditions that influence the transition from first drug use to risk of becoming drug dependent, and how are these genetic susceptibilities modified by environmental conditions and processes? These are questions for a 'human envirome project' to complement the ongoing human genome project and its new proteomics developments (Anthony et al., 1995; Yang and Khoury, 1997; Anthony, 2001).

Suspected Prenatal and Perinatal Influences on Risk. Within the field of human growth and development, there is a broad consensus that adult behavior and behavioral disturbances are more readily predicted from behavioral and performance characteristics measured in middle to late childhood (ages 5–13), and in adolescence, than from behavior exhibited during infancy and the early childhood (Collins, 1986). For this reason, and also because of major problems of logistics and cost, drug dependence researchers generally have not sought to link very early life experiences and infant development to later risk of drug dependence in adulthood. Instead, they have focused attention primarily on the adolescent years. Nonetheless, in recent drug dependence research there has been some progress in relation to risk-associated characteristics that are observable in the prenatal and perinatal periods and in childhood (e.g., see Glantz, 1992).

For example, preclinical laboratory studies show how prenatal and perinatal drug exposures can alter later drug action and drug-taking behavior. In addition, a human embryo or fetus continually exposed *in utero* to cocaine or heroin will develop drug dependence and will show signs of drug withdrawal within a few hours of delivery. By extension, it is plausible that *in utero* drug exposure might be an early predisposing factor for drug dependence later in life. This hypothesis now is under investigation as cocaine babies and other prenatally drug-exposed infants are being followed in studies of growth and development (e.g., Mayes et al., 1998;

Bandstra et al., 2001; Morrow et al., 2001). Studies of the effects of prenatal tobacco and alcohol exposure also are under way, and already have produced some new and interesting findings that perhaps the early drug involvement of offspring has been increased in response to prenatal alcohol or tobacco exposure (e.g., see Yates et al., 1998; Kandel et al., 1998).

When human research on neurobehavioral responses to prenatal drug exposure is evaluated in relation to principles of epidemiological research, there is an immediate methodological challenge. In these studies, investigators generally have used multiple regression models to hold constant alternative sources of variation in the responses under study. Prominent in the lists of alternative sources of variation are maternal behaviors such as the mother's level of alcohol, tobacco, and marijuana use during pregnancy, as well as the results of maternal behavior such as the number of visits for prenatal care. By using standard regression models to adjust for these alternative sources of variation, the investigators seek to learn whether the neurobehavioral response in any way depends upon prenatal cocaine exposure, *independent* of the other sources of variation. The methodological challenge is introduced because of reciprocities that are likely to exist between the use of cocaine during pregnancy and the use of other drugs during pregnancy, and because maternal characteristics such as the number of visits for prenatal care also depend to some extent upon whether the mother is a cocaine user. Because these behaviors and characteristics are *endogenous* with respect to the mother's cocaine use, regression adjustment for these characteristics, in general, will produce a downward bias in the estimates of cocaine influence on the neurobehavioral responses of the offspring. In effect, what is being controlled is a potential intermediate variable in the pathway that leads from prenatal cocaine exposure to the neurobehavioral response of the offspring (e.g., see Weinberg, 1993, 1994).

Methodological challenges of this type will become increasingly important as the generation of cocaine-exposed children enter the adolescent years when they are exposed to opportunities to try tobacco, cocaine, and other drugs. Even if there is no effect of prenatal cocaine exposure on impulsive, dysregulated, sensation seeking, or aggressive behavior, it will be important to discover whether there are effects on the lag times from first opportunity to first use, from first use to multiple uses, and from first use to the occurrence of drug dependence syndromes. An intriguing possibility is that this type of cocaine effect will be limited to psychostimulant drugs, perhaps due to a change in what Ralph Tarter has called a vector of influence on the ontogenetic trajectory that leads toward drug use. Alternately, the effect of prenatal cocaine exposure might be generic in nature, affecting the trajectories of involvement with alcohol, marijuana, and other drugs, in addition to effects on cocaine, amphetamine, and other psychostimulant drugs.

Building from early work on a continuum of reproductive casualty identified by Pasamanick, Knobloch, and Lilienfeld, several research teams have sought complications of pregnancy and delivery that might produce psychiatric disorders, including disturbances of behavior as well as drug dependence. Several inquiries along these lines are under way, some of them using a nonconcurrent prospective research design to study newborns assessed between 1960 and 1966 for the multisite National Collaborative Perinatal Project (NCPP), with follow-up assessments in young adulthood. To date, the NCPP follow-up studies have not identified prenatal or perinatal causes of drug dependence, but the early evidence points toward a possibly protective effect of chronic fetal hypoxia. Among young adults followed to ages 18–27 years, the occurrence of DIS/DSM-III drug dependence or abuse was observed to be 0.7 times lower among subjects who had experienced chronic fetal hypoxia, as compared to subjects without pregnancy or delivery complications. The investigators have suggested that the protective effect might be due to poor health or functional status of the hypoxia group, with secondary impact to make them less out-going, more sheltered by parents, and thereby less likely to become cases of drug dependence or abuse (Buka et al., 1993). Additional followup of these NCPP samples is underway; this research has produced some new findings on parent-child relationships (e.g., attachment behavior) and the subsequent risk of illegal drug problems (e.g., Windham and Chilcoat, 2001), which have resonance with a still-evolving body of evidence on a possibly protective influence of parent-child mutual attachment during the childhood years and adolescence, as reviewed recently by Brook et al. (2000a).

In summary, until more inquiries have been completed, it will not be possible to speak confidently about the impact of prenatal or immediate postnatal factors on the risk of later drug dependence. Nonetheless, as suggested by the NCPP investigators, early life experiences such as chronic fetal hypoxia theoretically are capable of reducing the risk of later drug dependence by virtue of their more proximal impact on childhood behavior and then by secondary parental or school responses to the child's behavior.

The next several sections of this chapter shed additional light on the importance for drug dependence research of the work that maps human environments and exposures from early embryonic development through gestation and birth and onward toward childhood and later stages of development.

Suspected Determinants of Risk as Observed in Childhood. Seeking the root causes of drug dependence, many investigators have turned to the period of childhood and adolescent development, and the result has been several classic studies on the hypothesis that childhood deviance, misbehavior, and aggression might be important behavioral causal factors for later drug dependence, especially for males. The balance of evidence on this matter now favors a possibly causal predictive linkage between early misbehavior and later serious drug involvement, implicating not only drug dependence and drug abuse syndromes, but also intravenous drug use. This suspected causal association has received generally consistent support from a variety of research designs, including a nonconcurrent prospective study, a concurrent prospective study, an application of the epidemiologic case-base strategy, and a growing number of both longitudinal and retrospective studies (e.g., see Robins, 1966; Kellam et al., 1983; Tomas et al., 1990; White, 1992).

The base of evidence linking childhood misbehavior and conduct problems to later serious drug involvement now has become so strong that randomized field trials are underway to test the hypothesized linkage. In these trials, experimental school-based programs are being tested to determine whether they first reduce childhood misbehavior and conduct problems and then whether they reduce risk of later drug involvement and drug dependence. Using this approach, investigators hope to translate the observational research findings into practical public health action against drug dependence (e.g., see Kellam et al., 1991; Hawkins et al., 1991; Dolan et al., 1993). For example, Kellam and Anthony (1998) have described promising results from a randomized prevention trial to evaluate the "Good Behavior Game," which can be used by a teacher to reinforce rule-abiding behavior and to reduce the occurrence of rule breaking in first and second grade classrooms: boys randomly assigned to "Good Behavior Game" classrooms in this trial were some 30%–50% less likely to start smoking tobacco by their early teen years. A second replication of this experiment produced consistent estimates (Kellam and Anthony, 1998). This type of experimental test of the hypothesized causal link from rule breaking to later drug involvement and drug dependence is important because the strengths of a randomized design have been used to constrain the potential influence of genetic or acquired liabilities that might link rule breaking with risk of drug involvement, as discussed by Cadoret et al. (1995a, b).

Several recent retrospective studies and a few longitudinal studies have implicated child psychiatric syndromes other than conduct disorder and the later risk of drug problems (e.g., Boyle et al., 1993; Kandel et al., 1997; Brook et al., 1998a, b; Weinberg and Glantz, 1999). Some prominence has been given to Attention Deficit Hyperactivity Disorder (e.g., see Biederman et al., 1997; Chilcoat and Breslau, 1999) and to a more general hyperactivity syndrome of attentional difficulties, impulsivity, and hyperactive behavior in childhood for drug dependence, separate from conduct problems. There now are mixed results from studies on hyperactivity and drug use, but the most definitive inquiries to date suggest that hyperactive boys without early aggressive behavior are more likely to have developed DSM-III drug dependence and/or abuse in the early years of adulthood, that is, between ages 23 and 30 . Boys whose hyperactive behavior, impulsivity, or attentional difficulties persisted into adulthood seem to be an especially high prevalence group for drug dependence and/or abuse (Mannuzza et al., 1993). There are a variety of possible mechanisms to account for this finding, including potentially reciprocal interplay between drug use, impulsivity, and attentional difficulties once drug experimentation has begun. The same issue of reciprocal interplay has been raised in relation to the dimensional personality constructs of sensation seeking and openness, which have modest correlations with hyperactivity. Namely, it can be argued that sensation seeking, openness to new experiences, and other behavioral tendencies displayed in childhood are determined by both inherited and experiential factors and that these behavioral tendencies in turn bring the child into contact with later experiences and environments that promote the reinforcing functions of subsequent drug use. In this way, inherited and situational conditions may transact reciprocally with one another, leading toward greater risk of drug dependence. This transactional model of the interplay between inherited predispositions and situational circumstances is a theme of increasing importance in psychopathologic research, including studies of alcoholism and drug dependence as well as other forms of behavioral and mental disorders (e.g., see Sameroff and Fiese, 1989; Tarter et al., 1990; Tarter and Mezzich, 1992; Kendler and Prescott, 1998a, b; Vanyukov and Tarter, 2000). In a recent etiologically oriented model, Giancola et al. (1998) have stressed a possible risk-enhancing effect associated with dysregulation of executive cognitive functioning in childhood (i.e., impairments in higher order cognitive abilities such as abstract reasoning and planning), and the model accommodates a possibility that drug exposure might become a cause of greater dysregulation of executive functioning once drug use begins.

The academic prowess of children remains somewhat of a puzzle in relation to initiation of drug use and risk of later, more serious drug involvement. In some research, the very capable children initiated drug use earlier than their less capable classmates, perhaps in connection with status as leaders in diffusion of innovations, although early academic competence did not signal increased probability of more serious drug involvement (Fleming et al., 1982). In other research, an improvement in academic performance in later childhood and adolescence has seemed to afford some protection against what otherwise would be a higher risk trajectory toward serious drug involvement (Brook et al., 1986; Hawkins et al., 1992). However, in a recently published long-term followup of a controlled trial, illegal drug involvement was not reduced while heavy drinking was reduced among students who had the benefit of a primary school intervention intended to strengthen school bonding and performance. That is, the impact on illegal drug involvement was not as predicted by current conceptual models of prevention, neither with respect to school bonding and academic performance, nor with respect to the link from heavy drinking to potentially more serious illegal drug involvement (Hawkins et al., 1999).

There also is some evidence to suggest that risk of developing drug problems is greater when drug use starts early, for example, in middle to late childhood (e.g., see Robins and Przybeck, 1985). This relationship does not appear to be due simply to the fact that early starters accumulate more years of drug use, although more prospective evidence on this topic is needed (e.g., see Anthony and Petronis, 1995; Tarter et al., 1999).

Recently, Brook et al. (1998a, b) have offered a synthetic model that attempts to integrate facets of social and psychological development in the etiology of drug involvement from childhood through adulthood, but gives little attention to macrosocial and mesosocial influences that are experienced outside the domains of family, school, and peer groups. In contrast, Szapocznik and Coatsworth (1999) specify an ecodevelopmental trajectory model that is true to the suspected multilevel influences of community, family, and peer groups across stages of development, but this model fails to integrate basic biological and maturational processes that may be of importance. Dawes et al. (2000) have advanced a conceptual model in which liability to drug dependence problems is characterized in relation to cognitive, affective, and behavioral dysregulation, with links to neuroadaptational substrates such as cortisol reactivity. This synthesis is attractive because it draws together many of the above-mentioned threads, including the influence of parental drinking and drug use, rule breaking and other forms of behavioral dysregulation, disruptions of attention and other dysregulated executive functioning, traits of temperament such as irritability (which might mediate the influence of parental drinking or drug use per Blackson et al., 1994), and precocious or delayed maturation (e.g., see Newcomb, 1992). In a study previously mentioned for an inverse and possibly protective association between childhood drug involvement and church and religion-related behaviors, Johanson et al. (1996) described a separate facet of precocious development and risk of becoming an early onset drug user. Namely, younger children who had assumed adult-like social roles (working for pay, taking care of children, housekeeping) were more likely to have become early-onset drug users; older children who had yet not assumed these adult-like social roles were less likely to have become early-onset drug users.

Finally, for some (but not all) investigators in this arena, an early thematic focus on childhood behavioral and temperamental characteristics has begun to shift toward aspects of childhood environment, especially modifiable aspects of childhood environment. For example, there is an accumulation of evidence from a variety of studies that lapses in parental supervision and monitoring in middle to late childhood might signal increased risk of initiating drug use and perhaps increased risk of later drug dependence (e.g., Barnes and Farrell, 1992; Chassin et al., 1993; Chilcoat et al., 1995; Chilcoat and Anthony, 1996). Of course, it also is possible for the adolescents to shape the practices of their parents, including parental supervision and monitoring (e.g., see Niederhiser et al., 1999), but this reciprocity does not gainsay the potential benefits of increased parental supervision and monitoring of children with respect to later drug involvement. Storr et al. (in press) have reported promising early results from a field experiment to prevent early onset drug use via improvements in parenting practices in the early primary school years, including improved parental supervision and monitoring.

In new epidemiologic research on suspected determinants of risk that can be observed in childhood, it will be important to use field experiments and other rigorous forms of program evaluation to probe causal inferences derived from theory or from the systematically replicated evidence of observational studies. In some instances, these field experiments can be mounted by extending evaluation research now underway to test elementary school drug prevention programs and efforts to improve childhood education. For example, if these drug prevention programs are shown to delay onset of drug experimentation, then it will be important to determine whether they also lead to reduced risk of later, more serious drug involvement. In a similar fashion, programs of large-scale experimental evaluations of new changes in the elementary school curriculum can be made into a foundation for epidemiologic inquiries into whether experimentally induced improvements in academic performance yield later reduced risk of drug dependence (e.g., see Kellam, 1994, and Mrazek and Haggerty, 1994, for discussions of theory-based preventive interventions).

In this respect, a prevailing shift away from psychological and behavioral constructs toward modifiable aspects of childhood environment has an added appeal. Having discovered that a childhood behavioral or temperamental characteristic signals an increased risk of drug dependence, it is necessary to undertake an additional lengthy program of research to identify changes in the childhood environment that might alter this characteristic or dampen its risk-enhancing impact. For example, whereas early childhood misbehavior has been identified as a risk indicator for later serious drug involvement, we still do not know which early interventions directed toward misbehavior are most effective. In addition, it will not suffice simply to probe whether the intervention changes the early risk indicator; evidence of impact on later risk of drug dependence is required before we mount large-scale public health actions in the name of preventing drug dependence. In contrast, an orientation to modifiable aspects of childhood environment can be guided by a focus on environments that are known to be responsive to existing interventions or with moderate adaptation of those interventions (e.g., see Davis and Tunks, 1990, 1991).

Parent monitoring offers a case in point. To be sure, the evidence on poor monitoring and risk of drug dependence must be strengthened by systematic replication in a series of epidemiologic studies. Nonetheless, by virtue of prior research on parent monitoring and childhood conduct problems, the intervention programs known to improve parent monitoring already are in existence so that the portfolio of studies for systematic replication can be balanced in favor of rigorous field experiments versus strictly observational studies.

Suspected Determinants of Risk as Observed in Adolescence. We already have remarked on the striking association between age and drug dependence and on the observation that risk of serious drug involvement increases sharply between middle and late adolescence. These observations have provided a strong rationale for investigators to study the developmental period of adolescence in relation to drug use and drug problems (e.g., see Chassin et al., 1996). In addition, many of the world's epidemiological surveillance operations are directed toward the drug-taking experiences of school-aged youths, and this orientation helps promote a concentration on this developmental period (e.g., see Johnston et al., 2001).

Some of the themes discussed in relation to childhood determinants of risk also appear in research on adolescence and drug use, particularly those concerning sensation seeking, impulsivity, conduct problems, delinquency, and low academic achievement. Other risk indicators with some supportive evidence include religiosity, emotionality, depressed mood, low self-esteem, and self-derogation, as well as a domain of psychological constructs that involve expectancies about the functions to be served by alcohol and other drug use, as well as the perceived risks of drug taking (Johnston et al., 2001). That is, in some work, early assessments of teens' expectations for what can be gained by consuming drugs have signaled later, more intensive drug involvement; use of cocaine and other controlled drugs has occurred less often among those who rate drug use as an especially risky behavior (e.g., see Weinberg et al., 1998).

In some instances, a longitudinal research design has helped to test hypotheses about the precursors of these psychological characteristics, as well as co-occuring psychiatric disorders, including, for example, (1) suspected linkages between uncontrollable negative life events, followed by secondary mood disturbances, and then followed by drug use in adolescence; and (2) a possible sequence from parental alcoholism toward adolescent drug use via three hypothesized mediators: lapses in parent monitoring and control over adolescent offspring, levels of stress and negative mood states in the offspring, and emotionality in the offspring (e.g., see Hawkins et al., 1992; Clayton, 1992; Kaplan and Johnson, 1992; Chassin et al., 1993). With respect to adolescent psychiatric disorders, a growing body of evidence indicates that these disorders are not generally powerful causal influences on later risk of youthful drug involvement or drug dependence, but that drug involvement in early-to-mid-adolescence might influence later risk of psychiatric disturbances in adolescence and young adulthood (e.g., see Brook et al., 1998a; Wu and Anthony, 1999; Johnson et al., 2000). Johnson et al. (1997) anticipated an association between adolescent bipolar disorder and later drug dependence problems, but found no longitudinal association.

Applications of longitudinal latent growth curve models created for studies of human growth, psychological development, and educational achievement have started to penetrate epidemiological studies of these suspected influences on drug involvement. One recent illustration involves the work of a research group led by Judith Brook, previously mentioned in relation to studies of a possibly protective influence of parent–child mutual attachment and a hypothesized mediation of this influence via adolescent intolerance toward deviant behavior and reduced affiliation with deviant peers (Brook et al., 2000a). In order to probe the issue of adolescent intolerance of deviance in more detail, Brook and colleagues investigated whether this kind of "conventionality" or "unconventionality" might be related to a developmental trajectory of marijuana use across the developmental period from early adolescence through the late twenties. Drawing upon a longitudinal latent growth model that expresses developmental trajectories in terms of subject-specific intercepts and subject-specific slopes, the research team found evidence of original cross-sectional relationships between conventionality and reduced levels of marijuana involvement, plus evidence that declining levels of conventionality were associated with growth (i.e., steeper slope) in the trajectory of marijuana involvement from the early teen years to the later years of young adulthood (Brook et al., 2000a).

Notwithstanding some excellent studies on these suspected determinants of risk in the adolescent years (e.g., see Weinberg et al., 1998; Derzon and Lipsey, 1999), the affiliation with peer groups far and away is the most dominant focus of research on drug use in the teen years. This focus can be supported on theoretical grounds: peer interaction is central in the creation of exposure opportunities that bring youths into contact with drugs, and peers often are participating vectors in the sequence of movements that convey drugs out of the reservoir toward human populations. There now also is considerable empirical evidence on peer drug use and affiliation with deviant peers as strong indicators of risk for teenage drug involvement (e.g., see Kandel, 1996), including recent data on how affiliation with deviant peers might be facilitated by lapses in parent monitoring that are associated with parental alcoholism (e.g., see Hawkins et al., 1992; Chassin et al., 1993). Duncan et al. (1998) used latent growth curves to probe a social context model for adolescent drug involvement, with levels and accelerated rates of drug involvement expressed as a function of increases in parent–child conflict, affiliation with deviant peers, and academic difficulties. Brook et al. (2000a) have offered evidence that a previously mentioned protective influence of early parent–child mutual attachment might be mediated, in part, by development of less tolerant attitudes toward deviance in adolescence, which in turn may reduce affilation with deviant peers and later associated risks of illegal drug involvement. In addition to many observational studies on peer group affiliation and teen drug use, there now is supportive data from several field experiments to test interventions that increase peer resistance skills and other social competencies of adolescents (e.g., Ellickson and Bell, 1990; Hansen and Graham, 1991; Hansen, 1992; Botvin et al., 1995, 2000; Spoth et al., 1999; Scheier et al., 2001).

There remain four especially important gaps in the epidemiology of drug dependence in relation to adolescent peer groups. First, the experimental data on peer resistance and social skill training do not yet speak to whether these interventions reduce the risk of later drug dependence, although these data generally are balanced in favor of short-term and longer-term impact to delay initiation of drug use and some of the persistence of smoking (e.g., see Resnicow and Botvin, 1993; Ellickson et al., 1993a, b; Botvin et al., 1995, 2000). To date, there is promising but still meagre evidence that these interventions have reduced risk of progression from tobacco use to later more serious drug involvement, for example, use of cocaine or heroin (Ellickson et al., 1993b; Spoth et al., 1999; Botvin et al., 2000). Second, for adolescents who have already started to use drugs, the peer resistance and social skills training may boomerang and actually lead to increased drug use (Ellickson and Bell, 1990). This is a potentially adverse consequence of these intervention programs that now must be probed in more detail. Third, no more than a handful of studies now speak to the mechanisms by which the peer-focused intervention programs might exert a risk-reducing effect on later drug involvement, although there are some intriguing leads that implicate sensation seeking as a potentially modifying variable (e.g., see Clayton et al., 1991; Scheier et al., 2001). Finally, there continues to be a pressing need for more research on what determines adolescent peer affiliations, including studies that give more attention to aspects of childhood and adolescent environment, such as parent monitoring, in addition to a more traditional focus on childhood behavioral and temperamental characteristics such as sociability and self-derogation (e.g., see Kaplan and Johnson, 1992; Brown et al., 1993; Richardson et al., 1993; Brook et al., 2000a).

To some extent, research on these environmental conditions has been held back by impressions that in adolescence the influence of parents is superceded by that of peer groups. This impression was bolstered by reports that peer factors pre-empted parent and family factors in predictive models of adolescent drug taking, where the modeling strategy was that of stepwise regression, which neglects to account for the possibility that parenting is one of the determinants of peer affiliation. As such, controlling for peer drug use when seeking to test hypotheses about parental influence may represent an instance of inappropriate control of a suspected confounding variable in the model-building process, a topic that has been discussed thoroughly in the epidemiologic literature (Weinberg, 1993, 1994; Joffe and Greenland, 1994), and previously raised in this chapter's review of methodological challenges in research on prenatal drug exposures.

To some extent, the peer group research entails a shift from the domain of individual-level determinants of risk to a domain of group-level determinants. Other group-level or macro-social conditions of recent interest include (1) community norms and public attitudes for and against drug taking and (2) neighborhood deterioration as an indicator of exposure opportunity for contact with illicit drugs. Working from a theory that community norms and public attitudes are of central importance, the Partnership for a Drug-Free America and others have mounted a massive media campaign of counterprogramming against otherwise prevailing prodrug influences. The Partnership has produced reports on early time series analyses, based on a repeated sequence of cross-sectional surveys, that suggest not only that adolescents have seen and remembered the antidrug media announcements but also that the announcements have promoted lower prevalence of drug taking. These are important and promising results on an innovative public health strategy, but a more rigorous analysis by an independent evaluation team is needed.

Several lines of epidemiologic research are raising the possibility that some individual-level risk characteristics can be understood best in relation to community-level characteristics, including both demographic and economic indicators of neighborhood (e.g., percent living in single-family housing), as well as signs of neighborhood deterioration and other evidence of social capital and material wealth. For example, when African-American and white American teenagers living in the same neighborhood have been compared, there is either no difference in prevalence of crack smoking or the African-American teens appear to be at lower risk (e.g., see Lillie-Blanton et al., 1993). There also is some evidence that neighborhood deterioration might be an important risk-modifying condition. A preliminary report from one prospective study suggests that exposure opportunities for illicit drug use depend in part on prior levels of neighborhood deterioration assessed in relation to lack of nearby parks and recreational facilities, deteriorated housing, public intoxication, and related characteristics of the neighborhood of residence (Crum et al., 1994).

For most of the last three decades of the twentieth century, it was quite common to see community-level characteristics and neighborhood context embedded within theories to explain the occurrence of drug dependence problems. However, in empirical research, these higher-level conditions and processes either were neglected, or were incorporated as individual-level characteristics. For example, each study participant might be given an individual value, corresponding to a characteristic of his or her neighborhood, such as the delinquency rate (e.g., see Majumder et al., 1998). Recent developments in multilevel methods have made it possible to incorporate family, neighborhood, and community context variables within working conceptual models for epidemiological analysis (e.g., see Diez-Rouz, 1998; Greenland, 2000).

One family of multilevel methods is based upon so-called marginal or population-averaged models. To illustrate, one of the observable manifestations of the influence of neighborhood context is the clustering of drug-related behavior, which diffuses from person to person, and might do so within neighborhoods of residence. A marginal model known as "alternating logistic regression" uses a generalized estimating equations method to estimate clustering in the form of a pairwise cross product ratio (PWCPR). This PWCPR has properties similar to an odds ratio: upward deviations from a null value of 1.0 signify associations of note, and clustering: the larger the pairwise cross product ratio, the more clustering. In a series of applications of the alternating logistic regression method, epidemiological research on drug involvement has disclosed the following: (1) clustering of marijuana use and cocaine use has been observed as manifestations of city-level and neighborhood-level context; clustering of inhalant drug use has been observed as a manifestation of school-level context; (2) the magnitude of clustering tends to be larger for the more extreme forms of drug-taking behavior (e.g., daily or weekly marijuana use versus ever use of marijuana), (3) neighborhood context determines clustering associated with city context in the sense that once neighborhood context is taken into account, there is no palpable city-level clustering, (4) the magnitude of clustering differs across subgroups of the population (e.g., in relation to daily marijuana use, the clustering is stronger for women than for men), and (5) it is not just the drug-taking behavior that clusters; in addition, opportunities to try illegal drugs shows clustering within neighborhood contexts, and so do perceptions about the harmfulness or risk associated with illegal drug use (Bobashev and Anthony, 1998, 2000; Petronis and Anthony, 2000; Delva et al., 2000). As this line of research proceeds, there is an expectation that the studies will disclose links between clustering of perceived risks of cocaine use within neighborhoods, clustering of opportunities to try cocaine, and clustering of different levels of cocaine involvement, as well as the influence of social capital or other suspected contextual determinants of the clustering (Petronis and Anthony, 2000).

These methods might be used to evaluate media campaigns of the type described above. For example, within communities having greater exposure to media campaigns of this type, there should be greater clustering of individuals who espouse community norms and public attitudes that are not conducive to drug use (e.g., see Petronis and Anthony, 2000). Moreover, within neighborhoods, subgroups of individuals with antidrug attitudes should show less clustering of illegal drug involvement than subgroups with more ambivalent or prodrug attitudes (e.g., see Bobashev and Anthony, 2000). Research on these clustering hypotheses about media campaign effects has not yet been conducted.

Separate from the marginal models, another family of multilevel methods is based upon so-called subject-specific or "random effects" models. Duncan et al. (1998) provide an illustration of the use of this type of multilevel model in a longitudinal study of drinking by members of 435 families, each with at least one adolescent child between the ages of 11 and 15 years, and each with at least one parent, or one sib age 11 years or older, or both. Here, the context under study was that of the family, and one of the main research questions involved expressing initial levels and later trajectories of alcohol use of adolescent family members as a function of shared aspects of family context such as family socioeconomic status and parental presence (e.g., step-family, 1-parent only, etc.), as well as individual-level characteristics such as level of deviance or rule breaking, age, and sex (male vs female). In addition to anticipated findings on age and male–female differences, this model provided evidence in support of the possibility that increases in adolescent drinking occurred in connection with families experiencing parental transitions (i.e., step families), and in association with lower SES of the families. Advantages of this type of multilevel model may be readily apparent to readers who face complex family data with a varying number of multiple respondents per family, or other types of "nested structures" in their observational data on dependent happenings, even if the advantages of longitudinal latent growth curve models are not immediately clear.

As a final note in relation to epidemiologic research on determinants of risk for drug dependence in adolescence, we draw attention to the concept of a comprehensive community-based prevention strategy that has been developed in response to requests by American community leaders concerned about youthful drug taking. As the label states, the underlying concept is that a combination of concurrent intervention tactics will be required in order to bring about reduced prevalence of drug taking in the community. Some of these interventions involve mass media announcements (e.g., billboards, public service announcements on television and radio), police initiatives, and other tactics directed toward community norms and other community-level characteristics thought to reduce prevalence of drug taking. Concurrently, there are interventions directed toward parents (often, drug education programs for parents) and toward schools (for example, creation of the school neighborhood as a drug-free zone; establishment of an anti-tobacco smoking policy for the school students, faculty, and staff), as well as peer resistance training and other school-based interventions directed toward adolescents and their peers (e.g., see Johnson et al., 1990).

Early evaluation research on community prevention programming of this type showed promising results in relation to adolescent initiation of drug use, although inferences about program impact were constrained by nonequivalence of the community control group and lack of random assignment to intervention status (e.g., see MacKinnon et al., 1991). Nonetheless, as in the instance of peer resistance and social skills training, the evaluation has not yet clarified whether drug dependence and other serious drug involvement are being prevented or whether the interventions modify risk characteristics of adolescents unlikely to develop drug dependence even in the absence of an intervention program. Whereas there are promising findings from community-based prevention programs that are directed toward alcohol use or toward behaviors thought to influence risk of cardiovascular diseases (e.g., Farquhar et al., 1990), more research on this question is needed before we can be confident that comprehensive community drug abuse prevention programming merits application beyond current levels. In addition, once we see definitive evidence of total program impact, it will be necessary to conduct experiments to reveal which of the several tactics are basically inert resource-consuming activities and which deliver the observed impact.

Suspected Determinants of Risk as Observed in Late Adolescence and Early Adulthood. Many clinical observers trace the origins of drug dependence to the developmental periods of childhood and early to middle adolescence, neglecting the potential importance of suspected risk determinants that are not observed until late adolescence or adulthood. Nonetheless, there is some epidemiologic evidence about suspected determinants of risk during these later periods of development, in addition to what we already have reported concerning age, sex, and race.

An important finding about the later environmental determinants of drug dependence emerged from a study of 571 male Vietnam veterans returning to the United States in the early 1970s (mean age, 19 years), with urinalysis and DIS-like methods used to assess drug use and drug dependence, already mentioned earlier in this chapter. Studied retrospectively, only one veteran had a history of dependence on narcotic drugs (i.e., opioids) prior to enlistment, but a very large proportion, 19.5%, became dependent while serving in Vietnam, where opium, heroin, and other opioids often were available.

The 571 veterans were reassessed 10 months after returning to the United States, when only 0.9% were found to be opioid dependent, and again 2–3 years later, when an additional 1.8% were found to have become dependent. That is, upon return to the United States, the vast majority of the Vietnam veterans in this study did not remain or become dependent on heroin or other opioid drugs, despite a remarkably high prevalence of opioid dependence during the period of Vietnam service (Helzer, 1985; Robins, 1993).

Continued study of the post-Vietnam experience of these veterans has shown that residence in a large city was an important determinant of using opioids after return from Vietnam. Large-city residence also was implicated as a possible influence on the transition from opioid use to opioid dependence. Opioids seem to be more readily available to adults living in the larger cities of the United States, and this might account for the observed geographic distribution of the drug dependence cases among these veterans, just as availability of opioids was associated with occurrence of opioid use and dependence while they were in Vietnam (Helzer, 1985).

The study of veterans also found that having a nontraffic arrest was associated with making the transition from opioid use to opioid dependence upon return to the United States. This finding of a behavioral problem in adulthood in association with drug dependence is consistent with results from many retrospective and cross-sectional studies, as well as a separate prospective study, with a focus on adult-onset DSM-III drug dependence and/or abuse, based on 101 incident cases found in the ECA project and 342 controls matched for age and geographic location of residence. In the ECA analysis, a history of antisocial personality disorder had a strong association with risk of becoming an adult-onset case of drug dependence and/or abuse, even when the analyses controlled for prior illicit drug use (Anthony, 1991a). In a separate prospective study with an epidemiologic sample of drug users, persistence of cocaine use in adulthood also has been linked with level of adolescent deviance, at least among men (Kandel and Raveis, 1989). Thus, it is necessary to consider that general deviance or social maladaptation in the form of police trouble or long-standing behavioral problems might continue to exert an influence on risk and duration of drug dependence in adulthood, and not just in relation to earlier onset of drug dependence (see Anthony, 1991a).

Prior alcoholism and alcohol problems also appear consistently in the causal models developed for occurrence of drug disorders in the late adolescent period and prior to the middle-age years and also in cross-sectional studies. A considerable number of youths and young adults become cases of alcohol dependence or alcohol abuse and then later develop dependence on controlled substances such as marijuana and cocaine. In the study of veterans, opioid dependence occurred more than three times more often among men with alcohol problems after Vietnam. Based on multiple logistic regression analysis of the ECA data, adults with a history of DSM-III alcoholism were an estimated four times more likely to develop a DSM-III drug dependence or abuse syndrome in later adulthood (Helzer, 1985; V. Chen, unpublished doctoral dissertation; Anthony, 1991a).

Cross-sectional and retrospective studies lead to an impression that many other different types of psychiatric disturbances are present among cases of drug dependence, as reviewed by Anthony and Helzer (1991), among others. Nonetheless, the evidence from prospective studies is inconsistent, sometimes implicating mood disorders, especially depression, and other times implicating conditions such as agoraphobia (e.g., see Anthony, 1991a).

In attempts to unravel the patterns of co-occurring mental disorders, the insidious onset of drug dependence is a complicating influence. For example, it is plausible that early drug use develops out of a background of more general socially maladaptive behavior or deviance, and then the drug use is followed by feelings of depressed mood, irritability, sleep problems, and other complaints that are featured prominently in the case definitions for mood disorders (e.g., see Wu and Anthony, 1999; Brook et al., 2001). These mood-related complaints then might promote continued drug taking, with reciprocal relationships that build up insidiously toward drug dependence on the one hand and mood disorder on the other hand (e.g., see Kaplan and Johnson, 1992).

This notion of a reciprocal coinfluence model for different pairs of insidiously developing psychiatric disturbances is plausible and fits well with at least some of the available evidence from rigorous epidemiologic studies, as well as clinical observations. However, it is not a model that can be tested readily with cross-sectional or retrospective data on age at onset of different psychiatric symptoms. To test a coinfluence model of this type, it will be necessary to conduct longitudinal studies with frequently repeated assessments of the fine-grained time sequences that can link one episode of drug-taking to subsequent processes and episodes of subthreshold mental disorders, prospectively looking for the emergence of a fully formed mental disorder that meets all diagnostic criteria. Confident statements about co-occurrence of drug dependence with other disorders will require longitudinal data of this type, coupled with evidence from intervention studies to test whether incidence of drug dependence might be reduced by effective treatment of mood disorder and whether risk of depression might be reduced by effective treatment of drug dependence (Wittchen, 1996; Anthony, 1991b).

Suspected sociodemographic influences on risk that have been implicated in evidence from two or more prospective studies of the transition from illicit drug use to adult-onset drug dependence and/or abuse include marital status and educational achievement. In both the Vietnam veteran study and the ECA investigation, being married was associated with a lower risk, and poor educational achievement was associated with a higher risk. Persistence of marijuana and cocaine use at ages 28–29 years has not been found to be associated with either marital status in earlier adulthood or having been a high school dropout (Helzer, 1985; Kandel and Raveis, 1989; Anthony, 1991a).

Some of the ECA work on determinants of risk observed in the adult years was concentrated on adult occupations and job environments that might convey greater risk, especially psychosocial job characteristics such as the levels of physical hazards or psychosocial stressors associated with each job category, as well as a possible stress-buffering impact associated with conditions such as the level of decision-making autonomy on the job (e.g., C. Muntaner et al., 1995). These hypotheses build, in part, from cross-sectional analyses of the ECA prevalence data on alcohol and drug dependence found in different occupations. Taking into account age, sex, race, education, and recency of employment, these analyses have identified construction laborers, carpenters, transportation workers, waiters, and waitresses as working adults with an especially high prevalence of alcohol or drug disorders. Doctors and nurses have received special attention because their access to pharmaceutical products and their working conditions might promote occurrence of drug dependence. However, several studies based on the ECA data suggest that prevalence of alcohol and drug disorders is no different or lower among these health professionals compared with other adult workers (Anthony et al., 1992; Trinkoff et al., 1991).

DETERMINANTS OF DURATION: THE ROLE OF TREATMENT

Whereas organized efforts to prevent drug dependence focus mainly on the young, public health efforts to control drug dependence by reducing its duration focus mainly on adults. Methadone, oral naltrexone, LAAM, and buprenorphine are four medicines for which there is compelling evidence of efficacy in treatment and

TABLE 5. Treatment Agents

Medication	Approved Use	Potential Use	Status
For opiates			
Buprenorphine	Relieve pain	Opiate maintenance therapy	Phase III
Depot Naltrexone	None	Long-term opiate blockade	Phase I
LAAM	Opiate maintenance therapy	—	Clinical testing completed; now has FDA approval
For Cocaine			
Amantadine	Treat viral infection	Prevent relapse/prolong abstinence	Phase II
Bromocriptine	Treat Parkinson's	Prevent relapse/prolong abstinence	Phase II
Carbamazepine	Treat epilepsy	Facilitate abstinence	Phase II
Desiperamine	Treat depression	Facilitate abstinence	Phase II
Fluoxetine	Treat depression	Facilitate abstinence	Phase II
Flupenthixol	Treat psychosis	Facilitate abstinence	Phase II
Imipramine	Treat depression	Facilitate abstinence	Phase II
Mazindol	Treat obesity	Facilitate abstinence	Phase II
Methylphenidate	Treat attention deficit disorder	Prevent relapse/prolong abstinence	Phase II
Sertraline	None	Facilitate abstinence	Phase II

rehabilitation of opioid-dependent cases. At present, there is no corresponding medicine known to be effective for the treatment of cocaine dependence or dependence on other controlled substances, although new products are under development (e.g., see Kosten et al., 2000). Promising treatment agents are listed in Table 5; these drugs for treatment of opioid or cocaine dependence now are primarily in an intermediate phase of research and development, some years away from governmental approval for widespread medical usage.

Other treatment modalities, such as Narcotics Anonymous, therapeutic communities, behavior therapy, and contingency management, are also at an intermediate phase of evaluation, although there is no formal review process for these treatment programs as there is for pharmaceutical products. At present, the available evidence on these other forms of treatment for drug dependence appears promising, but all too often confidence in the results of treatment evaluation research has been undermined by limitations such as widespread loss of subjects during follow-up and lack of randomized allocation plans (e.g., see Onken et al., 1993; Manski et al., 2001).

While it might be argued that international drug control policies and associated police work now reduce both the risk and the duration of drug dependence, there is no compelling epidemiologic evidence to support this argument. Anecdotal evidence abounds, for example, in relation to police and regulatory actions to curtail amphetamine problems in Japan and Sweden. Nonetheless, rigorous evaluation studies to guide future policy and programmatic decisions are lacking within this arena (Bonnie, 1985; MacCoun and Reuter, 1997; Manski et al., 2001).

DIRECTIONS FOR FUTURE RESEARCH

Many gaps in knowledge remain in relation to the epidemiology of drug dependence, but this overview has mentioned several topics that deserve greater priority in new research. Having already discussed some directions for research in genetic epidemiology, we now draw specific attention to the need for a more deliberate plan of research on the different environmental conditions that are thought to affect risk of drug dependence in adolescence and adulthood.

At present, the range of relevant environmental conditions for which there are reliable and valid measurements is quite limited. For example, investigators studying monozygotic twin pairs discordant for drug dependence have had to craft their own assessments of these environmental conditions and have not been able to draw upon a well-researched array of measurement tools. One specific goal of new research should be creation of tools and methods for assessing environmental conditions that are comparable to the array of measurement tools now available for studying different aspects of cognitive performance.

Concurrent with development of these tools, it should be possible to construct a map of environmental conditions that affect risk and/or duration of drug dependence, leading toward more effective prevention and control initiatives of the future. This map of environmental conditions can be juxtaposed with new evidence from the human genome mapping project in order to guide the search for environmental conditions that might modify the expression of specific genetic liabilities and thereby reduce the risk of drug dependence, a research agenda originally mentioned by Anthony et al. (1995) and discussed in more detail by Anthony (2001).

The construction of these maps for human genes and human environments will depend on epidemiologic research that makes a bridge from laboratory and clinical studies to large-scale population research. Effective bridging across the disciplines engaged in these studies implies a sharing of conceptual models and assessment methods not only in relation to the occurrence of drug dependence but also in relation to the suspected causal hypotheses. That is, in future laboratory and clinical research, we hope to see a more prevalent application of concepts and methods developed as part of large-scale epidemiologic studies, and in future epidemiologic studies we hope to see reciprocal progress and application of laboratory and clinical approaches to the study of drug dependence.

In conclusion, future epidemiologic research on drug dependence can build on a substantial body of evidence that has accumulated quite rapidly since the end of World War II, beginning with retrospective studies of clinical cases and continuing through recent large-sample prospective studies. The prospects for future advances in relation to the epidemiology of drug dependence will be determined in large part by greater attention to the environmental conditions that are independent causal determinants for drug dependence, concurrent with attention to environmental conditions that might modify genetic vulnerabilities to this important psychiatric disturbance. Given the multifactorial complexity of conceptual models now used to account for drug involvement and the risk of drug dependence, one may expect a continuing interplay between methodological advances in measurement and analysis, and substantive advances in the content of drug dependence epidemiology. Future directions will include a continued elaboration of multilevel

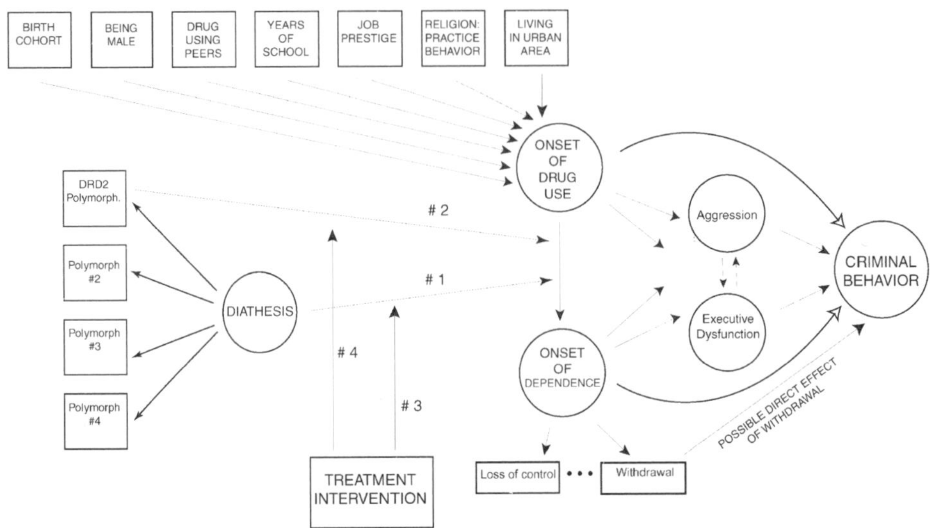

Figure 3. Illustration of a conceptual model for research on gene–environment interactions that are pertinent to the transition from first drug use to onset of drug dependence and subsequent criminal behavior. Here we see a hypothesized genetic diathesis or general susceptibility factor allowed to influence the probability of making the transition from onset of drug use to onset of drug dependence, via Path 1. In addition, there is a hypothesized specific influence of a DRD2 polymorphism on that transition, via Path 2. An environmental condition or process, in the form of an early treatment intervention is hypothesized to influence the relationship between the genetic susceptibility and the transition from drug use to drug dependence, either by acting upon the generic diathesis (Path 3) or on the specific influence of the DRD2 polymorphism (Path 4). To the right is an elaboration to link drug use and drug dependence with later criminal behavior, either via direct paths or via mediational pathways involving aggression and dysregulated executive cognitive functioning. Aggression and executive function are allowed to influence one another in reciprocity. The profile of exogenous conditions that is arrayed along the top of the figure is meant to be illustrative rather than exhaustive. In addition, for simplicity, there are paths drawn only to the onset of drug use. Some of these covariates might be expected to influence onset of drug dependence or criminal behavior as well, and might be influenced by the genetic susceptibility factor. (Copyright © 2001, James C. Anthony)

and growth models of the type described in this chapter, as well as advances in statistical methods required to study gene-environment interactions in detail and to examine mediational pathways that cut across developmental periods or stages in the natural history and clinical course of drug dependence.

Figure 3 provides an illustration for one type of mediational model that may prove to be important in future epidemiological studies of genetic susceptibility and risk of making a transition from drug use to drug dependence. The figure shows a profile of antecedent conditions that might influence risk of initiating drug use (as well as risk of progressing from first use to dependence). It also shows possible impact of preventive or therapeutic interventions designed to disrupt the expression of either a general susceptibility or a specific gene effect. To the right of the figure is a set of relationships between drug use, drug dependence, and

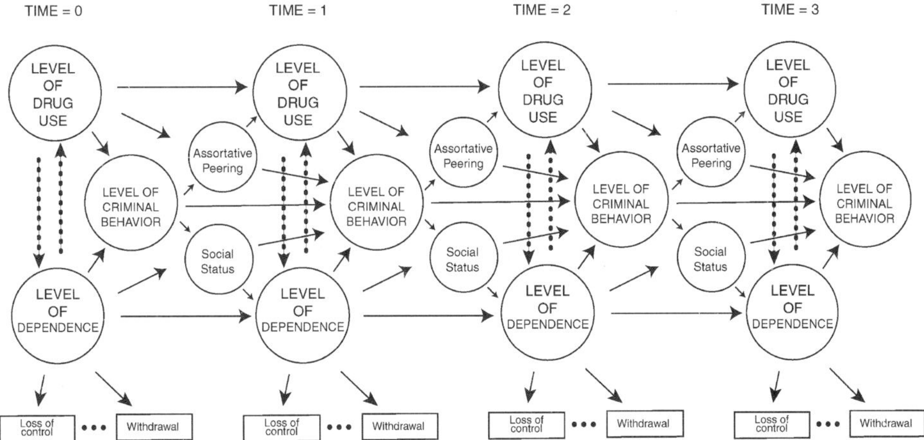

Figure 4. Illustration of a conceptual model for research on relationships linking level of drug use and level of drug dependence with later levels of criminal behavior. Mediational pathways involving social status and "assortative peering" also are shown, as described in the accompanying text. Reciprocities between level of drug use and level of drug dependence are depicted, consistent with the idea that level of drug use influences level of drug dependence, and that in turn, level of drug dependence influences level of dru use. A question of interest is how might an intervention alter this system of longitudinal relationships, if at all? (Copyright © 2001, James C. Anthony)

criminal behavior, which is one of the major sources of public concern about drug taking. As shown, there is hypothesized influence of drug use and dependence on criminal behavior via mediational pathways that involve both aggression and dysregulation of executive cognitive functions.

Figure 4 represents a longitudinal elaboration of a portion of the conceptual model offered in Figure 3. Here, the focus is upon over-time relationships linking drug use, drug dependence, and criminal behavior. Intermediate conditions and processes include not only social status of the drug user (e.g., whether employment is maintained; upward or downward mobility with respect to SES) but also affiliation with drug-using or deviant peers (termed "assortative peering" by analogy with assortative mating in the genetics literature).

Evaluating these models with respect to future directions for research, readers will appreciate that future epidemiological studies of drug dependence call upon a mastery of concepts, principles, and methods beyond those of standard case–control and cohort research designs. This is not to say that progress requires complex conceptual models or sophisticated statistical methods. To be sure, there is much work to be done with standard epidemiological surveillance procedures, and in the context of epidemiological field surveys described in the first sections of this chapter. Nonetheless, standard case–control and cohort study designs will not always serve well if the task is to probe gene–environment interactions or the suspected mediational causal pathways that link suspected causal influences to later drug dependence and to one another. Of course, drug dependence epidemiology is not unique in this respect; the same may be said for virtually all of the behavioral and psychiatric conditions reviewed elsewhere in this text book.

REFERENCES

American Psychiatric Association (1980): "Diagnostic and Statistical Manual of Mental Disorders," 3rd ed. Washington, DC: American Psychiatric Association.

American Psychiatric Association (1987): "Diagnostic and Statistical Manual for Mental Disorders," 3rd ed, revised. Washington, DC: American Psychiatric Association.

Anglin DM, Brecht ML, Woodward JA (1986): An empirical study of maturing out: Conditional factors. Int J Addictions 21:233–246.

Anthony JC (1982): Influence of federal drug law on the incidence of drug abuse. J Health Politics, Policy Law.

Anthony JC (1983): The regulation of dangerous psychoactive drugs. In Morgan JP, Kagan DV (eds): Society and Medication: Conflicting Signals for Prescribers and Patients. Lexington, MA: D.C. Health, pp 163–180.

Anthony JC (1991a): The epidemiology of drug addiction. In Miller NS (ed): "Comprehensive Handbook of Drug and Alcohol Addiction." New York: Marcel Dekker, Inc., pp 55–86.

Anthony JC (1991b): Epidemiology of drug dependence and illicit drug use. Curr Opin Psychiatry 4:435–439.

Anthony JC (1992): Epidemiological research on cocaine use in the USA. In: "Cocaine: Scientific and Social Dimensions," Proceedings of the CIBA Foundation Symposium 166. Chichester, England. Wiley, pp 20–39.

Anthony JC (1993): The scope of epidemiologic research on drug use: A rationale for change. In Monteiro MG, Inciardi JA (eds): Brasil–United States Binational Research. Sao Paulo, Brasil: CEBRID, pp 213–223.

Anthony JC, Arria AM (1999):. Epidemiology of psychoactive drug dependence in adulthood. In Tarter RE, Ammerman RT, Ott PJ, eds. "Sourcebook on Substance Abuse." Needham Heights, MA: Allyn and Bacon.

Anthony JC, Eaton WW, Mandell W (1992): Psychoactive drug dependence and abuse: More common in some occupations than others? J Employee Assistance Res 1:148–186.

Anthony JC, Helzer JE (1991): Syndromes of drug abuse and dependence. In Robins LN, Regier DA (eds): "Psychiatric Disorders in America." New York: The Free Press, pp 116–154.

Anthony JC, Petronis KR (1995): Early-onset drug use and risk of later drug problems. Drug Alcohol Depend. 40:9–15.

Anthony JC, Eaton WW, Henderson AS (1995) Looking to the future (in psychiatric epidemiology). Epidemiologic Reviews 17:1–8.

Anthony JC, Warner LA, Kessler RC (1994): Comparative epidemiology of dependence on tobacco, alcohol, controlled substances, and inhalants: Basic findings from the National Comorbidity Survey. Exp Clin Psychopharmacol 2:1–24.

Anthony JC, Neumark YD, Van Etten ML (2000): Do I do what I say? A perspective on self-report methods in drug dependence epidemiology. In Stone A, Turkan JS, Bachrach CA, Jobe JB, Kurtzman HS (eds.) "The Science of Self-Report: Implications for Research and Practice. New Jersey: Lawrence Erlbaum Associates.

Babor TF (1992): Nosological considerations in the diagnosis of substance use disorders. In Glantz M, Pickens R (eds): "Vulnerability to Drug Abuse." Washington, DC: American Psychological Association, pp 53–74.

Bandstra ES, Morrow CE, Anthony JC et al. (2001): Intrauterine growth of full-term infants: Impact of prenatal cocaine exposure. Pediatrics (to appear).

Barnes GM, Farrell MP (1992): Parental support and control as predictors of adolescent drinking, delinquency, and related problem behaviors. J Marriage Fam 54:763–776.

Beirut LJ, Dinwiddie SH, Begleiter H, et al. (1998): Familial transmission of substance dependence: Alcohol, marijuana, cocaine, and habitual smoking. Arch Gen Psychiatry 55:982–988.

Beiser M, Erickson D, Fleming JAE, Iacono WG (1993): Establishing the onset of psychotic illness. Am J Psychiatry 150:1349–1354.

Benjamin J, Li J, Patterson C, Greenberg BD, Murphy DL, Hamer DH (1996): Population and familial association between the D4 dopamine receptor gene and measures of novelty seeking. Nature Genetics. 12:81–84.

Berkson JA (1946). Limitations of the application of fourfold table analysis to hospital data. Biometrics. 2:47–53.

Berrettini WH, Persico AM (1996): Dopamine D2 receptor gene polymorphisms and vulnerability to substance abuse in African-Americans. Biol Psychiatry 40:144–147.

Biederman J, Wilens T, Mick E, Faraone SV (1997): Is ADHD a risk factor for psychoactive substance use disorders: Findings from a four-year prospective study. J Am Acad Child Adolesc Psychiatry 36:21–29.

Blackson TC, Tarter RE, Martin CS (1994): et al. Temperament-induced father-son family dysfunction: etiological implications for child behavior problems and substance abuse. Am J Orthopsychiatry. 64:280–292.

Bland RC, Newman SC, Orn H (1988a): Period prevalence of psychiatric disorders in Edmonton. Acta Psychiatr Scand 77 (Suppl 338):33–42.

Bland RC, Orn H, Newman SC (1988b): Lifetime prevalence of psychiatric disorders in Edmonton. Acta Psychiatr Scand 77(Suppl 338):24–32.

Blendy JA, Maldonado R (1998): Genetic analysis of drug addiction: The role of CAMP response element binding protein. J Molecular Medicine. 76:104–110.

Blum K, Noble EP, Sheridan PJ, et al. (1990): Allelic association of human dopamine D2 receptor gene in alcoholism. JAMA 263:2055.

Bobashev GV, Anthony JC (1998): Clusters of marijuana use in the United States. Am J Epidemiol 148:1168–1174.

Bobashev GV, Anthony JC (2000): Use of alternating logistic regression in studies of drug-use clustering. Substance Use Misuse. 35:245–267.

Bonnie R (1985): Efficacy of law as a paternalistic instrument. In Melton G (ed): "Nebraska Symposium on Human Motivation." Omaha: University of Nebraska, pp 131–2211.

Botvin GJ, Schinke SP, Epstein JA, Diaz T, Botvin EM (1995): Effectiveness of culturally focused and generic skills training approaches to alcohol and drug abuse prevention among minority adolescents: Two-year follow-up results. Psychology of Addictive Behaviors 9:183–194.

Botvin GJ, Griffin KW, Diaz T, Scheier LM, Williams C, Epstein JA (2000): Preventing illicit drug use in adolescents: Long-term follow-up data from a randomized control trial of a school population. Addictive Behaviors. 25:769–774.

Boustead C, Taber H, Idle JR, Cholerton S (1997): CYP2D6 genotype and smoking behaviour in cigarette smokers. Pharmacogenetics 7:411–414.

Boyd JH, Robins IN, Holzer CE III, Von Korff M, Jordan KB, Escobar JI (1985): Making diagnoses from DIS data. In Eaton WW, Kessler LG (eds): "Epidemiologic Field Methods in Psychiatry." New York: Academic Press, pp 209–234.

Boyle MH, Offord DR, Racine YA et al. (1993): Predicting substance use in early adolescence based on parent and teacher assessments of childhood psychiatric disorder. J Child Psychol Psychiatry 34:535–544.

Breslau N, Fenn N, Peterson EL (1993): Early smoking initiation and nicotine dependence in a cohort of young adults. Drug Alcohol Depend 33:129–138.

Brook JS, Cohen P, Brook DW (1998a): Longitudinal study of co-occurring psychiatric disorders and substance use. J Am Acad Child Adolesc Psychiatry 37:322–330.

Brook JS, Brook DW, de la Rosa M, et al. (1998b): Pathways to marijuana use among adolescents: cultural/ecological, family, peer, and personality influences. J Am Acad Child Adolesc Psychiatry. 37:759–766.

Brook JS, Whiteman M, Finch S, Cohen P (2000a): Longitudinally foretelling drug use in the late twenties: adolescent personality and social-environmental antecedents. J Genetic Psychol 161:37–51.

Brook JS, Whiteman M, Finch SJ, Morojele NK, Cohen P (2000b): Individual latent growth curves in the development of marijuana use from childhood to young adulthood. J Behavioral Med. 23: 464

Brook JS, Rosen Z, Brook DW. (2001): The effect of early marijuana use on later anxiety and depressive symptoms. NYS Psychologist. 35–40.

Brook JS, Whiteman MM, Gordon AS, Cohen P (1986): Dynamics of childhood and adolescent personality traits and adolescent drug use. Dev Psychol 22:403–414.

Brown BB, Mounts N, Lamborn SD, Steinberg L (1993): Parenting practices and peer group affiliation in adolescence. Child Dev 64:467–482.

Brunner HG, Nelen M, Breakefeld XO, Ropers HH, van Oost BA (1992): Science 262: 578.

Buck, AA, Sasaki TT, Hewitt JJ, Macrae AA. (1968): Coca chewing and health: An epidemiologic study among residents of a Peruvian village. Am J Epidemiol. 88:159–177.

Buka SL, Tsuang MT, Lipsitt LP (1993): Pregnancy/delivery complications and psychiatric diagnosis: A prospective study. Arch Gen Psychiatry 50:151–156.

Burke KC, Burke JD, Regier DA, Rae DS (1990): Age at onset of selected mental disorders in five community populations. Arch Gen Psychiatry 48:789–795.

Cadoret JR, Troughton E, O'Gorman TW, Heywood E (1986): An adoption study of genetic and environmental factors in drug abuse. Arch Gen Psychiatry 43:1131–1136.

Cadoret RJ (1992): Genetic and environmental factors in initiation of drug use and the transition to abuse. In Glantz M, Pickens R (eds): "Vulnerability to Drug Abuse." Washington, DC: American Psychological Association, pp 99–113.

Cadoret RJ, Cain CA, Grove WM (1980): Development of alcoholism in adoptees raised apart from alcoholic biologic relatives. Arch Gen Psychiatry 37:561–563.

Cadoret RJ, Yales WR, Troughton E, Woodworth G, Stewart MA (1995a): Genetic-environmental interaction in the genesis of aggressivity and conduct disorders. Arch Gen Psychiatry. 52:916–924.

Cadoret RJ, Yates WR, Troughton E, Woodworth G, Stewart MA (1995b): Adoption study demonstrating two genetic pathways to drug abuse. Arch Gen Psychiatry. 52:42–52.

Cadoret RJ, Yates WR, Troughton E, Woodworth G, Stewart MA (1996): An adoption study of drug abuse/dependency in females. Comp Psychiatry. 37:88–94.

Canino G, Anthony JC, Freeman DH, Shrout P, Rubio-Stipec M (1993): Drug abuse and illicit drug use in Puerto Rico. Am J Public Health 83:194–200.

Caris L, Anthony J (2000): Estimates of prevalence of cocaine and coca paste use among 8th to 12th grade students in Chile: Results of the 1999 national survey of students in Chile. Drug Alcohol Depend. S31, 89.

Carroll E (1977): Coca, the plant and its use. In Petersen RC, Stillman RC (eds): "Cocaine: 1977." NIDA Research Monograph 13. Washington, DC: U.S. Government Printing Office, pp 35–45.

Cases O, Seif I, Grimsby J, Gaspar P, Chen K, Pournin S, Muller U, Aguet M, Babinet C, Shih JC, de Maeyer E. (1995): Aggressive behavior and altered amounts of brain serotonin and norepinephrine in mice lacking MAOA. Science. 268:1763–1766.

Chassin L, Pillow DR, Curran PJ et al. (1993): Relation of parental alcoholism to early adolescent substance use: A test of three mediating mechanisms. J Abnorm Psychol 102:319.

Chassin L, Presson C, Rose J, Sherman S (1996): The natural history of cigarette smoking from adolescence to adulthood: demographic predictors of continuity and change. Health Psychol 15:478–484.

Chen K, Kandel DB (1995): The natural history of drug use from adolescence to the mid-thirties in a general population sample. Am J Public Health. 85:41–47.

Chilcoat HD, Anthony JC (1996): Impact of parent monitoring on initiation of drug use through late childhood. J Am Acad Child Adoles Psychiatry. 35:91–100.

Chilcoat HD, Dishion TJ, Anthony JC (1995): Parent monitoring and the incidence of drug sampling in urban elementary school children. Am J Epidemiol 141:114.

Chilcoat HD, Breslau N (1999): Pathways from ADHD to early drug use. J Am Acad Child and Adoles Psychiatry 38: 1347–1354.

Childress AR, Franklin T, McElgin W et al (2000): GABAergics may blunt limbic activation during cue-induced cocaine craving. Drug and Alcohol Dependence. 60 (Suppl 1): S36: 103.

Clayton RR (1992): Transitions in drug use: Risk and protective factors. In Glantz M, Pickens R (eds): "Vulnerability to Drug Abuse." Washington, DC: American Psychological Association, pp 15–51.

Clayton RR, Cattarello A, Walden KP (1991): Sensation seeking as a potential mediating variable for school-based prevention intervention: A two-year follow-up of DARE. Health Commun 3:229–239.

Cloninger CR, Adolfsson R, Svrakic NM (1996): Mapping genes for human personality. Nature Genetics. 12:81–84.

Collins WA (ed) (1986): Development During Middle Childhood: The Years From 6 to 12. Washington, DC: National Academy of Sciences.

Comings DE, Ferry L, Bradshaw-Robinson S, Burchette R, Chiu C, Muhleman D (1996): The dopamine D2 receptor (DRD2) gene: A genetic risk factor in smoking. Pharmacogenetics. 6: 73–79.

Comings DE (1998): Why different rules are required for polygenic inheritance: Lessons from studies of the DRD2 gene. Alcohol. 16:61.

Conneally PM (1991): Association between the D2 dopamine receptor gene and alcoholism: Comment. Arch Gen Psychiatry 48:664–666.

Crabbe JC, Belknap JK, Buck KJ (1994): Genetic animal models of alcohol and drug abuse. Science 264:1715–1723.

Croughan JL (1985): The contribution of family studies to understanding drug abuse. In Robins LN (ed): "Studying Drug Abuse." Series in Psychosocial Epidemiology, vol 6. New Brunswick, NJ: Rutgers University Press, pp 93–116.

Crum RM, Lillie-Blanton M, Anthony JC (1994): "Neighborhood Environment and the Opportunity To Use Cocaine." Baltimore, MD: Johns Hopkins University (to appear).

Cutronia CE, Cadoret RJ, Suhr JA, et al. (1994): Interpersonal variables in the prediction of alcoholism among adoptees: evidence for gene-environment interactions. Comp Psychiatry. 35:171–179.

Davis JR, Tunks E (1990, 1991): Environments and addiction: A proposed taxonomy. Intl J Addict 25:805–826.

Dawes MA, Antelman SM, Vanyukov MM, et al. (2000): Developmental sources of variation in liability to adolescent substance use disorders. Drug Alcohol Depend. 61:3–14.

de Alarcon R (1969): The spread of heroin abuse in a community. Bull Narc 21:17–22.

Delva J, Van Etten ML, Gonzalez GB, Cedeno MA, Penna M, Caris LH, Anthony JC (1999): First opportunities to try drugs and the transition to first drug use: Evidence from a national school survey in Panama. Subst Use Misuse 34:1451–1467.

Delva J. 2000.

Derzon JH, Lipsey MW (1999): Predicting tobacco use to age 18: A synthesis of longitudinal research. Addiction 94:995–1006.

Diez-Roux AV (1998): Bringing context back into epidemiology: variables and fallacies in multi-level analysis. Am J Public Health 88:216–222.

Dishion TJ, Andrews DW (1995): Preventing escalation in problem behaviors with high-risk young adolescents: immediate and 1-year outcomes. J Consult Clin Psychol. 63:538–548.

Dohrenwend BP. Levav I, Shrout PE et al. (1992): Socioeconomic status and psychiatric disorders. Science. 255:946–952.

Dolan LJ, Kellam SG, Brown C et al. (1993): The short-term impact of two classroom-based preventive interventions on aggressive and shy behaviors and poor achievement. J Appl Dev Psychol 14:317–345.

Duncan TE, Duncan SC, Hops H (1998): Latent variable modeling of longitudinal and multilevel alcohol use data. J Stud Alcohol 59:399–408.

Duncan SC, Duncan TE, Biglan A, Ary D (1998): Contributions of the social context to the development of adolescent substance use: A multivariate latent growth modeling approach. Drug and Alcohol Dependence. 50:57–71.

Eaton WW, Holzer CE, Von Korff MR, Anthony JC et al. (1984): The design of the ECA surveys: The control and measurement of error. Arch Gen Psychiatry 41:942–948.

Eaton WW, Kramer M, Anthony JC, Dryman A, Shapiro S, Locke BZ (1989): The incidence of specific DIS/DSM-III mental disorders: Data from the NIMH Epidemiologic Catchment Area Program. Acta Psychiatr Scand 79:163–178.

Ebstein RP, Novick O, Umansky R et al. (1996): Dopamine D4 receptor (D4DR) exon III polymorphism associated with the human personality trait of novelty seeking. Nature Genetics. 12:78–80.

Eddy NB, Halbach H, Isbell H, Seevers MH (1965): Drug dependence: Its significance and characteristics. Bull WHO 32:724–748.

Edwards G, Gross MM (1976): Alcohol dependence: Provisional description of a clinical syndrome. Br Med J 1:1058–1061.

Ellickson PL, Bell RM (1990): Drug prevention in junior high: A multi-site longitudinal test. Science 247:1299–1305.

Ellickson PL, Bell RM, McGuigan K (1993a): Preventing adolescent drug use: Long-term results of a junior high program. Am J Public Health 83:856–861.

Ellickson PL, Hays RD, Bell RM (1993b): Stepping through the drug use sequence: A Guttman scalogram analysis of adolescent drug use. J Abnorm Psychology 101:441–451.

Ellickson PL, Morton SC (1999): Identifying adolescents at risk for hard drug use: racial/ethnic variations. J Adolesc Health 25:382–395.

Farquhar J, Formann S, Flora J et al. (1990): Effects of community-wide education on cardiovascular disease risk factors: The Stanford Five-City Project. JAMA 264:359–365.

Fleming JP, Kellam SG, Brown CH (1982): Early predictors of age at first use of alcohol, marijuana and cigarettes. Drug Alcohol Depend 9:285–303.

Flewelling RL, Ennett ST, Rachal JV, Theisen AC (1993): Race/Ethnicity, Socioeconomic Status, and Drug Abuse: 1991. DHHS Publication No. (SMA) 93–2062. Washington, DC: U.S. Government Printing Office, 81 pp.

Frost WH (1927): Epidemiology. Nelson Loose-Leaf System. Public Health-Preventive Medicine. Volume 2, Chapter 7. New York: Thomas Nelson. Pp 163–190. Also available in Maxcy KF,(ed.) (1941): "Papers of Wade Hampton Frost, M.D.: Contribution to Epidemiological Method." New York: The Commonwealth Fund. pp. 493–542.

Furr-Holden CD. (2001): Unpublished manuscript..

Gelernter J, Kranzler H, Coccaro E, Siever L, New A, Mulgrew CL (1997): D4 dopamine receptor (DRD4) alleles and novelty seeking in subtance-dependent, personality-disorder, and control subjects. Am J Hum Genet. 61:1144–1152.

Gerlernter J, Goldman D, Risch N (1993): The A1 allele at the D2 dopamine receptor gene and alcoholism. JAMA 269:1673–1677.

Gerlernter J, Kranzler H (1999): D2 dopamine receptor gene (DRD2) allele and haplotype frequencies in alcohol dependent and control subjects: no association with phenotype or severity of phenotype. Neuropsychopharmacology 20:640.

Giancola PR, Mezzich AC, Tarter RE (1998): Disruptive, delinquent and aggressive behavior in female adolescents with a psychoactive substance use disorder: Relation to executive cognitive functioning. J Stud Alcohol 59:560–567.

Glantz M (1992): A developmental psychopathology model of drug abuse vulnerability. In Glantz M, Pickens R (eds): "Vulnerability to Drug Abuse." Washington, DC: American Psychological Association, pp 389–418.

Goldman D (1993): Genetic transmission. In Galanter M (ed): "Recent Developments in Alcoholism," Vol 11, "Ten Years of Progress." New York: Plenum Press, pp 232–248.

Golub A, Johnson BD (2001): Variation in youthful risk of progression from alcohol and tobacco to marijuana and hard drugs across generations. Am J Public Health. 91:225–232.

Grant BF (1997): Prevalence and correlates of alcohol use and DSM-IV alcohol dependence in the United States. J Stud Alcohol. 58:464–473.

Grant BF (1996): Prevalence and correlates of drug use and DSM-IV drug dependence in the United States: Results of the National Longitudinal Alcohol Epidemiologic Study. J Substance Abuse. 8:195–210.

Greenland S (2000): Principles of multi-level modeling. Int J Epidemiol 29:158–167.

Haastrup S (1973): Young Drug Abusers: 350 Patients Interviewed at Admission and Followed Up Three Years Later. Copenhagen: Munksgaard.

Hansen WB (1992): School-based substance abuse prevention: A review of the state of the art in curriculum, 1980–1990. Health Educ Res 7:403430.

Hansen WB, Graham JW (1991): Preventing alcohol, marijuana, and cigarette use among adolescents: Peer pressure resistance training versus establishing conservative norms. Prev Med 20:414–430.

Hanzi (Crider) R (1976): Diffusion of heroin use. Unpublished doctoral dissertation, submitted to Arizona State University, Tucson, AZ.

Harrison LD (1992): Trends in illicit drug use in the United States: Conflicting results from national surveys. Int J Addict 27:817–847.

Hawkins JD, Catalano RF, Miller JY (1992): Risk and protective factors for alcohol and other drug problems in adolescence and early adulthood: Implications for substance abuse prevention. Psychol Bull 112:64–105.

Hawkins JD, Von Cleve E, Catalano RF Jr (1991): Reducing early childhood aggression: Results of a primary prevention program. J Am Acad Child Adoles Psychiatry 30:208–217.

Hawkins JD, Catalano RF, Kosterman R, Abbott R, Hill KG (1999): Preventing adolescent health-risk behaviors by strengthening protection during childhood. Arch Pediatrics Adolesc Med 153:226–234.

Heath AC, Madden PAF (1995): Genetic influences on smoking behavior. In Turner JR, Cardon LR, Hewitt JK, (eds). Behavior Genetic Approaches in Behavioral Medicine. New York: Plenum, pp 45–66.

Helzer JE (1985): Specification of predictors of narcotic use versus addiction. In Robins LN (ed): "Studying Drug Abuse." Series in Psychosocial Epidemiology, vol 6. New Brunswick, NJ: Rutgers University Press, pp 173–197.

Helzer JE, Burnam MA, McEvoy LT (1991): Alcohol abuse and dependence. In Robins LN, Regier DA (eds): "Psychiatric Disorders in America." New York: The Free Press, pp 81–115.

Helzer JE, Canino GJ, Yeh E-K, Bland RC, Lee CK, Hwu HG, Newman S (1990): Alcoholism (2001): North America and Asia. Arch Gen Psychiatry 47:313–319. Hser et al.

Hughes JR, Oliveto AH, Helzer JE, Higgins ST, Bickel WK (1992): Should caffeine abuse, dependence, or withdrawal be added to DSM-IV and ICD-10? Am J Psychiatry 149:33–40.

Hughes PH, Canavan KP, Jarvis G, Arif A (1983): Extent of drug abuse: An international review with implications for health planners. World Health Stat Q 36:394–497.

Hwu HG, Yeh EK, Chang LY (1989): Prevalence of psychiatric disorders in Taiwan defined by the Chinese Diagnostic Interview Schedule. Acta Psychiatr Scand 79:136–147.

Joffe MM, Greenland S (1994): Toward a clearer definition of confounding. Letter to the Editor. Am J Epidemiol 139:962.

Johanson CE, Duffy F, Anthony JC (1996): Associations between drug use and behavioral repertoire in urban youths. Addiction 91:523–534.

Johnson CA, Pentz MA, Weber MD et al. (1990): The relative effectiveness of comprehensive community programming for drug abuse prevention with high-risk and low-risk adolescents. J Consult Clin Psychol 58:447–456.

Johnson R, Gerstein DR (1998): Initiation of use of alcohol, cigarettes, marijuana, cocaine, and other substances in US birth cohorts since 1919. Am J Pub Health 88:27–33

Johnson JG, Cohen P, Pine DS, Klein DF, Kasen S, Brook JS (2000): Association between cigarette smoking and anxiety disorders during adolescence and early adulthood. JAMA 284:2348–2351.

Johnson JG, Cohen P, Brook JS (1997): Associations between bipolar disorder and other psychiatric disorders during adolescence and early adulthood: A community-based longitudinal study. Am J Psychiatry 157:1679–1681.

Johnston LD (1985): Techniques for reducing measurement error in surveys of drug use. In Robins LN (ed): "Studying Drug Abuse." Series in Psychosocial Epidemiology, vol 6. New Brunswick, NJ: Rutgers University Press, pp 117–136.

Johnston LD, O'Malley PM, Bachman JG (2001): "Monitoring the Future: National Results on Adolescent Drug Use. Overview of Key Findings, 2000." Bethesda MD: National Institute on Drug Abuse.

Jones CP, Laveist TA, Lillie-Blanton M (1991): Race in the epidemiologic literature: An examination of the American Journal of Epidemiology. Am J Epidemiol 34:1079–1084.

Jones CP (2001): Invited Commentary: "Race," racism, and the practice of epidemiology. Am J Epidemiol. 154:299–304.

Kandel DB (1991): The social demography of drug use. Milbank Q 69:365–402.

Kandel DB (1992): Epidemiological trends and implications for understanding the nature of addiction. In O'Brien CP, Jaffe JH (eds): "Addictive States." New York: Raven Press, pp 23–40.

Kandel DB, Davies M (1992): Progression to regular marijuana involvement: Phenomenology and risk factors for near-daily use. In Glantz M, Pickens R (eds): "Vu-lnerability to Drug Abuse." Washington, DC: American Psychological Association, pp 211–254.

Kandel DB, Raveis VH (1989): Cessation of illicit drug use in young adulthood. Arch Gen Psychiatry 46:109–116.

Kandel DB, Yamaguchi K, Chen K (1992): Stages of progression in drug involvement from adolescence to adulthood: further evidence for the gateway theory. J Studies on Alcohol 53:447–457.

Kandel DB (1996) The parental and peer contexts of adolescent deviance: An algebra of interpersonal influences. J Drug Issues. 26:289–315.

Kandel DB, Johnson JG, Bird HR (1997): Psychiatric disorders associated with substance use among children and adolescents: Findings from the Methods for the Epidemiology of Child and Adolescent Mental Disorders (MECA) study. J Abnormal Child Psych. 25:121–132.

Kaplan HB, Johnson RJ (1992): Relationships between circumstances surrounding initial illicit drug use and escalation of drug use: Moderating effects of gender and early adolescent experiences. In Glantz M, Pickens R (eds): "Vulnerability to Drug Abuse." Washington, DC: American Psychological Association, pp 299–358.

Karkowski LM, Prescott CA, Kendler KS (2000): Multivariate assessment of factors influencing illicit substance use in twins from female–female pairs. Am J Med Genetics (Neuropsychiatric Genetics) 96:665–670.

Kaufman JS, Cooper RS (2001a): Commentary: Considerations in the use of racial/ethnic classification in etiologic research. Am J Epidemiol. 154:291–298.

Kaufman JS, Cooper RS (2001b): Kaufman and Cooper respond to "Race," racism, and the practice of epidemiology. Am J Epidemiol. 154:305–306.

Kelada SN, Shelton E, Kaufmann RB, Khoury MJ (2001): Gamma-aminolevulinic acid dehydratase genotype and lead toxicity: A HuGE review. Am J Epidemiol. 154:1–13.

Kellam SG (1994): Testing theory through developmental epidemiologically based prevention research. In Cazares A, Beatty LA (eds): "Scientific Methods for Prevention Intervention Research." NIDA Research Monograph No. 139, Washington, DC: U.S. Government Printing Office, pp 37–58.

Kellam SG, Anthony JC (1998): Targeting early antecedents to prevent tobacco smoking: findings from an epidemiologically base randomized field trial. Am J Public Health. 88:1490–1495.

Kellam SG, Werthamer-Larsson L, Dolan LJ, Brown CH, Mayer LS, Rebok GW, Anthony JC, Laudolff J, Edelsohn G, Wheeler L (1991): Developmental epidemiologically-based preventive trials: Baseline modeling of early target behaviors and depressive symptoms. Am J Community Psychol 19:563–584.

Kellam SK, Brown CH, Rubin BR, Ensminger MD (1983): Paths leading to teenage psychiatric symptoms and substance use: Developmental epidemiological studies in Woodlawn. In Guze SB, Earls FJ, Barrett JE (eds): "Childhood Psychopathology and Development" New York: Raven Press, pp 17–55.

Kendler KS, Gardner CO (1998): Twin studies of adult psychiatric and substance dependence disorders: Are they biased by differences in the environmental experiences of monozygotic and dizygotic twins in childhood and adolescence? Psychological Med. 28: 625–633.

Kendler KS, Neale MC, Prescott CA et al. (1996): Childhood parental loss and alcoholism in women: A causal analysis using a twin-family design. Psychological Med. 26:79–95.

Kendler KS, Prescott CA (1998b): Cannabis use, abuse, and dependence in a population-based sample of female twins. Am J Psychiatry. 155:1016–1022.

Kendler KS, Prescott CA (1998a): Cocaine use, abuse and dependence in a population-based sample of female twins. Brit J Psychiatry. 173:345–350.

Kendler KS, Karkowski LM, Neale MC, Prescott CA (2000): Illicit psychoactive substance use, heavy use, abuse, and dependence in a US population-based sample of male twins. Arch Gen Psychiatry 57:261–269

Kessler RC, McGonagle KA, Zhao S, Nelson C, Hughes M, Eshleman S, Wittchen H-U, Kendler K (1994): Lifetime and 12-month prevalence of DSM-IIIR psychiatric disorders in the United States: Results from the National Comorbidity Survey. Arch Gen Psychiatry 51:819.

Koob GF, Le Moal M. (2001): Drug addiction, dysregulation of reward, and allostasis. Neuropsychopharmacology 24:97–129.

Kosten TA, Kosten TR (1991): Criteria for Diagnosis. In Miller NS (ed): "Comprehensive Handbook of Drug and Alcohol Addiction." New York: Marcel Dekker, pp 263–283.

Kosten TR, Roberts JSC, Bond J et al. (2000): Longitudinal safety and immunogenicity of a therapeutic cocaine vaccine. Drug and Alcohol Dependence 60 (Suppl 1):S250, 704.

Kramer M (1989): Barriers to prevention. In Cooper B, Helgason T (eds): "Epidemiology and the Prevention of Mental Disorders." London: Routledge, pp 30–55.

Kramer M (1992a): Barriers to the primary prevention of mental, neurological, and psychosocial disorders of children: A global perspective. In Albee GW, Bard LA, Monsey TVC (eds): "Improving Children's Lives: Global Perspectives on Prevention." Newbury Park, CA: Sage Publications. pp 3–36.

Kramer M (1992b): Projected Changes in the population of the United States, 1990, 2000, and 2010: Implications for mental health and primary health care. Baltimore, MD: Johns Hopkins University School of Hygiene and Public Health, Department of Mental Hygiene, technical report, pp 1–27.

Kramer M, Von Korff M, Kessler LG (1980): The lifetime prevalence of mental disorders: Estimation, uses, and limitations. Psychol Med 10:429–435.

Labuda MC, Gottesman II, Pauls DL (1993): Usefulness of twin studies for exploring the etiology of childhood and adolescent psychiatric disorders. Am J Med Genet (Neuropsychiatric Genetics) 48:47–59.

Landry DW, Zhao K, Yang GX-Q, Glickman M, Georgiadis TM (1993): Antibody-catalyzed degradation of cocaine. Science 259:1899–1901.

Langenbucher J, Morgenstern J, Labouvie E, Nathan PE (1994): Lifetime DSM-IV diagnosis of alcohol, cannabis, cocaine and opiate dependence: Six-month reliability in a multi-site clinical sample. Addiction 89:1115–1127.

Langleben D, Maldjian J, McDonald S et al. (2000): Functional magnetic resonance imaging (fMRI) during "deception" and "gambling" paradigms in normals and in cocaine-dependent individuals. Drug and Alcohol Dependence. 60 (Suppl 1):S121, 345.

Lee CK, Kwak YS, Yamamoto J, Rhee H, Kim YS, Han JH, Choi JO, Lee YH (1990a): Psychiatric epidemiology in Korea: Part I. Gender and age differences in Seoul. J Nerv Ment Dis 178:242–246.

Lee CK, Kwak YS, Yamamoto J, Rhee H, Kim YS, Han JH, Choi JO, Lee YH (1990b): Psychiatric epidemiology in Korea: Part II. Urban and rural differences. J Nerv Ment Dis 178:247–252.

Leshner A (2001): NIDA Directors Address. Invited lecture. Annual Scientific Meeting of the College on Problems of Drug Dependence. Scottsdale, Arizona.

Lillie-Blanton M, Anthony JC, Schuster CR (1993): Probing the meaning of racial/ethnic group comparisons in crack cocaine smoking. JAMA 269:993–997.

Luthar SS, Anton SF, Merikangas KR, Rounsaville BJ (1992a): Vulnerability to drug abuse among opioid addicts siblings: Individual, familial, and peer influences. Comp Psychiatry 33:190–196.

Luthar SS, Anton SF, Merikangas KR, Rounsaville BJ (1992b): Vulnerability to substance abuse and psychopathology among siblings of opioid abusers. J Nerv Ment Dis 180:153–161.

Luthar SS, Rounsaville BJ (1993): Substance misuse and comorbid psychopathology in a high-risk group: A study of siblings of cocaine misusers. Int J Addictions 28:415–434.

Lyons MJ, Toomey R, Meyer JM et al. (1997): How do genes influence marijuana use? The role of subjective effects. Addiction. 92:409–417.

MacCoun R, Reuter P (1997): Interpreting Dutch cannabis policy: reasoning by analogy in the legalization debate. Science. 278:47–49.

MacKinnon DA, Johnson CA, Pentz MA, et al. (1991): Mediating mechanisms in a school-based drug prevention program: First year effects of the Midwestern Prevention Project. Health Psychol 10:164–172.

Maes HH, Woodard CE, Murrelle L et al. (1999): Tobacco, alcohol, and drug use in eight- to sixteen-year-old twins: the Virginia Twin Study of Adolescent Behavioral Development. Journal of Studies on Alcohol. 60:293–305.

Majumder PP, Moss HB, Murrelle (1998): Familial and non-familial factors in the prediction of disruptive behaviors in boys at risk for substance abuse. J Child Psycho Psychiatry 39:203–213.

Maldonado R, Blendy JA, Tzavara E, Gass P, Roques BP, Hanoune J, Schutz G (1996): Reduction of morphine abstinence in mice with a mutation in the gene encoding CREB. Science 273:657–659.

Mannuzza S, Klein RG, Bessler A, Malloy P, LePadula M (1993): Adult outcome of hyperactive boys: Educational achievement, occupational rank, and psychiatric status. Arch Gen Psychiatry 50:565–576.

Mayes LC, Grillon C, Granger R, Schottenfeld R (1998): Regulation of arousal and attention in preschool children exposed to cocaine prenatally Ann NY Acad Sci 846:126–143.

McCrae RR, Costa PRJ (1990): "Personality in Adulthood." New York. Guilford.

McGlothlin WH (1985): Distinguishing effects from concomitants of drug use: The case of crime. In Robins LN (ed): "Studying Drug Abuse." Series in Psychosocial Epidemiology, vol 6. New Brunswick, NJ: Rutgers University Press, pp 153–172.

McGue M, Elkins I, Iacono WG (2000): Genetic and environmental influences on adolescent substance use and abuse. Am J Med Genet (Neuropsychiatric Genetics) 96:671–677.

McGue M, Sharma A, Benson P (1996): Parent and sibling influence on adolescent alcohol use and misuse: Evidence from a U.S. adoption cohort. J Stud Alcohol 57:8–18.

Merikangas KR, Metha Rl, Molnar BE, Walters EE, Swendsen JD, Aguilar-Gaziola S, Bijl R, Borges G, Caraveo-Anduaga JJ, Dewit DJ, Kolodny B, Vega WA, Wittchen HU, Kessler RC (1998a): Comorbidity of substance use disorders with mood and anxiety disorders: Results of the International Consortium in Psychiatric Epidemiology. Addictive Behaviors 23:893–907.

Merikangas KR, Rounsaville BJ, Prusoff BA (1992): Familial factors in vulnerability to substance abuse. In Glantz M, Pickens R (eds): "Vulnerability to Drug Abuse." Washington, DC: American Psychological Association, pp 75–97.

Merikangas KR, Stolar M, Stevens DE et al. (1998b): Familial transmission of substance use disorders. Arch Gen Psychiatry 55:973–979.

Miles DR. van den Bree MBM, Gupman AE, Newlin DB, Glantz MD, Pickens RW (2001): A twin study on sensation seeking, risk taking behavior and marijuana use. Drug Alcohol Depend 62:57–68.

Mirin SM, Weiss RD, Griffin ML, Michael JL (1991): Psychopathology in drug abusers and their families. Comp Psychiatry 32:36–51.

Morrow CE, Bandstra ES, Anthony JC, Ofir AY, Xue L, Reyes ML (2001): Influence of prenatal cocaine exposure on full-term infant neurobehavioral functioning (to appear).

Mrazek PJ, Haggerty RJ (1994): "Reducing Risks for Mental Disorders. Frontiers for Preventive Intervention Research." Washington DC. National Academy Press.

Musto DF (1987): "The American Disease: Origins of Narcotic Control," 2nd ed. New York: Oxford University Press.

Musto DF (1990): Illicit price of cocaine in two eras: 1908–14 and 1982–89. Conn Med 54:321–326.

Musto DF (1991): Opium, cocaine, and marijuana in American history. Sci Am 265:40–47.

Myers JK, Weissman MM, Tischler GL et al. (1984): Six-month prevalence of psychiatric disorders in three communities. Arch Gen Psychiatry 41:959–967.

Nestler EJ, Landsman D (2001): Learning about addiction from the genome. Nature 409:834–835.

Neumark YD, Van Etten ML, Anthony JC (2001): "Drug dependence" and death: survival analysis of the Baltimore ECA sample from 1981 to 1995. Subst Use Misuse 35:313–327.

Newcomb MD (1992): Understanding the multidimensional nature of drug use and abuse: the role of consumption, risk factors, and protective factors. In Glantz M, Pickens R (eds): "Vulnerability to Drug Abuse." Washington, DC: American Psychological Association, pp 280–296.

Newlin DB, Miles DR, van den Bree MBM, Gupman AE, Pickens RW (2000): Environmental transmission of DSM-IV substance use disorders in adoptive and step families. Alcoholism: Clin Experimental Res 24:1785–1793.

Nurco DN, Hanlon TE, Kinlock TW, Duszynski KR (1989): The consistency of types of criminal behavior over preaddiction, addiction, and nonaddiction status periods. Comp Psychiatry 30:391–402.

Oakley-Browne MA, Joyce PR, Wells JE, Bushnell JA, Hornblow AR (1989): Christchurch Psychiatric Epidemiology Study, Part II: Six month and other period prevalences of specific psychiatric disorders. Aust NZ J Psychiatry 23:327–340.

O'Donnell JA (1985): Interpreting progression from one drug to another. In Robins LN (ed): "Studying drug abuse." New Jersey: Rutgers University Press 1985:137–151.

Onken LS, Blaine JD, Boren JJ (eds) (1993): "Behavioral Treatments for Drug Abuse and Dependence." NIDA Research Monograph No. 137. Washington, DC: U.S. Government Printing Office.

Pandina RJ, White HR, Yorke J (1981): Estimation of substance use involvement: Theoretical consideration and empirical findings. Int J Addict 16:124.

Pato CN, Macciardi F, Pato MT, Verga M, Kennedy JL (1993): Review of the putative association of dopamine D2 receptor and alcoholism: a meta-analysis. Am J Med Genetics. 48:78.

Petersen RC (1977): History of cocaine. In Petersen RC, Stillman RC (eds): "Cocaine: 1977." NIDA Research Monograph No. 13. Washington, DC: U.S. Government Printing Office, pp 17–34.

Petronis KR, Anthony JC. (2000): Perceived risk of cocaine use and experience with cocaine: Do they cluster within U.S. neighborhoods and cities. Drug Alcohol Depend 57:183–192.

Piannezza et al. (1998): Nature 393:750.

Pickens RW, Svikis DS, McGue M, Lykken DT, Heston LL, Clayton PJ (1991): Heterogeneity in the inheritance of alcoholism. Arch Gen Psychiatry 48:19–28.

Pickens RW, Thompson T, Muchow DC (1973): Cannabis and phencyclidine self-administration by animals. In Goldberg L, Hoffmeister F (eds): "Psychic Dependence." New York: Springer, pp 78–87.

Plomin R, Daniels D (1987): Why are children in the same family so different from one another? Behav Brain Sci. 10:1–16.

Prusoff BA, Merikangas KR, Weissman MM (1988): Lifetime prevalence and age of onset of psychiatric disorders: recall 4 years later. J Psychiatr Res 22:107–117.

Radel M, Goldman D (2001): Pharmacogenetics of alcohol response and alcoholism: the interplay of genes and environmental factors in thresholds for alcoholism. Drug Metabolism and Disposition. 29:489–494.

Rae BA, Braude MC (eds) (1989): "Women and Drugs: A New Era for Research." NIDA Research Monograph No. 65. Washington, DC: U.S. Government Printing Office.

Regier DA, Boyd JH, Burke JD, Rae DS, Myers JK, Kramer M, Robins LN, George LK, Karno M, Locke BZ (1988): One-month prevalence of mental disorders in the U.S.: Based on five epidemiologic catchment area sites. Arch Gen Psychiatry 45:977–986.

Reich T, Edenberg HJ, Goate A et al. (1998): Genome-wide search for genes affecting the risk for alcohol dependence. Am J Med Genet (Neuropsychiatric Genetics) 87:207–215.

Resnicow K, Botvin G (1993): School-based substance use prevention programs: Why do effects decay? Prev Med 22:484–490.

Richardson JL, Radziszewska B, Dent CW, Flay BR (1993): Relationships between afterschool care of adolescents and substance use, risk taking, depressed mood, and academic achievement. Pediatrics 92:32–38.

Robins LN (1966): "Deviant Children Grown Up." Baltimore, MD: Williams and Wilkins.

Robins LN (1977): Estimating addiction rates and locating target populations: How decomposition into stages helps. In Rittenhouse JD (ed): "The Epidemiology of Heroin and Other Narcotics." Washington, DC: U.S. Government Printing Office, pp 25–39.

Robins LN (1983): The consequences of recommendations of the U.S. Privacy Protection Study Commission for longitudinal studies. In Ricks DF, Dohwenrend BS (eds): "Origins of Psychopathology: Problems in Research and Public Policy." New York: Cambridge University Press, pp 175–186.

Robins LN (1993): The Sixth Thomas James Okey Memorial Lecture: Vietnam veterans rapid recovery from heroin addiction: A fluke or normal expectation? Addiction 88:1041–1054.

Robins LN, Helzer JE, Orvaschel H, Anthony JC, Blazer DG, Burnam A, Burke JD Jr (1985): The Diagnostic Interview Schedule. In Eaton WW, Kessler LG (eds): "Epidemiologic Field Methods in Psychiatry." New York: Academic Press, pp 143–170.

Robins LN, Przybeck TR (1985): Age of onset of drug use as a factor in drug and other disorders. In "Etiology of Drug Abuse: Implications for Prevention." National Institute on Drug Abuse Research Monograph No. 56. DHHS Publication No. (ADM)-85-1335 (Jones CL, Battjes RL (eds): Washington, DC: U.S. Government Printing Office, pp 178–192.

Rosenberg MF, Anthony JC (2001a): Aggressive behavior and opportunities to purchase drugs. Drug Alcohol Depend (to appear).

Rosenberg MF, Anthony JC (2001b): Pharmacothanatology: an epidemiological investigation of drug related deaths. Drug Alcohol Depend (to appear).

Rounsaville BJ, Kosten TR, Weissman MM, Prusoff BA, Pauls D, Foley S, Merikangas KR (1991): Psychiatric disorders in the relatives of probands with opioid addiction. Arch Gen Psychiatry 48:33–42.

Rutter M (1991): Protective factors: Independent or interactive? J Am Acad Child Adolesc Psychiatry 30:151–152.

Sameroff AJ, Fiese BH (1989): Conceptual issues in prevention. In Shaffer D, Philips I, Enzer NB, Silverman MM, Anthony V (eds): "Prevention of Mental Disorders, Alcohol and Other Drug Use in Children and Adolescents." Office of Substance Abuse Prevention, Monograph No. 2. Rockville, MD: Office of Substance Abuse Prevention, pp 23–53.

Sapira JD, Ball JC, Penn H (1970): Causes of death among institutionalized narcotic addicts. J Chronic Dis 22:733–742.

Scheier LM, Botvin GJ, Griffin KW (2001): Preventive intervention effects on developmental progression in drug use: structural equation modeling analyses using longitudinal data. Prevention Science 2:91–112.

Sellers EM, Hoffmann E, Rao Y et al. (2000): Ethnic variation in CYP2A6: Impact on smoking and health consequences. Drug Alcohol Depend 60 (Suppl 1):S250, 706.

Sells SB (1977): Reflections on the epidemiology of heroin and narcotic addiction from the perspective of treatment data. In Rittenhouse JD (ed): "The Epidemiology of Heroin and other Narcotics." Washington, DC: U.S. Government Printing Office, pp 147–176.

Shillington AM, Clapp JD (2000): Self-report stability of adolescent substance use: Are there differences for gender, ethnicity and age? Drug Alcohol Depend 60:19–27

Shillington AM, Cottler LB, Mager DE, Compton WM 3rd (1995): Self-report stability for substance use over 10 years: data from the Epidemiologic Catchment Study. Drug Alcohol Depend 40:103–109

Smart R (1992): The problems perspective: Implications for prevention policies. In Lader M, Edwards G, Drummond DC (eds): "The Nature of Alcohol and Drug Related Problems." Society for the Study of Addiction, Monograph No. 2. New York: Oxford University Press, pp 167–177.

Smart RG (1977): Comments on Sells paper: Reflections on the epidemiology of heroin and narcotic addiction from the perspective of treatment data. In Rittenhouse JD (ed): "The Epidemiology of Heroin and Other Narcotics." Washington, DC: U.S. Government Printing Office, pp 177–182.

Smith SS, O'Hara BF, Persico AM, Gorelick DA, Newlin DB, Vlahov D, Solomon L, Pickens R, Uhl GR (1992): Genetic vulnerability to drug abuse. Arch Gen Psychiatry 49:723–727.

Sonnedecker G (1962): Emergence of the concept of opiate addiction. J Mondial Pharmacie 3:279–290.

Spoth R, Reyes ML, Redmond C, Shin C (1999): Assessing a public health approach to delay onset and progression of adolescent substance use: Latent transition and log-linear analyses of longitudinal family preventive intervention outcomes. J Consult Clin Psychol 67:619–630.

Stenbacka M, Allebeck P, Rmelsj A (1993): Initiation into drug abuse: The pathway from being offered drugs to trying cannabis and progression to intravenous drug abuse. Scand J Social Med 21:31–39.

Suarez BK, Parsian A, Hampe CL, Todd RD, Reich T, Cloninger CR (1994): Linkage disequilibrium at the D2 dopamine receptor locus (DRD2) in alcoholics and controls. Genomics 19:12.

Szapocznik J, Coatsworth JD (1999): An ecodevelopmental framework for organizing the influences on drug abuse: A developmental model of risk and protection. In Glantz MD, Hartel CR, (eds). "Drug Abuse: Origins and Interventions." Washington DC. American Psychological Association, pp 331–366.

Swift W, Hall W, Teesson M (2001): Characteristics of DSM-IV and ICD – 10 cannabis dependence among Australian adults: Results from the National Survey of Mental Health and Wellbeing. Drug Alcohol Depend 63:147–153.

Tanaka E (1999): Update: genetic polymorphisms of drug metabolizing enzymes. J Clin Pharm Ther 24:323–329.

Tarter RE, Laird SB, Kabene M, Bukstein O, Kaminer Y (1990): Drug abuse severity in adolescents is associated with magnitude of deviation in temperament traits. Br J Addict 85:1501–1504.

Tarter RE, Mezzich AC (1992): Ontogeny of substance abuse: Perspectives and findings. In Glantz M, Pickens R (eds): "Vulnerability to Drug Abuse." Washington, DC: American Psychological Association, pp 149–177.

Tarter RE, Vanyukov M, Giancola P et al. (1999): Etiology of early age onset substance abuse: a maturational perspective. Dev Psychopathol. 11:657–683.

Tomas JM, Vlahov D, Anthony JC (1990): The association between intravenous drug use and early childhood misbehavior. Drug Alcohol Depend 25:79–89.

Trinkoff AM, Eaton WW, Anthony JC (1991): The prevalence of substance abuse among registered nurses. Nursing Res 40:172–175.

Trostle JA, Sommerfeld J (1996): Medical anthropology and epidemiology. Ann Rev Anthropol 25:253–274.

True WR, Heath A, Scherrer JF, Waterman B, Goldberg J, Lin N, Eisen SA, Lyons MJ, Tsuang MT (1997): Genetic and environmental contributions to smoking. Addiction. 92:1277–1287.

Tsuang MT, Lyons MJ, Eisen SA et al. (19xx): Co-occurrence of abuse of different drugs in men. Arch Gen Psychiatry. 55:967–972.

Tsuang MT, Lyons MJ, Eisen SA, et al. (1996): Genetic influences on DSM-III-R drug abuse and dependence: A study of 3,372 twin pairs. Am J Med Genet 67:473–477.

Turner E, Ewing J, Shilling P, Smith TL, Irwin M, Schuckit M, Kelsoe JR (1992): Lack of association between an RFLP near the D2 dopamine receptor gene and severe alcoholism. Biol Psychiatry 31:285–290.

Turner WM, Cutter HSG, Worobec TG, O'Farrell TJ, Bayog RD, Tsuang MT (1993): Family history models of alcoholism: Age of onset, consequences and dependence. J Study Alcohol 54:164–171.

Uhl GR, Persico AM, Smith SS (1992): Current excitement with D2 dopamine receptor gene alleles in substance abuse. Arch Gen Psychiatry 49:157–160.

United States. Department of Health and Human Services. (2001): National Institutes of Health. National Institute on Drug Abuse. Community Epidemiology Work Group. "Epidemiologic Trends in Drug Abuse." vol. I: Proceedings of the Community Epidemiology Work Group. Highlights and Executive Summary. December 2000. NIH Publication Number 01–4916. Rockville MD: National Institute on Drug Abuse.

United States. Department of Health and Human Services. (1994): Public Health Service. National Institutes of Health. National Institute on Drug Abuse. "Assessing Drug Abuse

Among Adolescents and Adults: Standardized Instruments." Clinical Report Series. NIH Publication Number 94–3757. Rockville, MD.

United States Substance Abuse and Mental Health Services Administration (1993): "Preliminary Estimates from the 1992 National Household Survey on Drug Abuse." Washington, DC: U.S. Government Printing Office.

United States Substance Abuse and Mental Health Services Administration (2000): "Preliminary Estimates From the 1999 National Household Survey on Drug Abuse." Washington, DC: U.S. Government Printing Office.

Vaillant GE (1966): A twelve-year followup of New York narcotic addicts: IV. Some characteristics and determinants of abstinence. Am J Psychiatry 123:573–584.

Van Etten ML, Anthony JC (2001): Male–female differences in transitions from first drug opportunity to first use: searching for sub-group variation by age, race, region, and urban status. J Women's Health and Gender-Based Med (to appear).

Van Etten ML, Neumark YD, Anthony JC (1997): Initial opportunity to use marijuana and the transition to first use: United States, 1979 to 1994. Drug Alcohol Depend 49:1–7.

Vandenbergh DJ, Rodriguez LA, Hivert E et al. (2000): Long forms of the dopamine receptor (DRD4) gene VNTR are more prevalent in substance abusers: no interaction with functional alleles of the catechol-o-methyltransferase (COMT) gene. Am Jo Med Genet (Neuropsychiatric Genetics). 96:678–683.

Vandenbergh DJ, Rodriguez LA, Miller IT et al. (1997): High-activity catechol-o-methyltransferase allele is more prevalent in polysubstance abusers 74:439–442.

Vanyukov MM, Moss HB, Ling MY, Tarter RE, Deka R (1995): Preliminary evidence for an association of a dinucleotide repeat polymorphism at the MAOA gene with early onset alcoholism/substance abuse. Am J Med Genet (Neuropsychiatric Genetics). 60:122–126.

Vanyukov MM, Tarter RE (2000): Genetic studies of substance abuse. Drug Alcohol Depend 59:101–123.

Vanyukov MM (1999): Association between a functional polymorphism at the DRD2 gene and the liability to substance abuse. Am J Med Genet (Neuropsychiatric Genetics). 88:446–447.

Warner LA, Kessler RC, Hughes M, Anthony JC, Nelson CB (1995): Prevalence and correlates of drug use and dependence in the Uniteds States: Results from the National Comorbidity Survey. Arch Gen Psychiatry. 52:219–229.

Weinberg CR (1993): Toward a clearer definition of confounding. Am J Epidemiol 137:18.

Weinberg CR (1994): Letter to the Editor. Am J Epidemiol 139:962–963.

Weinberg NZ, Glantz MD (1999): Child psychopathology risk factors for drug abuse: An overview. J Clinical Child Psychol 28:290–297.

Weinberg NZ, Rahdert E, Colliver J, Glantz MD (1998): Adolescent substance abuse: a review of the past 10 years. J Am Acad Child Adolesc Psychiatry 37: 252–261.

Wells JE, Bushnell JA, Hornblow AR, Joyce PR, Oakley-Browne MA (1989): Christchurch Psychiatric Epidemiology Study. Part I. Methodology and lifetime prevalence for specific psychiatric disorders. Aust NZ J Psychiatry 23:315–326.

White HR (1992): Early problem behavior and later drug problems. J Res Crime Delinq 29:412–429.

Windham AJ, Chilcoat HD (2001): Paper presented at the Annual Scientific Meeting of the College on Problems of Drug Dependence. Scottsdale, AZ.

Wittchen HU, Burke JD, Semler G, Pfister H, Von Cranach M, Zaudig M (1989): Recall and dating of psychiatric symptoms. Test-retest reliability of time-related symptom questions in a standardized psychiatric interview. Arch Gen Psychiatry 46:437–443

Wittchen H-U, Essau CA, von Zerssen D, Krieg J-C, Zaudig M (1992): Lifetime and six-month prevalence of mental disorders in the Munich Follow-up Study. Eur Arch Psychiatry Clin Neurosci 241:247–258.

Wittchen HU (1996): Critical issues in the evaluation of comorbidity of psychiatric disorders. Br J Psychiatry 30 Suppl:9–16

Wittchen HU, Lachner G, Wunderlich U, Pfister H (1998): Test-retest reliability of the computerized DSM-IV version of the Munich-Composite International Diagnostic Interview (M-CIDI). Soc Psychiatry Psychiatr Epidemiol 33:568–578

Wittchen HU, Ustun TB, Kessler RC (1999): Diagnosing mental disorders in the community. A difference that matters? Psychol Med 29:1021–1027

Wong AHC, Buckle CE, Van Tol HHM (2000): Polymorphisms in dopamine receptors: what do they tell us? Eur J Pharmacol 410:183–203.

Woody G, Schuckit M, Weinrieg R, Yu E (1993): A review of the substance use disorders section of the DSM-IV. Recent Adv Addictive Disord 16:21–32.

World Health Organization (1992): "The ICD–10 Classification of Mental and Behavioural Disorders: Clinical Descriptions and Diagnostic Guidelines." Geneva: World Health Organization.

World Health Organization (2000): Department of Mental Health and Substance Dependence. "International Guide for Monitoring Alcohol Consumption and Related Harm. WHO/MSD/MSB/00.4". Geneva: World Health Organization.

Wu Li-Tzy, Anthony JC (1999): Am J Public Health.

Yang Q, Khoury M (1997): Evolving methods in genetic epidemiology: III. Gene-environment interaction in epidemiolical research. Epidemiol Rev 19:33–43.

Yates WR, Cadoret RJ, Troughton EP, Stewart M, Giunta TS (1998): Effect of fetal alcohol exposure on adult symptoms of nicotine, alcohol, and drug dependence. Alcoholism: Clin Experimental Res 22:914–920.

CHAPTER 21

Personality Disorders: Epidemiological Findings, Methods, and Concepts

MICHAEL J. LYONS and BETH A. JERSKEY

Department of Psychology, Boston University (M.J.L., B.A.J.); Harvard Institute of Psychiatric Epidemiology and Genetics (M.J.L.)

INTRODUCTION

With the advent of the third edition of the *Diagnostic and Statistical Manual* (DSM-III) (American Psychiatric Association, 1980), the personality disorders were assigned their own axis (axis II) in the diagnostic nomenclature. DSM-III was a major impetus for clinical and research interest in the personality disorders because it provided explicit diagnostic criteria for their diagnosis. It included 11 specific disorders, some of which were relatively unknown. Many of the personality disorders, unlike axis I disorders such as schizophrenia and depression, did not have long histories as subjects of clinical attention or systematic observation. In an important way, one may mark the advent of systematic studies of personality disorders by the publication of DSM-III in 1980. This is not the case for all of the personality disorders, such as antisocial personality disorder, but it is for many of them.

Personality traits are described in the fourth edition of the DSM (DSM-IV; American Psychiatric Association, 1994) as "enduring patterns of perceiving, relating to, and thinking about the environment and oneself, and are exhibited in a wide range of important social and personal contexts" (p. 630). DSM-IV defines *personality disorders* as inflexible and maladaptive personality traits that cause either significant functional impairment or subjective distress. Personality disorders are conceptualized as long-term characteristics of individuals that are likely to be evident by adolescence and continue through adulthood. Based on the current conceptualization of the personality disorders, key features for diagnosis include: early onset, stability and persistence, pervasiveness, interpersonal focus and impairment (Hirschfeld, 1993). The diagnosis of personality disorder should not be made if the characteristics only occur during episodes of an axis I disorder. The

Textbook in Psychiatric Epidemiology, Second Edition, Edited by Ming T. Tsuang and Mauricio Tohen.
ISBN 0-471-40974-X

DSM-IV suggests that a personality disorder may become less obvious in middle and later life.

In addition to specifying ten individual personality disorders (passive–aggressive personality disorder was dropped), DSM-IV groups the personality disorders into three clusters. Cluster A includes paranoid, schizoid, and schizotypal personality disorders; the basis for this cluster is the odd or eccentric characteristics common to individuals with each of these three disorders. Cluster B includes antisocial, borderline, histrionic, and narcissistic personality disorders. This cluster is characterized by dramatic, emotional, or erratic features. Cluster C includes avoidant, dependent, and obsessive–compulsive personality disorders. This has been designated the "anxious" or "fearful" cluster.

This chapter is divided into three primary sections. The first describes substantive findings with an emphasis on the prevalence of personality disorders in different settings. The second section of the chapter discusses conceptual issues, such as categorical versus dimensional approaches to classifying personality disorders. The third section addresses methodological issues that are important for studying the epidemiology of personality disorders.

SUBSTANTIVE FINDINGS

Compared to many axis I disorders, such as schizophrenia, there are less extensive data available on the prevalence of axis II disorders. To a great extent, this is due to a much shorter history of empirical work on most of the constructs embodied in the personality disorders. In the case of schizophrenia, the definition formulated by Kraepelin (1919/1971) shortly after the turn of the century is relatively similar to the criteria in DSM-III, DSM-III-R, and DSM-IV. In general, the personality disorders, with the possible exception of antisocial personality disorder (and its related progenitors, moral insanity, psychopathy, sociopathy, etc.), have not been the object of empirical, let alone epidemiological, research for very long. In this section a brief description of findings predating the publication of DSM-III will be provided. The largest part of this section will review findings bearing on the "true prevalence" of personality disorders, that is, rates of the disorders in representative community and nonclinical samples. Available data will be presented for the prevalence of having any personality disorder and for individual disorders.

True Prevalence Studies

Pre-DSM-III. In the Midtown Manhattan study, Srole et al. (1962) reported a prevalence rate of 6% for sociopathy. In the Stirling County study using DSM-I diagnoses, Leighton (1963) reported that 11% of males and 5% of females received a sociopathic diagnosis. Merikangas and Weissman (1991) reviewed the prevalence rates for personality disorder reported in pre-DSM-III studies that permitted the exclusion of alcoholism and drug abuse (which were classified as personality disorders in some older systems) from other personality disorders (Bremer, 1951; Essen-Moller et al., 1956; Langner and Michael, 1963; Leighton, 1959). They concluded that, in spite of nonuniformity in diagnostic definition, the reported rates were quite similar. Approximately six to nine percent of the samples were characterized as having a major personality disturbance. In these early data reviewed by Merikangas and Weissman, there is an indication that the overall sex ratio for personality disorders is about equal, with differences for specific disorders. Prevalence is fairly even across age groups with a slight increase in later life, higher rates in urban than rural populations, and higher rates in lower socioeconomic groups compared to higher groups.

Post-DSM-III. Since the publication of DSM-III in 1980 there have been several studies that provided data on the prevalence of having any personality disorder. Nestadt and his coworkers, in a series of reports (1990, 1991, 1992) detailed the results of a follow-up assessment for personality disorders of the Epidemiologic Catchment Area (ECA) study. At the Baltimore site of the ECA, a total of 3,481 individuals were interviewed with the Diagnostic Interview Schedule (Robins et al., 1981), the General Health Questionnaire (Goldberg, 1974), and the Mini-Mental Status Exam (Folstein et al., 1975) as part of the ECA. Subsequent to the ECA data collection, the Clinical Reappraisal was carried out and included all subjects who had been "screened positive" for psychopathology and a random sample of 17% of the 3,481 original respondents. Of the 1,086 subjects selected for inclusion in the Clinical Reappraisal, 810 agreed to participate for a response rate of 75%. Board-certified or board-eligible psychiatrists, blind to first stage information, interviewed the subjects. The psychiatrists used the Standardized Psychiatric Examination (SPE), a semistructured interview that averaged one and one-half to three hours to complete. The authors described the SPE as assessing personal history, medical and psychiatric problems and present mental status; it includes an inventory and direct question approach. Nestadt et al. (1993) reported a prevalence of 5.9% for a definite diagnosis of personality disorder and a prevalence of 9.3% for their combined "definite" plus "provisional" diagnostic categories.

Zimmerman and Coryell (1989a) reported the rates of DSM-III personality disorders assessed through the use of the Structured Interview for DSM-III Personality Disorders (SIDP) (Stangl et al., 1995) among a nonpatient sample of 797 individuals. There are several features of the study that qualify somewhat the interpretation of their results. The sample that they studied was a mixture of relatives of normal controls (n = 185), relatives of schizophrenic probands (n = 131), relatives of probands with psychotic depression (n = 247), relatives of probands with nonpsychotic depression (n = 235), and relatives of probands with other psychiatric disorders (n = 10). Eleven individuals refused the SIDP interview, yielding the final sample size of 797. Their sample is problematic because certain personality disorders may have a familial relationship to axis I disorders. To the extent that a personality disorder has a familial relationship to an axis I disorder, the rate of the personality disorder among first-degree relatives of probands with the axis I disorder will be elevated and results may not generalize to the general population. Therefore, the prevalence of some personality disorders may be inflated in the sample that Zimmerman and Coryell studied. Approximately three-fourths of the sample was interviewed by telephone (72.9%) and one-fourth by face-to-face interviews (27.1%). The authors found no difference in the frequency of axis II diagnoses between telephone and face-to-face interviews. The prevalence of any DSM-III personality disorder diagnosis using the SIDP, including mixed personality disorder, was 17.9%. These investigators also administered the Personality Diagnostic Questionnaire (Hyler, 1983) to their subjects (Zimmerman and Coryell, 1990). Prevalence rates were fairly similar, but the PDQ produced higher rates of schizotypal, compulsive, dependent, and borderline personality disorders. The SIDP yielded higher rates of antisocial and passive–aggressive personality disorders. More individuals were diagnosed with a personality disorder by the SIDP, but the PDQ diagnosed multiple personality disorders more often. The results of the PDQ are not tabulated separately because the same sample was utilized for both instruments.

Casey and Tyrer (1986) carried out a study of 200 randomly selected community residents in the United Kingdom. They administered the Present State Examination (9th edition) (Wing et al., 1974) for axis I disorders and the Personality Assessment Schedule (PAS; Tyrer et al., 1979) for the assessment of personality disorders. The PAS obtains information from an informant as well as the subject. Ordinal ratings are made on 24 personality traits. A computer algorithm is applied to determine personality disorder diagnoses according to the International Classification of Diseases (World Health Organization, 1978). Personality disorders were diagnosed in 26 of their subjects (13%). The personality disorder with the highest prevalence was explosive personality, which probably corresponds most closely to the DSM-III diagnoses of antisocial personality disorder or intermittent explosive disorder on axis I. There were no differences in prevalence between their urban and rural samples and males and females did not differ in the overall rate of personality disorder; women had a higher prevalence of asthenic personality disorder. They did not find a relationship between neurotic depression or the combined category of neuroses and personality disorder. Subjects with a personality disorder were found to have significantly poorer social functioning.

Reich and colleagues (1989) conducted a random mailed survey of the adult population of Iowa City, Iowa. Surveys were mailed to 401 subjects; 240 surveys were returned for a response rate of 62.1%. Data were collected using the Personality Diagnostic Questionnaire (Hyler et al., 1983). Diagnoses were based on meeting the requisite number of criteria for a given personality disorder and meeting the impairment distress scale criterion for the presence of a disorder. The rate for receiving any axis II disorder was 11%.

Maier and his coworkers (1992) studied a sample of 452 subjects in the mixed urban–rural Rhein-Main area of Germany. Subjects were recruited to serve as controls in a family study of affective disorders and schizophrenia. The sample of control probands (n = 109) was selected randomly without regard to psychiatric status and was stratified by age, sex, residential area, and educational status. Maier et al.'s sample included the probands, their mates, and all first-degree relatives over age 20 who agreed to take part in face-to-face interviews, for a total of 452. Subjects were administered the Schedule for Affective Disorders and Schizophrenia: Lifetime Version (Mannuzza et al., 1986) for axis I diagnoses and the Structured Clinical Interview for DSM-III Axis II (Spitzer et al., 1987) for axis II diagnoses. The rate of receiving any personality disorder diagnosis was 10.0%. They followed DSM-III-R diagnostic criteria with the exception of exclusionary criteria; for example, schizotypal personality disorder could be diagnosed in the presence of schizophrenia.

We recently administered the SIDP-IV to a sample of 693 male twins who were members of the Vietnam Era Twin (VET) Registry. The SIDP-IV yields DSM-IV diagnoses. The sample was randomly selected from the VET Registry (details of construction of the Registry have been reported elsewhere, Eisen et al., 1989; Henderson et al., 1990). The men were between the ages of 45 and 55 years. The sample is limited because it includes only males, participants were screened for mental health at military induction during early adulthood, and the observations of members of a twin pair are not statistically independent. The prevalence of having any DSM-IV personality disorders among these men was 7.6%. These data are presented here for the first time and are identified in the tables as "Lyons and Jerskey."

Developmental Issues

Personality disorder diagnoses may be applied to children or adolescents in those unusual instances in which the maladaptive traits appear to be pervasive, persistent and unlikely to be limited to a particular developmental stage. However, it should be recognized that traits that appear in childhood may not persist into later adulthood (American Psychiatric Association, 1994). For diagnosis, the features of the personality disorder must be present for at least one year, with the exception of antisocial personality disorder, which cannot be diagnosed until after the age of eighteen.

To investigate longevity of personality disorders diagnosis in childhood, Bernstein and colleagues (1993) performed a cross-sectional prevalence analysis across the age span from late childhood to early adulthood, as well as a longitudinal assessment of the stability of personality disorder diagnoses. Subjects were a random sample of children from families in two upstate counties in New York. A single child was selected from each of the 976 families that agreed to participate in the study, after which an interview with the mother of the child was conducted. Follow-up assessments were conducted on the families that were located eight and ten years later (n = 724 and n = 733). The findings suggested that there is a high proportion of adolescents not referred for treatment that meet DSM-III-R criteria for a personality disorder diagnosis. Longitudinal data revealed substantial stability. However, less then half the subjects receive the same diagnosis at follow-up.

Johnson et al. (2000) reported three different kinds of information about the development and course of personality disorders in adolescents. First, they reported that significant declines (28%) in personality disorder traits were observed between early adolescence and early adulthood. They also found that stability in these traits ranged from low to moderate over a six-year interval that began in middle adolescence. Finally, they reported that adolescents with diagnoses of personality disorders tended to have elevated disordered traits in their early adult years. It is important to recognize that diagnostic criteria were originally designed to diagnose personality disorders in adults and not younger populations. Further investigation may be warranted to see if modifications of the criteria are needed to appropriately assess younger individuals.

On the other end of the developmental continuum, Abrams and Horowitz (1996) performed a meta-analysis of the literature concerning the frequency and distribution of personality disorders in older adults. Their review of eleven articles

TABLE 1. Post-DSM-III Community Studies of Prevalence of Any Personality Disorder

Authors (year)	Population	Instrument and DX System	Prevalence (%) of any PD	Comments
Nestadt et al. (1993)	810 subjects from the Clinical Reappraisal at Baltimore ECA site	DSM-III by SPE administered by psychiatrist	5.9 (definite) 9.3 (definite plus provisional)	
Zimmerman and Coryell (1989)	797 nonpatient relatives of normal controls and probands with schizophrenia and depression	DSM-III by SIDP	17.9	Sample limits generalizability telephone 72.9 face-to-face 27.1
Casey and Tyrer (1986)	200 urban and rural residents, selected randomly	Personality Assessment Schedule, ICD	13.0	Not DSM based
Reich et al. (1989)	235 community residents, selected randomly	Personality Diagnostic Questionnaire, DSM-III	11.0	Required criteria plus impairment/ distress for diagnosis
Maier et al. (1992)	452 probands and relatives from randomly selected families in Germany	DSM-III-R by SCID	10.0	Did not use DSM-III-R exclusionary criteria
Bernstein et al. (1993)	733 adolescences and their mothers selected randomly	Ten diagnostic scales combined including structured interviews and self-report questionnaires	31.2 moderate) 17.2 (severe)	Not all criteria were matched by protocol items
Abrams and Horowitz (1996)	meta-analysis of eleven studies, samples ranging from 30–547 (SD = 214.53)	Structured interviews, clinician consensus, and chart review	10.0	Settings of subjects varied
Lenzenweger et al. (1997)	1646 college students	DSM-III-R by International Personality Disorder Examination	6.7 (definite) 11.0 (definite + probable)	Results are estimated from a two-stage case identification procedure
Lyons and Jerskey	693 male twins from the Vietnam Era Twin Registry	DSM-IV by SIDP	7.6	Males only

published from 1980 through 1994 found that the overall prevalence for that age group of 50 years and older was 10%. However, the prevalences ranged from 6% to 33% based upon the setting in which participants were recruited (e.g., senior citizen center, psychiatric inpatients, psychiatric outpatients) and methods of assessment (e.g., structured interviews, consensus of clinicians, and retrospective chart reviews).

Treated Prevalence

Merikangas and Weissman (1991) pointed out the hazards of using treated rates for drawing inferences about true prevalence of personality disorders. They identified a number of factors that could lead to bias in treated samples: (1) differences in the availability of treatment; (2) the role of cultural factors in help-seeking behavior; (3) differences in the severity of the disorder; (4) the potential influence of other comorbid psychiatric disorders; and (5) differences among the personality disorders in the likelihood of seeking treatment. However, the importance of personality disorders in clinical practice makes their prevalence in such settings valuable information in its own right.

Dahl (1986) reported results of the systematic assessment of DSM-III personality disorders in 231 consecutive admissions to a psychiatric inpatient unit in Norway. Chronic patients and those with organic disorders were excluded. Approximately 45% of the sample received a personality disorder diagnosis (40% of females and 49% of males). Forty-four percent of those with a personality disorder received one diagnosis, 36% had two diagnoses, 15% had three diagnoses, and 5% had four diagnoses. Schizotypal, histrionic, antisocial, and borderline personality disorders were each present in approximately 20% of the sample. Avoidant personality disorder was diagnosed in 9% of the sample and the remaining personality disorders were diagnosed much less frequently. In a series of 100 patients admitted with major psychiatric disorders (affective disorders, schizophrenia, and other functional psychosis), Cutting et al. (1986) found that 44% had an "abnormal personality" based on informant interviews about the period preceding the acute episode.

Oldham and Skodol (1991) investigated the prevalence of personality disorders among the 129,268 patients treated in New York state mental health facilities in 1988. Using the system's centralized database, they found that 10.8% received a personality disorder diagnosis. The personality disorder diagnosis was the primary diagnosis of 1.2% of patients and only 0.2% of patients received more than one personality disorder diagnosis. The most common diagnosis was borderline personality disorder; 17.2% of the patients with any personality disorder received a diagnosis of borderline personality disorder. These authors concluded that the standard record-keeping procedures underestimated the prevalence of personality disorders and that personality disorders were not being systematically assessed.

The prevalence of personality disorders has also been examined in nonpsychiatric medical populations. Casey and her coworkers reported on the prevalence of personality disorders in British clinical settings using the ICD classification (Casey et al., 1984; Casey et al., 1985). They found a 34% prevalence of personality disorder in primary care settings; anxiety states and alcohol abuse were the conditions most commonly associated with personality disorders. In a rural general practice, they found a prevalence rate for personality disorders of 20%. Reich et al. (1989) found a significant positive association between the presence of personality disorder and the probability of being hospitalized for a nonpsychiatric medical illness.

As is the case for both axis I and axis II disorders, treated rates shed little light on the prevalence of disorders in untreated samples. However, because personality disorders have important implications for service provision, it is useful to consider their frequency in various clinical populations. Obviously, the nature of the setting in which the disorders are studied and the method by which they are studied will influence the findings. The treated rates of the individual personality disorders will be included in the next section. [Data on treated rates are drawn primarily from a review by Widiger (1991)].

Prevalence of Specific DSM-III, DSM-III-R, or DSM-IV Personality Disorders

In this section, each of the personality disorders will be presented, starting with the essential features of the disorder according to the DSM-IV criteria published by the American Psychiatric Association in 1994. Available data about prevalence in clinical and nonclinical populations will be presented. For several personality disorders, such as antisocial personality disorder, there are a number of studies that have reported prevalence. For many of the personality disorders, however, there have been very few reports of true prevalence. The length of each section is somewhat proportional to the amount of epidemiological data that is available about the disorder. In some cases a single study provided data on a number of individual personality disorders. To avoid redundancy, the methodology of the study is mentioned only once.

Paranoid Personality Disorder. The essential feature of paranoid personality disorder is a "pervasive distrust and suspiciousness of others such that their motives are interpreted as malevolent" (American Psychiatric Association, 1994). All four nonclinical studies of paranoid personality disorder reported prevalence rates less than 2.0%. The rates in clinical samples reported in Widiger (1991) ranged from 1.0% to 36% with a median prevalence of 6.0%. Reich (1987a) found an excess of paranoid personality disorder among males compared to females in an outpatient sample. The DSM-IV reports rates in the general population to be between 0.5% to 2.5%, in inpatient psychiatric settings 10% to 30%, and in outpatient mental health clinics 2.5% to 10% (APA, 1994).

Schizoid Personality Disorder:. The essential feature of this disorder is a "pervasive pattern of detachment from social relationships and a restricted range of expression of emotions in interpersonal settings" (APA, 1994). In general, schizoid personality disorder has been a very infrequent diagnosis in clinical settings. For example, Zanarini et al. (1987) found no cases in a clinical sample of 97 patients and Koenigsberg et al. (1985) reported no cases on the basis of chart review in a sample of 2,462 patients. The prevalences in nonclinical samples reported in Table 2 are 1.0% or lower. The rates in clinical samples reported in Widiger (1991) ranged from 0.0% to 8% with a median prevalence of 1.0%. Comparison studies using DSM-III-R criteria report higher prevalence rates than DSM-III criteria. Morey (1988) compared the two sets of criteria on the same group of patients; rates were substantially higher using the DSM-III-R criteria. Individuals with schizoid personality disorder may be less likely to seek treatment as a function of their disorder. It may also be that the diagnosis of schizotypal personality disorder is applied to a number of individuals that might have been characterized as schizoid before DSM-III or that the current criteria are inadequate (Zanarini et al., 1987).

TABLE 2. Prevalence of Cluster A Personality Disorders

Authors (year)	Population	Instrument	Prevalence (%)	Comments
Paranoid PD				
Zimmerman and Coryell (1989)	797 nonpatient relatives of normal controls and probands with schizophrenia and depression	DSM-III by SIDP telephone 72.9% face-to-face 27.1%	0.9	Sample limits generalizability
Reich et al. (1989)	235 community residents, selected randomly	Personality Diagnostic Questionnaire, DSM-III	0.9	Required criteria plus impairment/ distress for diagnosis
Maier et al. (1992)	452 probands and relatives from randomly wselected families in Germany	DSM-III-R by SCID	1.8	Did not use DSM-III-R exclusionary criteria
Lyons and Jerskey	693 male twins from the Vietnam Era Twin Registry	DSM-IV by SIDP	0.4	Males only
Schizoid PD				
Zimmerman and Coryell (1989)	797 nonpatient relatives of normal controls and probands with schizophrenia and depression	DSM-III by SIDP: telephone 72.9% face-to-face 27.1%	0.9	Sample limits generalizability
Casey and Tyrer (1986)	200 urban and rural residents, selected randomly	Personality Assessment Schedule, ICD	1.0	Not DSM based
Reich et al. (1989)	235 community residents, selected randomly	Personality Diagnostic Questionnaire, DSM-III	0.9	Required criteria plus impairment/ distress for diagnosis
Maier et al. (1992)	452 probands and relatives from randomly selected families in Germany	DSM-III-R by SCID	0.4	Did not use DSM-III-R exclusionary criteria
Lyons and Jerskey	693 male twins from the Vietnam Era Twin Registry	DSM-IV by SIDP	0.9	Males only
Schizotypal PD				
Zimmerman and Coryell (1989)	797 nonpatient relatives of normal controls and probands with schizophrenia and depression	DSM-III by SIDP; telephone 72.9% face-to-face 27.1%	2.9	Sample limits generalizability

(*Continued*)

TABLE 2. (*Continued*)

Authors (year)	Population	Instrument	Prevalence (%)	Comments
Schizotypal				
Baron et al. (1985)	376 relatives of control subjects in a family study	DSM-III by Schedule for Interviewing Borderlines; 70% interviews 30% family history	2.2	Adjustment for sensitivity of family history method
Reich et al. (1989)	235 community residents, selected randomly	Personality Diagnostic Questionnaire, DSM-III	5.1	Required criteria plus impairment/ distress for diagnosis
Maier et al. (1992)	452 probands and relatives from randomly selected families in Germany	DSM-III-R by SCID	0.7	Did not use DSM-III-R exclusionary criteria
Lyons and Jerskey	693 male twins from the Vietnam Era Twin Registry	DSM-IV by SIDP	0.3	Males only

Schizotypal Personality Disorder:. The essential feature of schizotypal personality disorder is a "pervasive pattern of social and interpersonal deficits marked by acute discomfort with, and reduced capacity for, close relationships as well as by cognitive or perceptual distortions and eccentricities of behavior" (APA, 1994). These characteristics must be present by early adulthood in various contexts. The symptoms must not be severe enough to warrant a diagnosis of schizophrenia. The DSM-III diagnostic criteria for schizotypal personality disorder were drawn from the definition for the diagnosis of borderline schizophrenia in the Danish Adoption study (Kety et al., 1978). A number of studies have indicated a familial relationship between schizotypal personality disorder and schizophrenia. However, a number of studies have failed to find an excess risk for schizophrenia among the relatives of schizotypal probands.

Baron et al. (1985) conducted a family study of the transmission of schizotypal and borderline personality disorder. They identified a control group of 90 subjects and subsequently included 376 of their relatives. Their findings on the relatives of controls is relevant for inferring prevalence in a nonclinical sample. Seventy percent of the relatives of controls were personally interviewed by mental health professionals using the Schedule for Affective Disorders and Schizophrenia (Spitzer and Endicott, 1978) for axis I and with the Schedule for Interviewing Borderlines (Gunderson, 1982) which yields diagnoses for DSM-III schizotypal and borderline personality disorders. Data were obtained on 30% of the relatives using a family history version of the Schedule for Interviewing Borderlines (the family history method refers to obtaining information from an informant rather than through a direct interview). Seventy-five percent of the relatives of controls were studied blind to the diagnostic status of the proband. Baron and colleagues did not find differences in outcome between subjects rated in the blind versus nonblind conditions. The risk to relatives was age corrected using the Stromgren method for schizotypal but not for borderline personality disorder. The authors also adjusted the morbidity risks to compensate for the inferior sensitivity of the family history method compared to direct interview. Although this procedure applied across all relative groups in their study may help the comparison of relatives of different types of probands, it also makes epidemiological inferences from these data somewhat tentative.

In a small study of consecutive outpatient admissions, Bornstein et al. (1988) reported that patients with schizotypal personality disorder were more likely to receive a diagnosis of substance abuse or dependence and major affective disorder than nonschizotypal patients in their series. The prevalences in nonclinical samples reported in Table 2 range from 0.3% to 5.1% with a median value of about 3.0%. The rates in clinical samples reported in Widiger (1991) ranged from 2.0% to 64% with a median prevalence of 17.5%.

Antisocial Personality Disorder:. The essential feature of antisocial personality disorder is a "pervasive pattern of disregard for and violation of the rights of others" (APA, 1994). The DSM-III and DSM-III-R criteria were heavily influenced by the work of Robins (1984) and place an emphasis on antisocial and criminal behavior. In prison populations the prevalence of DSM-III-R antisocial personality disorder may be over 50%. Reich (1987a) found an excess of males with antisocial personality disorder among an outpatient sample.

Antisocial personality disorder was one of the DSM-III personality disorders about which Nestadt and his coworkers reported results. They found a positive association between the number of criteria for antisocial PD and the risk for an alcohol use disorder diagnosis. Swanson and colleagues (1994) found that 90.4% of their sample of individuals with antisocial personality disorder had at least one other DSM-III lifetime psychiatric diagnosis. Moran (1999a, b) found several sociodemographic predictors of antisocial personality disorder. Males outnumbered females by as much as 8:1 and younger age groups and people with limited education were at higher risk. In a follow-up study of 500 psychiatric outpatients, Martin et al. (1985) found that the mortality rates for patients with antisocial personality disorder was almost four times greater than the comparison population.

Using DSM-I criteria, Leighton et al. (1963) reported a prevalence of 11% in men and 5% for women for a sociopathic diagnosis. Weissman et al. (1978) reported results from a systematic survey of households in New Haven, Connecticut. Their diagnostic data were collected in an eight-year follow-up of the sample. The original sample was 1,095 individuals; the diagnostic sample included 511 of the original sample. The follow-up sample differed from the original sample on the basis of race and class; the follow-up included a higher proportion of whites and a lower proportion of the lowest social class. Diagnostic data were collected with the SADS and diagnoses were based on the Research Diagnostic Criteria. The rate of current antisocial personality disorder was 0.2%.

Antisocial personality disorder was the only personality disorder included in the ECA study and the National Comorbidity Survey (Kessler et al., 1994). Data are presented in Table 3. Compton et al. (1991) applied the methodology of the ECA study to a community-based sample in Taiwan. The prevalences in nonclinical

TABLE 3. Prevalence of Cluster B Personality Disorder

Authors (year)	Population	Instrument	Prevalence (%)	Comments
Antisocial PD				
Robins et al. (1984)	9,543 subjects strict probability sampling at 3 sites	DIS	2.5	Very rigorous sampling
Compton et al. (1991)	11,004 community residents in Taiwan; strict probability sample	DIS	0.2	Very rigorous sampling and methodology
Zimmerman and Coryell (1989)	797 nonpatient relatives of normal controls and probands with schizophrenia and depression	DSM-III by SIDP telephone 72.9% face-to-face 27.1%	3.3	Sample limits generalizability
Casey and Tyrer (1986)	200 urban and rural residents, selected randomly	Personality Assessment Schedule, ICD	6.0	(included explosive personality) not DSM based
Nestadt et al. (1990)	810 subjects from the Clinical Reappraisal at Baltimore ECA site	DSM-III by SPE administered by psychiatrist	1.5	
Weissman et al. (1978)	511 systematically identified community residents	Research Diagnostic Criteria; RDC	0.2	Significant sample attrition is a problem
Reich et al. (1989)	235 community residents, selected randomly	Personality Diagnostic Questionnaire, DSM-III	0.4	Required criteria plus impairment/ distress for diagnosis
Oakley-Browne (1989)	1,498 New Zealand	DIS	3.1	
Maier et al. (1992)	452 probands and relatives from randomly selected families in Germany	DSM-III-R by SCID	0.2	Did not use DSM-III-R exclusionary criteria
Swanson et al. (1994)	3258 (Edmonton, Canada)	DIS	3.7	Weighted prevalence rate
Kessler et al. (1994)	8098 Strict probability sample	DSM-III-R by CIDI	3.5	National Comorbidity Survey
Lyons and Jerskey	693 male twins from the Vietnam Era Twin Registry	DSM-IV byz SIDP	0.9	Males only

TABLE 3. *(Continued)*

Authors (year)	Population	Instrument	Prevalence (%)	Comments
Borderline				
Zimmerman and Coryell (1989)	797 nonpatient relatives of normal controls and probands with schizophrenia and depression	DSM-III by SIDP telephone 72.9% face-to-face 27.1%	1.6	Sample limits generalizability
Baron et al. (1985)	376 relatives of control subjects in a family study	DSM-III by Schedule for Interviewing Borderlines; 70% interviews 30% family history	1.7	Unorthodox adjustment for sensitivity of family history method
Reich et al. (1989)	235 community residents, selected randomly	Personality Diagnostic Questionnaire, DSM-III	0.4	Required criteria plus impairment/ distress for diagnosis
Swartz et al. (1990)	1,541 community residents from the Duke ECA site	DIS/Borderline Index, DSM-III	1.8	Included subjects between ages 19 and 55
Maier et al. (1992)	452 probands and relatives from randomly selected families in in Germany	DSM-III-R by SCID	1.1	Did not use DSM-III-R exclusionary criteria
Lyons and Jerskey	693 male twins from the Vietnam Era Twin Registry	DSM-IV by SIDP	1.2	Males only
Histrionic PD				
Zimmermanand Coryell (1989)	797 nonpatient relatives of normal controls and probands with schizophrenia and depression	DSM-III by SIDP telephone 72.9% face-to-face 27.1%	3.0	Sample limits generalizability
Nestadt et al. (1990)	810 subjects from the Clinical Reappraisal at Baltimore ECA site	DSM-III by SPE administered by psychiatrist	2.2	
Reich et al. (1989)	235 community residents, selected randomly	Personality Diagnostic Questionnaire, DSM-III	2.1	Required criteria plus impairment/ distress for diagnosis
Maier et al. (1992)	452 probands and relatives from randomly selected families in Germany	DSM-III-R by SCID	1.3	Did not use DSM-III-R exclusionary criteria
Lyons and Jerskey	693 male twins from the Vietnam Era Twin Registry	DSM-IV by SIDP	0.0	Males only

(Continued)

TABLE 3. (*Continued*)

Authors (year)	Population	Instrument	Prevalence (%)	Comments
Narcissistic PD				
Zimmerman and Coryell (1989)	797 nonpatient relatives of normal controls and probands with schizophrenia and depression	DSM-III by SIDP telephone 72.9,% face-to-face 27.1%	0.0	Sample limits generalizability
Reich et al. (1989)	235 community residents, selected randomly	Personality Diagnostic Questionnaire, DSM-III	0.4	Required criteria plus impairment/ distress for diagnosis
Maier et al. (1992)	452 probands and relatives from randomly selected families in in Germany	DSM-III-R by SCID	0.0	Did not use DSM-III-R exclusionary criteria
Lyons and Jerskey	693 male twins from the Vietnam Era Twin Registry	DSM-IV by SID	0.9	Males only

samples reported in Table 3 range from 0.2% in a Taiwanese population to over 3% with a median value of about 2.0%. The rates in clinical samples reported in Widiger (1991) ranged from 0.0% to 37% with a median prevalence of 7%. DSM-IV reports prevalence estimates in clinical settings ranging from 3% to 30% depending on the predominant characteristics of the populations that are sampled, with higher rates being associated with substance abuse treatment settings and prison and forensic settings (APA, 1994).

Borderline Personality Disorder. The essential feature of borderline personality disorder is a "pervasive pattern of instability of interpersonal relationships, self-image, affects, and control over impulses" (APA, 1994). Swartz et al. (1990) derived a diagnostic algorithm for diagnosing BPD from the Diagnostic Interview Schedule (Robins et al., 1981). Using a cutoff of 11 items from their 24-item index, they classified 1.8% of their sample (from the Duke site of the ECA study) between ages 19 and 55 as having borderline personality disorder. Merikangas and Weissman (1986) estimated the prevalence of borderline personality disorder to be between 1.7% and 2.0% based on community studies carried out before the diagnostic criteria for borderline personality disorder were codified in DSM-III.

Borderline personality disorder is the most common personality disorder seen in most psychiatric settings and is overrepresented in clinical populations because of the tendency toward help-seeking (Galenberg, 1987). Nurnberg et al. (1991) found that 82% of patients with a diagnosis of borderline personality disorder received at least one other axis II diagnosis, among a sample of outpatients with personality disorder and no concurrent axis I disorder. They concluded that borderline personality disorder characterizes a general personality disorder construct.

Widiger and Weissman (1991) and Widiger and Trull (1992) reviewed the epidemiology of borderline personality disorder. They reported an average prevalence of 8.0% in studies of outpatients and 15% in studies of inpatients. Among studies of patients with personality disorder, the average prevalence among outpatients was 27% and among inpatients, 51%. These authors concluded that BPD is the most common personality disorder diagnosis given in clinical samples, with prevalence rates of up to 70% found among inpatient samples (Standage and Ladha, 1988).

Akhtar, Byrne, and Doghramji (1986) reviewed 23 studies of borderline personality disorder to investigate associations between borderline personality disorder and demographic characteristics. All of the studies that they reviewed used clinical samples, mostly inpatients. They only included studies that utilized one of several widely used criteria sets to define the disorder. They pooled data across the samples of borderlines and compared these data to pooled comparison group data from the same studies. They found that patients receiving a diagnosis of borderline personality disorder tended to be young, with a mean age in the mid-twenties. A significantly higher percentage of borderline patients (77%) were female. The samples of borderline patients were disproportionally white; the mean percentage of blacks in the borderline samples was 10%, while the mean percentage of blacks in the comparison samples was 20%, a statistically significant difference. Reich (1987a) did not find an excess of borderline personality disorder among female outpatients.

The prevalences in nonclinical samples reported in Table 3 range from 0.4% to 1.8% with a median value of about 1.6%. The rates in clinical samples reported in Widiger (1991) ranged from 11% to 70% with a median prevalence of 31%.

Histrionic Personality Disorder. The essential feature of histrionic personality disorder is a "pervasive pattern of excessive emotionality and attention-seeking" (APA, 1994). The term "hysterical personality" has been used in other classifications. There has been relatively little empirical work done on histrionic personality disorder (Pfohl, 1991). When structured diagnostic assessments have been utilized, no sex difference in histrionic personality disorder has been observed, however, there is some suggestion that clinicians may more frequently apply the diagnosis to females (Pfohl, 1991).

Histrionic personality disorder was one of the DSM-III Personality disorders about which Nestadt and his coworkers (described above) reported results from the Clinical Reappraisal of the ECA Baltimore site. There were no differences in prevalence by sex (males, 2.2%; females, 2.1%), race, or education. The prevalence declined with age in males but not in females. There was a higher rate of histrionic personality disorder among separated and divorced subjects than among married subjects. There was also an increase in depressive disorder, suicide attempts, and the occurrence of three or more unexplained medical symptoms in females associated with histrionic personality disorder. In males there was an increase in substance use disorders associated with histrionic personality disorder. Subjects with histrionic personality disorder were significantly more likely to seek medical and psychiatric treatment than subjects without.

The prevalences in nonclinical samples reported in Table 3 range from 0.0% to 3.0% with a median value of about 2.2%. The rates in clinical samples reported in

Widiger (1991) ranged from 2.0% to 45% with a median prevalence of 19%. Rates in inpatient and outpatient mental health settings have been reported to be between 10% to 15% when a structured assessment has been conducted (APA, 1994).

Narcissistic Personality Disorder. The essential feature of this disorder is a "pervasive pattern of grandiosity (in fantasy or behavior), need for admiration, and lack of empathy" (APA, 1994). There has not been a great deal of empirical work done on narcissistic personality disorder in general, and very little epidemiological work in particular. Although there is considerable clinical interest in the disorder, it has only recently been included in official nomenclatures. Narcissistic personality disorder became part of the American nomenclature in 1980 with DSM-III and there is no counterpart to it in ICD-10.

Gunderson et al. (1991b) reviewed several studies that reported the prevalence of DSM-III-R narcissistic personality disorder in clinical populations (Dahl, 1986; Frances et al., 1984; Skodol, 1989; Zanarini et al., 1987) and reported prevalence rates ranging from 2.0% to 16%. The prevalences in nonclinical samples reported in Table 3 range from 0.0% to 0.4% with a median value of about 0.2%. The rates in clinical samples reported in Widiger (1991) ranged from 2.0% to 35% with a median prevalence of 6.0%.

Avoidant Personality Disorder. The essential feature of avoidant personality disorder is a "pervasive pattern of social inhibition, feelings of inadequacy, and hypersensitivity to negative evaluation" (APA, 1994). An important issue in the epidemiology of avoidant personality disorder is its potential overlap with an axis I disorder: generalized social phobia. Turner et al. (1991) studied axis II comorbidity in a sample of individuals with social phobias. Avoidant personality disorder was present in 22.1% of the sample and an additional 52.9% of the sample had avoidant features that fell short of meeting the diagnostic threshold. Schneier et al. (1991) studied a sample of 50 patients with social phobias. They found that 70% of patients with social phobia met criteria for avoidant personality disorder and 89% of patients with generalized social phobia received a diagnosis of avoidant personality disorder. Herbert et al. (1992) found that 61% of patients in their series with generalized social phobia also met criteria for avoidant personality disorder. Holt et al. (1992) found that 50% of their sample with generalized social phobia met criteria for avoidant personality disorder. Schneier et al. (1991) suggested that generalized social phobia and avoidant personality disorder may define a single psychopathological entity.

The prevalences in nonclinical samples reported in Table 4 range from 0.0% to 2.3% with a median value of about 1.1%. The rates in clinical samples reported in Widiger (1991) ranged from 5.0% to 55% with a median prevalence of 16%.

Dependent Personality Disorder. The essential feature of dependent personality disorder is a "pervasive and excessive need to be taken care of, leading to submissive and clinging behaviors and fears of separation" (APA, 1994). Dependent personality disorder was recently reviewed by Hirschfeld et al. (1991). They pointed out that dependent personality disorder derives from psychoanalytic theory, social psychological theory, and ethological theory. The construct of dependent personality disorder overlaps with borderline, avoidant, and histrionic personality disorders. In studies of clinical samples reviewed by Hirschfeld et al. (1991),

TABLE 4. Prevalence of Cluster C Personality Disorders

Authors (year)	Population	Instrument	Prevalence (%)	Comments
Avoidant PD				
Zimmerman and Coryell (1989)	797 nonpatient relatives of normal controls and probands with schizophrenia and depression	DSM-III by SIDP: telephone 72.9%, face-to-face 27.1%	1.3	Sample limits generalizability
Reich et al. (1989)	235 community residents, selected randomly	Personality Diagnostic Questionnaire, DSM-III	0.0	Required criteria plus impairment/distress for diagnosis
Maier et al. (1992)	452 probands and relatives from randomly selected families in Germany	DSM-III-R by SCID	1.1	Did not use DSM-III-R exclusionary criteria
Lyons and Jerskey	693 male twins from the Vietnam Era Twin Registry	DSM-IV by SIDP	2.3	Males only
Dependent PD				
Zimmerman and Coryell (1989)	797 nonpatient relatives of normal controls and probands with schizophrenia and depression	DSM-III by SID: telephone 72.9% face-to-face 27.1%	1.8	Sample limits generalizability
Reich et al. (1989)	235 community residents, selected randomly	Personality Diagnostic Questionnaire, DSM-III	5.1	Required criteria plus impairment/distress for diagnosis
Maier et al. (1992)	452 probands and relatives from randomly selected families in Germany	DSM-III-R by SCID exclusionary criteria	1.5	Did not use DSM-III-R
Lyons and Jerskey	693 male twins from the Vietnam Era Twin Registry	DSM-IV by SIDP	0.1	Males only

(Continued)

TABLE 4. (*Continued*)

Authors (year)	Population	Instrument	Prevalence (%)	Comments
Obsessive-Compulsive PD				
Zimmerman and Coryell (1989)	797 nonpatient relatives of normal controls and probands with schizophrenia and depression	DSM-III by SIDP: telephone 72.9%, face-to-face 27.1%	2.0	Sample limits generalizability
Nestadt et al. (1990)	810 subjects from the Clinical Reappraisal at Baltimore ECA site	DSM-III by SPE administrated by psychiatrist	1.7	Male rate 5 times female rate
Reich et al. (1989)	235 community residents, selected randomly	Personality Diagnostic Questionnaire, DSM-III	6.4	Required criteria plus impairment/ distress for diagnosis
Maier et al. (1992)	452 probands and relatives from randomly selected families in Germany	DSM-III-R by SCID	2.2	Did not use DSM-III-exclusionary criteria
Lyons and Jerskey	693 male twins from Vietnam Era Twin Registry	DSM-IV by SIDP	2.3	Males only

substantial overlap with other personality disorders was reported. The greatest degree of overlap was with borderline personality disorder (over 50 in most studies), followed by avoidant, histrionic, and schizotypal personality disorders. Hirschfeld and associates discussed the issues of sex differences and possible sex bias in the diagnosis of dependent personality disorder. They pointed out that dependent personality disorder was diagnosed more frequently in females when assessment was not carried out using standardized instruments. When standardized instruments were used, males and females did not differ in the frequency of the diagnosis. This suggests that clinicians, rather than the standardized diagnostic criteria, may be responsible for observed differences in male and female rates. Individuals with a depressive disorder may be more likely to display dependent personality traits (Overholser, 1991). According to the DSM-IV, dependent personality is among the most frequently reported of the personality disorders encountered in mental health clinics (APA, 1994).

The prevalences of dependent personality disorder in nonclinical samples reported in Table 4 range from 0.1% to 5.1% with a median value of about 1.8%. The rates in clinical samples reported in Widiger (1991) ranged from 2.0% to 55% with a median prevalence of 20%.

Obsessive–Compulsive Personality Disorder:. The essential feature of obsessive–compulsive personality disorder is a "pervasive pattern of preoccupation with orderliness, perfectionism, and mental and interpersonal control, at the expense of flexibility, openness, and efficiency" (APA, 1994). Compulsive personality disorder was one of the DSM-III personality disorders about which Nestadt and his coworkers (described above) reported results from the Clinical Reappraisal of the ECA Baltimore site. Males had a significantly higher prevalence (3.0%) than females (0.6%). White respondents had a significantly higher prevalence than black respondents. There was no association between age and risk of the disorder. The diagnosis of compulsive personality disorder was associated with higher education, greater likelihood of being employed, and greater likelihood of being married as against being widowed, separated, divorced, or never married. Subjects with compulsive personality disorder had a higher income than those without after correcting for age and sex. Nestadt et al. (1992) found that compulsive traits were associated with greater risk of generalized anxiety disorder and simple phobia and lower risk of alcohol use disorder.

Turner et al. (1991) studied axis II comorbidity in a sample of individuals with social phobias. Obsessive–compulsive personality disorder was present in 13.2% of the sample and an additional 48.5% of the sample had obsessive–compulsive traits that fell short of meeting the diagnostic threshold. Baer et al. (1990) studied 96 patients with obsessive–compulsive disorder (OCD), which is an anxiety disorder recorded on axis I. Only 6% of the patients received a diagnosis of obsessive–compulsive personality disorder; of the six patients receiving the obsessive–compulsive personality disorder diagnosis, five had onset of obsessive–compulsive symptoms before age 10. Pfohl et al. (1990) found that among patients with OCD, 30% met criteria for obsessive–compulsive personality disorder. (To put this finding in context, in the same study they found dependent personality disorder in 46% of their OCD subjects and passive–aggressive personality disorder in 49%.) Reich (1987a) found an excess of males with obsessive–compulsive personality disorder among an outpatient sample in comparison to females.

The prevalences in nonclinical samples reported in Table 4 range from 1.7% to 6.4% with a median value of about 2.0%. The rates in clinical samples reported in Widiger (1991) ranged from 1.0% to 20% with a median prevalence of 9%.

CONCEPTUAL ISSUES

Probably the primary conceptual issue with implications for investigating the epidemiology of personality disorders is the question of whether personality disorders are best considered to be categories or whether they should be considered to represent extreme standings on universally occurring dimensions of personality.

Models of Personality Disorder

The issue of the relative merits of categorical versus dimensional approaches cuts across most domains of psychopathology. However, in the domain of personality disorders it is especially significant, in part, because of the long tradition of research in personality psychology based on dimensional models. Currently, clinicians using DSM-IV must decide whether a patient meets criteria for one or more personality disorders, each considered a separate and distinct category.

If the true nature of personality disorders is dimensional, it would suggest that the most appropriate epidemiological approach might be to determine the mean and standard deviation of the population on the appropriate dimension. Consistent with such an approach, prevalence could be regarded as the proportion of the population that exceeds a threshold associated with impairment and/or distress.

The *DSM-IV Options Book* (American Psychiatric Association, 1991) described the strengths and weaknesses of the current categorical system. The *Options Book* pointed out that a dimensional approach would improve flexibility, possibly improve reliability and validity for certain disorders, and save information lost in categorical classification. The inclusion of a dimensional approach in an appendix of DSM-IV was proposed (American Psychiatric Association, 1991). However, lack of consensus about the dimensions to include was a disadvantage of adopting a dimensional approach (American Psychiatric Association, 1991) and DSM-IV continues to use a categorical system.

Costa and McCrae (1990) suggested that personality disorders, at least as they are assessed by the scales created by a number of different investigators, represent an extreme standing or a configuration of extreme standings on the dimensions of normal personality. This might be termed the "defining model," in which the disorder results from exceeding the threshold on some dimension (or dimensions); the dimension is causally related to the disorder and exceeding the threshold is a sufficient cause. A medical example of this model would be cases of essential hypertension without a demonstrable underlying pathophysiological cause for elevated blood pressure. That is, the factors that go into determining the blood pressure of the afflicted individuals are the same as those for the general population. Blood pressure, in general, is normally distributed in the population and some individuals, for the same multifarious genetic and environmental factors that determine the blood pressure of human beings in general, fall at the high end of the distribution. Because blood pressure at the high end of the distribution is associated with excess morbidity and mortality, it is justifiably considered a disorder: hypertension. The defining model of personality disorder is similar to this example. Some individuals, due to the same genetic and environmental factors that influence everyone, are at the high or low end of a dimension or dimensions of personality and this standing defines (it *is*) their personality disorder.

The defining model, however, does not describe the only possible manner in which dimensions of normal personality may relate to personality disorders. There are at least two other models that are equally plausible. In the "descriptive (trivial) model" the disorder can be described in terms of a dimension (or dimensions), but the relationship is not causal and is uninformative for understanding the disorder. A medical example of the descriptive model would be explaining Downs syndrome in terms of the "universally occurring" dimensions of height and IQ. That is, individuals with Downs syndrome could be described as being at the low end of the continuum of height and at the low end of the continuum of IQ. However, this is an uninformative approach. A telling question would be, "Are people with Downs syndrome short for the same reason that short people without Downs syndrome are short?" If the answer is no, then trying to understand Downs syndrome through the mechanism that determines height for most people would not be informative. Individuals with Downs syndrome differ qualitatively from the general population. If a personality disorder is caused by some factor or factors that are independent of "normal" personality, it still might be described in these terms but such a procrustean approach will be counterproductive for understanding the nature of the phenomenon.

In the "predisposing model," exceeding a threshold on the relevant dimension is a risk factor for the disorder and could be a necessary cause, but it is not a sufficient cause. Phenylketonuria (PKU) can serve as a medical example of this model. An individual who is homozygous for a defective gene that leads to the production of phenylalanine hydroxylase is vulnerable to the development of PKU. Such a genotype is a necessary but not sufficient cause. In order for the individual to manifest PKU, he or she must be exposed to dietary phenylalanine. If such an individual ingests phenylalanine, damage to the nervous system results. Without such exposure, there is no damage to the nervous system. For example, schizotypal personality disorder could be due to an extreme position on a universal continuum of introversion: extroversion plus possessing a schizophrenia genotype. In this example, introversion is necessary but not sufficient to produce schizotypal personality disorder.

Block and Ozer (1982) discussed a similar issue with regard to the use of typologies in the study of personality. They made a distinction between *type-as-label* and *type-as-distinctive-form.* Type-as-label refers to the practice of establishing categories by classifying individuals above some threshold on an underlying continuum as being in the category. The category so established is then given a name or label. The defining model discussed above corresponds to type-as-label. The alternative definition of "category" or "type" described by Block and Ozer is stronger and more implicative. Type-as-distinctive-form refers to "a subset of individuals characterized by a reliably unique or discontinuously different pattern of covariation ... with respect to a specifiable (and nontrivial) set of variables" (Block, 1971). The use of a dimensional approach to personality disorders is not appropriate if these disorders fit the type-as-distinctive-form model. Meehl (1979) made a similar distinction between a communicative taxon and a "true" taxon.

It seems likely that some aspects of personality disorders are related to deviation within normal dimensions of personality while other features are best considered categorical. It is unlikely that any single model will adequately describe all personality disorders. For example, Gunderson et al. (1991) have suggested that the more severe personality disorders (e.g., schizotypal, paranoid, and borderline) may be discrete clinical syndromes with discrete etiological pathways, while less severe personality disorders (e.g., compulsive, avoidant, and dependent) represent extremes of normally occurring traits. It is conceivable that certain types of personality pathology represent a "common final pathway" for a number of different etiological factors, while others might be uniquely related to a specific standing on universal dimensions of personality.

It is unlikely that the diagnostic system will be changed because personality disorders *can* be described in dimensional terms; change is only likely to occur if it is demonstrated that personality disorders *should* be described dimensionally. The result of solely descriptive or clinical research is unlikely to be decisive in resolving the issue of categorical versus dimensional approaches. Research on etiology and pathophysiology may be more promising for adducing the type of evidence required. For example, data from genetic studies might shed light on whether factors contributing to conscientiousness and neuroticism in the general population are responsible for the occurrence of compulsive personality disorder. Another example of such an approach would be to determine whether the relationship between MAO activity and sensation seeking seen in normal populations could predict risk for antisocial personality disorder. A delineation of relationships between dimensions of normal personality and personality disorders is an important step towards acquiring the knowledge required to create a diagnostic system that accurately reflects the nature of personality disorders.

Distinguishing Axis I from Axis II Disorders

DSM-III introduced the distinction between clinical disorders on axis I and personality disorders on axis II. DSM-IV states that this distinction is made to foster consideration of the presence of personality disorders that may be overlooked if attention is directed to more florid axis I disorders. Personality disorders are suggested to be more stable than axis I disorders. However, there are reasonable questions about whether personality disorders are sufficiently different from other mental disorders to warrant their own axis. It has been suggested that the distinction between axis I and axis II is not supported by empirical evidence. However, in clinical practice the term "axis II disorder" has become synonymous with "personality disorder" and it is unlikely that any proposal to eliminate axis II would receive enough support to change the current diagnostic system in the near future.

METHODOLOGICAL ISSUES

Diagnostic Issues

As in other areas of psychiatric research, the reliability and validity of diagnosis has been a central issue in research on personality disorders. Also, as in other areas of psychopathology, there is no "gold standard" that can be used to validate diagnoses. However, the problem seems to be greater for personality disorders than for axis I disorders. There are a number of issues that probably contribute to the difficulty in reliably and validly diagnosing personality disorders. One important factor is that axis II symptomatology is often less florid and dramatic than axis I symptomatology.

Skodol et al. (1990) identified a number of issues that contribute to the difficulty in assessing personality disorders. In comparison to axis I disorders, personality disorders are more likely to be ego syntonic. This means that to the individual with a personality disorder, his or her symptomatology is not experienced as alien to his or her usual experience of self. The story is often different for axis I disorders. For example, a panic attack is typically experienced as being distinctively different from normal experience. The nature of personality disorders may make it more difficult for the individual to describe symptoms to an interviewer. The symptoms of personality disorder may be more recognizable and troublesome to individuals in the environment of the person with the disorder than to the person him or herself. Clinicians may be inclined to rely more on their own observations than on the patient's reports when assessing the presence of personality disorder. In the type of assessment of personality disorder typically used in research, the respondent is asked a series of questions about symptoms and answers are generally taken to be veridical. There is usually some provision for the diagnostician to override the subject's self-report if there is contradictory information. Given that personality disorders are defined as long-standing stable characteristics, one time, cross-sectional assessment may not be ideal. If the person has a concurrent axis I disorder, the symptoms of that disorder may influence the report of axis II symptoms.

Zanarini and her colleagues (1987) also identified a number of issues that contribute to the difficulty of making reliable and valid diagnoses of personality disorders. Many of the DSM diagnostic criteria are not clearly operationalized, necessitating clinical interpretation. Some symptoms, such as low self-esteem, have a very high base rate and may require significant clinical judgment as to whether they achieve clinical significance. Many diagnostic criteria (e.g., vanity or criminal behavior) reflect traits that are generally held to be negative, and may be denied on the basis of social desirability. Reporting certain traits may require a level of insight that is absent in some individuals.

Another central issue in diagnosing personality disorders is the occurrence of certain spectrum relationships that exist between personality disorders and axis I disorders, which are thought to represent phenotypic variations of the same underlying pathology. Such relationships have been suggested to exist between borderline personality disorder and depression, depressive personality disorder and depression, schizotypal personality disorder and schizophrenia, avoidant personality disorder and social phobia, cluster B personality disorders and substance use, cluster B and C personality disorders and eating disorders, cluster C personality disorders and anxiety disorders and cluster A and schizophrenia (Tyrer et al., 1997). There is evidence that the co-occurrence of personality disorders with axis I disorders predicts worse outcome than an axis I disorder alone (Reich and Green, 1991) and that personality disorders may impair subsequent axis I treatment response. However, acknowledgement of the relationship in devising treatment options could influence the delivery and type of treatment and therefore possible subsequent success (Oldham, 1994).

Methods for Collecting Diagnostic Information

There are a number of methods that may be utilized to collect data on which to base a diagnosis of personality disorders. These methods range from relatively unstructured clinical interviews to self-report questionnaires. There is no compelling evidence for the superiority of any single approach to the diagnosis of personality disorders (Skodol et al., 1990). However, as is the case for axis I disorders, the most widely accepted methodology for epidemiological applications is the structured diagnostic interview.

Chart Review/Records. It has been suggested that clinicians often do not systematically assess their patients for the presence of personality disorders (Kass et al., 1985). When clinicians do assess personality disorder, they often diagnose only one (Oldham and Skodol, 1991), while systematic evaluation suggests that an individual who meets criteria for one personality disorder will usually meet criteria for at least one other personality disorder (Widiger et al., 1990). Obviously, the quality of clinical diagnoses contained in medical records may vary dramatically from one setting to another. But given the fact that an acute axis I disorder is typically more florid than any accompanying personality disorder, it is quite likely that in most clinical settings the sensitivity of diagnoses of personality disorders will be poorer than for axis I disorders. Especially for diagnoses made at admission, the axis II diagnosis is often deferred and may or may not be added to the record at a later time.

Informants. Because the symptomatology of personality disorder may be subtle, ego syntonic, socially undesirable to acknowledge, and not obvious to the subject because of lack of insight, it has been suggested that information should be sought from another person who is familiar with the individual being diagnosed. However, in most cases it is not clear how to combine and weight information from an informant relative to that provided by the subject or observed by the diagnostician (Widiger and Frances, 1987).

Zimmerman et al. (1986) administered a structured interview to 82 patients and also interviewed a close friend or relative about the patient's normal personality. Adding the informant's information to that obtained from the patient led to changes in whether a personality disorder was judged to be present or absent in approximately 20% of the cases. In most cases, the informant information indicated more personality pathology. Zimmerman et al. (1988) also reported a comparison of information obtained from patients with information from informants using the SIDP in both groups. Significantly more of the criteria for all personality disorders were rated positively based on the informant [criteria positive by informant = 23.0 ($\pm$15.1) vs. criteria positive by subject = 17.1 ($\pm$13.4)]. Only antisocial personality disorder was diagnosed more frequently using subject data. The κ coefficient between patients and informants for the presence of any personality disorder was 0.13, and the κ's for every one of the individual personality disorders was below 0.35. The rate of personality disorders in the patients based on their own report was 36.4%; the rate based on informants was 57.6%. Zimmerman and colleagues concluded that patients and informants differed "markedly" in their descriptions of personality and that informants reported more personality pathology than did the patients themselves. Bernstein et al. (1997) carried out a similar study. Results replicated the previous findings, suggesting that the agreement between patient interview and informant interview is poor. However, in contrast to previous work, Bernstein et al. found that the addition of informant data to information given by the patient resulted in slight and nonsignificant increases in the final diagnostic decision.

Clinical Interview. Perry (1992) suggested that structured diagnostic interviews may emphasize reliability to the point that validity is degraded. He proposed that the clinical interview, with its emphasis on history, important stories from the subject's life, and the discernment of longstanding patterns of behavior in historical context, may be very useful for the identification of personality disorder. Perry advocated several steps to ensure the quality and comparability of information obtained from clinical interviews: (1) the use of guidelines for the interview; (2) a compendium of good case examples; and (3) good training procedures.

Structured Interviews. Reich (1987b) reviewed the most widely used instruments for diagnosing personality disorders and may be consulted for more detailed information about these instruments. Because of potential confounding between reported personality traits and axis I disorders, it is good practice to assess the presence of axis I disorders when assessing personality disorders. Empirical evidence indicates that the assessment of personality disorders may be influenced by changes in the status of an axis I disorder (Hirschfeld et al., 1983). This section will review the most widely utilized structured interviews for making diagnoses of all DSM personality disorders. There are not striking differences in the κ's reported for interrater agreement and test–retest reliability of these broad-spectrum diagnostic interviews. There will also be a brief description of several interviews intended to assess only one or several personality disorders.

The Structured Clinical Interview for DSM-IV Personality Disorders (First et al., 1994) is a semistructured interview. It was developed to accompany the Structured Clinical Interview for DSM-IV, which diagnoses axis I disorders. Criteria are rated on a three-point scale. Questions are organized by disorder and the interviewer is encouraged to ask clarifying questions for responses that require it. The number of criteria rated as present can also be summed to provide dimensional scores.

The Structured Interview for DSM-IV Personality Disorders (Pfohl et al., 1994) includes 160 questions. Questions are grouped into topical sections (e.g., egocentricity, unemotional), which facilitates a natural flow to the interview. At the end of each section, the relevant diagnostic criteria are rated on a three-point scale. The use of a knowledgeable informant is encouraged.

The International Personality Disorders Examination (World Health Organization, 1995) contains questions that are grouped by topical areas rather that by disorder. Positive responses may be followed up by probes and requests for examples.

In the Diagnostic Interview for DSM-IV Personality Disorders (Zanarini et al., 1996) each DSM-IV criterion is assessed by separate questions scored on a three-point scale. It is designed to be administered by interviewers trained to make clinical judgments. The interview provides follow-up probes, but also encourages the interviewer to be flexible and to employ clinical judgment. Interviewers should have substantial clinical experience and familiarity with DSM, but not necessarily formal graduate training.

A practical issue that will confront anyone planning to use a structured interview in an epidemiological study is whether to use a broad-spectrum interview that includes all of the personality disorders or to select a specialized interview. The decision will depend on the purpose of the study. If one particular disorder is the subject of study, then it may be desirable to collect the type of detailed information provided by a specialized interview. If the purpose of the study is to investigate all of the personality disorders, then the obvious choice would be one of the more general interviews. There are quite a number of structured and semistructured interviews for specific personality disorders, such as the Diagnostic Interview for Borderlines (Gunderson et al., 1981) and the Structured Interview for Schizotypy (Kendler, 1985). It is beyond the scope of this chapter to describe them individually.

Self-Report Questionnaires. There are several self-report instruments available for assessing personality disorders. The Personality Diagnostic Questionnaire, Revised (PDQ-IV; Hyler et al., 1987) is a self-report questionnaire with a true/false format. The items reflect the criteria for all of the DSM-IV personality disorders. Diagnoses reflect endorsement of symptom items plus the presence of impairment or distress. The internal consistency reliabilities of the original PDQ-R scales ranged from 0.56 to 0.84 with a median alpha of 0.69 (Hyler et al., 1989). Hyler et al. (1990) reported κ values ranging from 0.23 to 0.63 (mean = 0.41) in a comparison of the PDQ-R to the SCID-II. Comparing the PDQ-R to the PDE yielded κ's from −0.02 to 0.54 (mean = 0.33). The Millon Clinical Multiaxial Inventory (MCMI; Millon, 1983) is a self-report questionnaire designed to measure the dimensions underlying the DSM-III personality disorders. The questionnaire does not inquire directly about the presence of the diagnostic criteria, but there is a method for using responses to assign DSM diagnoses. Test–retest reliability as assessed by correlations between two administrations separated by eight weeks ranged from 0.60 to 0.89 (median = 0.75). Two studies have been reported comparing the MCMI to the SIDP; Hogg et al. (1990) reported a median κ of 0.14 and Jackson et al. (1991) a median κ of 0.18. The Schedule for Nonadaptive and Adaptive Personality (SNAP; Clark, 1993) is a self-report questionnaire that uses 375 true–false items to provide scores on 34 scales, covering 12 traits and 3 temperaments and including 6 validity and 13 diagnostic scales. There is a system for recombining items to provide a measure of DSM personality disorders. Clark (1993) reported one-week retest correlations ranging from 0.68 to 0.89 in a sample of state hospital patients. Internal consistency reliability coefficients ranged from 0.68 to 0.90 in a patient sample. Neal et al. (1997) developed a computerized self-report instrument based on the DSM-III-R and validated it against the Structured Clinical Interview for DSM-III-R Axis II (SCID-II) in part to reduce the time needed to administer and score standard tests of personality disorders. As an assessment instrument, it demonstrated moderate validity (mean κ coefficient = 0.47).

Bodlund and associates (1998) used the DSM-IV and ICD-10 Personality Questionnaire (DIP-Q) to screen personality disorders in three clinical populations, including general and forensic psychiatric patients and candidates for psychotherapy as well as healthy volunteers (n = 587). The DIP-Q is a 140-item self-report questionnaire that is used to asses the ten DSM-IV and eight ICD-10 personality disorders. Analyses showed that the prevalence rate for any personality disorder was 14% among volunteers, 59% in the general psychiatric sample, 68% in the forensic sample and up to 90% in the candidates for psychotherapy. When compared to a clinical assessment, the DIP-Q reported higher prevalence rates (DIP-Q reported 70% prevalence across clinical samples, while the clinical assessment reported 55% prevalence). Although the instrument discriminated well between the clinical samples, the results suggest that the DIP-Q may be overinclusive of certain disorders such as paranoid, obsessive–compulsive and possibly borderline personality disorders.

Rating Scales. The Personality Assessment Form (PAF; Shea et al., 1987) uses a prototypical rating approach to assess DSM personality disorders. The PAF includes a paragraph describing the diagnostic features of each personality disorder. The clinician uses data from available clinical sources to rate the long-term personality functioning of the subject on a six-point scale ("not at all" to "to an extreme degree") for each personality disorder. Shea et al. (1990) reported interrater reliability assessed by κ for the diagnosis of any personality disorder and any cluster C personality disorder as 0.48 and 0.47, respectively.

Recent Developments in the Assessment of Personality Disorders

Lenzenweger and colleagues (1997) applied the type of two-stage procedure advocated by Dohrenwend and Shrout (1981) to study the prevalence of personality disorders. In this procedure, subjects are administered a less intensive screening instrument (e.g., a self-report questionnaire or an interview that does not require the individual administering it to have considerable clinical expertise) at the first stage and then those who screen positive and only a sample of those who screen negative are administered a more intensive assessment (e.g., an interview by an experienced clinician) at the second stage. Lenzenweger et al. administered the International Personality Disorder Examination Screen to a sample of 1646 undergraduate students during the first stage of data collection. In the second stage, experienced clinicians administered a diagnostic interview, the International Personality Disorder Examination, to 258 subjects selected from the first stage. This procedure achieved very good sensitivity; no subject classified as negative for a personality disorder in the first stage was found to have a personality disorder at the second stage. This approach could make epidemiological studies more efficient by permitting first-stage, relatively inexpensive screening of large samples, while allowing for the final diagnostic determination to be based on information collected by skilled clinicians.

One of the major impediments to personality disorder research may be reliance on self-reported symptoms. Because the symptoms of personality disorders may be more subtle, more ego syntonic, and less socially acceptable to acknowledge than the symptoms of axis I disorders, it may be important to collect information from sources other than the subject himself or herself. Two alternatives to self-reported information have recently been described. The first approach, developed by Westen and Shedler, uses information from a treating clinician to diagnose personality disorders. The Shedler-Westen Assessment Procedure-200 (SWAP-200; Westen and Shedler 1999a, b; 2000) is a 200-item Q-sort designed to assess personality and personality pathology. A Q-Sort is a set of statements printed on separate index cards, in this case, statements about personality and personality dysfunction. Using the SWAP-200, an experienced clinical observer sorts (rank-orders) the statements into categories (piles), from those that are not descriptive of the patient to those that are highly descriptive, with intermediate placement of items that apply to varying degrees. Clinician-judges can sort the items based on the Clinical Diagnostic Interview (Westen et al., 1997) or on knowledge of the patient over the course of treatment. Oltmanns et al. (1998) have proposed a technique in which peer assessments are utilized to identify the symptoms of personality disorder. This procedure capitalizes on naturally occurring social groupings by using members of a group to "nominate" peers with characteristic features of personality disorders. Peers may be better able and more willing to identify socially undesirable traits. Weston and Shedlers Q-sort procedure and Oltmann et al.'s peer nomination procedure may provide very valuable alternatives to reliance on self-reports of personality disorder symptoms. However, logistical considerations in implementing these approaches in large, representative samples might limit their utility in epidemiological research.

Diagnostic Agreement

Although it does not directly address the issue of validity, it is certainly desirable that different instruments used to assess personality disorders yield similar, if not identical, results. Before the advent of DSM-III, the interrater reliability of personality disorders was poor. Based on a review of reported results, Spitzer and Fleiss (1974) reported that the average pre-DSM-III κ was 0.32 for clinical diagnosis. In the DSM-III field trials, a κ for the presence of any personality disorder of 0.61 was reported when both diagnosticians rated the same interview; when two separate interviews were conducted, κ was 0.54 (Spitzer et al., 1979).

Perry (1992) reviewed results from eight studies that reported results from different structured interviews or self-report questionnaires on the same individuals. Perry concluded that the reliability of the individual instruments assessed by interrater reliability is in the fair-to-high range. As mentioned earlier, there is no clear-cut criterion for validity available. However, an important consideration, while pertaining neither to validity nor reliability, is the level of agreement between different instruments. If these instruments are all measuring constructs validly, then they should lead to similar diagnostic conclusions. Perry found that agreement across instruments was poor. One way that Perry summarized agreement between different instruments was to determine the median κ for the individual disorders between the two instruments being considered. When he examined the highest κ between disorders from each study, he found a median κ of 0.54. For the lowest κ between disorders from each study, he found a median κ of 0.0. Finally, he determined the median κ from each study and computed a "median of medians," which yielded a κ value of 0.25, in the poor range. When Perry separated studies that compared two interviews from those that compared self-report questionnaires with interviews there were minor changes in the results. The median highest κ from studies comparing two interviews was 0.61, the median lowest κ was 0.09, and the median of medians was 0.25. The results were somewhat poorer for studies comparing self-report questionnaires to interview. The median highest κ was 0.50, the median lowest κ was 0.01, and the median of medians was 0.16. Perry suggested that demonstrating acceptable reliability for the individual instruments leaves unanswered questions about assessment validity. Perry concluded that the different instruments for assessing personality disorders, on average, agree with one another at a level that is only slightly better than chance and often reach different conclusions.

Comorbidity and Diagnostic Overlap

If the diagnosis of more than one personality disorder in an individual is seen as reflecting the actual presence of two or more personality disorders, then this section could be considered to be about comorbidity. To the extent that current assessment techniques and diagnostic criteria fail to differentiate phenomena due to methodological shortcomings, it could be considered to be about "overlap."

Zimmerman and Coryell (1989b) in their nonpatient sample of relatives of normal controls and probands with schizophrenia and depressive disorders found that approximately one-fourth of subjects with any personality disorder met criteria for more than one. Fossati and colleagues (2000) reported that the co-occurrence rate was greater then 50% for all DSM-IV personality disorders in a population of 431 consecutively admitted psychiatric patients with various axis I diagnoses, excluding psychotic disorders. Oldham and his co-workers (Oldham et al., unpublished data described in Skodol et al,, 1990), in a study of 100 patients with suspected character pathology, reported an average of 3.4 personality disorders in patients with at least one personality disorder. Zanarini et al. (1987) reported 2.8 diagnoses per patient, Widiger et al. (1990) reported 3.75, and Skodol et al. (1988) reported 4.6.

Widiger and Rogers (1989) suggested that patterns of comorbidity between personality disorders and axis I may best be understood in terms of the DSM-III clusters. The odd–eccentric cluster should be associated with psychotic disorders, the dramatic–impulsive cluster should be associated with affective disorders, and the anxious–fearful cluster should be associated with anxiety disorders. Pfohl et al., (1990) reviewed findings on the comorbidity of axis I and axis II disorders. They included studies that employed patient samples with major depression, obsessive–compulsive disorder (OCD), and panic disorder. The hospitalized depressed patients had an increased risk for dramatic–impulsive cluster (cluster B) personality disorders. The OCD and panic disorder samples were more likely to receive a diagnosis from the anxious–fearful cluster (cluster C). OCD subjects were also more likely to receive a diagnosis from the odd–eccentric cluster (cluster A) than either depressed or panic patients.

Bollinger et al. (2000) examined the prevalence of personality disorders in combat veterans diagnosed with post-traumatic stress disorder. The personality disorders were assessed using the Structured Clinical Interview for DSM-III Personality Disorders; nearly 80% of the sample received a diagnosis of at least one personality disorder, with 29.9%receiving a diagnosis of one, 21.5% receiving a diagnosis of two, 15.9% receiving a diagnosis of three and 12.1% receiving a diagnosis of four or more. The most frequent diagnoses were avoidant, paranoid, obsessive–compulsive and antisocial personality disorder.

A meta-analysis of twenty-five studies published since the 1980s by Corruble et al. (1996) found that 20–50% of inpatients and 50–85% of outpatients with current major depression have an associated personality disorder. Furthermore,

Skodol et al. (1999) found that certain clinical characteristics of major depressive disorder and dysthymia disorder predicted personality disorder co-occurrence. For major depression, the greater the number of prior episodes, the more likely the patient was to receive a diagnosis of borderline personality disorder. However, dependent personality disorder was associated with fewer episodes. Earlier onset dysthymia also signified an increased likelihood of borderline personality disorder; however, no evidence was found that early onset of major depressive disorder increased the likelihood of any other personality disorders.

When a personality disorder is found to be highly comorbid with another disorder there are several possibilities to consider: (1) there may be some significant association between the two, such that one disorder is a risk factor for the other, or both disorders share some underlying risk factor, vulnerability, or pathophysiological process; (2) the two diagnoses may describe only one disorder (e.g., avoidant personality disorder and generalized social phobia might be the same disorder); or (3) the diagnostic criteria for the disorders may include overlapping features that promote individuals with certain symptomatology to receive both diagnoses.

FUTURE DIRECTIONS

In comparison to the major axis I disorders, there is considerably less epidemiological information about the personality disorders. There are a number of factors that have contributed to this state of affairs. Before DSM-III was published in 1980, there was less of a consensus about how to define the individual personality disorders (as well as disagreement about which disorders to include under the heading) than there was for the major axis I disorders. The most ambitious studies of true prevalence, the ECA study and the NCS, included most of the important axis I disorders, but only antisocial personality disorder was included from axis II. There is good evidence that personality disorders are strongly associated with use of mental health services, use of medical services (Reich et al., 1989), prognosis and responsiveness to treatment of axis I disorders (Reich and Green, 1991), and substantial impairment in functioning and subjective distress. There are important questions that remain unanswered about the true prevalence of most of these disorders, about the stability of these disorders, their natural course, as well as risk and protective factors for their development.

ACKNOWLEDGMENTS

The work presented here was supported by NIAAA research grant AA10586. The authors acknowledge the assistance of Ms. Catherine Hynds and Ms. Christa Laib in the preparation of this chapter.

REFERENCES

Abrams RC, Horowitz SV (1996): Personality disorders after age 50: A meta-analysis. J Personality Disord 10:271–281.

Akhtar S, Byrne JP, Doghramji K (1986): The demographic profile of borderline disorder. J Clin Psychiatry, 47:196–198.

American Psychiatric Association (1980): "Diagnostic and Statistical Manual of Mental Disorders" 3rd ed. Washington, DC: American Psychiatric Association.

American Psychiatric Association (1987). "Diagnostic and Statistical Manual of Mental Disorders" 3rd ed. revised, Washington, DC: American Psychiatric Association.

American Psychiatric Association, Task Force on DSM-IV (1991): "DSM-IV Options Book: Work in Progress." Washington, DC: American Psychiatric Association.

American Psychiatric Association (1994): "Diagnostic and Statistical Manual of Mental Disorders" 4th ed. Washington, DC: American Psychiatric Association.

Baer L, Jenike MA, Ricciardi JN, Holland AD, Seymour RJ, Minichiello WE, Buttolph ML (1990): Standardized assessment of personality disorders in obsessive-compulsive disorder. Arch Gen Psychiatry 47:826–830.

Baron M, Gruen R, Asnis L, Lord S (1985): Familial transmission of schizotypal and borderline personality disorders. Am J Psychiatry 142:927–934.

Bernstein DP, Cohen P, Velez CN, Schwab-Stone M (1993): Prevalence and stability of the DSM-III-R personality disorders in a community-based survey of adolescents. Am J Psychiatry 150:1237–1243.

Bernstein DP, Kasapis C, Bergman A, Weld E, Mitropoulou V, Horvath T, Klar HM, Silverman J, Siever LJ (1997): Assessing Axis II disorders by Informant interview. J Personality Disorders 11:158–167.

Block J (1971): Lives Through Time. Berkeley, CA: Bancroft.

Block J, Ozer DJ (1982): Two types of psychologists: Remarks on the Mendelsohn, Weiss, and Feimer contribution. J Personality and Social Psychology 42:1171–1181.

Bodlund O, Grann M, Ottosson H, Svanborg C (1998): Validation of the self-report questionnaire DIP-Q in diagnosing DSM-IV personality disorders: A comparison of three psychiatric samples. Acta Psychiatrica Scandinavica 97:433–439.

Bollinger AR, Riggs DS, Blake DD, Ruzek JI (2000): Prevalence of personality disorders among combat veterans with posttraumatic stress disorder. J Traumatic Stress 13:255–270.

Bornstein RF, Klein, DN, Mallon JC, Slater JF. (1988): Schizotypal personality disorder in an outpatient population: incidence and clinical characteristics. J Clin Psychology 44:322–325.

Bremer J (1951): A social psychiatric investigation of a small community in Northern Norway. Acta Psychiatr Neurol Scand, Suppl 62:10–166.

Casey PR, Tyrer PJ (1986): Personality, functioning and symptomatology. J Psychiatric Res 20:363–374.

Casey PR, Tyrer PJ, Dillon S (1984): The diagnostic status of patients with conspicuous psychiatric morbidity in primary care. Psycho Med 14:673–681.

Casey PR, Tyrer PJ, Platt SP (1985): The relationship between social functioning and psychiatric symptomatology in primary care. Social Psychiatry 20:5–9.

Clark LA (1993): "Schedule for Nonadaptive and Adaptive Personality (SNAP): Manual for Administration, Scoring and Interpretation." Minneapolis, Minnesota: University of Minnesota Press.

Compton WM, Helzer JE, Hwu HG, Yeh EK, McEvoy L, Tipp JE, Spitznagel EL (1991): New methods in crosscultural psychiatry: psychiatric illness in Taiwan and the United States. Am J Psychiatry 148:1697–1704.

Corruble E, Ginestet D, Guelfi JD (1996): Comorbidity of personality disorders and unipolar major depression: A review. J Affec Disorders 37:157–170.

Costa PT, McCrae RR (1990): Personality disorders and the five factor model of personality. J Personality Disorders 4:362–371.

Cutting J, Cowen PJ, Mann AH, Jenkins R (1986): Personality and psychosis: Use of the standardized assessment of personality. Acta Psychiatr Scand 73:87–92.

Dahl AA (1986): Some aspects of DSMIII personality disorders illustrated by a consecutive sample of hospitalized patients. Acta Psychiatrica Scandinavica 73(Suppl 328):61–66.

Dohrenwend BP, Shrout PE (1981): Toward the development of a two-stage procedure for case identification and classification in psychiatric epidemiology. Research in Community Mental Health 2:295–323.

Eisen S, Neuman R, Goldberg J, Rice J, True W (1989): Determining zygosity in the Vietnam Era Twin Registry. Clin Genetics 35:423–434.

Essen-Moller E, Larsson H, Uddenberg CE, et al. (1956): Individual traits and morbidity in a Swedish rural population. Acta Psychiatrica Neurol Scand Suppl. 100.

Folstein MF, Folstein SE, McHugh PR (1975): Mini mental state: a practical method for grading the cognitive state of patients for the clinician. J Psychiatr Res 12:189–198.

First MB, Spitzer RL, Gibbon M, Williams JBW, Benjamin L (1994): Structured Clinical Interview for the DSM-IV Axis II Personality Disorders (SCID-II) (Version 2.0). New York: Biometrics Research Department, New York State Psychiatric Institute.

Fossati A, Maffei C, Bagnato M, Battaglia M, Donati D, Donini M, Fiorilli M, Novella L, Prolo F (2000): Patterns of covariation of DSM-IV personality disorders in a mixed psychiatric sample. Comprehensive Psychiatry 41:206–215.

Frances A, Clarkin J, Gilmore M, et al. (1984): Reliability of criteria for borderline personality disorder: a comparison of DSMIII and the diagnostic interview for borderline patients. American Journal of Psychiatry 141:1080–1084.

Galenberg AJ (1987): Introduction: The borderline patient. J Clin Psychiatry 48(Suppl):3–11.

Goldberg D (1974): "The Detection of Psychiatric Illness by Questionnaire: A Technique for the Identification and Assessment of Nonpsychotic Psychiatric Illness." London: Oxford University Press.

Gunderson JG (1982): "Diagnostic Interview for Borderline Patients." New York: Roerig Pfizer.

Gunderson JG, Kolb JE, Austin V (1981): The diagnostic interview for borderline patients. Am J Psychiatry 138:896–903.

Gunderson JG, Links PS, Reich JH (1991): Competing models of personality disorders. J Personality Disorders 5:60–68.

Gunderson JG, Ronningstam E, Smith LE (1991b): Narcissistic personality disorder: A review of data on DSMIIIR descriptions. J Personality Disord 5:167–177.

Henderson WG, Eisen SE, Goldberg J, True WR, Barnes JE, Vitek M (1990): The Vietnam Era Twin Registry: A resource for medical research. Public Health Reports 105:368–373.

Herbert JD, Hope DA, Bellack AS (1992): Validity of the distinction between generalized social phobia and avoidant personality disorder. J Abnorm Psychol 101:332–339.

Hirschfeld RMA (1993): Personality disorders: Definition and diagnosis. J Personality Disord Suppl., 9–17.

Hirschfeld RMA, Klerman GL, Clayton PJ, et al. (1983): Assessing personality: Effects of the depressive state on trait measurement. Am J Psychiatry 140:695–699.

Hirschfeld RMA, Shea MT, Weise R (1991): Dependent personality disorder: Perspectives for DSMIV. J Personality Disord 5:135–149.

Hogg B, Jackson HJ, Rudd RP, Edwards J (1990): Diagnosing personality disorder in recent-onset schizophrenia. J Nervous and Mental Disorders 178:194–199.

Holt CS, Heimberg RG, Hope DA (1992): Avoidant personality and the generalized subtype in social phobia. J Abnormal Psychology 101:318–325.

Hyler SE, Rieder RO, Williams JBW, Spitzer RL (1983): "Personality Diagnostic Questionnaire" (PDQ). New York: New York State Psychiatric Institute, Biometrics Research.

Hyler SE, Rieder RO, Williams JBW, Spitzer RL, Lyons M, Hendler J (1989): A comparison of clinical and self-report diagnoses of DSMIII personality disorders in 552 patients. Comprehensive Psychiatry 30:170–178.

Hyler SE, Rieder RO, Williams JBW, et al. (1987): The Personality Diagnostic Questionnaire Revised (PDQR) . New York: New York State Psychiatric Institute, Biometrics Research.

Hyler SE, Skodol AE, Kellman HD, Doidge N (1990): Validity of the Personality Diagnostic Questionnaire-Revised: Comparison with two structured interviews. Am J Psychiatry 147:1043–1048.

Jackson HJ, Gazis J, Rudd RP, Edwards J (1991): Concordance between two personality disorder instruments with psychiatric inpatients. Comprehensive Psychiatry 32:252–260.

Johnson JG, Cohen P, Kasen S, Skodol AE, Hamagami F, Brook JS (2000): Age-related change in personality disorder trait levels between early adolescence and adulthood a community-based longitudinal investigation. Acta Psychiatrica Scandinavica 102:265–275.

Kass F, Skodol AE, Charles E, Spitzer RL, Williams JBW (1985): Scaled ratings of DSMIII personality disorders. Am J Psychiatry 142:627–630.

Kendler K (1985): "The Structured Interview for Schizotypy (SIS)" 1.5 ed. Richmond, VA.: Medical College of VA Hospitals .

Kessler RC, McGonagle KA, Zhao S, Nelson CB, Hughes M, Eshelman S, Wittchen H-U, Kendler KS (1994): Lifetime and 12-month prevalence of DSM-III-R psychiatric disorders in the United States. Arch Gen Psychiatry 51:8–19.

Kety SS, Rosenthal D, Wender PH, et al. (1978): The biologic and adoptive families of adopted individuals who became schizophrenic: Prevalence of mental illness and other characteristics. In Wynne LC, Cromwell RL, Matthysse S (eds): "The Nature of Schizophrenia: New Approaches to Research and Treatment" New York: Wiley.

Koenigsberg HW, Kaplan RD, Gilmore MM, Cooper AM (1985): The relationship between syndrome and personality disorder in DSM-III: experience with 2462 patients. Am J Psychiatry 142:207–212.

Kraepelin E (1919/1971): "Dementia Praecox and Paraphrenia," Krieger R, Barclay RM (eds), Huntington, New York: Robert E Krieger.

Langner TS, Michael ST (1963): Life Stress and Mental Health. The Midtown Manhattan Study. London: Collier, Macmillan.

Leighton A (1959): My name is legion: The Stirling County study. Am J Psychiatry 119:1021–1026.

Leighton DC, Harding JS, Macklin MA, Hughes CC, Leighton AH (1963): Psychiatric findings of the Stirling County Study. Am J Psychiatry 119:1021–1026.

Lenzenweger MF, Loranger AW, Korfine L, Neff C (1997): Detecting personality disorders in a nonclinical population. Arch Gen Psychiatry 54:345–351.

Maier W, Lictermann D, Klingler T, Heun R, Hallmayer J (1992): Prevalences of personality disorders (DSM-III-R) in the community. J Personality Disord 6:187–196.

Mannuzza S, Fyer AJ, Klein DF, Endicott J (1986): Schedule for Affective Disorders and Schizophrenia–Lifetime Version modified for the study of anxiety disorders (SADS-LA): Rationale and conceptual development. J Psychiatric Res 20:317–325.

Martin RL, Cloninger CR, Guze SB, Clayton PJ (1985): Mortality in a follow-up of 500 psychiatric outpatients. II. Cause specific mortality. Arch Gen Psychiatry 42:58–66.

Meehl PE (1979): A funny thing happened to us on the way to the latent entities. J Personality Assessment 42:1157–1170.

Merikangas KP, Weissman MM (1986): "The epidemiology of DSM-III axis II personality disorders." In Frances AJ, Hales RE (eds), APA Annual Review, Vol. 5, "Psychiatry Update," 258–278. Washington, DC: American Psychiatric Press.

Merikangas KR, Weissman MM (1991): Epidemiology of DSM-III Axis II Personality Disorders. Oldham, J (ed): In "Personality Disorders: New Perspectives on Diagnostic Validity" Washington, DC: American Psychiatric Association.

Millon T (1983): "Millon Clinical Multiaxial Inventory Manual," Minneapolis: National Computer Systems.

Moran P (1999a): "Antisocial Personality Disorder: An Epidemiological Perspective." Geskell, London.

Moran P (1999b): The epidemiology of antisocial personality disorder. Social Psychiatry and Psychiatric Epidemiology 34:231–242.

Morey L (1988): Personality disorders in the DSM-III and DSM-III-R: Convergence, coverage, and internal consistency. Am J Psychiatry 145:573–577.

Neal LA, Fox C, Carroll N, Holden M, Barnes P (1997): Development and validation of a computerized screening test for personality disorders in DSM-III-R. Acta Psychiatr Scand 95:351–356.

Nestadt G, Samuels JF, Romanoski AJ, Folstein MF, McHugh PR (1993): "DSM-III Personality Disorders in the Population" No. NR500. Washington, DC: American Psychiatric Association Annual Meeting .

Nestadt G, Romanoski AJ, Brown CH, Chahal R, Merchant A, Folstein MF, Gruenberg EM, McHugh PR (1991): DSMIII compulsive personality disorder: An epidemiological survey. Psychol Med 21:461–471.

Nestadt G, Romanoski AJ, Chahal R, Merchant A, Folstein MF, Gruenberg EM, McHugh PR (1990): An epidemiological study of histrionic personality disorder. Psychol Med 20:413–422.

Nestadt G, Romanoski AJ, Samuels JF, Folstein MF, McHugh PR (1992): The relationship between personality and DSMIII axis I disorders in the population: results from an epidemiological survey. Am J Psychiatry 149:1228–1233.

Nurnberg HG, Raskin M, Levine PE, Pollack S, Siegel O, Prince R (1991): The co-morbidity of borderline personality disorder and other DSM-III-R Axis II personality disorders. Am J Psychiatry 148:1371–1377.

Oakley-Browne MA, Joyce PR, Wells E, Bushnell JA, Hornblow AR (1989): Christchurch psychiatric epidemiology study, part II: Six-month and other period prevalences of specific psychiatric disorders. Aust N Zeal J Psychiatry 23:327–340.

Oldham JM (1994): Personality disorders. Current perspectives. J Amer Med Assoc 272:1770–1776.

Oldham J M, Skodol AE (1991): Personality disorders in the public sector. Hosp Community Psychiatry 42:481–487.

Oltmanns TF, Turkheimer E, Strauss ME (1998): Peer assessment of personality traits and pathology in college students. Assessment 5:53–65.

Overholser JC (1991): Categorical assessment of the dependent personality disorder in depressed inpatients. J Personality Disord 5:243–255.

Perry JC (1992): Problems and considerations in the valid assessment of personality disorders. Am J Psychiatry 149:1645–1653.

Pfohl B (1991): Histrionic personality disorder: A review of available data and recommendations for DSM-IV. J Personality Disorder 5:150–166.

Pfohl B, Black DW, Noyes R, et al. (1990): Axis I and axis II co-morbidity findings: implications for validity. In "Personality Disorders: New Perspectives on Diagnostic Validity." Washington, DC: American Psychiatric Press.

Pfohl B, Blum N, Zimmerman M (1994): "Structured Interview for DSM-IV Personality Disorders." Iowa City: University of Iowa Hospitals and Clinics.

Reich J (1987a): Sex Distribution of DSM-III Personality Disorders in Psychiatric Outpatients. Am J Psychiatry 144:485–488.

Reich J (1987b): Instruments measuring DSM-III and DSM-III-R personality disorders. J Personality Disord 1:220–240.

Reich J, Boerstler H, Yates W, Nduaguba M (1989): Utilization of medical resources in persons with DSM-III personality disorders in a community sample. Int J Psychiatry Med 19:1–9.

Reich JH (1989): Familiality of DSM-III dramatic and anxious personality clusters. J Nerv Ment Dis 177:96–100.

Reich JH, Green AI (1991): Effect of personality disorders on outcome of treatment. J Nerv Ment Dis 179:74–82.

Reich JH, Yates W, Nduaguba M (1989): Prevalence of DSM-III personality disorders in the community. Social Psychiatry Psychiatr Epidemiol 24:2–16.

Robins LN, Helzer JE, Croughan J, Williams JBW, Spitzer RL (1981): "N.I.M.H. Diagnostic Interview Schedule," Version III. Rockville, MD: National Institute of Mental Health.

Robins LN, Helzer JE, Weissman MM, Orvaschel H, Gruenberg E, Burke JD Jr, Regier DA (1984): Lifetime prevalence of specific psychiatric disorders in three sites. Arch Gen Psychiatry 41:949–958.

Schneier FR, Fyer AJ, Martin LY, Ross D et al. (1991): A comparison of phobic subtypes with panic disorder. J Anxiety Disord 5:65–75.

Shea MT, Glass DR, Pilkonis PA, Watkins J, Docherty JP (1987): Frequency and implications of personality disorders in a sample of depressed outpatients. J Personality Disord 1:27–42.

Shea MT, Pilkonis PA, Beckham E, Collins JF, Elkin I, Sotsky SM, Docherty JP (1990): Personality disorders and treatment outcome in the NIMH Treatment of Depression Research Program. Am J Psychiatry 147:711–718.

Skodol A (1989): Cooccurrence and diagnostic efficiency statistics (unpublished).

Skodol AE, Rosnick L, Kellman D, et al. (1988): Validating structured DSM-III-R personality disorder assessments with longitudinal data. Am J Psychiatry 145:1297–1299.

Skodol AE, Rosnick L, Kellman D, Oldham JM, Hyler S (1990): Development of a procedure for validating structured assessments of Axis II. In Oldham J (ed): "Personality Disorders: New Perspectives on Diagnostic Validity." Washington, DC: American Psychiatric Association.

Skodol AE, Stout RL, McGlashan TH, Grilo CM, Gunderson JG, Shea MT, Morey LC, Zanarini M.C, Dyck IR, Oldham JM (1999): Co-Occurrence of Mood and Personality Disorders: A report from the collaborative longitudinal personality disorders study (CLPS). Depression and Anxiety 10:175–182.

Spitzer RL, Endicott J (1978): "Schedule for Affective Disorders and Schizophrenia." New York: NIMH, Clinical Research Branch Collaborative Program on the Psychobiology of Depression.

Spitzer RL, Fleiss JL (1974): A reanalysis of the reliability of psychiatric diagnosis. Br J Psychiatry 125:341–347.

Spitzer RL, Forman JBW, Nee J (1979): DSM-III field trials. I. Initial inter-rater diagnostic reliability. Am J Psychiatry 136:815–817.

Spitzer RL, Williams JBW, Gibbon M (1987): "Structured Clinical Interview for DSM-III-R Personality Disorders (SCID-II)." New York: Biometric Research Department New York State Psychiatric Institute.

Srole L et al. (1962): "Mental Health in the Metropolis: The Midtown Manhattan Study." New York: McGrawHill.

Standage K, Ladha N (1988): An examination of the reliability of the Personality Disorders Examination and a comparison with other methods of identifying personality disorders in a clinical sample. J Personality Disord 2:267–271.

Stangl D, Pfohl B, Zimmerman M, Bowers W, Corenthal C (1985): A structured interview for the DSM-III personality disorders. A preliminary report. Arch Gen Psychiatry 42:591–596.

Swanson MCJ, Bland RC, Newman SC (1994): Antisocial personality disorders. Acta Psychaitr Scand 89 (suppl. 376):63–70.

Swartz M, Blazer D, George L, Winfield I (1990): Estimating the prevalence personality disorder in the community. J Personality Disord 4:257–272.

Turner SM, Beidel DC, Borden JW, Stanley MA, Jacob RG (1991): Social Phobia: Axis I and II correlates. J Abnorm Psychology 100(1):102–106.

Tyrer P, Alexander MS, Cicchetti D, Cohen MS, Remington M (1979): Reliability of a schedule for rating personality disorders. Br J Psychiatry 135:168–174.

Tyrer P, Gunderson J, Lyons M, Tohen M (1997): Extent of comorbidity between mental state and personality disorders. J Personality Disord 11:242–259.

Weissman MM, Myers JK, Harding PS (1978): Psychiatric disorders in the U.S. urban community: 1975–1976. Am J Psychiatry 135:459–462.

Westen D, Shedler J (1999a): Revising and assessing Axis II. Part 1: Developing a clinically and empirically valid assessment method. Am J Psychiatry 156:258–272.

Westen D, Shedler J (1999b): Revising and assessing Axis II. Part 2: Toward an empirically based and clinically useful classification of personality disorders. Am J Psychiatry 156:273–285.

Westen D, Shedler J (2000): A prototype matching approach to personality disorders: Toward DSM-V. J Personality Disord 14:109–126.

Westen D, Shedler J (2001): The factor structure of personality pathology. Unpublished manuscript, Boston University.

Westen D, Muderrisoglu S, Fowler C, Shedler J, Koren D (1997): Affect regulation and affective experience: Individual differences, group differences, and measurement using a Q-sort procedure. J Consulting Clin Psychology 65:429–439.

Widiger T, Frances AJ, Harris M, et al. (eds) (1990): Co-morbidity among Axis II Disorders, in Personality Disorders: New Perspectives on Diagnostic Validity. Washington, DC: American Psychiatric Press.

Widiger TA (1991): DSMIV reviews of the personality disorders: Introduction to special series. J Personality Disord 5:122–134.

Widiger TA, Frances A (1987): Interviews and inventories for the measurement of personality disorders. Clin Psychology Rev 7:49–75.

Widiger TA, Rogers JH (1989): Prevalence and co-morbidity of personality disorders. Psychiatr Ann 19:132–136.

Widiger TA, Trull TJ (1992): Personality and psychopathology: An application of the five factor model. J Personality 60:363–393.

Widiger TA, Weissman MM (1991): Epidemiology of borderline personality disorder. Hosp Community Psychiatry 42:1015–1021.

Wing JK, Cooper JE, Sartorius N (1974): "Measurements and Classification of Psychiatric Symptoms." New York: Cambridge University Press.

World Health Organization (1978): "Mental Disorders: Glossary and Guide to Their Classification in Accordance with the Ninth Revision of the International Classification of Diseases (ICD9)." Geneva: World Health Organization.

World Health Organization. (1995): "The International Personality Disorder Examination (IPDE): DSM-IV Module." Washington, DC: American Psychiatric Association.

Zanarini MC, Frankenberg FR, Chauncey DL, Gunderson JG (1987): The diagnostic interview for personality disorders: interviewer and test-retest reliability. Compr Psychiatry 28:467–480.

Zanarini MC, Frankenburg FR, Sickel AE, Yong L (1996): "The Diagnostic Interview for DSM-IV Personality Disorders." Belmont, MA: McLean Hospital Laboratory for the Study of Adult Development.

Zimmerman M, Coryell W (1989a): DSM-III personality disorder diagnosis in a nonpatient sample: Demographic correlates and comorbidity. Arch Gen Psychiatry 47:527–531.

Zimmerman M, Coryell W (1989b): The reliability of personality disorder diagnoses in a non-patient sample. J Personality Disord 3:53–57.

Zimmerman M, Coryell WH (1990): Diagnosing personality disorders in the community: A comparison of selfreport and interview measures. Arch Gen Psychiatry 47:527–531.

Zimmerman M, Pfohl B, Coryell W, Stangl D, Corenthal C (1988): Diagnosing personality disorder in depressed patients: A comparison of patient and informant interviews. Arch Gen Psychiatry 45:733–737.

Zimmerman M, Pfohl B, Stangl D, Corenthal C (1986): Assessment of DSMIII Personality Disorders: The Importance of Interviewing an informant. J Clin Psychiatry 47:261–263.

PART IV

Epidemiology of Special Populations

CHAPTER 22

Epidemiology and Geriatric Psychiatry

CELIA F. HYBELS and DAN G. BLAZER

Department of Psychiatry and Behavioral Sciences and Center for the Study of Aging and Human Development, Duke University Medical Center, Box 3003, Durham NC 27710

INTRODUCTION

Geriatric psychiatry has emerged during the last two decades as a specialty field within the discipline of psychiatry (Blazer, 1998). The emergence of the field is due, in part, to the growing numbers of individuals age 65 or older, and in particular the increasing numbers of persons 80 or over. Demographers in the United States coined the term "oldest old" in 1984 to identify a fast growing group of individuals 85 or older. In 1993, approximately 2.9% of the population was 80 years or older, and the percentage is projected to be 4.3% by 2025 (Fries and Ribbe, 1999). Life expectancy at age 80 in the Unites States is now 9.1 years for white women and 7.0 years for white men (Manton and Vaupel, 1995). Geriatric psychiatry is gaining attention because of increased understanding of mental disorders that are common in late life, such as Alzheimer's disease and depression, as well as the growing body of knowledge suggesting the psychiatric nomenclature may be less applicable for older adults for disorders such as major depression (Blazer, 1994).

Epidemiology, as the study of the distribution and determinants of disease frequency in populations (MacMahon and Pugh, 1970), has much to offer geriatric psychiatry. First, epidemiology informs us how a case is defined, as well as how cases are distributed across different subgroups of the older population. Second, epidemiology informs how risk factors are related to the onset of mental illness in late life, as well as how factors influence the progression of the illness and associated outcomes.

In this chapter, we present data on the epidemiology of psychiatric disorders in older adults, with a particular focus on two prevalent syndromes: dementia and depressive disorders. Key data are presented in the context of the essential tasks of an epidemiologist: the identification and distribution of cases within the population of interest, the etiology of these disorders and the identification of risk factors

Textbook in Psychiatric Epidemiology, Second Edition, Edited by Ming T. Tsuang and Mauricio Tohen.
ISBN 0-471-40974-X

which affect disease occurrence, outcomes associated with these disorders, historical trends in the prevalence of these disorders, and the impact of disease on the health care system (Morris, 1975).

WHAT IS A CASE?

Identifying and describing psychiatric disorders is of critical importance in psychiatric epidemiology. This task is particularly problematic in elderly individuals, however, because of factors such as comorbidity with medical illness and the presentation of symptoms as a consequence of medication use. In addition, elders often fail to meet the specific diagnostic criteria for a particular illness, yet the syndrome is significantly related to decreased functioning and quality of life.

The *Diagnostic and Statistical Manual of Mental Disorder*, Fourth Edition, DSM-IV, (American Psychiatric Association, 1994), and its predecessors (American Psychiatric Association, 1980) and DSM-III-R (American Psychiatric Association, 1987), operationalizes case identification by the presentation of specific symptoms. This operationalization has made possible the development of specific instruments such as the Diagnostic Interview Schedule (DIS) (Robins et al., 1981) and the Composite International Diagnostic Interview (CIDI) (World Health Organization, 1990) which can be administered by clinicians and lay persons to capture the lifetime and current prevalence of disorders both in clinical and community populations. Other diagnostic systems have been developed for some late life psychiatric disorders, specifically Alzheimers disease. A widely accepted diagnostic system is the National Institute of Neurologic, Communicative Diseases and Stroke—Alzheimer's Disease and Related Disorders Association (NINCDS-ADRDA) work group diagnoses (McKhann et al., 1984). In this system, clinical examination and the results of laboratory tests and imaging studies such as computerized topography or magnetic resonance imaging scans are utilized.

Numerous scales have also been used by community and clinical epidemiologists as either screening instruments or for case identification without regard to specific DSM criteria. For example, the Mini-Mental State Exam (MMSE) (Folstein et al., 1975) is often used by clinicians and epidemiologists to screen for cognitive impairment. The Center for Epidemiologic Studies—Depression Scale (CES-D) (Radloff, 1977) is widely used to screen for depression symptoms. For each of these instruments, a somewhat arbitrary cutpoint or threshold has been identified, above which signifies more severe symptomatology. The correspondence between these thresholds and DSM disorders is less established.

While DSM-IV has been of much assistance in case classification in psychiatric epidemiology, it has failed to account for less severe but clinically important presentation of symptoms such as subsyndromal depression and mild memory loss. Both of these are particularly relevant for older adults. For example, across all age groups, there is a growing body of evidence focusing on cases of depression that do not meet DSM criteria for major depression, but are clinically significant (Pincus et al., 1999). The lifetime prevalence of minor depression reported from the National Comorbidity Study of adults 18–55 was 10% (Kessler et al., 1997). The one-year prevalence of subsyndromal depression, defined as depressive symptomatology not meeting the criteria for either major or minor depression, in adults 18 or older in the ECA study was 11.8%, higher than for all DSM-III mood disorders combined (Judd et al., 1994). In a sample of community dwelling elders, the prevalence of significant depressive symptomatology was 14.7%, while the prevalence of major depression was only 3.7% (Blazer and Williams, 1980). These and similar findings combined with the low prevalence of DSM depression in older adults suggest the current diagnostic criteria for depression may be less applicable for older adults (Blazer, 1994) (Ernst and Angst, 1995). The prevalence and importance of subthreshold depression in late life will be addressed in more detail in the next section.

Another limitation of the current diagnostic criteria for older adults is comorbidity of mental disorders. While there are many examples of comorbidity of mental disorders among older adults, we will discuss in a later section as an example the comorbidity of depression and dementia. Comorbid depression and dementia is by far the most common problem of comorbidity encountered by clinicians treating neuropsychological disorders in older adults and distinguishing between the two disorders is difficult (Blazer, 2002).

In summary, the issue of case classification is complex for older individuals whose symptoms do not fit into the DSM criteria. The identification of geriatric syndromes that potentially lead to functional impairment, frailty, and decreased quality of life, rather than focusing on specific psychiatric disorders, may be a more important issue in determining what is a case (Blazer, 2000).

THE DISTRIBUTION OF CASES

The Epidemiologic Catchment Area (ECA) program was established by the National Institute of Mental Health (NIMH) to determine the prevalence of specific DSM disorders in community and institutional populations (Regier et al., 1984). Five community surveys were funded from 1980–1984 and the Diagnostic Interview Schedule (DIS) (Robins et al., 1981) was used to identify participants who met criteria for specific DSM disorders. A total of 18,571 persons were interviewed, including a total of 5,702 persons 65 or older. Although these data were collected a number of years ago, the ECA surveys remain the landmark study for addressing DSM disorders in those 65 or older in the United States. Figure 1 presents the age-specific one-month prevalence across all five sites of specific disorders (Regier et al., 1988).

For all disorders, with the exception of severe cognitive impairment, the prevalence was lowest among those 65 or older compared to younger adults. With the exception of alcohol and drug abuse and dependence, the prevalence of all disorders was higher in women. A total of 12.3% of those 65 or older had one or more DIS disorders within the month prior to interview. The most prevalent disorder in the 65 or older age group was an anxiety disorder (5.5%), primarily due to the high prevalence of phobic disorder in this group (4.8%). The prevalence of severe cognitive impairment was 4.9%. The ECA studies did not identify specific categories of dementia.

The prevalence of DSM major depression in the ECA in those 65 or older was 0.7%, which was lower than the prevalence in those 18–24 (2.2%), 25–44 (3.0%) and those 45–64 (2.0%). The ECA finding that the prevalence of major depression

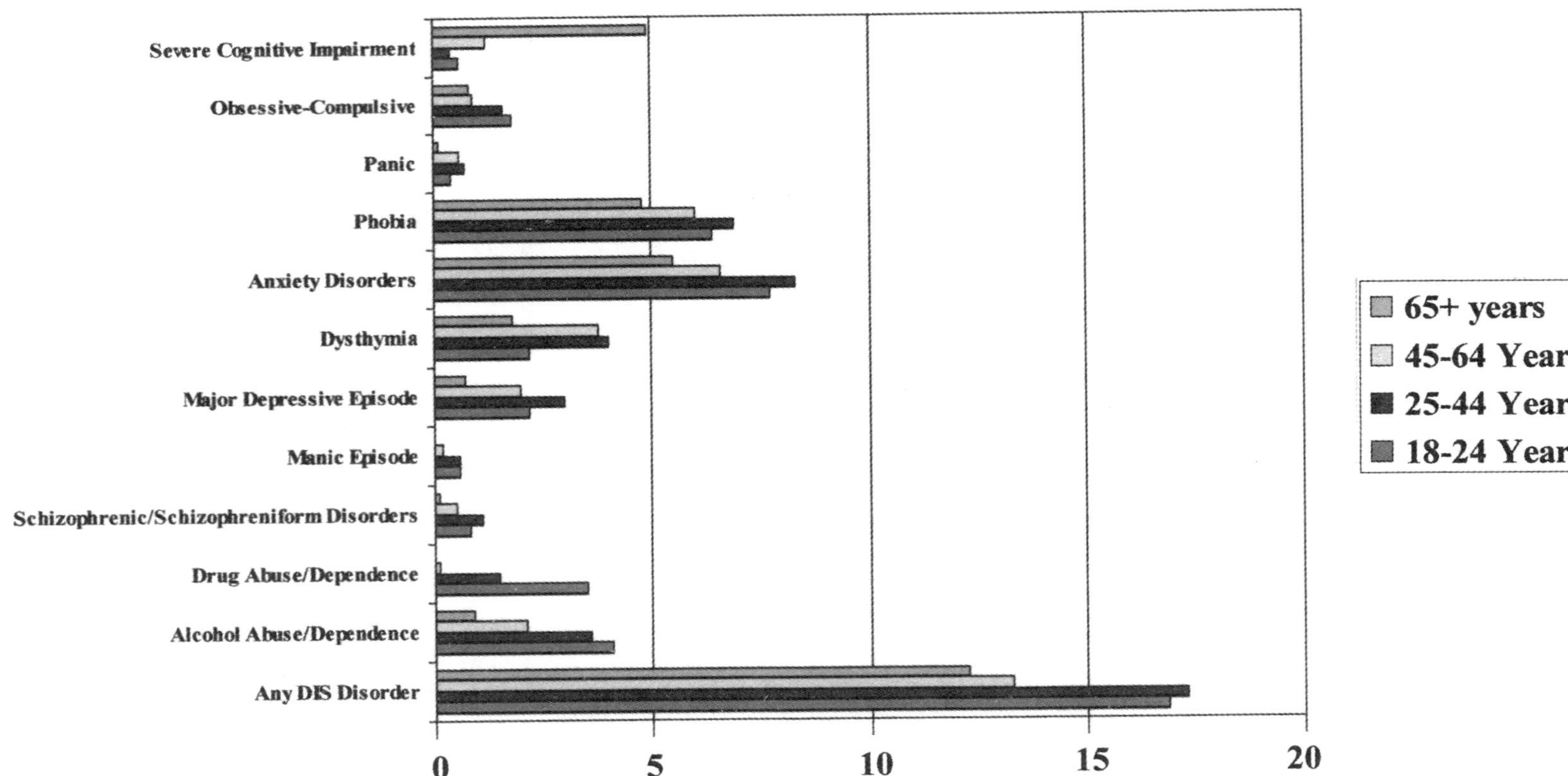

Figure 1. Standardized one-month prevalence of DIS/DSM-III disorders for all ECA sites combined.

was lower in older adults was surprising, since elders were thought to have more risk factors such as loss of roles and reduced income through retirement as well as loss of friends and family. In addition, older adults are high users of psychotropic medications (Blazer et al., 2000a, b).

Explanations for why the prevalence of psychiatric disorders, with the exception of cognitive impairment, is lower in older adults generally fall into three categories: (1) methodological or sampling errors, (2) cohort or period effects, and (3) older persons may be relatively protected against psychiatric disorders. In the section following, we review these arguments with regard to the low prevalence of depression in late life.

Methodological arguments include the suggestion that older adults are less likely to report depressive symptoms or to report depressive symptoms in somatic terms or in a way that makes it difficult to fit into the criteria for major depression (Blazer, 1989; Henderson, 1994). Using structural equation modeling, Christensen et al. found a direct effect of age on both anxiety and depression items, suggesting a differential probability of endorsement by age for certain symptoms such as somatic items. That is, the nature of the depression may differ qualitatively between older and younger adults (Christensen et al., 1999). It is also plausible that although the symptoms are greater in number, they are not distributed across the categories necessary to meet DSM criteria for major depression. Whether older adults are less likely to report depressive symptoms overall is not known, but older adults may deny reporting the symptoms (Blazer, 1989; Henderson, 1994).

Selection bias may also contribute to the reduced prevalence of depression among older adults. It is possible that elders with depression are less likely to participate in mental health studies or answer questions about their mood in the context of a general survey (Blazer, 1989). Individuals with a lifetime history of depression may not survive to old age (selective survival). Elders with comorbid depression and physical illness may not be physically able to participate in a research study and objective information may be collected from a proxy informant. Subjective information, such as depressive symptoms, is not collected from proxy respondents in standard survey procedures. Each one of these possibilities would lead to an underestimate of the true prevalence of depression. The elderly may have a similar incidence of depression, but the duration may be shorter, which would result in a lower prevalence (Henderson, 1994). Finally, in studies such as the ECA, the data were from community samples. Older adults in institutions were not included in the analysis.

Most epidemiologists agree that the contribution of methodologic and sampling bias to the low prevalence of depression in late life is quite small (Blazer, 1989). A more plausible explanation is a cohort effect. That is, those individuals born in the early twentieth century are psychologically healthier than those born in more recent years. Elders are experiencing fewer disorders today because as a cohort they have always been healthy. A related explanation is that of a period effect. Many of the cohorts of older adults lived through the Great Depression and World War II and have experienced hard times. Today's standard of living is likely to be by comparison more comfortable. Remembering poorer times may change the current perspective and result in a less depressed mood. Similarly, younger adults are less likely to have seen economic depression and war, and any current difficulties may result in a depressed mood. These effects are discussed later in the context of historical trends in the prevalence of disorders. The possibility of a true protective effect conferred by age cannot be dismissed, but discussion of this possibility is beyond the scope of this chapter.

Prevalence of Depressive Disorders

Recent community longitudinal studies have provided the opportunity to examine the prevalence and outcomes associated with depressive disorders in older adults. The Established Populations for Epidemiologic Studies of the Elderly (EPESE) in the United States is one such study. The EPESE program was a set of longitudinal studies sponsored by the National Institute on Aging to identify risk factors associated with mortality, morbidity and health services utilization in individuals 65 or older (Cornoni-Huntley et al., 1986). EPESE surveys were conducted in four sites and depression was measured using the Center for Epidemiologic Studies—Depression scale (CES-D) (Radloff, 1977). The prevalence of significant depressive symptomatology was 9.0% in the North Carolina sample (Blazer et al., 1991) and 15.1% in the New Haven sample (Cornoni-Huntley et al., 1986). In controlled analyses of the North Carolina data, depression was not associated with age. Specifically, the oldest old suffered fewer depressive symptoms when factors known to be associated with depression were simultaneously controlled (Blazer et al., 1991). A similar prevalence of 11.3% of depressive illness in adults over 65 was found in Liverpool (Copeland et al., 1987).

The prevalence of major depression as identified by the DIS was 1.2% among adults 65 or older in Edmonton (Bland et al., 1988). In the Longitudinal Aging Study Amsterdam (LASA), a study of adults 55–85 years of age conducted in the Netherlands, the prevalence of DIS defined major depression was 2.02%. The prevalence increased with age, from 1.3% in those subjects ages 55–59 to 2.7% in those 80–85. Among the LASA participants, the prevalence of clinically relevant depression was 14.9% (Beekman et al., 1995b). Henderson et al. reported from Australia the point prevalence of depressive episodes as defined by draft ICD-10 criteria in persons 70 or older was 3.3%. The prevalence of DSM-III-R major depression was 1.0%. The number of depressive symptoms did not increase with age (Henderson et al., 1993). Steffens et al. recently reported the prevalence of DSM-IV major depression in older adults was 4.4% in women and 2.7% in men (Steffens et al., 2000). Higher levels of DSM depression were also reported from the Hobart, Tasmania study. The prevalence was 6.3% in those 70–79 and 15.5% in those 80 or older (Kay et al., 1985). In summary, there is a range in the reported prevalence of depression depending on the criteria used. In addition, studies have provided mixed results concerning the relationship between depression and age.

The prevalence of depression in clinical settings is higher than that reported from community studies. In a review of the epidemiology of depression in primary care, Katon and Schulberg (1992) concluded that the prevalence of major depression increases linearly as studies move from the community to the primary care clinic to the inpatient medical ward. In a sample of primary care patients 60 years of age or older, the prevalence of major depression was 6.5%, while the prevalence of minor depression was 5.2% (Lyness et al., 1999a). In a study of HMO patients 65 or older, 14% met criteria for CES-D depression (Unutzer et al., 2000).

The prevalence of major depression in male veterans hospitalized with medical illness was 11.5%–13.3%, while the prevalence of minor depression was 23.0%–29.2% (Koenig et al., 1988, 1991). The prevalence of major depression was lower than that in veterans under 40, but the prevalence of minor depression was higher (Koenig et al., 1991). In another study, Koenig et al. reported the prevalence of major depression in male and female hospitalized adults 60 or older was 10% to 21%, depending on the diagnostic scheme used. The prevalence of minor depression varied from 14% to 25% (Koenig et al., 1997).

Among 708 aged nursing home and congregate apartment residents, the prevalence of possible major depression was 12.4%. Another 30.5% reported less severe depressive symptoms. Possible major depression was more prevalent among newly admitted residents, while long-term residents were more likely to report minor depression (Parmelee et al., 1989).

The incidence, or onset, of depression in late life, though important, has been less studied. In a study of 875 nondepressed older adults with a mean age of 85, the incidence of depression was 4.1%. The incidence of first onset depression was 1.4% per person year (0.8% for males and 1.5% for females). Characteristics at baseline associated with incidence of depression were having a dementia, insufficient social network, and having more than two depressive symptoms at baseline (Forsell and Winblad, 1999). A lower incidence of 133.49 per 1000 person years at risk was reported in another study of adults 85 or older in Munich (Meller et al., 1996). A similar incidence was reported from Australia in a sample of community dwelling elders 70 or older followed for three to six years. Of those nondepressed, 2.5% had become cases of major depression during the follow up period (Henderson et al., 1997). In a sample of adults 55 or older in The Netherlands followed for one year, the incidence was much higher. A total of 16% suffered an incident depression (Beekman et al., 1995a).

Subsyndromal Depression

The concept of subsyndromal depression has received much attention in the last decade. Data from community studies of the elderly have found depressive symptoms not meeting DSM criteria may be clinically significant. Minor depression that is clinically significant may be more common in older adults, suggesting that "major" depression does not fully capture the spectrum of depression seen in late life (Blazer, 1994). In elders from the North Carolina ECA study, the overall prevalence of depressive symptoms was 27%; the prevalence of DIS/DSM-III major depression was 0.8%, mixed depression and anxiety syndrome was 1.2%, dysthymia 2%, symptomatic depression 4% and mild dysphoria 19% (Blazer et al., 1987). Those with symptomatic depression not meeting DSM-III criteria were more likely than the dysphoric group to complain of poor health and to report benzodiazepine use in the past year. Additionally, one-fourth reported their depression to be associated with the death of a loved one, with the experience of social isolation, with fear of being in crowds, and with feeling useless. In a sample of primary care patients age 60 or older, the prevalence of subsyndromal depression was 9.9%, while the prevalence was 6.5% for major depression, 5.2% for minor depression, and 0.9% for dysphoria. Subsyndromal depression was associated with functional disability and medical comorbidity similar to major and minor depression (Lyness et al., 1999b).

In the recently conducted study of community dwelling elderly, the Longitudinal Aging Study Amsterdam (LASA), the prevalence of minor depression, classified as cases above the CES-D cut-point of 16 but not meeting DIS/DSM-III criteria for major depression, was 12.9% (Beekman et al., 1995b). The prevalence of minor depression increased with age, from 9.4% in those 55–59 to 16.7% in those 80–85 years of age. In the LASA data, minor depression shared a similar risk factor profile to major depression. In addition, however, lower level of education, urbanicity, chronic physical illness, cognitive impairment and smaller social network were associated with minor depression but not major depression. Using data from the Duke EPESE, even depressive symptomatology below the traditional cut point of the CES-D has recently been shown to be prevalent in older adults and associated with decreased quality of life (Hybels et al., 2001). Like CES-D depression, subthreshold depression was associated with impairment in physical functioning. disability days, poorer self-rated health, the use of psychotropic medications, perceived low social support, female gender, and being unmarried. In summary, the demographic and social and physical health predictors of subthreshold depression were similar to the predictors of CES-D depression.

Prevalence of Dementing Disorders

Among a sample of 1070 community dwelling elders aged over 65 in Liverpool, the prevalence of probable dementia was 5.2%. The prevalence increased with age (Copeland et al., 1987). Using data from the Duke EPESE. Fillenbaum et al. reported the prevalence of dementia in persons 68 or older was 0.070 for blacks and 0.072 for whites. The prevalence of dementia was higher for black men than black women, but higher for white women than white men. Race and gender differences were not significant. The prevalence of dementia increased to age 84 and then tapered off (Fillenbaum et al., 1998). In the Canadian Study of Health and Aging in adults 65 or older, the prevalence of dementia was 8.0%. The age-standardized rate ranged from 2.4% among those 65 to 74 to 34.5% among those 85 or older (Canadian Study of Health and Aging Working Group, 1994). Jorm et al. (1987) reviewed studies of dementia and found the prevalence varied as a function of methods. They concluded the relationship between age and dementia was consistent across studies, with rates doubling every 5.1 years.

As with depression, the prevalence of dementia has also been shown to vary by criteria used. Henderson et al. (1994) found the point prevalence of dementia was lower when using ICD-10 criteria compared to DSM-III-R. However, both criteria showed the expected increase in prevalence with age. Similarly, the prevalence of dementia was estimated using six classifications in the Canadian Study of Health and Aging. The prevalence of dementia ranged from 3.1% using ICD-10 criteria to 29.1% using DSM-III criteria (Erkinjuntti et al., 1997).

As expected, the prevalence of Alzheimer's disease is lower than that of dementia. In the Canadian Study of Health and Aging of adults 65 or older, the prevalence was 5.1% (Canadian Study of Health and Aging Working Group, 1994), while in the Liverpool study of adults over 65, the prevalence was 3.3% (Copeland et al., 1992). Data from the East Boston EPESE suggest the prevalence may be much higher. Specifically, the overall prevalence of probable Alzheimer's disease was 10.3%. The prevalence was 3.0% in those 65 to 74, 18.7% in those 75–84, and 47.2% among those 85 or older (Evans et al., 1989).

The incidence of dementia also increases with age. Five-year incidence data from the Framingham Study found the incidence ranged from 7.0 per 1000 at ages 65 to 69 to 118.0 per 1000 at ages 85 to 89. A similar increase in incidence with age for Alzheimer's disease was noted: 3.5 at ages 65 to 69 and 72.8 at ages 85 to 89 years (Bachman et al., 1993). An increase in incidence of dementia with age was also reported from two studies in Britain (Clarke et al., 1996; Paykel et al., 1994). Similarly, the estimated annual incidence of Alzheimers disease among those 65 to 69 in the East Boston EPESE was 0.6%, compared to 1.0% for persons 70 to 74, 2.0% for persons 75–79, 3.3% for those 80–84, and 8.4% for those 85 or older (Hebert et al., 1995).

The three-year incidence of dementia in the Duke EPESE was 0.058 for blacks and 0.062 for whites, but race and gender differences in incidence were not significant (Fillenbaum et al., 1998). In a prospective study of 1135 persons 70 or older, incident dementia was associated with age and level of cognitive performance at baseline, but not with rate of decline. Decline is almost universal in at least one cognitive area among those over the age of 85 (Korten et al., 1997). In a review of the incidence of dementia, Jorm and Jolley (1998) concluded the incidence of dementia rises exponentially up to the age of 90. They did not find a gender difference in incidence, but women tended to have a higher incidence of Alzheimer's disease at older ages, while men tended to have a higher incidence of vascular dementia at younger ages. Finally, Hendrie et al. has studied the prevalence and incidence of dementia in two communities with similar ethnic origins using the same research methods. The prevalence in a Nigerian community of dementia was 2.29% compared to 4.82% in a community sample of African-Americans in Indianapolis. Similar differences were reported for Alzheimer's disease: 1.41% in Nigeria compared to 3.69% in Indianapolis (Hendrie et al., 1995). Age-standardized incidence rates were also lower in Nigerian Africans compared to African Americans (Hendrie et al., 2001).

In the Canadian Study of Health and Aging, both community and institutional samples were included. As expected, the prevalence of dementia in the institutional sample was much higher (569 per 1000 population) that the prevalence in the community sample (42 per 1000 population) (Canadian Study of Health and Aging Working Group, 1994). In their review of the prevalence of dementia, Jorm et al. noted that studies including institutionalized elders did not report higher rates than those covering community residents only. While a higher proportion of institutionalized older adults are demented, institutionalized elders make up only a small proportion of all older adults (Jorm et al., 1987).

ETIOLOGIC STUDIES

In identifying determinants of disease, epidemiology offers the opportunity to look for both correlates of psychiatric disorders as well as risk factors for onset of the disorder. In the sections following, we will present results from etiologic studies identifying risk factors for both dementia and depressive disorders in late life. In addition, we present a summary of studies which identify factors which may not necessarily put the individual at risk for developing the disorder, but are associated with the prevalence of the disorder. Therefore, the term "risk factor" is used here to include both etiologic factors as well as correlates of depression and dementia.

Risk Factors for Depression

Blazer et al. reported from the Duke EPESE that in bivariate analysis, CES-D depression was associated with increased age, being female, lower income, physical disability, cognitive impairment, and having no close relatives. When these potential confounders were simultaneously controlled, however, the association between age and depressive symptoms reversed, with the oldest old suffering fewer symptoms than those younger (Blazer et al., 1991). Henderson et al. reported from a general population sample of persons 18 to 79 years of age that depressive symptoms declined with age in both men and women, due only in part to the decline in prevalence of factors known to be associated with depression (Henderson et al., 1998). In a study of community dwelling adults 70 or older in Canberra, the number of depressive symptoms did not increase with age, but was correlated with neuroticism, poor physical health, disability, and a history of previous depression (Henderson et al., 1993). In a study from the Netherlands, depressive symptoms were associated with dysfunction, poor health perception, and poorer life satisfaction and well being in late middle-aged and older persons (Ormel et al., 1998).

Other cross-sectional studies have found a similar profile of factors correlated with depression. In the LASA study, major depression was associated with being unmarried, having one or more functional limitations, perceived health as fair or good, not receiving instrumental support, perception of loneliness, and internal locus of control (Beekman et al., 1995b). In the Duke ECA data, major depression in older adults was associated with recent negative life events and poor social relations (Blazer et al., 1987).

The LASA data showed a differential relationship between depression and physical health by number of depressive symptoms. Specifically, in controlled analyses, minor depression was related to physical health, defined as the presence of chronic disease, while DIS major depression was not (Beekman et al., 1997b). Both major and minor depression, however, were associated with disability in cross-sectional analyses, controlling for chronic disease and functional limitations (Beekman et al., 1997a).

Risk factors that lead to incident depression are less understood. Disability may lead to depression because of decreased capability. In a two-year follow-up of 1457 community residents 65 or older, increasing disability and declining health preceded the emergence of depressive symptoms, while the number of medical conditions, social support, life events, and demographic characteristics contributed little (Kennedy et al., 1990). In a sample of physically disabled adults age 18 or older, the disabled were at increased risk of depressive symptoms, with eventful stress, chronic strain, mastery, and social support significant determinants. The risk of depression in those 65 or older was higher than that in younger adults (Turner and Noh, 1988).

Some biological variables have been explored to determine their relationship with depression. An association between lower cholesterol level and a higher prevalence of depressive symptoms in middle-aged men has been reported (Steegmans et al., 2000), and there is evidence that serum cholesterol levels may be associated with variations in mental state or personality (Boston et al., 1996). Studies of the relationship between APOE genotype and depression have resulted in mixed findings. Krishnan et al. (1996) found an association between the APOE 3 and 4 alleles and late onset major depression. However, no association was observed between APOE genotype and change in depressive symptoms in a five-year longitudinal study of community-dwelling older adults (Mauricio et al., 2000). Similarly, depression was not strongly associated with APOE polymorphism in a sample of 806 persons aged 78 or older (Forsell et al., 1997).

Risk Factors Associated with Dementia

Cross-sectional studies have shown cognitive dysfunction to be associated, in addition to age, with depressive symptoms (Yaffe et al., 1999), self-rated health but not physical conditions (Christensen et al., 1994), physical functioning as measured by activities of daily living (Christensen et al., 1994), and level of education (Inouye et al., 1993).

In longitudinal studies, many risk factors for cognitive decline have been studied and/or identified. In the Rancho Bernardo Study, where 800 women and 551 men were followed from 1972/1974 to 1988/1991, no gender differences were found in decline in cognitive function with age (Barrett-Conner and Kritz-Silverstein, 1999). In a study of 5781 mostly white women 65 or older followed for four years, depressive symptoms were associated with subsequent cognitive decline (Yaffe et al., 1999). Similarly, in a study of 1070 men and women aged 60 or older followed for five years, depressed mood at baseline was associated with an increased risk of incident dementia, after adjusting for age, gender, education, language, and baseline functioning (Devanand et al., 1996). Depressive symptomatology was a predictor of three-year cognitive decline in the Duke EPESE (Blazer et al., 1997). Other research has shown the association between depression and cognitive decline is related to level of functioning. In the New Haven EPESE, depressive symptoms were predictive of cognitive decline among elders with moderate cognitive impairment, but not among elders with intact cognitive functioning (Bassuk et al., 1998). Finally, data from two studies in The Netherlands found depression was associated with an increased risk of cognitive decline and Alzheimers disease, but only in subjects with higher education (Geerlings et al., 2000). Cognitive complaints have not been found to be associated with cognitive decline (Blazer et al., 1997) (Jorm et al., 1997).

Education has been found to be a predictor of cognitive decline. In cross-site analysis of the ECA data, Farmer et al. found among individuals with higher cognitive performance at baseline that fewer years of education was a predictor of one-year cognitive decline, not only in elderly subjects but also in younger adults. Among those with worse cognitive scores at baseline, education did not predict cognitive decline (Farmer et al., 1995). Evans et al. found in the East Boston EPESE that fewer years of formal education was associated with a three-year decline in cognitive functioning, independently of age, birthplace, language, occupation and income (Evans et al., 1993). Using data from the Iowa EPESE, Colsher and Wallace found lower levels of education were predictive of more rapid cognitive decline in women (Colsher and Wallace, 1991).

Over the last decade, numerous environmental risk factors have been examined as possible risk factors for Alzheimer's disease. Studies of the association between prior head trauma and risk of Alzheimer's disease have been inconclusive. Mortimer et al. (1991) analyzed data from eleven case-control studies and found the pooled relative risk of head trauma as a risk factor for Alzheimer's disease was 1.82 (95% confidence interval: 1.26–2.67). Mehta et al. (1999) found, however, in the prospective Rotterdam Study, that mild head trauma was not a major risk factor for dementia or Alzheimer's disease. Studies of the protective effect of estrogen have also yielded mixed results. Kawas et al., (1997) using data from the Baltimore Longitudinal Study of Aging, found that after adjusting for education, the relative risk of Alzheimer's disease in female estrogen users compared to nonusers was 0.46 (95% confidence interval: 0.209–0.997), indicating a reduced risk for women who had used estrogen. Other studies, however, have not found an association between estrogen use and risk of Alzheimer's disease in women (Brenner et al., 1994; Fillenbaum et al., 2001). Finally, an inverse relationship between Alzheimer's disease and nonsteroidal anti-inflammatory use has been reported (Anthony et al., 2000, Breitner et al., 1994, 1995).

Both prevalent and incident cognitive dysfunction has been associated with the E4 allele of APOE (Evans et al., 1997; Saunders et al. 1993). Therefore, the E4 allele can be viewed as a general risk factor for Alzheimer's disease though the mechanisms have not been identified. (The E2 allele has a corresponding protective effect). The E4 allele is a susceptibility gene in that not all (or even most) persons with the allele eventually develop overt dementia. There have been other genetic correlates of dementia, but these are rare and are usually associated with clearly familial Alzheimer's disease. Only the E4 allele has been associated with the sporadic onset of Alzheimer's disease.

Comorbidity of Depression and Dementia

Many studies have emerged estimating the comorbidity of depression and dementia (primarily Alzheimers disease) in the elderly. Virtually all report similar ranges of prevalence. Reifler et al. found that 20% of Alzheimer's disease patients admitted to an outpatient memory disorders clinic experienced major depression. Depression was more severe in the less cognitively impaired (Reifler et al., 1989). Patterson et al. found that 18% of Alzheimer's patients in an outpatient setting had mild-to-moderate symptoms of depression (Patterson et al., 1990). Lazarus et al. found mild depression in 40% of the patients with Alzheimers disease compared with 12% of the controls (Lazarus et al., 1987). Merriam et al. found depressive disorders in 87% of Alzheimer's disease patients (yet this included all varieties of depressive disorders) (Merriam et al., 1988). As with Reifler et al., they found that severe depressive symptoms were greater in the less cognitively impaired.

Alexopoulas et al. (1993) studied a group of severely depressed elders, some of whom experienced cognitive dysfunction in the midst of their depression and some who did not. All were treated and the depression remitted. In addition, the cognitive function after treatment in both groups was similar after treatment. Over five years of follow-up they found that the elders who experienced cognitive dysfunction during their depressive episode were much more likely to develop dementia. This finding suggests either that a severe depression "unmasks" a dementia or that the pathophysiological changes in depression and dementia are similar, that is, these elders experienced one disease, not two.

Other investigators have been interested in the past history and family history of depression in Alzheimer's disease. Pearlson et al. (1990), when comparing depressed with nondepressed Alzheimer patients, found that the lifetime risk for major depression was greater in the first-degree relatives of an index case of Alzheimer's disease, suggesting that depression in Alzheimer's disease is genetically related to primary mood disorders. Rovner et al. (1989) found that 30% of depressed Alzheimer's patients had a previous history of psychiatric illness and 70% had a history of major depression.

OUTCOME STUDIES

Both depressive disorders and dementia have been shown to be associated with adverse outcomes in late life, particularly increased mortality and disability.

Outcomes Associated with Depressive Disorders

Depression in late life has been linked to both physical illness and decline in physical and cognitive functioning as well as mortality (Sevick et al., 2000). The risk for adverse outcomes may be due, in part, to the chronicity of depression in late life. In a small sample of depressed community residents followed for one year, 32% remitted without relapse, 25% remitted but relapsed during the year, and 43% were chronically depressed (Beekman et al., 1995a). In their five-year study of outcomes of depression, Sharma et al. (1998) found only 22% of those depressed at baseline had recovered. A total of 30% were cases at one of the follow-ups, 24% were cases at two of the follow-ups, and 24% were cases at each of the three follow-up waves. Chronic depression (present for at least six years) has been linked with incident cancer (Penninx et al., 1998b).

One of the major strengths of longitudinal studies is the ability to establish temporality. This is particularly relevant to the relationship between physical health and depression. As discussed above, depression has been shown in cross-sectional studies to be associated with impairments in physical functioning and overall poorer physical health. As discussed earlier, disability is a risk factor for depression. It is plausible that depression is a risk factor for physical decline. Specifically, because of the depression, individuals may become less physically active and become over time more vulnerable to physical decline. Depression in older women has been linked to falls and fractures (Whooley et al., 1999). Penninx et al. (1999b) followed a cohort of 6247 subjects 65 or older and free of disability from three communities of the EPESE for six years. They found compared with the nondepressed, subjects who were depressed at baseline had an increased risk for incident disability in both activities of daily living and mobility, controlling for baseline chronic conditions and sociodemographic factors. Less physical activity and fewer social contacts among depressed persons further explained part of the increased disability risk.

It is not just more symptomatic depression that puts elders at risk for disability and physical decline. Depressive symptoms and minor depression have also been linked to decline in physical functioning. In a longitudinal study of community dwelling elders, the likelihood of becoming disabled increased with each additional symptom of depression. In addition, as the number of depressive symptoms increased, the likelihood of recovering from a physical disability decreased. These effects were not accounted for by age, gender, level of educational attainment, body mass index, or chronic health conditions (Cronin-Stubbs et al., 2000). Similarly, in a four-year follow-up of 1286 persons 71 years of age or older, increasing levels of depressive symptoms predicted decline in physical performance, after adjustment for level of functioning at baseline, health status, and sociodemographic status. Even among those at the high end of the physical functioning spectrum, depressed mood predicted subsequent decline (Penninx et al., 1998a).

As mentioned earlier, whether depressive symptoms are associated longitudinally with cognitive decline is inconclusive. Data from the Study of Osteoporatic Fractures showed depressive symptoms were associated with cognitive decline in older women (Yaffe et al., 1999). Henderson et al. (1997) found depressive symptoms did not predict subsequent cognitive decline or dementia in a 3–6 year follow-up. Other research has found depressive symptoms are related to cognitive decline among elders with moderate cognitive impairment at baseline, but not among cognitively intact elders (Bassuk et al., 1998).

Results from studies in older adults of the association between depression and mortality have been inconsistent. Bruce and Leaf (1989) found among a U.S. sample of community residents 55 or older a four-fold increase risk of death over 15 months if an individual had experienced a mood disorder at baseline. Similarly, depression was significantly associated with six-year mortality in a study of 5201 men and women 65 or older in four U.S. communities, controlling for sociodemographic factors, clinical disease and subclinical indicators, as well as biological and behavioral risk factors (Schulz et al., 2000). Similar results have been reported from Australia (Henderson et al., 1997), Finland (Pulska et al., 1998), and England (Sharma et al., 1998). However, using the Duke ECA data, Fredman et al. (1989) found neither major depression nor depressive symptoms were associated with mortality in persons 60 years of age or older followed for two years. Thomas et al. (1992) followed a sample of 1855 community residents for three years and classified subjects according to their stability or direction of change in depression status. Symptoms of depression were not related to mortality.

One reason for conflicting results has been the different sets of control variables investigators have used in the models. Those with more variables suggest depression is associated with mortality through different independent mechanisms, such as chronic disease, functional impairment, and social support (Blazer et al., 2001). Black and Markides (1999) found, in 2489 older Mexican Americans followed for two years, a high number of depressive symptoms, when comorbid with chronic medical conditions, increased the risk of mortality. In a six-year follow-up of community-dwelling women age 65 or older, Fredman et al. (1999) found the risk of mortality increased with the number of depressive symptoms. However, depressive symptoms were only associated with mortality among women in poor health, suggesting the association between depression and mortality is affected by physical health.

Another reason for the mixed results concerning the relationship between depression and mortality in elders is whether major or minor depression is used as the predictor variable. In a recently published report using the LASA data, Penninx et al. (1999a) reported major depression was associated with four year mortality for both men and women, after adjustment for sociodemographic variables, health status, and health behaviors such as smoking history and physical inactivity. Minor depression, however, was only associated with mortality in men. Similar gender differences were noted in the Amsterdam Study of the Elderly (AMSTEL). Major depressive symptoms were associated with six-year mortality in men and women, but mild depression was only associated with mortality in men (Schoevers et al., 2000).

The association between depression and cause of death, particularly cardiovascular death, in older adults has been studied. Whooley et al. (1998) followed a sample of 7518 white women 67 years of age or older for seven years and found depressive symptoms were a significant risk factor for cardiovascular and non-cancer as well as noncardiovascular mortality, but not cancer mortality. There was an increased risk of mortality as the number of depressive symptoms increased. Barefoot and Schrell (1996) followed middle-aged and older men and women for 27 years, and found high levels of depressive symptomatology were associated with increased risk of myocardial infarction and mortality, 1996). In contrast, Coryell et al. (1999) followed 903 patients who sought treatment for depression for an average of 11 years, and found patients whose depressive symptoms were most persistent were no more likely to die of cardiovascular causes than those with the fewest weeks of illness.

Studies examining the relationship between depression and mortality have also been conducted with inpatients. In a study of 573 patients age 70 or older, depressive symptoms were associated with three-year mortality, after adjusting for potential confounders (Covinsky et al., 1999). Similarly, in a sample of 667 medically ill adults age 60 or older, depressive symptoms predicted one-year mortality, independent of medical illness or disability. The odds of mortality for mild depression were 1.64 and moderate depression 2.49 (Arfken et al., 1999). In a study of institutionalized elderly residents, there was increased mortality among those with major depression six to eighteen months earlier. However, the risk was not statistically significant when physical health, functional ability, and cognitive status were simultaneously controlled, suggesting the effects of depression on mortality appear to be attributable to the correlation between depression and poorer health (Parmelee et al., 1992).

Outcomes Associated with Dementia

Witthaus et al. (1999) reported the burden of dementia in the general population has been shown to be similar to that of lung cancer or stroke. The authors used data from the Rotterdam study and compared lost life years in a demented population to lost life years in a healthy population. Fifty-five-year-old men were estimated to lose 1.2 life years due to morbidity and mortality due to dementia. Women lose an estimated 3.1 years to dementia. Lanska (1998) reported in the last year of life, most demented patients require assistance with activities of daily living (ADL), have severe impairments in cognitive functioning, and receive some hospital care. Poorer cognitive functioning has been linked to decline in physical functioning in longitudinal community studies. In the New Haven EPESE among persons who were free of limitations in physical functioning at baseline, individuals who scored more errors on a short cognitive screening measure were more likely to report incident ADL limitations three years later, independently of age, race, history of chronic health conditions, incident health conditions, and type of residence (Moritz et al., 1995). Similar findings were reported from Sweden. In a study of 1745 elders 75 or older followed for three years, age and dementia were strongly associated with the development of functional dependence and decline. The population-attributable risk percentage of dementia in the development of functional dependence was 49% (Aguero-Torres et al., 1998).

Much research has examined mortality as an outcome of cognitive decline. Bruce et al. (1998) examined nine-year mortality using data from the New Haven ECA project. Poorer performance on cognitive assessments at baseline decreased the risk of survival. The effect was stronger for younger respondents than older participants. Evans et al., (1991), using data from the East Boston EPESE, found persons with probable Alzheimer's disease had a relative risk of death 1.44 times that of the nondiseased when followed for 4.9 years. In a study of 1855 community residents 65 or older in New York followed for four years, the survival probability for the cognitively unimpaired was 0.85, 0.69 for the mildly impaired, and 0.51 for the severely impaired (Kelman et al., 1994). Poor cognitive functioning was linked to 3–4 year mortality in a sample of 897 adults 70 or older in Australia (Korten et al., 1999).

In the Dutch Longitudinal Study Among the Elderly 211 Dutch adults 65–84 years of age were followed for eight years. The rate of decline in cognitive function was associated with survival time in those 70 or older, with a large decline having a shorter survival time. This association was not found in those 65–69 at baseline (Deeg et al., 1990). In the LASA data, cognitive functioning predicted morality independent of age, sex, education, and depressive symptoms. When physical health was taken into account, information processing speed, fluid intelligence, proportion of information retained, remained predictors of mortality, but general cognitive functioning and learning were not predictors (Smits et al., 1999). In a study of adults 75 or older followed for five years, the risk of death for subjects with Alzheimer's disease after adjustments for age and sex was 1.53 compared to those free of dementia. The study also found a greater risk of death for males with Alzheimer's disease compared to females (Jagger et al., 1995). Research in Sweden found the mortality rate for dementia was 2.4 per 100 person years. After controlling for sociodemographic variables and comorbidity, the risk of death among the demented was twice as high as that for the nondemented (Aguero-Torres et al., 1999).

Clinical studies have also found a relationship between cognitive decline and mortality. Among a sample of medically ill older adults, cognitive impairment predicted one-year mortality independent of medical illness and disability (Arfken et al., 1999). In an eight-year follow-up of 606 nursing home dementia patients, comorbidity and severity of dementia were independent predictors of mortality (van Dijk et al., 1996).

Finally, research from the Life Events and Senile Dementia Study in England has suggested social factors may influence the outcome of dementia. Specifically, while the experience of life events did not appear to affect outcome, having social support was associated with increased survival from dementia. Receiving meals on wheels, higher dependency, and poorer physical health were associated with poorer survival in patients with dementia (Orrell et al., 2000).

HISTORICAL TRENDS IN THE EPIDEMIOLOGY OF PSYCHIATRIC DISORDERS IN LATE LIFE

One of the contributions of epidemiology to medicine is studying changes in the distributions of disease over time. For example, the incidence of a childhood disease such as measles was much higher prior to the development of a vaccine. In the case of psychiatric epidemiology, studying historical trends involves documenting the prevalence of psychiatric disorders at different periods in history. The prevalence of a disorder may be affected by factors such as current events. For example, the prevalence of a disorder such as post-traumatic stress disorder may be higher in the years following a catastrophic event such as a war, or a disorder such as depression may be less prevalent in times of economic prosperity. The prevalence of disorders may also be affected by the nomenclature in place at the time the data are examined. For example, the prevalence rates of specific disorders in the ECA were different from those obtained in the National Comorbidity Study less than ten years later, and the differences were due in part to changes in the DSM criteria for the disorder (Regier et al., 1998).

Suicide in older adults has received much attention in psychiatric research as it has become apparent the rates of suicide in late life are high. In the United States, suicide rates tend to rise with age and are highest among white men age 65 or older. About 20% of suicide deaths are in older adults although elders make up only 13% of the population. Older adults make fewer suicide attempts than younger adults do, but the attempts are more successful (Centers for Disease Control, 2000). In a study of completed suicides in primary care patients, completed suicides were associated with depressive illness, physical illness burden, and functional limitations and were more likely to have been prescribed antidepressants, anxiolytic agents, and narcotic analgesics (Conwell et al., 2000).

From 1980 to 1986, the suicide rates in the United States for persons 65 or older increased by 21%. Rate increase ranged from 9% in those 65–69 years old to 38% in those in the 80–84 years age group (Meehan et al., 1991). Allebeck et al. (1996) observed suicide rates in Sweden from 1952–1992 and noted a marked decline in suicide rates in men aged 60–70 years during this period, with the rates among women more stable. A decline in suicide rates was observed for elderly men and women in England and Wales during the period 1985–1996. The authors note the suicide rates decreased as the elderly population increased (Hoxey and Shah, 2000).

One reason for these varying rates may be the concept of a cohort effect, as introduced earlier in this chapter. Just as different cohorts may exhibit different rates of psychiatric illness, they may exhibit different rates of suicide at comparable ages because of generational effects. Blazer et al. studied suicide rates in white males in successive cohorts at different points in time. Birth cohort was found to be a strong predictor of suicide rates. Different birth cohorts were found to have consistent suicide rates across time, with significant increases in rates after age 75 (Blazer et al., 1986).

In summary, when comparing prevalence or incidence of a disorder or syndrome over time, it is important to note both measurements used and possible generational effects.

THE IMPACT OF MENTAL ILLNESS IN OLDER ADULTS ON THE HEALTH CARE SYSTEM

Many elderly adults with psychiatric disorders do not receive treatment. For example, in the Camberwell Needs for Care Survey, 10% of the general population were identified as having a need for treatment of a psychiatric condition. Less than half of all potentially meetable needs were met (Bebbington et al., 1997). In the Duke ECA study, only 0.5% of 1300 persons with depression aged 60 or older reported having seen a psychiatrist in the past 6 months, but 1.5% sought help from a minister or religious counselor and 6.6% from a general medical physician (Blazer et al., 1987). A total of 86% of the subjects in the Canberra, Australia study had had at least one consultation with a general health practitioner in the six months prior to the interview and depressive symptoms significantly predicted consulting a practitioner after controlling for self-reported health problems (Henderson et al., 1993).

In a study of 2558 Medicare enrollees in an HMO, only 4–7% of older adults were treated for depression. The proportion receiving treatment was higher among those with probable depressive disorders, 12 to 25%, but most of the individuals with probable depression were not treated. Predictors of treatment included being female, severity and persistence of depressive symptoms, and severity of comorbid medical illness (Unutzer et al., 2000). In the Cache County Study, only 35.7% of those older adults with major depression were taking an antidepressant. A total of 27.4% of those with major depression were taking a sedative or hypnotic (Steffens et al., 2000). Finally, while many older adults with clinically significant depression remain untreated, a large proportion of older adults continue to use psychotropic medications, and the use of antidepressants has increased over the last two decades (Blazer et al., 2000a, b).

ACKNOWLEDGMENTS

The preparation of this manuscript was supported by a National Institute on Aging Training Grant 5T32 AG00029 (Dr. Hybels) and by National Institute on Aging Grant R01-AG17559 (Dr. Blazer).

REFERENCES

Aguero-Torres H, Fratiglioni L, Guo Z, Viitanen M, Winblad B (1999): Mortality from dementia in advanced age: A 5-year follow-up study of incident dementia cases. J Clin Epidemiol 52:737–743.

Aguero-Torres H, Fratiglioni L, Guo Z, Vittanen M, von Strauss E, Winblad B (1998): Dementia is the major cause of functional dependence in the elderly: 3-year follow-up data from a population based study. Am J Public Health 88:1452–1456.

Alexopoulas GS, Meyers BS, Young RC (1993): The course of geriatric depression with "reversible dementia": A controlled study, Am J Psychiatry 150:1693–1699.

Allebeck P, Brandt L, Nordstrom P, Asgard U (1996): Are suicide trends among the young reversing?, Acta Psychiatr Scand 93:43–48.

American Psychiatric Association (1980): DSM-III: "Diagnostic and Statistical Manual of Mental Disorders" Washington, DC: American Psychiatric Association.

American Psychiatric Association (1987): DSM-III-R: "Diagnostic and Statistical Manual of Mental Disorders" Washington DC: American Psychiatric Association.

American Psychiatric Association (1994): DSM-IV: "Diagnostic and Statistical Manual of Mental Disorders" (Washington DC: American Psychiatric Association).

Anthony JC, Breitner JC, Zandi PP, Meyer MR, Jurasova J, Norton MC, Stone SV (2000): Reduced prevalence of AD in users of NSAIDs and H2 receptor antagonists: the Cache County Study. Neurology, 54:2066–2071.

Arfken CL, Lichtenberg PA, Tancer ME (1999): Cognitive impairment and depression predict mortality in medically ill older adults. J Gerontol A Biol Sci Med Sci 54A:M152–M156.

Bachman DL, Wolf PA, Linn RT, Knoefel JE, Cobb JL, Belanger AJ, White LR, D'Agostino RB (1993): Incidence of dementia and probable Alzheimer's disease in a general population: The Framingham Study. Neurology 43:515–519.

Barefoot JC, Schroll M (1996): Symptoms of depression, acute myocardial infarction, and total mortality in a community sample. Circulation 93:1976–1980.

Barrett-Conner E, Kritz-Silverstein D (1999): Gender differences in cognitive function with age: The Rancho Bernardo Study. J Am Geriatr Soc 47:159–164.

Bassuk SS, Berkman LF, Wypij D (1998): Depressive symptomatology and incident cognitive decline in an elderly community sample. Arch Gen Psychiatry 55:1073–1081.

Bebbington PE, Marsden L, Brewin CR (1997): The need for psychiatric treatment in the general population: the Camberwell Needs for Care Survey. Psychol Med, 27:821–834.

Beekman ATF, Deeg DJH, Braam AW, Smit JH, van Tilberg, W (1997a): Consequences of major and minor depression in later life: A study of disability, well-being, and service utilization, Psychol Med 27:1397–1409.

Beekman ATF, Deeg DJH, Smit JH, van Tilberg, W (1995a): Predicting the course of depression in the older population: results from a community-based study in the Netherlands, J Affect Disord 34:41–49.

Beekman ATF, Deeg DJH, van Tilberg T, Smit JH, Hooijer C, van Tilberg W (1995b): Major and minor depression in later life: a study of prevalence and risk factors. J Affect Disord 36:65–75.

Beekman ATF, Penninx BWJH, Deeg DJH, Ormel J, Braam AW, van Tilberg W (1997b): Depression and physical health in later life: Results from the Longitudinal Aging Study Amsterdam (LASA). J Affect Disord 46:219–231.

Black SA, Markides KS, (1999): Depressive symptoms and mortality in older Mexican Americans Ann Epidemiol 9:45–52.

Bland RC, Newman SC Orn, H (1988): Prevalence of psychiatric disorders in the elderly in Edmonton. Acta Psychiatr Scand (Supp) 338:57–63.

Blazer D (1989): The epidemiology of depression in late life. J Geriatr Psychiatry 22:35–52.

Blazer D (1998): Geriatric psychiatry matures: Advantages and problems as the psychiatry of old age grows older. Curr Opin Psychiatry 11:401–403.

Blazer D, Burchett B, Service C George LK (1991): The association of age and depression among the elderly: An epidemiologic exploration. J Gerontol A Biol Sci Med Sci 46:M210–M215.

Blazer D, Hughes DC, George, LK (1987): The epidemiology of depression in an elderly community population. Gerontologist 27:281–287.

Blazer D, Williams CD (1980): Epidemiology of dysphoria and depression in an elderly population. Am J Psychiatry 137:439–444.

Blazer DG (1994): Is depression more frequent in late life? An honest look at the evidence. Am J Geriatr Psychiatry 2:193–199.

Blazer DG (2000): Psychiatry and the oldest old. Am J Psychiatry 157:1915–1924.

Blazer DG (2002): "Depression in late life" New York: Springer, pp. 349–374.

Blazer DG, Bachar JR, Manton, KG (1986): Suicide in late life. J Am Geriatr Soc 34:519–525.

Blazer DG, Hays JC, Fillenbaum GG, Gold DT (1997): Memory complaint as a predictor of cognitive decline. J Aging Health 9:171–184.

Blazer DG, Hybels CF, Pieper CF (2001): The association of depression and mortality in the elderly: A case for multiple, independent pathways. J Gerontol A Biol Sci Med Sci 56A:m505–m509.

Blazer DG, Hybels CF, Simonsick E, Hanlon JT (2000a): Marked differences in antidepressant use by race in an elderly community sample: 1986–1996. Am J Psychiatry 157:1089–1094.

Blazer DG, Hybels CF, Simonsick E, Hanlon JT (2000b): Sedative, hypnotic and anti-anxiety medication use in an aging cohort over ten years: A racial comparison. J Am Geriatr Soc 48:1073–1079.

Boston PF, Dursun, SM, Reveley MA (1996): Cholesterol and mental disorder. Br J Psychiatry 169:682–695.

Breitner JC, Gau BA, Welsh KA, Plassman BL, MCDonald WM, Helms MJ, Anthony JC (1994): Inverse association of anti-inflammatory treatments and Alzheimer's disease: Initial results of a co-twin control study. Neurology 44:227–232.

Breitner JC, Welsh KA, Hlems MJ, Gaskell PC, Gau BA, Roses AD, Pericak-Vance MA, Saunders AM (1995): Delayed onset of Alzheimer's disease with nonsteroidal anti-inflammatory and histamine H2 blocking drugs. Neurobiol Aging 16:523–530.

Brenner DE, Kukull WA, Stergachis A, van Belle G, Bowen JD, MCCormick WC, Teri L, Larson EB (1994): Postmenopausal estrogen replacement therapy and the risk of Alzheimer's disease: A population-based case control study. Am J Epidemiol 140:262–267.

Bruce ML, Hoff RA, Jacobs SC, Leaf PJ (1995): The effects of cognitive impairment on 9-year mortality in a community sample. J Gerontol B Psychol Sci Soc Sci 50B:P289–P296.

Bruce ML, Leaf PJ (1989): Psychiatric disorders and 15-month mortality in a community sample of older adults. Am J Public Health 79:727–730.

Canadian Study of Health and Aging Working Group (1994): Canadian Study of Health and Aging: Study methods and prevalence of dementia. Can Med Assoc J 150:899–912.

Centers for Disease Control (2000): "Suicide and Suicidal Behavior: Fact Book for the Year 2000" National Center for Injury Prevention and Control. http://www.cdc.gov/ncipc/pub-res/FactBook/suicide.htm

Christensen H, Jorm AF, Henderson AS, MacKinnon AJ, Korten AE, Scott LR (1994): The relationship between health and cognitive functioning in a sample of elderly people in the community. Age Ageing 23:204–212.

Christensen H, Jorm AF, MacKinnon AJ, Korten AE, Jacomb PA, Henderson AS, Rodgers B (1999): Age differences in depression and anxiety symptoms: a structural equation modelling analysis of data from a general population sample. Psychol Med 29:325–339.

Clarke D, Morgan K, Lilley J, Arie T, Jones R, Waite J, Prettyman R (1996): Dementia and "borderline dementia" in Britain: 8-year incidence and post-screening outcomes. Psychol Med 26:829–835.

Colsher PL, Wallace RB (1991): Longitudinal application of cognitive function measures in a defined population of community-dwelling elders. Ann Epidemiol 1:215–230.

Conwell Y, Lyness JM, Duberstein P, Cox C, Seidlitz L, DiGiorgio A, Caine E (2000): Completed suicide among older patients in primary care practices: A controlled study. J Am Geriatr Soc 48:23–29.

Copeland JRM, Davidson IA, Dewey ME, Gilmore C, Larkin BA, McWilliam C, Saunders PA, Scott A, Sharma V Sullivan C (1992): Alzheimer's disease, other dementias, depression, and pseudodementia: Prevalence, incidence, and three-year outcome in Liverpool. Br J Psychiatry 161:230–239.

Copeland JRM, Dewey ME, Wood N, Searle R, Davidson IA, McWilliam C (1987): Range of mental illness among the elderly in the community: Prevalence in Liverpool using the GMS-AGECAT package. Br J Psychiatry 150:815–823.

Cornoni-Huntley J, Brock D, Ostfeld A, et al. (1986): "Established Populations for Epidemiologic Studies of the Elderly: Resource Data Book." Bethesda, MD: National Institute on Aging.

Coryell W, Turvey C, Leon A, Maser J, Solomon D, Endicott J, Muleller, T Keller M (1999): Persistence of depressive symptoms and cardiovascular death among patients with affective disorder. Psychosom Med 61:755–761.

Covinsky KE, Kahana E, Chin MH, Palmer RM, Fortinsky RH, Landefeld CS (1999): Depressive symptoms and 3-year mortality in older hospitalized medical patients. Ann Intern Med 130:563–569.

Cronin-Stubbs D, Mendes de Leon CF, Beckett LA, Field TS, Glynn RJ, Evans DA (2000): Six-year effect of depressive symptoms on the course of physical disability in community-living older adults. Arch Intern Med 160:3074–3080.

Deeg DJH, Hofman A, van Zonneveld, RJ (1990): The association between change in cognitive function and longevity in Dutch elderly. Am J Epidemiol 132:973–982.

Devanand DP, Sano M, Tang M-X, Taylor S, Gurland LJ, Wilder D, Stern Y, Mayeux, R (1996): Depressed mood and the incidence of Alzheimer's disease in the elderly living in the community. Arch Gen Psychiatry 53:175–182.

Erkinjuntti T, Ostbye T, Steenhuis R Hachinski V (1997): The effect of different diagnostic criteria on the prevalence of dementia. N Engl J Med 337:1667–1674.

Ernst C, Angst, J (1995): Depression in old age. Is there a real decrease in prevalence? A review. Eur Arch Psychiatry Clin Neurosci 245:272–287.

Evans DA, Beckett LA, Albert MS, Hebert LE, Scherr PA, Funkenstein HH, Taylor JO (1993): Level of education and change in cognitive function in a community population of older persons. Ann Epidemiol 3:71–77.

Evans DA, Beckett LA, Field, T (1997): Apolipoprotein E e4 and incidence of Alzheimer's disease in a community population of older persons. JAMA 277:822–824.

Evans DA, Funkenstein H, Albert MS, Scherr PA, Cook NR, Chown MJ, Hebert LE, Hennekens CH, Taylor JO (1989): Prevalence of Alzheimer's disease in a community population of older persons: Higher than previously reported. JAMA 262:2551–2556.

Evans DA, Smith LA, Scherr PA, Albert MS, Funkenstein HH, Hebert L (1991): Risk of death from Alzheimer's disease in a community population of older persons. Am J Epidemiol 134:403–412.

Farmer ME, Kittner SJ, Rae DS, Bartko JJ, Regier DA (1995): Education and change in cognitive function: The Epidemiologic Catchment Area Study. Ann Epidemiol 5:1–7.

Fillenbaum GG, Hanlon JT, Landerman LR, Schmader, KF (2001): Impact of estrogen use on decline in cognitive function in a representative sample of older community-resident women. Am J Epidemiol 153:137–144.

Fillenbaum GG, Heyman A, Huber MS, Woodbury MA, Leiss J, Schmader KE, Bohannon A, Trapp-Moen B (1998): The prevalence and 3-year incidence of dementia in older black and white community residents. J Clin Epidemiol 51:587–595.

Folstein MF, Folstein SE, McHugh, P (1975): Mini-mental state: A practical method for grading the cognitive state of patients for clinicians. J Psychiatr Res 12:189–198.

Forsell Y, Corder EH, Basun H, Lannfelt L, Viitanen M, Winblad B (1997): Depression and dementia in relation to apolipoprotein E polymorphism in a population sample age 75 + . Biol Psychiatry 42:898–903.

Forsell Y, Winblad B (1999): Incidence of major depression in a very elderly population. Int J Geriatr Psychiatry 14:368–372.

Fredman L, Magaziner J, Hebel JR, Hawkes W, Zimmerman SI (1999): Depressive symptoms and 6-year mortality among elderly community-dwelling women. Epidemiology 10:54–59.

Fredman L, Schoenbach VJ, Kaplan BH, Blazer DG, James SA, Kleinbaum DG, Yankaskas B (1989): The association between depressive symptoms and mortality among older participants in the Epidemiologic Catchment Area-Piedmont Health Survey. J Gerontol B Psychol Sci Soc Sci 44:S149–156.

Fries B, Ribbe M (1999): Cross-national aspects of geriatrics: comparisons of nursing home residents. Hazzard WR, Blass JP, Ettinger WH, Halter JB, Ouslander JG (eds): in "Principles of Geriatric Medicine and Gerontology." (New York: McGraw-Hill.

Geerlings MI, Schoevers RA, Beekman ATF, Jonker C, Deeg, DJH Schmand, B Ader, HJ, Bouter LM, van Tilberg W (2000): Depression and risk of cognitive decline and Alzheimer's disease. Br J Psychiatry 176:568–575.

Hebert LE, Scherr PA, Beckett lA, Albert mS, Pilgrim DM, Chown MJ, Funkenstein HH, Evans DA (1995): Age-specific incidence of Alzheimer's disease in a community population. JAMA 273:1354–1359.

Henderson AS (1994): Does ageing protect against depression? Soc Psychiatry Psychiatr Epidemiol 29:107–109.

Henderson AS, Jorm AF, Korten AE, Jacomb P, Christensen H, Rodgers B (1998): Symptoms of depression and anxiety during adult life: Evidence for a decline in prevalence with age. Psychol Med 28:1321–1328.

Henderson AS, Jorm AF, MacKinnon A, Christensen H, Scott LR, Korten AE, Doyle C (1993): The prevalence of depressive disorders and the distribution of depressive symptoms in later life: A survey using Draft ICD-10 and DSM-III-R. Psychol Med 23:719–729.

Henderson AS, Jorm AF, MacKinnon A, Christensen H, Scott LR, Korten AE, Doyle C (1994): A survey of dementia in the Canberra population: experience with ICD-10 and DSM-III-R criteria. Psychol Med 24:473–482.

Henderson AS, Korten AE, Jacomb PA, MacKinnon AJ, Jorm AF, Christensen H, Rodgers B (1997): The course of depression in the elderly: a longitudinal community-based study in Australia. Psychol Med 27:119–129.

Hendrie HC, Ogunniyi A, Hall KS, Baiyewu O, Unverzagt FW, Gureje O, Gao S, Evans RM, Ogunseyinde AO, Adeyinka AO, Misick B, Hui SL (2001): Incidence of dementia and Alzheimer disease in 2 communities. JAMA 285:739–747.

Hendrie HC, Osuntokun BO, Hall KS, Ogunniyi AO, Hui SL, Unverzagt FW, Gureje O, Rodemberg CA, Baiyewu O, Musick BS, Adeyinka A, Farlow MR, Oluwole SO, Class CA, Komolafe O, Brashear A, Burdine V (1995): Prevalence of Alzheimer's disease and dementia in two communities: Nigerian Africans and African Americans. Am J Psychiatry 152:1485–1492.

Hoxey K, Shah A (2000): Recent trends in elderly suicide rates in England and Wales, Int J Geriatr Psychiatry 15:274–279.

Hybels CF, Blazer DG, Pieper CF (2001): Toward a threshold for subthreshold depression: An analysis of correlates of depression by severity of symptoms using data from an elderly community sample. Gerontologist 41:357–365.

Inouye SK, Albert MS, Mohs R, Sun K, Berkman LF (1993): Cognitive performance in a high-functioning community dwelling elderly population. J Gerontol A Biol Sci Med Sci 48:M146–M151.

Jagger C, Clarke M, Stone A (1995): Predictors of survival with Alzheimer's disease: A community-based study. Psychol Med 25:171–177.

Jorm AF, Christensen H, Korten AE, Henderson AS, Jacomb PA, MacKinnon A (1997): Do cognitive complaints either predict future cognitive decline or reflect past cognitive decline? A longitudinal study of an elderly community sample. Psychol Med 27:91–98.

Jorm AF, Jolley D (1998): The incidence of dementia: A meta-analysis. Neurology 51:728–733.

Jorm AF, Korten AE, Henderson AS (1987): The prevalence of dementia: A quantitative integration of the literature. Acta Psychiatr Scand 76:465–479.

Judd LL, Rapaport MH, Paulus MP, Brown JL (1994): Subsyndromal symptomatic depression: A new mood disorder? J Clin Psychiatry (Suppl):18–28.

Katon W, Schulberg H (1992): Epidemiology of depression in primary care. Gen Hosp Psychiatry 14:237–247.

Kawas C, Resnick S, Morrison A, Brookmeyer R, Corrada M, Zonderman A, Bacal C, Donnell Lingle D, Metter E (1997): A prospective study of estrogen replacement therapy and the risk of developing Alzheimer's disease: The Baltimore Longitudinal Study of Aging. Neurology 48:1517–1521.

Kay DWK, Henderson AS, Scott R, Wilson J, Rickwood D, Grayson DA (1985): Dementia and depression among the elderly living in the Hobart community: The effect of the diagnostic criteria on the prevalence rates. Psychol Med 15:771–788.

Kelman HR, Thomas C, Kennedy GJ, Cheng J (1994): Cognitive impairment and mortality in older community residents. Am J Public Health 84:1255–1260.

Kennedy GJ, Kelman HR, Thomas C (1990): The emergence of depressive symptoms in late life: The importance of declining health and increasing disability. J Community Health 15:93–103.

Kessler RC, Zhao S, Blazer DG, Swartz M (1997): Prevalence, correlates, and course of minor depression and major depression in the national comorbidity survey. J Affect Disord 45:19–30.

Koenig HG, George LK, Peterson BL, Pieper CF (1997): Depression in medically ill hospitalized older adults: Prevalence, characteristics, and course of symptoms according to six diagnostic schemes. Am J Psychiatry 154:1376–1383.

Koenig HG, Meador KG, Cohen HJ, Blazer DG (1988): Depression in elderly hospitalized patients with medical illness. Arch Intern Med 148:1929–1936.

Koenig HG, Meador KG, Shelp F, Goli V, Cohen HJ, Blazer DG (1991): Major depressive disorder in hospitalized medically ill patients: An examination of young and elderly male veterans. J Am Geriatr Soc 39:881–890.

Korten AE, Henderson AS, Christensen H, Jorm AF, Rodgers B, Jacomb P, MacKinnon AJ (1997): A prospective study of cognitive function in the elderly. Psychol Med 27:919–930.

Korten AE, Jorm AF, Jiao Z, Letenneur L, Jacomb PA, Henderson AS, Christensen H, Rodgers B (1999): Health, cognitive, and psychosocial factors as predictors of mortality in an elderly community sample. J Epidemiol Community Health 53:83–88.

Krishnan KRR, Tupler LA, Ritchie JC, McDonald WM, Knight DL, Nemeroff CB, Carroll BJ (1996): Apolipoprotein E-e4 frequency in geriatric depression. Biol Psychiatry 40:69–71.

Lanska DJ (1998): Dementia mortality in the United States: Results of the 1986 National Mortality Followback Survey. Neurology 50:362–367.

Lazarus LW, Newton N, Cohler B, Lesser J, et al. (1987): Frequency in presentation of depressive symptoms in patients with primary degenerative dementia. Am J Psychiatry 144:41–45.

Lyness JM, King DA, Cox C, Yoediono Z, Caine EC (1999a): The importance of subsyndromal depression in older primary care patients: Prevalence and associated functional disability. J Am Geriatr Soc 47:647–652.

Lyness JM, King DA, Cox C, Yoediono Z, Caine ED (1999b): The importance of subsyndromal depression in older primary care patients: Prevalence and associated functional disability. J Am Geriatr Soc 47:647–652.

MacMahon B, Pugh TF (1970): "Epidemiology: Principles and Methods" Boston: Little, Brown.

Manton KG, Vaupel JW (1995): Survival after the age of 80 in the United States, Sweden, France, England, and Japan. N Engl J Med 333:1232–1235.

Mauricio M, O'Hara R, Yesavage JA, Friedman L, Kraemer HC, Van de Water M, Murphy GM (2000): A longitudinal study of apolipoprotein-E genotype and depressive symptoms in community-dwelling older adults. Am J Geriatr Psychiatry 8:196–200.

McKhann G, Drachman D, Folstein M et al. (1984): Clinical diagnosis of Alzheimer's disease: Report of the NINCDS-ADRDA Work Group under the auspices of Department of Health and Human Service Task Force on Alzheimer's Disease. Neurology 34:939–944.

Meehan PJ, Saltzman LE, Sattin RW (1991): Suicides among older United States residents: Epidemiologic characteristics and trends. Am J Public Health 81:1198–1200.

Mehta KM, Ott A, Kalmijn, S Slooter, A van Duijn, CM Hofman, A Breteler, M (1999): Head trauma and risk of dementia and Alzheimer's disease: The Rotterdam Study. Neurology 53:1959–1962.

Meller I, Fichter MM, Schroppel H (1996): Incidence of depression in octo- and nonagenerians: results of an epidemiologial follow-up community study. Eur Arch Psychiatry Clin Neurosci 246:93–99.

Merriam AE, Aronson MK, Gaston P, Wey SL, Katz L (1988): The psychiatric symptoms of Alzheimer's disease. J Am Geriatr Soc 36:7–12.

Moritz, DJ, Kasl, SV, Berkman, LF (1995): Cognitive functioning and the incidence of limitations in activities of daily living in an elderly community sample. Am J Epidemiol 141:41–49.

Morris JN (1975): "Uses of Epidemiology" London: Churchill Livingstone.

Mortimer JA, van Duijn CM, Chandra V, Fratiglioni L, Graves AB, Heyman A, Jorm AF, Kokmen E, Kondo K, Rocca WA, et al. (1991): Head trauma as a risk factor for Alzheimer's disease: A collaborative re-analysis of case-control studies. EURODEM Risk Factors Research Group. Int J Epidemiol 20(Suppl):S28–35.

Ormel J, Kempen GIJM, Deeg DJH, Brilman EI, van Sondersen E, Relyveld J (1998): Functioning, well-being, and health perception in late middle-aged and older people:

Comparing the effects of depressive symptoms and chronic medical conditions. J Am Geriatr Soc 46:39–48.

Orrell M, Butler R, Bebbington P (2000): Social factors and the outcome of dementia. Int J Geriatr Psychiatry 15:515–520.

Parmelee PA, Katz IR, Lawton MP (1989): Depression among institutionalized aged: Assessment and prevalence estimation. J Gerontol A Biol Sci Med Sci 44:M22–M29.

Parmelee PA, Katz IR, Lawton MP (1992): Depression and mortality among institutionalized aged. J Gerontol B Psychol Sci Soc Sci 47:P3–P10.

Patterson MB, Schnell AH, Martin RJ, Mendez MF, Smyth KA et al. (1990): Assessment of behavioral and affective symptoms in Alzheimer's disease. J Geriatr Psychiatry 3:21–30.

Paykel ES, Brayne C, Huppert FA, Gill C, Barkley C, Gehlhaar E, Beardsall L, Girling DM, Pollitt P, O'Conner D (1994): Incidence of dementia in a population older than 75 years in the United Kingdom Arch Gen Psychiatry 51:325–332.

Pearlson GD, Ross CA, Lohr WD, et al. (1990): Association between family history of affective disorder and the depressive syndrome of Alzheimer's disease Am J Psychiatry 147:452–456.

Penninx BWJH, Geerlings SW, Deeg DJH, van Eijk JTM, van Tilberg W, Beekman ATF (1999a): Minor and major depression and the risk of death in older persons. Arch Gen Psychiatry 56:889–895.

Penninx BWJH, Guralnick JA, Ferrucci L, Simonsick EM, Deeg DJH, Wallace RB (1998a): Depressive symptoms and physical decline in community-dwelling older persons. JAMA, 279:1720–1726.

Penninx BWJH, Guralnick JM, Pahor M, Ferrucci L, Cerhan JR, Wallace RB, Havlik RJ (1998b): Chronically depressed mood and cancer risk in older persons. J Natl Cancer Inst 90:1888–1893.

Penninx BWJH, Leveille S, Ferrucci L, van Eijk JTM, Guralnick JM (1999b): Exploring the effect of depression on physical disability: Longitudinal evidence from the Established Populations for Epidemiologic Studies of the Elderly. Am J Public Health 89:1346–1352.

Pincus HA, Davis WW, McQueen LE (1999): "Subthreshold" mental disorders: A review and synthesis of studies on minor depression and other "brand names." Br J Psychiatry 174:288–296.

Pulska T, Pahkala K, Laippala P, Kivela S-L (1998): Major depression as a predictor of premature deaths in elderly people in Finland: a community study. Acta Psychiatr Scand 97:408–411.

Radloff LS (1977): The CES-D scale: A self-report depression scale for research in the general population. Appl Psychol Meas 1:385–401.

Regier DA, Boyd JH, Burke JD, Rae DS, Myers JK, Kramer M, Robins LN, George LK, Karno M, Locke BZ (1988): One-month prevalence of mental disorders in the United States. Arch Gen Psychiatry 45:977–986.

Regier DA, Kaelber CT, Rae DS, Farmer ME, Knauper B, Kessler RC, Norquist GS (1998): Limitations of diagnostic criteria and assessment instruments for mental disorders: Implications for research and policy. Arch Gen Psychiatry 55:109–115.

Regier DA, Myers JK, Kramer M, Robins LN, Blazer DG, Hough RL, Eaton WW, Locke BZ (1984): The NIMH Epidemiologic Catchment Area Program: Historical context, major objectives and study population characteristics. Arch Gen Psychiatry 41:934–994.

Reifler BV, Teri L, Raskind M, Veith R, Bames R, et al. (1989): Double-blind trial of imipramine in Alzheimer's disease patients with and without depression. Am J Psychiatry 146:45–49.

Robins LN, Helzer JE, Croughan J, Ratcliff K (1981): National Institute of Mental Health Diagnostic Interview Schedule: Its history, characteristics, and validity. Arch Gen Psychiatry 38:381–389.

Rovner BW, Broadhead J, Spencer M, Carson J (1989): Depression and Alzheimer's disease. Am J Psychiatry 146:350–353.

Saunders AM, Schmader K, Breitner J (1993): Apolipoprotein E epsilon 4 allele distributions in late-onset Alzheimer's disease and in other amyloid forming disease. Lancet 342:710–711.

Schoevers RA, Geerlings MI, Beekman ATF, Penninx BWJH, Deeg DJH, Jonker C, van Tilberg W (2000): Association of depression and gender with mortality in old age. Br J Psychiatry 177:336–342.

Schulz R, Beach SR, Ives DG, Martire LM, Ariyo AA Kop WJ (2000): Association between depression and mortality in older adults: the Cardiovascular Health Study. Arch Intern Med 160:1761–1768.

Sevick MA, Rolih C, Pahor M (2000): Gender differences in morbidity and mortality related to depression: A review of the literature. Aging (Milano) 12:407–416.

Sharma VK, Copeland JRM, Dewey ME, Lowe D, Davidson I (1998): Outcome of the depressed elderly living in the community in Liverpool: A 5-year follow-up. Psychol Med 28:1329–1337.

Smits CHM, Deeg DJH, Kriegsman DMW, Schmand B (1999): Cognitive functioning and health as determinants of mortality in an older population. Am J Epidemiol 150:978–986.

Steegmans PH, Hoes AW, Bak AA, van der Does E, Grobbee DE (2000): Higher prevalence of depressive symptoms in middle-aged men with low serum cholesterol levels. Psychosom Med 62:205–211.

Steffens DC, Skoog I, Norton M, Hart AD, Tschanz JT, Plassman BL, Wyse BW, Welsh-Bohmer KA, Breitnet JCS (2000): Prevalence of depression and its treatment in an elderly population: The Cache County Study. Arch Gen Psychiatry 57:601–607.

Thomas C, Kelman HR, Kennedy GJ, Ahn C, Yang C-y (1992): Depressive symptoms and mortality in elderly persons. J Gerontol B Psychol Sci Soc Sci 47:S80–87.

Turner RJ, Noh S (1988): Physical disability and depression: A longitudinal analysis. J Health Soc Behav 29:23–37.

Unutzer J, Simon G, Belin T, Datt M, Katon W, Patrick D (2000): Care for depression in HMO patients aged 65 or older. J Am Geriatr Soc 48:871–878.

van Dijk PTM, Dippel DWJ, van dee Meulen JHP, Habbema JDF (1996): Cormorbidity and its effect on mortality in nusring home patients with dementia. J Nerv Ment Dis 184:180–187.

Whooley MA, Browner WS, for the Study of Osteoporatic Fractures Research Group (1998): Association between depressive symptoms and mortality in older women, Arch Intern Med 158:2129–2135.

Whooley MA, Kip KE, Cauley JA, Ensrud KE, Nevitt MC, Browner WS, for the Study of Osteoporatic Fractures Research Group (1999): Depression, falls, and risk of fracture in older women. Arch Intern Med 159:484–490.

Witthaus E, Ott A, Barendregt JJ, Breteler M, Bonneu L (1999): Burden of mortality and morbidity from dementia. Alzheimer Dis Assoc Disord 13:176–181.

World Health Organization (1990): "Composite International Diagnostic Interview" (CIDI, Version 1.0). Geneva, World Health Organization.

Yaffe K, Blackwell T, Gore R, Sands L, Reus V, Browner WS (1999): Depressive symptoms and cognitive decline in nondemented elderly women. Arch Gen Psychiatry 56:425–430.

CHAPTER 23

The Epidemiology of Child and Adolescent Mental Disorders

STEPHEN L. BUKA, MICHAEL MONUTEAUX, and FELTON EARLSI
Harvard School of Public Health, Boston, MA 02115

INTRODUCTION

Considerable scientific ground has been covered regarding the epidemiologic study of child and adolescent psychopathology in the past twenty years. Most notably, much more is known about the measurement, community study, prevalence and risk factors for psychiatric disorders, particularly those of older children and adolescents. This was not the case in 1980 when our earlier review noted "there are few published accounts of investigations which attempt to replicate and refine existing techniques in populations different from [the ones in which they] were originally developed" (Earls, 1980a). It was then noted that among the largest and most influential epidemiologic studies in child psychiatry there was little overlap in terms of definition of psychopathology, sources of information (parents, teachers or children), measurement instruments, or procedures for case definition. This is clearly not the case in 2002, where common nosology, instruments, study designs, and statistical procedures have been developed, implemented, and replicated. This chapter reviews some of the major accomplishments and milestones in our field over the past twenty years, while identifying notable challenges that remain.

Evidence that the mental health of children and adolescents is an area warranting continued scientific and public health attention is well documented, most recently by the Office of the U.S. Surgeon General (USDHHS, 1999, 2001), the World Health Organization and the National Institute of Mental Health (NIMH, 2001). Epidemiologic data suggest that roughly 20% of children ages 1–18 are in need of mental health services in the United States, half of which have mental illnesses severe enough to cause some level of impairment (Burns et al., 1995; Shaffer et al., 1996). Despite the high prevalence among children and adolescents, only about 5–7% have received services for their disability (NIMH, 2001). This number varies greatly by the child's age with 2% of preschoolers, 6–8% of children

Textbook in Psychiatric Epidemiology, Second Edition, Edited by Ming T. Tsuang and Mauricio Tohen.
ISBN 0-471-40974-X

ages 6–11 and 8–9% of adolescents ages 12–17 receiving services (NIMH, 2001) This unmet need for services has raised concerns as children with emotional and behavior problems are at increased risk for dropping out of school, being in trouble with the law and having an overall lower quality of life. Furthermore, mental disorders, particularly if left untreated, are likely to persist into adulthood. According to the 2001 Surgeon Generals Conference on Children's Mental Health, about 74% of 21-year olds with mental disorders had prior mental health problems.

In addition to these social costs, there is a high fiscal burden associated with child and adolescent mental disorders. A study in California found that 8.1% of hospital discharges for children ages 6–12 were for mental illness and that these children accounted for close to 90,000 days of hospitalization and 85 million dollars in hospital charges in 1992 (Chabra, Chavez, and Harris, 1999). A national estimate of child mental health expenditures was recently produced by Sturm and colleagues (2000). In 1998, the total treatment expenditures for child and adolescent mental health were 11.75 billion dollars including inpatient, outpatient, and medication costs. This, too, varied by age group with adolescents accounting for roughly 60% of the total expenditures. Unfortunately, the negative impact of poor child and adolescent mental health is felt worldwide and is likely to get worse. Based on recent data, the WHO predicts that by the year 2020, childhood neuropsychiatric disorders will become one of the leading causes of morbidity, mortality, and disability among children worldwide (USDHHS, 1999).

This summary of the global burden associated with child and adolescent mental disorder underscores the need for and utility of epidemiologic methods and data. Epidemiologic investigations in child psychiatry have been described as having three major purposes (Kellam and Ensminger, 1980). For public health planning purposes, epidemiology provides critical information regarding the prevalence of disorders, service utilization, treatment outcome, and costs. As epidemiology is the study of the distribution, determinants and causes of disease in human populations, a second purpose of epidemiologic investigations is to advance understanding of the origins and course of child psychiatric illness and disorder. This includes understanding the significance of early circumstances, both biological and social, that contribute to the etiology and progression of psychiatric diseases. Such data ideally lead to the third major application of epidemiology, the design and assessment of preventive and treatment interventions.

This chapter has been designed to provide to provide an introduction to and overview of some of the major developments in the epidemiologic study of child and adolescent mental disorders of the past twenty years. We summarize several of the current measures available for use with community samples, major community studies of the past decade, resulting information on the prevalence of and risk factors for child and adolescent disorders, and some concluding observations on future directions.

CLASSIFICATION AND MEASUREMENT

As noted in our previous review (Earls, 1980a), epidemiologic research in child psychiatry has generally assumed either a clinical or statistical approach to diagnosis and classification. Clinically oriented studies assume that cases of psychiatric disorder existing in the general population are broadly similar to declared cases in a clinic population (Ingham and Miller, 1976) and that the same tools that guide clinical diagnosis should be applied in epidemiologic studies. Such an orientation was applied in the classic Isle of Wight study, in which a series of reliability and validity studies based on the capacity of parent and child interview methods to select cases (children attending a psychiatric facility) from controls preceded application of this technique to a general population (Rutter and Graham, 1968). This clinical orientation has been accelerated by the refinement of diagnostic classification systems in adult and child psychiatry, most notably the publication of the modern *Diagnostic and Statistical Manuals for the Classification of Mental Disorders* (DSM-III, IIIR, and IV), beginning in 1980.

An alternative approach to measurement and classification derives from studies originating from a basic social science orientation, in which previous clinical practice and conditions are not taken as the starting point for definitional purposes. "The definition of disorder in these studies is arrived at as a *result* of carrying out a survey in a nonclinical population and not on *a priori* assumptions of what constitutes a psychiatric disorder" (Earls, 1980a, p. 8). This approach has yielded several self-report scales and symptom checklist inventories administered to parents, teachers, and youth, that query about a host of problem behaviors that may be indicative of underlying psychopathology. Such measures have been used both to generate categorical diagnoses and provide continuous, dimensional values for constructs such as depression, conduct problems, and the like. Below, we review some of the most commonly used measures of child and adolescent psychopathology in contemporary epidemiologic studies. These can be divided into two categories according to the quantitative approach utilized: categorical assessments and dimensional assessments.

Categorical Assessments

Categorical assessments are measures that provide discrete classifications of psychopathology according to prespecified diagnostic criteria, most often the DSM. These measures are usually in the form of structured interviews (see Chapter 11 for a more general discussion of structured interviews and their application). In general, these tools require an interviewer to present scripted questions to a research participant that elicit either a yes/no or more detailed response. These questions usually correspond to the symptoms of a specific disorder as defined by DSM criteria. Additional questions can be asked regarding ages of onset and offset, associated functional impairment, and treatment. Thus, these interviews typically consist of a series of modules addressing DSM-defined disorders, and generate diagnostic classifications for each. Specific interviews incorporate variations on the general format described above, and will be illustrated with each in turn. Those chosen for review below were selected based on their frequency of use in the literature and the variation in mode of data collection (interviewer-based versus respondent based). There are other well-designed interviews beyond those reviewed here, including the Diagnostic Interview for Children and Adolescents (DICA), Reich, 2000; Childrens Interview for Psychiatric Symptoms Syndromes (ChIPS), Weller at al., 2000; Interview Schedule for Children and Adolescents (ISCA), Sherrill and Kovacs, 2000. These are described further in a recent summary of this topic (McClellan and Werry, 2000).

Diagnostic Interview Schedule for Children (DISC). The DISC is a fully structured diagnostic interview designed to be administered by highly trained lay interviewers, covering 31 DSM diagnoses that can occur in childhood. Sponsored by the National Institute of Mental Health (NIMH), the measure has gone through several major revisions over the years, starting with the original (Costello et al., 1984), followed by a version still tied to DSM-III (DISC-R, Shaffer et al., 1993), through iterations congruent with DSM III-R (DISC-2.1, Fisher et al., 1993, Jensen et al., 1995; DSIC-2.3, Shaffer et al., 1996, Schwab-Stone et al., 1996), and, presently, with a version covering DSM-IV diagnoses (DISC-IV, Shaffer et al., 2000). The following discussion pertains to this most recent edition.

The questions of the DISC-IV are scripted to be read by the interviewer exactly as written, and are for the most part are designed to elicit a yes/no response. Interviewers are trained to record the response of the subject without interpretation. Questions can be divided into three categories. There are stem questions that ask about the fundamental aspects of symptoms, and are designed to be sensitive to symptom detection. Endorsed stem questions are followed by contingent questions, which determine whether the stem meets the DSM-defined clinical criteria. Finally, there are additional questions that ask about age of onset, impairment, and treatment. For example, after each diagnostic section there is a set of questions assessing the presence and severity of impairment in several domains of functioning, such as relationships with caregivers, participation in peer activities, and academic functioning. Parallel versions of the measure are available for use with both parents and youth.

The interview itself is organized into six modules, which consist of related diagnoses. It assesses the diagnostic status of participants in the past year as well as the past month. Computer-scored algorithms are used to determine if diagnostic criteria are met in order to define cases, strictly adhering to the requirements of DSM-IV. Level of impairment, in addition to symptom criteria, can also be incorporated into the diagnostic algorithm. To combine information from parent and child reports, a symptom criterion is treated as positive if met by either report.

The psychometric properties of the various versions of the DISC have been assessed in multiple reports (Shaffer, et al., 2000). The performance of the DISC-IV was assessed in one such study, involving 84 parents and 82 children. The children were a clinical sample recruited from outpatient psychiatric clinics. The test–retest reliability (mean interval between administration was 6.6 days) for 1-year diagnoses was considered comparable to earlier versions of the instrument. Specifically, κ statistics for major depressive episode, separation anxiety, and conduct disorder were 0.66, 0.58, and 0.43 for parent reports, respectively. The same diagnoses yielded reliability estimates of 0.92, 0.46, and 0.65 for youth reports, respectively. In a community sample of 247 parent-child pairs, the reliability of the DISC-2.3 was deemed moderate-to-good for parent combined reports; youth reports were less reliable in general (see Schwab-Stone et al., 1996 for details). There has been no validity testing of the DISC-IV to date.

There are alternate versions of the DISC-IV. The parent version is designed to assess youth aged 6–17, while the youth version can be used with participants aged 9–17. There is a computer version available (C-DISC-4.0), and it is recommended that this be used for studies assessing multiple diagnoses. The complex branching and skipping instructions coupled with the need to keep track of responses to multiple symptoms makes this administration format attractive. There is also a Spanish version available.

Child and Adolescent Psychiatric Assessment (CAPA). The CAPA (Angold and Costello, 1995a; 2000) is an interviewer-based lay-administered structured diagnostic interview designed to assess the presence of a large number of psychiatric diagnoses in children and adolescents, using DSM-III-R, ICD-10, or DSM-IV criteria.

The CAPA utilizes a different system to elicit information from respondents as compared to the DISC. The CAPA can be termed interviewer-based, which indicates that it is the responsibility of the CAPA interviewer to determine if a given symptom is present or not based on information provided by the subject. This is in contrast to the DISC, which are respondent based, as described above. So, the onus of the response is taken out of the hands of the subject and placed solely on the interviewer, who is required to combine scripted screening questions with probing questions until he or she can determine whether a symptom is present. Screening questions are akin to the stem questions described above, meant to identify subjects who may meet full criteria for a given diagnosis. These screening questions are followed by mandatory probes and discretionary probes, used to determine the presence of a symptom, based on elaborate symptom definitions. These definitions are encapsulated in a detailed glossary, which includes criteria for coding symptom severity in terms of intensity, frequency and duration, and psychosocial impairment.

The interview is organized into several sections covering psychiatric symptoms as well as other domains, such as sociodemographic information and family functioning. The CAPA is restricted to the three-month time period prior to the interview, to increase accuracy of recall. Computer-scoring algorithms convert interview data and generate diagnoses according to the criteria of the desired diagnostic system (DSM-III-R, ICD-10, or DSM-IV). In addition, impairment and symptom scale scores are calculated.

The psychometric properties of the CAPA have been investigated. In a study of 77 clinically referred children aged 10 to 16, test–retest reliability was assessed. Kappa statistics were calculated and were good to moderate. Specifically, κ's were 0.9, 0.74, 0.55, and 1.0 for major depression, overanxious disorder, conduct disorder, and substance abuse/dependence, respectively. With the recognition that no "gold standard" exists to assess criterion validity, an effort to examine the construct validity of the CAPA has been undertaken. The performance of the CAPA was reviewed in the light of what is empirically known about the construct of child and adolescent psychiatric diagnoses. Considering age and gender distributions of disorders, patterns of comorbidity and impairment, service utilization and treatment, familial patterns of disorders, and prediction of negative outcomes, the CAPA was deemed to have good construct validity (Angold and Costello, 2000).

There are several versions of the CAPA available. The primary version is meant for children aged 9–17 and can be administered to both parents and youth. There is also a young adult version (YAPA—Young Adult Psychiatric Assessment) designed for persons aged 18 and older, and a preschool version to be administered to parents of children aged 3–6 (PAPA—Preschool-Age Psychiatric Assessment). There is a Spanish version of the CAPA, and also a special shortened version designed to assess two children at once, to be used for twins. A computerized version is currently being developed.

Schedule of Affective Disorders and Schizophrenia, Epidemiological Version (K-SADS-E). The K-SADS-E (Orvashel, 1985; Ambrosini, 2000) is a semistructured interviewer-based diagnostic interview covering DSM-III-R and DSM-IV diagnoses, designed to be administered by clinician interviewers. It is part of a family of K-SADS interviews (K-SADS-P/L, K-SADS-P IVR) that are subtly different, mostly in terms of symptom scoring and diagnostic coverage. Only the K-SADS-E will be reviewed here.

The semistructured format of the K-SADS-E is similar to the format of the interviewer-based CAPA. The questions are scripted and interviewers are not allowed to deviate from them, as in the DISC. However, unlimited probing is allowed to elicit additional information about the presence and severity of symptoms, similar to the CAPA. The final response is based on the clinicians clarification of the respondents report. The interview itself is organized into modules, one for each diagnostic category. Each interview is ideally administered twice—once with the parent and once with the child. The interviewer then constructs a clinical consensus for each symptom, taking into account all the information.

The interview assesses lifetime as well as current (in the past month) diagnostic status. Lifetime symptoms are assessed as present or not, while current symptoms are additionally rated on a severity scale. In contrast to the interviews described above, a computer diagnostic algorithm is not used to define caseness, in part because only DSM symptoms are used to make a diagnosis. Diagnostic status is hand-coded after the interview. The hierarchical system for assigning diagnoses employed by the DSM is not used in the K-SADS-E.

Ambrosini (2000) has reported on the psychometric properties of the K-SADS-E. Interrater reliability was assessed in a sample of 72 children (no further information on the subjects was presented). Kappa statistics were moderate to good, with major depression, separation anxiety and conduct disorder yielding values of 0.73, 0.65, and 0.68, respectively. Validity was appraised in a variety of ways. Evidence for predictive validity was established by comparing the K-SADS-E depression diagnoses with ratings from dimensional scales designed to measure depression. Also, the construct validity of the K-SADS-E was supported when findings indicated that children and adolescents diagnosed with MDD by the K-SADS-E have abnormal neurobiological values, a family history of affective disorders, and clinically relevant psychosocial impairment.

How to Choose an Instrument

Sources of Measurement Error. The advantage of the interviewer-based system of the CAPA and K-SADS-E is the reduction of intersubject error that arises when each individual's response varies according to the subject's interpretation or understanding of the question. The meaning and intention of each question is meant to be held relatively constant as the interviewer is trained to understand the questions and determine what the answer should be, based on information provided by the subject. This is an intractable problem for the DISC. The disadvantage of this interviewer-based approach is the introduction of a new source of error, namely, interinterviewer error stemming from differences in probing for information, understanding of symptoms, and coding of responses. The DISC is largely designed to avoid this difficulty (particularly problematic in large-scale studies with multiple interviewers). Thus, when choosing an interview for a study, it is necessary to consider which source of error would be the least damaging to the reliability and validity of the assessment.

Cost. The costs of the interviews reviewed here vary. The K-SADS-E and the CAPA are comparably priced, at $75 and $50, respectively (Ambrosini, 2000; Angold and Costello, 2000). The DISC is more expensive, with costs ranging from $150 for students and educators to $2000 for projects funded by the Department of Health and Human Services (Shaffer et al., 2000). However, the cost of the actual interview programs and materials are not the only consideration. The cost of training and maintaining an interview staff is an important consideration, and varies depending on whether the interview is interviewer-based or respondent-based. That is, it is more time consuming and labor intensive to train a staff to administer the interviewer-based assessments, because of the detailed probing and clinical judgement required. This is particularly true for the K-SADS-E, which is designed to be administered by clinicians, in contrast to the CAPA and DISC which can be administered by well-trained undergraduate-level staff. Thus, in terms of training and supporting an interviewer staff, the DISC (undergraduate-level personnel requiring some training) is generally the least expensive, followed by the CAPA (undergraduate-level personnel requiring extensive training) and the K-SADS-E (graduate level personnel requiring extensive training), all other factors being equal (length of employment, number of subjects, and so on).

Coverage. All three schedules cover the same common diagnostic categories (major depression, conduct disorder, separation anxiety, etc.). The differences lie in the coverage of other, less common diagnoses and the assessment of other parameters (see Ambrosini, 2000, Angold and Costello, 2000, and Shaffer et al., 2000 for details). For example, the CAPA assesses family structure, peer–adult relationships and psychosocial impairment. Also, it provides symptom severity ratings, as does the K-SADS-E (current symptoms only). The DISC assesses impairment, but not at the symptom level.

Diagnostic Time Frame. There are differences across the interviews in what time periods are covered. The DISC assesses the past year as well as the past month (there is a "whole-life" module in the DISC-IV, but this piece has not yet been psychometrically scrutinized). The CAPA covers the three-month period preceding the time of the interview, while the K-SADS-E assesses the lifetime and current (past month) diagnoses.

Choosing an Interview for Your Study. Considering the sound psychometric properties of all three interviews, the decision of which to select depends on the resources, goals, and designs of the study in question. For example, the DISC was designed to be used in large-scale epidemiological studies where a large interview staff is necessary (Shaffer et al., 2000). However, the lifetime diagnostic assessment of the K-SADS-E is ideal for family genetic studies of psychiatric disorders. The

CAPA has a specialized module assessing family functioning, such as parent–child relationships and parenting style, as well as a module that evaluates the frequency, type, cost, accessibility, and effectiveness of mental health services, providing useful data largely unique to this instrument (Costello et al., 1996a, b). Finally, when selecting an instrument that is most appropriate to a given study, one should consider the other interviews not reviewed here as well [Diagnostic Interview for Children and Adolescents (DICA), Reich, 2000; Childrens Interview for Psychiatric Symptoms Syndromes (ChIPS), Weller et al., 2000; Interview Schedule for Children and Adolescents (ISCA), Sherrill and Kovacs, 2000]. A special section of the *Journal of the American Academy of Child and Adolescent Psychiatry* most recently reviewed these issues in further detail (McClellan and Werry, 2000).

Dimensional Assessments

Dimensional assessments, typically in the form of self-report scales, questionnaires and symptom checklist inventories, also permit the researcher to generate continuous measures of psychopathology (often in addition to categorical assessment). These measures usually consist of a series of questions pertaining to a related construct that can be aggregated to provide an overall score. They can be interview administered or self-administered by parents, teachers, other adults, children and adolescents. For some of these assessments, an individuals score can be standardized by age and/or gender by comparing it to population norms, which can also provide percentiles. There are numerous scales of this type used in child psychology and psychiatry (see Mental Measurements Yearbook, 2001), but this section will be limited to one of these most amenable to epidemiological applications.

Child Behavior Checklist (CBCL). The parent-reported CBCL (Achenbach, 1991a) and parallel versions for child, youth, and teacher report are among the most commonly used scales assessing child and adolescent psychopathology, in both the clinical and research realms. This measure incorporates a series of questions covering a wide range of problematic behaviors, with items scored as 0 (not true), 1 (somewhat or sometimes true), or 2 (very true or often true). The respondent is asked to answer each question as it describes the child presently or in the past six months. For these problematic behaviors, statistical methods of data reduction were used to group items that tended to correlate with each other. These grouped items were then designated as syndromes, which were named according to the overall content of the items. Examples of syndromes include anxious/depressed, delinquent behavior, attention problems and social problems. These syndromes were further grouped into the broad categories of externalizing and internalizing problems. Finally, a measure of total problems can be taken, which is the sum of all items. A child's score on any syndrome is simply the sum of item scores of all the questions designated as part of that syndrome. Norms have been made available, so that the scores of any individual child can be compared to population standards by age and gender. The author has provided cut-offs for classifying children as Borderline and Clinical for each syndrome scale and the composite scales, allowing for categorical measurement as well.

The CBCL also assesses adaptive behavior and functioning. A series of questions record the frequency and performance of the child relative to peers of the same age in activities such as sports, hobbies, clubs, and chores, on a three-point scale (less than average, average, more than average). Also, additional questions cover the amount and quality of the child's social relationships with peers and family. Finally, academic performance is assessed by an evaluation of the child's grades in a series of academic subjects, as well as attendance in a special class, grade retention, or other problems in school. A similar hierarchical taxonomy and scoring procedure is in place for these items of adaptive behaviors, using similar methods of data reduction. There are versions of the CBCL available to be filled out by teachers (Teacher Report Form, TRF, Achenbach, 1991b) and children themselves (Youth Self Report, YSR, Achenbach, 1991c), also scored and normed using the same methodology.

The reliability and validity of the CBCL has been well documented. Statistics on interinterviewer and test–retest reliabilities of the item scores and scale scores have been supportive of good reliability. Also, interparent agreement has been demonstrated (Achenbach, 1991a). Additionally, there is a large literature documenting the reliability and stability of the CBCL (McConaughy et al., 1992; Verhulst and van der Ende, 1992a, b). The validity of the CBCL is supported by findings documenting the ability of the measure to significantly differentiate between referred and community children, adjusting for demographic features. The CBCL also correlates highly with other instruments purported to measure similar constructs (Achenbach, 1991a).

Harm to Children from Interviews

It is possible to speculate that the experience of being interviewed or completing a self-report behavior checklist could be upsetting to children. Some have suggested that having a stranger ask questions about sensitive experiences and emotions could prove harmful to youth in some way, possibly eliciting anxiety or shame, causing them to ruminate over problems such as bedwetting, or even introducing ideas about substance use, suicide attempts, and the like. Herjanic and colleagues (1976) addressed these questions in an early study entitled "Does interviewing harm children?" These authors recontacted 121 families who had been interviewed in the previous four years with a structured diagnostic interviews for research purposes. The follow-up survey asked parents and youth about their recollection and perceptions of and feelings about the structured interview, such as whether it bothered or worried them, if it helped them, would they do it again, and so on. Follow-up responses were provided by 121 parents and 78 youth (ages 6–17). The vast majority of respondents (92%) either did not recall the structured psychiatric interview or reported that there had been neither concerns nor benefits resulting from the interview. Sixteen percent reported that they had benefited from the interview, and only four subjects (three mothers and one child) reported a negative effect of the interview. All four "bad effects" were reported by psychiatric patients (none among the comparison sample selected from a general pediatric clinic). One child noted that the interview made her worried about herself. One parent felt that the interview had put ideas into the head of her 10-year-old boy, a second reported that her 9-year-old boy was "upset about psychiatry" and the third felt that her child did not require such a thorough evaluation. The authors comment that "none of the bad effects seem to be of such a serious nature as to contradict the use of interviews" (p. 531). These authors also interviewed a separate sample of 88 children immediately following completion of a structured psychiatric interview. Unlike the longer-term recall, immediately after being interviewed 17 children (19%) did report concerns about the interview, which were mostly related to embarrassment from questions about drugs, sex, and suicide. It is noteworthy that while almost 20% of youth interviewed reported some concerns immediately following an interview, these seem to dissipate over time.

As expected, these results suggest, for the most part, that there is no detrimental effect of participating in structured psychiatric interviews, aside from the occasional transient embarrassment. All of the participants who reported negative effects were families seeking psychiatric care; it is not at all evident that the adverse effects reported emanate from the research procedures rather than the experience of receiving psychiatric treatment. Although this evidence is reassuring, future research should periodically monitor the effect of interviewing on children and parents.

Two other studies have since investigated subject reactions to structured psychiatric interviews. Zahner (1991) administered the Diagnostic Interview Schedule for Children, Version R, to a community sample of 144 preadolescents and their parents residing in New Haven, Connecticut. Following the interview, subjects were asked if they found the interview enjoyable, whether they would tell a friend to participate, and whether they found some parts of the interview too personal. The responses (weighted to represent general population rates) indicated that over 90% of parents and 80% of children reported that they found the interview enjoyable. Almost all (96%) parents reported that they would tell a friend to participate in a similar interview, as did 98% of children who reported low levels of symptomatology. Only three-quarters of children who scored above a clinical threshold for problem behavior symptoms had a similar response. Only 4% of parents reported that they found some parts of the interview too personal, although 12% of children had this reaction.

The final entry in this brief literature was a follow-up survey of 50 parents and 72 children who had previously been interviewed with the Diagnostic Interview for Children and Adolescents, a fully structured diagnostic interview (Reich and Kaplan, 1994). These authors reported results similar to the two previous studies. Parents and children were asked if the children had been upset by the interview experience or affected in any negative way. No serious negative effects were reported by either parents or children. All of the parents reported that they were not offended by the questions and were willing to be reinterviewed. Only two children reported that they had not liked the interview or had been made uncomfortable by questions. One was made uncomfortable by the vocabulary test and the second was upset over questions about his fathers drinking. In sum, the available evidence indicates that children and parents do not appear to be adversely affected by structured psychiatric interviews and, to the contrary, generally enjoy their interview experience. A minority of children and youth do report some discomfort immediately following the interview, but these responses seem to dissipate over time. In balance, the cost–benefit of epidemiologic studies with direct interviews of parents and children appear to lean heavily on the side of benefit.

POPULATION-BASED STUDIES

As noted in the Introduction, psychiatric disorders among children and adolescents is widespread. Research of the past 20–30 years have applied the diagnostic measures reviewed above (as well as others) in a number of important community-based investigations, enriching our understanding of the prevalence of specific forms of psychopathology. Angold and Costello (1995b) summarized many of these, including major investigations in the United States, the United Kingdom, Germany, and New Zealand. Sample sizes ranged from 399 to 2,734 (mean N = 1363). It was found that the 6-month prevalence rate for any psychiatric disorder ranged from 17 to 27% across all the studies reviewed. The most common categories of psychopathology were anxiety disorders, behavior disorders, and mood disorders, in that order (Angold and Costello, 1995b). A similar review by Friedman et al. (1996) also concluded that the prevalence rate of any diagnosable disorder in youth aged 9–17 years is 20%, consistent with the estimate above. These authors also presented summary prevalence estimates for disorders with functional impairment. The rate of serious emotional disturbance with substantial functional impairment ranged from 9 to 13%, while the prevalence of serious emotional disturbance with extreme functional impairment ranged from 5 to 9%.

In the following section, we review several of the major community studies of child and adolescent mental disorders that have contributed to this body of knowledge on prevalence, followed by a synthesis of findings. Due to developing diagnostic taxonomies and methods, we emphasize more recent studies.

Isle of Wight/Inner London Borough Study

In a landmark study, Rutter and colleagues (1975) reported on the prevalence of psychiatric disorder in a sample of ten-year-old male and female children from two geographic areas of England—an innercity London borough (ILB) and the Isle of Wight (IOW). These areas were considered similar in social composition but discrepant in terms of living conditions. All ten-year-old children attending local schools in both areas were screened using a teacher questionnaire covering emotional and behavioral problems, in order to identify a subsample that was likely to have a psychiatric disorder. A random sample of children so identified were recruited (n = 93 from IOW, n = 148 from ILB), as well as a random sample of the children not indicated as having a disorder (n = 93 from IOW; n = 80 from ILB). The mothers of these children were interviewed by a trained clinician using a standardized method to assess psychiatric disorders (Graham and Rutter, 1968). The interview covered the past year and recorded the frequency and severity of each symptom. The presence of psychiatric disorders was recorded only if symptomatology as well as impaired function were reported.

The prevalence of any psychiatric disorder in the ILB (25.4%) was significantly greater than in the IOW (12%). Due to sample size constraints, the prevalence of specific diagnoses can only be considered in a relative sense (ILB versus IOW), not in absolute terms. As such, the ILB had significantly increased rates of "emotional disorder," "disturbance of conduct," and "other" (enuresis or hyperkinetic syndrome) as compared to IOW children. Further analyses went on to identify a set of factors that were associated with childhood psychopathology, regardless of the study locale: family discord, parental psychopathology, and social disadvantage. The authors concluded that the higher rates of disorder in the ILB children can be at least partly attributed to the relatively greater presence of these risk factors in the ILB, as compared to the IOW (Rutter et al., 1975).

Ontario Child Health Study

This study sought to examine the prevalence of mental health problems and the utilization of mental health and social services among a sample of 4–16-year-old children residing in Ontario, Canada. See Boyle et al. (1987) and Offord et al. (1987) for detailed methodology. Briefly, a multistep random sampling scheme was used to ascertain a representative sample of male and female children residing in Ontario, Canada, using the 1981 Census of Canada. Four disorders were selected for study, based on their frequency and burden of suffering: conduct disorder, attention deficit disorder with hyperactivity, emotional disorder, and somatization. The presence of these psychiatric disorders was based on four rating scales complied by the authors, consisting of a subset of items from the Child Behavior Checklist (CBCL). Respondents were asked to consider the past six months when answering each item. Each of these scales was meant to operationalize specific DSM-III criteria for a disorder or set of disorders. Specifically, items in the hyperactivity, conduct disorder, and somatization scales were based on DSM-III criteria for ADHD and CD, and current somatic symptoms without organic cause, respectively. Items in the emotional disorder scale were designed to reflect the DSM-III criteria for affective disorder, overanxious disorder, and obsessive–compulsive disorder. To define cases for each disorder, each scale was dichotomized at a threshold that maximized its agreement with psychiatrists ratings of that disorder. These threshold scores for each scale were decided by having psychiatrists determine the presence or absence of each scale item to a clinically meaningful degree in a random subsample of children from the study.

The prevalence of any disorder (conduct disorder, hyperactivity, emotional disorder or somatization) was 18.1% (95% CI: 16.4%, 19.8%). The prevalence of all disorders and any disorder were higher in urban areas relative to rural areas, and this difference reached statistical significance for hyperactivity and any disorder. Rates of conduct disorder and hyperactivity were greater in males. A significant age by gender interaction was found for emotional disorder, with the rate in boys declining with age (10.2% in 4–11-year olds to 4.9% in 12–16-year olds) and the rate in girls increasing with age (10.7% in 4–11-year olds to 13.6% in 12–16-year olds). A similar interaction effect was noted with the rate of any disorder, increasing with age in girls (13.5% to 21.8%), while remaining relatively constant in boys (19.5% to 18.8%). Disturbingly, it was also found that only 16.1% of children with any disorder received mental health or social service attention in the six months prior to the study, despite a rate of 59% for routine or emergency medical care. Based on these results, the authors caution against recommending an increase in the availability of mental health services as a solution, and instead suggest efforts be focused on community primary prevention programs.

National Comorbidity Survey

The National Comorbidity Survey (NCS) was a congressionally mandated national survey of a representative sample of noninstitutionalized people aged 15–54 years in the continental United States. It was primarily designed to study the prevalence of psychiatric disorders in adults, but the lower age bound was set to 15 to minimize the effect of recall biases in the reporting of lifetime information. Thus, data was gathered on a subsample of adolescents, aged 15 to 17. As such, this study will be briefly reviewed.

The NCS interviewed a representative sample of 8,098 persons meeting the above criteria between September 1990 and February 1992. The prevalence estimates were adjusted with statistical weighting procedures to account for nonresponse error, variation within and between households, and national population distributions of major demographic factors. Psychiatric diagnoses were based on the DSM-III-R and derived using the Composite International Diagnostic Interview (CIDI), a fully structured assessment tool designed to be administered by trained lay interviewers (Kessler et al., 1994). For 15–17-year olds, a prevalence estimate for any psychiatric disorder with "substantial impairment" was reported as 8.7% (Friedman et al., 1996). The NCS is being readministered in 2001, including subjects aged 12 and above.

Great Smoky Mountain Study

The Great Smoky Mountains Study of Youth (GSMS; Costello et al., 1996a, b) was designed to investigate the need, utilization, and development of mental health services for children and adolescents. This study utilized a sophisticated sampling scheme designed to simultaneously allow for the study of children with mental health care needs as well as to allow for the estimation of the prevalence of mental disorders in the population. See Costello et al. (1996a, b) for detailed methodology. Briefly, out of the 12,000 children aged 9, 11, or 13 years in the public school database of the Appalachian Mountain region of North Carolina, 4500 were selected for screening through a multistep probability sampling procedure. This parent-reported screening tool consisted of a modified version of the Externalizing Problems composite scale items of the Child Behavior Checklist (Achenbach, 1991a). A study sample was constructed, consisting of the eligible children who scored above a predefined cutoff point on the screening measure, as well as a random sample of those who did not. A statistical weighting procedure was employed to allow for population prevalence estimates. The final sample consisted of 1015 children aged 9, 11 or 13 who were administered the Child and Adolescent Psychiatric Assessment (CAPA, Angold and Costello, 1995b). (Several other outcomes were examined in this study, such as mental health service use and impaired functioning (Costello et al., 1996a, b; Burns et al., 1995). However, only the findings related to psychiatric diagnoses will be reviewed here.)

The prevalence rate ($\pm$SE) for any DSM-III-R in the GSMS disorder was 20.3% $\pm$ 1.7%. This estimate includes many diagnoses not usually considered in other community studies (i.e., tic disorders and enuresis). Thus, it is useful to consider other summary measures of psychiatric morbidity. The prevalence rate for any anxiety disorder was 5.7% ± 1.0%, while the prevalence rate for any behavioral disorder was 6.6% ± 0.8%. The prevalence rate of any emotional (any anxiety disorder or any depressive disorder) or behavioral disorder was 11.9% ± 1.3%.

Other findings are noteworthy. It is clear from these findings that the children of this sample presented with a considerable degree of psychiatric comorbidity. Almost a third of the children with any diagnosis exhibited comorbidity, with depressive disorders being most likely to co-occur with another diagnosis. Males were at higher risk for any disorder, mostly due to higher rates of behavioral disorders. Aside from predictable differences in separation anxiety, tics, and enuresis, there were no differences between 9-year olds and older children. No significant findings were noted with regard to race. Finally, a strikingly consistent pattern of results was found in regards to income: children from the lowest income bracket were at increased risk for any disorder and for *every specific disorder* except tic disorder. No differences between urban and rural children were found after income was controlled.

Methods for the Epidemiology of Child and Adolescent Mental Disorders

The Methods for the Epidemiology of Child and Adolescent Mental Disorders (MECA) was an NIMH sponsored project designed to improve and develop the methodology for community psychiatric epidemiological studies of children and adolescents. Specifically, the study was intended to provide valid, reliable, and feasible methods for the study of the prevalence of mental disorders, risk factors for psychopathology, and mental health service utilization among youth aged 9–17 in large epidemiological community studies. The study was conducted across four sites (Westchester County, NY, New Haven, CT, Atlanta, GA, Puerto Rico), with the target population consisting of all children aged 9–17 residing within the predetermined geographic study areas at the time of subject enumeration. Since this study was not meant to provide a representative sample but to explore various methodological techniques, each site implemented its own specific method for subject selection (see Lahey et al., 1996, for details). Each site employed the Diagnostic Interview Schedule for Children, version 2.3 (DISC 2.3), a fully structured diagnostic interview designed to be administered by trained lay interviewers, to assess for the presence of DSM-III-R mental disorders in the six months prior to the interview. Both the child and a primary caregiver (usually the mother) were interviewed. These data were combined by considering a symptom positive if endorsed by either the child or the caregiver. The final sample consisted of 1,285 pairs of children and caregivers were aggregated across the four sites.

Shaffer and colleagues (1996) presented prevalence estimates for the MECA study across several levels of global functional impairment in addition to impairment specific to a particular given diagnosis. They note that prevalence estimates decrease, markedly in some cases, as impairment criteria become more stringent. Indeed, under the DSM-III-R nosology, it is possible to receive a diagnosis through satisfying symptomatic criteria without demonstrating significant functional impairment. The DSM-IV has modified this standard by requiring significant impairment as part of criteria for many diagnoses. Thus, the authors choose to define caseness as meeting DSM criteria with a Childrens Global Assessment of Scale (CGAS) score of less than or equal to 70 as well as diagnosis-specific impairment at home, school or with peers. Shaffer et al. (1996) also point out that these estimates are not meant to represent the likely prevalence of mental disorders in the United States, but the relative differences between prevalence rates and the effect of including impairment criteria on prevalence.

Using the authors definition of caseness, the prevalence of any disorder as derived from the combined parent–child report was 20.9%. Interestingly, this estimate dropped to 12.3% if only the youth report is considered, and 10.2% if only the caregiver report is used. Also, the prevalence of the combined parent-child report for any disorder decreased to 11.5% and 5.4% as the impairment criteria increased in severity. The prevalence rates of any anxiety disorder, any depression, and any disruptive disorder from the combined parent–child report were 13.0%, 6.2%, and 10.3%, respectively. Overall, it was noted that the reducing effect on prevalence estimates of increasing impairment criteria was greatest for anxiety disorders, intermediate for mood disorders, and inconsequential for conduct and oppositional-defiant disorders. Also, the limited agreement between parent and child reports was evident in these data, as the combined estimates were frequently at least equal to the sum of cases reported by youth and caregivers separately.

Project on Human Development in Chicago Neighborhoods

The Project on Human Development in Chicago Neighborhoods (PHDCN) is an ongoing, interdisciplinary study aimed at deepening our understanding of the multilevel pathways to child and adolescent criminal behavior, psychiatric disorder, and prosocial behavior among a sample of families living in Chicago (Earls and Buka, 1997). The study integrates neighborhood-level assessment of the neighborhoods and communities in which families reside, along with a longitudinal cohort study of the health and development of approximately 7000 youth, ages 0–18. Sampling for PHDCN occurred in two stages. First, 847 census tracts within the city of Chicago were examined for naturally occurring clusters of city blocks that were geographically compact as well as similar in socioeconomic and ethnic mix, housing density, and family structure. Through statistical analyses of census data, a total of 343 neighborhood clusters (NCs) were identified. Reflecting the high level of racial and ethnic segregation in Chicago, it was possible to group NCs by seven levels of race or ethnicity composition and three levels of average socioeconomic status (SES) into 21 cells. A random, stratified sample of 80 NCs were chosen for intensive study, representing all race and ethnic and SES types. These 80 NCs were assessed for a variety of contextual factors hypothesized to affect child and youth development, including formal and informal social control, cohesion, collective efficacy, community norms, safety, and the like. Four measurement techniques were used at the neighborhood level: (1) the Community Survey was a random probability household survey of residents aged 18 and above; (2) the Systematic Social Observation involved direct observation (videotapes) of over 27,000 street blocks, with coding of the lifestyle and behaviors of residents, along with measures of the physical environment (parks, playgrounds, litter, liquor stores, housing type, etc.); (3) open-ended qualitative interviews with approximately 3000 "neighborhood experts" representing key spheres of influence on child and adolescent development such as business, clergy, recreation, police and the like; and (4) administrative records including vital health statistics (birth and death data), crime and arrest rates, economic information and the like.

Embedded within this neighborhood study is a longitudinal cohort study of approximately 7000 children, youth, and their families. To draw on this random household sample, approximately 40,000 dwelling units households were screened to determine household composition. The ages and gender of household members within the 80 selected neighborhoods were used to identify households with children within six months of one of six target cohort ages (0, 3, 6, 9, 12, 15, 18 years), including all pregnancies. All eligible participants within a selected household were invited to participate. At least one primary caregiver of each child enrolled was also recruited, except for those in the 18-year-old cohort. Children and one primary caregiver were each assessed during a baseline interview, and two subsequent follow-up assessments (each with an interval of approximately two years). Mental health data was collected at all waves of assessment, using the Achenbach Child Behavior Checklist, and Youth Self-Report, and portions of the Diagnostic Interview Schedule for Children, both child and parent report versions. Substance use and abuse information was collected with a variety of measures, including portions of the NIDA National Household Survey on Drug Abuse battery, and others. Relevant articles from this project include Sampson, Raudenbush and Earls, 1997; Buka et al., 2001; Molnar et al., 2001; Reardon, Brennan and Buka, 2001.

Summary

Angold and Costello have summarized recent epidemiologic studies for major psychiatric disorders from middle childhood through adolescence (1995b). These studies generally report 6-month prevalence rates for psychiatric disorder ranging between 17 to 27%. The most prevalent disorders are the anxiety disorders, followed by conduct and oppositional disorders, attention deficit and depressive disorders. While these prevalence estimates consider any persons meeting diagnostic criteria, others have attempted to estimate the prevalence of "serious" and "severe" mental illness, in which the condition results in notable impairment in functioning. An expert task force assembled by the federal Center for Mental Health Services (CMHS) estimates that the 12-month prevalence of serious emotional disturbance in children and adolescents (aged 9–17 years) is 9–13% and that severe conditions are on the order of 5–9 %. (Friedman, 1997). As discussed below, in the absence of a single national survey, these estimates vary according to the samples and sites studied, the diagnostic measures used, and the criteria applied to define "functional impairment."

Taken together, these studies provide fertile ground for practical conclusions about childhood psychopathology, as well as directions for further research. For instance, a consistent finding across most of these studies, as well as those reviewed by Angold and Costello (1995b) is an overall prevalence rate of any disorder of about 20%. This is the case despite different sampling schemes, methods of diagnostic assessment, calendar year of study, and geographic location. This consistency of results in the face of variability of methods, time, and place is a strong testament to the validity of the findings.

However, a notable exception to this pattern is the NCS, with a prevalence estimate of 8.7%. Several factors could account for this discrepancy. First, this study utilized a diagnostic instrument designed for adults (the CIDI), and may not have been sensitive to disorders as they are manifested in childhood, a point supported by the differing diagnostic criteria for the same disorders (i.e., mania and depression) across adult and child structured interviews. Additionally, the CIDI did not assess diagnoses that are considered to be first diagnosed in childhood, such as attention deficit hyperactivity disorder and enuresis (APA, 1994). These diagnostic categories are responsible for a considerable amount of the psychopathology in the other studies reviewed here. Furthermore, the parents of these adolescents were not interviewed, a common practice in child psychiatric epidemiological studies (see section on multiple reporters); this omission could account for a nontrivial amount of missed cases. Finally, and possibly most important, the NCS prevalence estimate incorporated an impairment criteria that most likely reduced the prevalence estimate. In support of this notion is the report by Friedman et al. (1996) that notes that when functional impairment is taken into account, the rate of serious emotional disturbance with substantial functional impairment in children ranged from 9 to 13%.

The community studies reviewed above have involved both single stage and two-stage designs. The Isle of Wight, Ontario Child Health Study, and the Great Smoky Mountain Study all used screening tools as the first stage in a two stage design (in which a subsample is then interviewed at a second stage with a full diagnostic measure). These screening methods are typically based on the assumption that persons with probable diagnoses would have high symptom counts and are considered a cost-effective way of assessing specific diagnoses in large population samples. In earlier studies, second stage diagnoses were often determined by clinicians. However as it became increasingly evident that clinician interviewing failed to produce evidence of sound reliability, researchers were prone to rely on the structured methods of assessment. This has led to the more recent designs, in which structured interviews, typically administered by nonclinicians, are used both as the second stage of the two-stage designs and for entire populations in single stage designs. In the absence of biological markers for disease, these structured interview methods, despite their limitations, are heavily relied upon in population studies.

The importance of considering functional impairment when measuring the prevalence of mental disorders in children should not be underestimated. Functional impairment is a key feature of the diagnostic criteria of most disorders in the DSM-IV (APA, 1994; Shaffer et al., 1996) and is also a fundamental component of the definition of "serious emotional disturbance," as established by the Center for Mental Health Services of the U.S. federal government (U.S Government, 1993, p. 29425). Despite the importance of this construct, there is not a consensus in the field regarding how to quantitatively operationalize functional impairment associated with child and adolescent psychopathology. Costello and colleagues (1998) undertook an effort to this end. Their reanalysis of several community prevalence studies defined functional impairment in two ways: (a) the lowest 10% of a global functioning scale, and (b) the lowest 10% on one or more domain-specific functioning scales. They found that the median prevalence of serious emotional disturbance (a diagnosis plus functional impairment) was 5.4%, but this estimate climbed to 10.3% if the cutoff used to define impairment was raised to 20%. Thus, the estimated prevalence of child and adolescent psychopathology in the community depends greatly on the definition of functional impairment, and the authors note that more work is needed in this area.

RISK FACTORS

A multitude of risk factors for child and adolescent psychiatric disorders have been identified. In this section we summarize some of the major findings in this area, concluding with recommendations for future research.

Genetic Risk

An important objective in epidemiological studies is to determine if a disorder is familial in nature. Once established, the next step is to examine its mode of transmission. The fact that many types of disorders do exhibit familial patterns requires research designs that can both partition genetic and environmental contributions as well as suggest mechanisms in which such factors interact. Twin and adoption designs have so far guided the understanding of these issues to date. Advances in molecular biology are rapidly providing the capacity to identify genes associated with specific disorders. As this is achieved, the path will be open to study the mechanisms characterizing genetic risks and the integration of genetic and environmental determinants. Research of this nature may serve as a basis for further development of specific prevention and therapeutic interventions for a wide range of psychiatric morbidities.

The genetic risk associated with many psychiatric disorders in childhood is undeniable (State et al., 2000). The findings from twin and adoption studies have firmly established the contribution of genetics to the occurrence of disorders in children such as conduct disorder (Brennen et al., 1991); attention deficit hyperactivity disorder (Faraone and Biederman, 1994; Gillis et al., 1992); autism (Bailey et al., 1995; Steffenburg et al., 1989); depression (Jellinek and Snyder, 1998); and Tourettes disorder (Price et al., 1985).

An important caveat to these findings is the realization among researchers that psychiatric disorders are not transmitted through simple mendelian pathways; the mechanism of inheritance is more complex (State et al., 2000). However, a crucial point to remember is that the heritability estimate of each childhood psychiatric disorder is less than one. For example, heritiability estimates for attention deficit hyperactivity disorder have been estimated to range from 54% to 82%, depending on the study and method of assessment. Conduct disorder and oppositional defiant disorder were found to be heritable, with some estimates reaching considerable proportions (21%–74%). Estimates of heritiability for depression varied substantially depending on the informant: 60%–72% with parent reports and 11% when children report (Wamboldt and Wamboldt, 2000). The etiology of autism is distinguished by particularly high genetic influences, with a 100- to 200-fold increased risk for the disorder in family members of cases relative to family members of controls. The concordance rate in MZ twins for Tourettes disorder has been estimated at 55%–100%, with the concordance rate in DZ being only 20%

(State et al., 2000). Taken together, these results make a clear case for the conclusion that a substantial proportion of the variance in childhood psychopathology remains to be explained, either by environmental factors or the interaction between genes and environment.

An important objective in epidemiological studies is to determine if a disorder is familial in nature. Once established, the next step is to examine its mode of transmission. The fact that many types of disorders do exhibit familial patterns requires research designs that can both partition genetic and environmental contributions as well as suggest mechanisms in which such factors interact. Twin and adoption designs have so far guided the understanding of these issues to date. Advances in molecular biology are rapidly providing the capacity to identify genes associated with specific disorders. As this is achieved, the path will be open to study the mechanisms characterizing genetic risks and the integration of genetic and environmental determinants. Research of this nature may serve as a basis for more development of specific prevention and therapeutic interventions for a wide range of psychiatric morbidities.

Parental Psychopathology

Studies have consistently found that psychopathology in parents is associated with mental disorders in offspring (Angold and Costello, 1995b). Of course, without adoption study methodology, it is extremely difficult to separate the genetic effect from the environmental effect when studying the impact of parental psychopathology. Nevertheless, it is informative to note findings that document the association between parent and offspring mental illness. For instance, it is a well-replicated finding that children of parents with substance use disorders are at increased risk for delinquency (West and Prinz, 1987) and alcohol use themselves (Jackson, 1997; Day, 1995a, b). Also, it was found that parental alcoholism was associated with attention deficit hyperactivity disorder, and conduct disorder, while antisocial personality disorder plus alcoholism was associated with oppositional-defiant disorder, adjusting for gender, age, and socioeconomic status (Kuperman et al., 1999).

Research on the effect of parental psychopathology is not limited to behavioral disruptive disorders of childhood. It has been reported that children of parents with affective disorders are up to three times as likely to manifest depression, marked by an earlier age of onset and a longer duration (Beardslee et al., 1993). Anxiety disorders in parents have been linked to childhood anxiety disorders in offspring (Rosenbaum et al., 1991; Turner et al., 1987). While it is probable that genetic effects account for a nontrivial portion of these findings, the fact that twin and adoption studies consistently yield heritability estimates below one leaves room for the suggestion that exposure to parental psychopathology is an independent, and potentially modifiable, risk factor.

Socioeconomic Status

Since the well-known study conducted in Chicago by Faris and Dunham (1939) that documented an inverse association between the rate of schizophrenia and socioeconomic status (SES), researchers in psychiatry and psychiatric epidemiology have investigated the role of SES in the etiology of mental disorders. Rutter and colleagues (1975) documented the malignant role that socioeconomic deprivation can play in the occurrence of psychiatric disorders in children residing in two distinct areas, an industrialized urban center and a rural countryside. In a recent study by Kuperman et al. (1999), low SES was significantly associated with conduct disorder, an association that had been found several times previously (Loeber et al., 2000). Costello et al. (1996a, b), in a representative sample of 9, 11, and 13-year olds, found that children below the federal poverty line were three times more likely to meet criteria for any DSM-III-R psychiatric disorder, relative to children above the cutoff. Also, children below the poverty line were more likely to meet criteria for every individual diagnosis except tic disorder. A notable exception to these findings can be found in studies of substance use, where increases in the use of alcohol and drugs are seen at the upper end of the socioeconomic ladder (Hawkins et al., 1992). These findings suggest that the relationship between substance use and SES for adolescents may resemble a U-shaped curve; further research is needed in this area.

Debate has raged over the nature of this remarkably consistent relationship between social class and mental disease: do people with mental disorders slip down the social ladder due to their condition (social drift hypothesis), or does low social status play a causal role in the pathogenesis of psychopathology (social causation hypothesis) (Murphy et al., 1991)? For adults, a notable study by Dohrenwend et al. (1992) found that the social drift phenomenon appears to be more important in the occurrence of schizophrenia while the social causation mechanism is a superior explanation for the occurrence of depression in women and antisocial personality and substance use disorders in men. Questions about the etiology of psychopathology in children and adolescents await similar analytical efforts. Our Chicago neighborhoods project has been designed in part to address another key question about the association between social status and mental disease: to what extent is this association dependent upon one's individual social circumstance, and/or the level of social advantage of ones neighborhood and community?

Prenatal Exposures or Complications

There have been several links made between prenatal exposures and prenatal and perinatal complications (PPCs) and psychiatric disorders in children, adolescents, and adults (Buka, Lipsitt, and Tsuang, 1993). The evidence is greatest for schizophrenia, and includes several recent chart and interview-based case control studies (Kunugi et al., 1996; Hultman et al., 1997; Smith et al., 1995), large prospective cohort studies (Cannon, 1996; Jones et al., 1998) and a detailed meta-analysis on this topic (Geddes and Lawrie, 1995). Most reach the conclusion that prior PPCs are twice as common among individuals with schizophrenia, although there are notable exceptions that fail to report any such association (Kendell et al., 2000). A major meta-analysis estimated that, if PPCs have a causal role in schizophrenia, they could account for 22% of adult cases (Geddes and Lawrie, 1995). There has been some evidence suggesting a link between complications during pregnancy and birth and later delinquency, but conflicting results preclude a firm conclusion (Buka and Earls, 1993; Raine, 1993). There is a well-established relationship between prenatal exposure to alcohol and several negative outcomes, including mental retardation (Bee, 1995), attentional problems, and conduct disorder (Steinhausen et al., 1993; Streissguth, 1994). There has also been research delineating the possible effect of maternal smoking during pregnancy and the risk for attention deficit or hyperactivity disorder (Milberger et al., 1996).

Neighborhood and Contextual Effects

In the past decade there has been a renewed interest in the influence of neighborhood and other social contexts on the growth, development and health, including mental health, of children and youth. A growing body of literature has demonstrated that neighborhood conditions can affect the health and well-being of children, especially young children, as well as families. (Brooks-Gunn et al., 1997; Melton, 1992; Leventhal and Brooks-Gunn, 2000). Economic disadvantage and inequality have been shown to predict rates of community violence, as well as dimensions of social exchange and interaction, such as the willingness of neighborhood residents to work jointly to reduce social disorder (Sampson, Raudenbush and Earls, 1997). Less has been written about the impacts of neighborhood features on mental health, *per se*. In an earlier study on this topic, Wechsler and Pugh (1967) found that residents of communities in which there were fewer neighbors of the same age group experienced higher rates of mental illness than residents of communities with a higher density of same-age peers. Wandersman and Nation (1998) recently reviewed the literature on urban neighborhoods and mental health. They note four general attributes of urban neighborhoods that have been theorized to impact mental health: structural characteristics; neighborhood social disorder; environmental stressors (including youth exposure to violence); and "socially toxic neighborhoods." While interest in this topic is high, empirical evidence of contextual influences on mental health is quite limited, with most known regarding antisocial behavior and suicidality, and continuous measures of behavior problems and far less about psychiatric diagnoses. See Leventhal and Brooks-Gunn (2000) for an excellent review of this topic.

The literature reviewed above is merely a sample of the research that has been conducted investigating the relationship between child psychiatric disorders and risk factors. Other risk factors that have received attention in the literature include lead exposure, infectious agents, brain injuries, chronic medical illnesses, and psychological trauma, to name just a few. Space limitations prohibit further review here.

Beyond this survey of individual risk factors, the past decade has witnessed growing discussion of the aggregation of risk factors and likelihood of psychopathology. Studies by Rutter and colleagues (Rutter et al., 1975, 1977) have shown that the risk for mental disorders in children increased as the number of risk factors increased, regardless of which specific factors they were. Other more recent studies have found similar results (Blantz et al., 1991; Biederman et al., 1995; Sameroff, 1998). Interpretation of these findings should be cautious, however, as the association between increasing environmental adversity and increasing risk for psychopathology could be confounded by other, unmeasured factors, rather than a causative dose-response relationship.

For researchers and public health officials, it is important to keep in mind that the associations between risk factors and psychopathology do not necessarily imply a causative relationship, an error that surprisingly is still made (Wandersman and

Nation, 1998; Aneshensel and Sucoff, 1996). These associations are merely that—associations. This emphasizes the need for future research that moves toward experimental study designs to determine which risk factors are truly causal and which merely confounding (Hawkins, et al., 1992).

CONCLUSION

At the outset of this chapter, we reviewed three major purposes of epidemiologic investigations in child psychiatry: (1) to provide information on prevalence, service utilization, and cost of public health planning purposes; (2) to advance understanding of the origins and course of child psychiatric illness and disorder; and (3) to contribute to the design and assessment of preventive and treatment interventions. The material summarized above discusses some of the major developments of the past twenty years, including advances in nosology, instrumentation, community studies, prevalence data, and information on major risk factors. We have only touched lightly on some of the major methodologic challenges that have been partially resolved in reaching this state. While considerable progress has been made, these challenges are far from mastered and future advances in this area will be required to move beyond the current state of knowledge. Key issues requiring continued methodologic attention include: (1) refinement of the basic nosology or classification of major mental disorders of children and adolescents; (2) development of reliable and, in particular, valid measures to assess these conditions in treated and community populations; (3) determining optimal sources and types of information for such assessments (e.g., reporter: parent, child, teacher and source: interview, questionnaire, administrative data), which most likely will result in different solutions for different conditions and age groups; (4) methods for combining information from multiple sources; (5) the extremely challenging matter of classification and assessment of psychopathology for preschool and early school-age children; (6) methods for determining the degree of functional impairment associated with a given condition, with resulting implications for diagnosis and classification. With continued attention to these key methodologic concerns and maintained investment in population-based studies which are the cornerstone of the epidemiologic method, the next twenty years should witness even more dramatic advances in knowledge of the etiology, course, treatment, and prevention of mental disorders of children and youth.

REFERENCES

Achenbach TM (1991a): Manual for the Child Behavior Checklist/4-18 and 1991 Profile. Burlington: University of Vermont, Department of Psychiatry.

Achenbach TM (1991b): Manual for the Teachers Report Form and 1991 Profile. Burlington: University of Vermont, Department of Psychiatry.

Achenbach TM (1991c): Manual for the Youth Self Report and 1991 Profile. Burlington: University of Vermont, Department of Psychiatry.

Ambrosini PJ (2000): Historical development and present status of the Schedule for Affective Disorders and Schizophrenia for School-Age Children (K-SADS). J Am Acad Child Adolesc Psychiatry 39:49–58.

American Psychiatric Association. (1994) Diagnostic and Statistical Manual of Mental Disorders, 4th ed. Washington, DC: American Psychiatric Association.

Aneshensel DC, Sucoff CA (1996): The neighborhood context of mental health. J Health Soc Behavior 37:293–310.

Angold A, Costello EJ (1995a): A test–retest reliability study of child-reported psychiatric symptoms and diagnoses using the Child and Adolescent Psychiatric Assessment (CAPA-C). Psycholo Med 25:755–762.

Angold A, Costello EJ (1995b): Developmental epidemiology. Epidemiolo Rev 17:74–82.

Angold A, Costello EJ (2000): The Child and Adolescent Psychiatric Assessment (CAPA). J Am Acad Child Adolesc Psychiatry 39:39–48.

Bailey A, LeCouteur A, Gottesman I, et al. (1995): Autism as a strongly genetic disorder: Evidence from a British twin study. Psycholo Med 25:63–77.

Beardslee WR, Keller MB, Lavori PW, Staley J, Sacks N (1993): The impact of parental affective disorder on depression in offspring: a longitudinal follow-up in a nonreferred sample. J Am Acad Child Adolesc Psychiatry 32:723–30.

Bee, H (1995): "The Developing Child." New York: Harper Collins, pp 58–59.

Biederman J, Milbeger S, Faraone SV, et al. (1995): Family-environment risk factors for attention-deficit hyperactivity disorder: A test of Rutters indicators of adversity. Arch Gen Psychiatry 52:464–470.

Blantz B, Schmidt MH, Esser G (1991): Familial adversities and child psychiatric disorders. J Child Psycholo Psychiatry Disord 32:939–950.

Boyle MH, Offord DR, Hofmann HG, et al. (1987): Ontario Child Health Study I. Methodology. Arch Gen Psychiatry 44:826–831.

Brennen PA, Mendick SA, Gabrielli WF (1991): Genetic influences and criminal behavior. In Tsuang M, Kendler K, Lyons M, (eds): "Genetic Issues in Psychosocial Epidemiology." New Brunswick, NJ: Rutgers University Press, pp 231–246.

Brooks-Gunn J, Duncan GJ (1997): The effects of poverty on children. Future of Children 7:55–71.

Buka SL, Earls FE (1993): Early determinants of delinquency and violence. Health Affairs 12:46–64.

Buka SL, Lipsitt LP, Tsuang MT (1993): Perinatal complications and psychiatric diagnosis. Arch Gen Psychiatry 50:151–156.

Buka SL, Stichick TL, Birdthistle I, Earls FJ (2001): Youth exposure to violence: prevalence, risks and consequences. Am J Orthopsychiatry 71:298–310.

Burns BJ, Costello EJ, Angold A, Tweed DL, Stangl DK, Farmer EMZ, Erkanli A (1995): Childrens mental health service use across service sectors. Health Affairs 14:147–159.

Cannon TD (1996): Abnormalities of brain structure and function in schizophrenia: implications for aetiology and pathophysiology. Finnish Med Soc Ann Med 28:533–539.

Chabra A, Chavez GF, Harris ES (1999): Mental illness in elementary-school-aged children. Western J Med 170:28–34.

Costello EJ, Angold A, Burns BJ, Erkanli A, Stangl DK, Tweed DL (1996a): The Great Smoky Mountains study of youth: functional impairment and severe emotional disturbance. Arch Gen Psychiatry 53:1137–1143.

Costello EJ, Angold A, Burns BJ, Stangl DK, Tweed DL, Erkanli A, Worthman CM (1996b): The Great Smoky Mountains study of youth: Goals, design, methods and the prevalence of DSM-III-R disorders. Arch Gen Psychiatry 53:1129–1136.

Costello EJ, Messer SC, Bird HR, Cohen P, Reinherz HZ (1998): The prevalence of serious emotional disturbance: A re-analysis of community studies. J Child Family Studies 7:411–432.

Costello EJ, Edelbrock CS, Dulcan MK, Kalas R, Klaric SH (1984): Report on the NIMH Diagnostic Interview Schedule for Children (DISC): Pittsburgh, PA: Department of Psychiatry, University of Pittsburgh.

Day NL (1995a): Alcohol use, abuse, and dependence. In Tsuang M, Tohen M, Zahner G (eds): "Textbook in Psychiatric Epidemiology." New York: Wiley, pp 345–360.

Day NL (1995b): Research on the effects of prenatal alcohol exposure—a new direction. Am J Public Health 85:1614–5.

Dohrenwend BP, Levav I, Shrout PE, Schwartz S, Naveh G, Link BG, Skodol AE, Stueve A (1992): Socioeconomic status and psychiatric disorders: The causation-selection issue 255:946–52.

Earls F (1980a): Epidemiologic methods for research in child psychiatry. In Earls F (ed): "Studies of Children." New York: Prodist, pp 145–180.

Earls F (1980b): Prevalence of behavior problems in 3-year-old children. A cross-national replication. Arch Gen Psychiatry 37:1153–7.

Earls F, Buka SL (1997): Project on Human Development in Chicago Neighborhoods: Technical Report . Rockville, MD: National Institute of Justice.

Faraone SV, Biederman J (1994): Genetics of attention-deficit hyperactivity disorder. Child Adolesc Psychiatric Clin North America 3:285–302.

Faris REL, Dunham HW (1939): "Mental Disorders in Urban Areas: An Ecological Study of Schizophrenia and Other Psychoses." Chicago: University of Chicago Press.

Fisher P, Shaffer D, Piacentini J, et al. (1993): Sensitivity of the Diagnostic Interview Schedule for Children, 2nd ed. (DISC 2.1) for specific diagnoses of children and adolescents. J American Acad Child Adolesc Psychiatry 32:666–673.

Friedman EH (1997): Behavioral inhibition, attachment, and anxiety in children of mothers with anxiety disorder. Canad J Psychiatry 42:980.

Friedman RM, Katz-Leavy JW, Manderscheid RW, Sondheimer DL (1996): Prevalence of serious emotional disturbance in children and adolescents. In Manderscheid RW, Sonnerschein MA (eds). "Mental Health, United States." Rockville, MD: SAMHSA, Center for Mental Health Services, pp 71–89.

Geddes JR, Lawrie SM (1995): Obstetric complications and schizophrenia: A meta-analysis. Br J Psychiatry 67:786–793.

Gillis JJ, Gilger JW, Pennington BF, Defires JC (1992): Attention deficit disorder in reading-disabled twins: Evidence for a genetic etiology. J Abn Child Psychology 20:303–315.

Graham P, Rutter M (1968): The reliability and validity of the psychiatric assessment of the child: II. Interview with the parent. Br J Psychiatry, 114:581–592.

Hawkins DJ, Catalano RF, Miller JY (1992): Risk and protective factors for alcohol and other drug problems in adolescence and early adulthood: Implications for substance abuse prevention. Psycholo Bull 112:64–105.

Herjanic B, Hudson R, Kotloff K (1976): Does interviewing harm children? Res Commun Psychology, Psychiatry Behavior 4:523–531.

Hultman CM, Ohman A, Cnattingius S, Wieselgren IM, Lindstrom LH (1997): Prenatal and neonatal risk factors for schizophrenia. Br J Psychiatry 170:128–133.

Ingham JG, Miller P (1976): The concept of prevalence applied to psychiatric disorders and symptoms. Psycholo Med 6:217–225.

Jackson C (1997): Initial and experimental stages of tobacco and alcohol use during late childhood: Relation to peer, parent, and personal risk factors. Addictive Behavior 22:685–698.

Jellinek MS, Snyder JB (1998): Depression and suicide in children and adolescents. Pediatric Rev 19:255–264.

Jensen P, Roper M, Fisher P et al. (1995): Test–retest reliability of the Diagnostic Interview Schedule for Children (Version 2.1): Parent, child, and combined algorithms. Arch Gen Psychiatry 52:61–71.

Kellam SG, Ensminger ME (1980): Theory and method in child psychiatric epidemiology. In Earls F (ed): "Studies of Children." New York: Prodist, 1980:145–180.

Kendell RE, McInneny K, Juszczak E, Bain, M (2000): Obstetric complications and schizophrenia. Two case-control studies based structured obstetric records. Br J Psychiatry 176:516–522.

Kessler RC, McGonagle KA, Zhao S, et al. (1994): Lifetime and 12-month prevalence of DSM-III-R psychaitric disorders in the United States. Arch Gen Psychiatry 51:8–19.

Kunugi H, Nanko S, Takei N, Saito K, Muray R, Hirose T (1996): Perinatal complications and schizophrenia. J Nervous Mental Disease 184:542–546.

Kuperman S, Schlosser SS, Lidral J, Reich W (1999): Relationship of child psychopathology to parental alcoholism and antisocial personality disorder. J Am Acad Child Adolescent Psychiatry 38:686–692.

Lahey BB, Flagg EW, Bird HR et al. (1996): The NIMH methods for the Epidemiology of Child and Adolescent Mental Disorders (MECA) study: Background and methodology. J Am Acad Child Adolesc Psychiatry 35:855–864.

Leventhal T, Brooks-Gunn J (2000): The neighborhoods they live in: the effects of neighborhood residence on child and adolescent outcomes. Psycholo Bull 126:309–337.

Loeber R, Burke JD, Lahey BB, Winters A, Zera M (2000): Oppositional defiant and conduct disorder: A review of the past 10 years. Part I. J Am Acad Child Adolesc Psychiatry 39:1468–1484.

McClellan JM, Werry (2000): Research psychiatric diagnostic interviews for children and adolescents. J Am Acad Child Adolesc Psychiatry 39:19–27.

McConaughy SH, Stanger C, Achenbach TM (1992): Three-year course of behavioral/emotional problems in a national sample of 4 to 16-year olds. I. Agreement among informants. J Am Acad Child Adolesc Psychiatry 31:932–940.

Melton GB (1992): It's time for neighborhood research and action. Child Abuse Neglect 16:909–913.

Mental Measurements Year book (14th Ed.) Eds: Barbara S. Plake and James C. Impara (2001): University of Nebraska Press.

Milberger S, Biederman J, Faraone SV, Chen L, Jones J (1996): Is maternal smoking during pregnancy a risk factor for attention deficit hyperactivity disorder in children? Am J Psychiatry 153:1138–1142.

Molnar BE, Buka SL, Kessler RC (2001): Child sexual abuse and subsequent psychopathology: Results from the National Comorbidity Survey. Am J Public Health 91:753–760.

Murphy JM, Olivier DC, Monson RR, Sobol AM, Federman EB, Leighton AH (1991): Depression and anxiety in relation to social status. A prospective epidemiologic study. Arch Gen Psychiatry 48:223–229.

National Institute of Mental Health (2001): "Blueprint for Change: Research on Children and Adolescent Mental Health." Washington, DC: National Advisory Mental Health Council Workgroup on Child and Adolescent Mental Health Intervention Development and Deployment.

Offord DR, Boyle MH, Szatmari P, et al. (1987): Ontario Child Health Study II. Six month prevalence of disorder and rates of service utilization. Arch Gen Psychiatry 44:832–836.

Orvaschel H (1985): Psychiatric interviews suitable for use in research with children and adolescents. Psychopharmacol Bull 21:737–745.

Price RA, Kidd KK, Cohen DJ, Pauls DL, Leckman JF (1985): A twin study of Tourette syndrome. Arch Gen Psychiatry 42:815–820.

Raine A (1993): Features of borderline personality and violence. J Clin Psycholo 49:277–281.

Reardon SF, Brennan R, Buka SL (2001): Does neighborhood context affect age of onset of cigarette use? Multiv Behavioral Res (in press).

Reich W (2000): Diagnostic Interview for Children and Adolescents (DICA). J Am Acad Child Adolesc Psychiatry 39:59–66.

Reich W, Kaplan K (1994): The effects of psychiatric and psychosocial interviews on children. Comprehensive Psychiatry 35:50–53.

Rosenbaum JF, Biederman J, Hirshfeld DR, Bolduc EA, Chaloff J. (1991): Behavioral inhibition in children: A possible precursor to panic disorder or social phobia. J Clin Psychiatry 52:Suppl:5–9.

Rutter M, Cox A, Tupling C, Berger M, Yule W (1975): Attainment and adjustment in two geographic areas: I. The prevalence of psychiatric disorder. Br J Psychiatry 126:493–509.

Rutter M, Graham P. (1968): The reliability and validity of the psychiatric assessment of the child. I. Interview with the child. Br J Psychiatry 114:563–579.

Rutter M, Quinton D (1977): Psychiatric disorder: ecological factors and concepts of causation. In McGurk H (ed.): "Ecological Factors in Human Development." Amsterdam: North-Holland, pp 173–187.

Rutter M, Yule B, Quinton D, Rowlands O, Yule W, Berger M (1975): Attainment and Adjustment in two geographic areas. III. Some factors accounting for area differences. Br J Psychiatry 126:520–533.

Sampson RJ, Raudenbush SW, Earls F (1997): Neighborhoods and violent crime: a multilevel study of collective efficacy. Science 277:918–924.

Schwab-Stone ME, Shaffer D, Dulcan MK, et al. (1996): Criterion validity of the NIMH Diagnostic Interview Schedule for Children Version 2.3 (DISC 2.3). J Am Acad Child Adolesc Psychiatry 35:865–877.

Shaffer D, Schwab-Stone ME, Fisher P, et al. (1993): The Diagnostic Interview Schedule for Children—Revised Version (DISC-R), I: Preparation, field testing, interrater reliability, and acceptability, J Am Acad Child Adolesc Psychiatry 32:643–650.

Shaffer D, Fisher P, Dulcan MK, et al. (1996): The NIMH Diagnostic Interview Schedule for Children Version 2.3 (DISC 2.3): Description, acceptability, prevalence rates, and performance in the MECA study. J Am Acad Child Adolesc Psychiatry 35:865–877.

Shaffer D, Fisher P, Lucas, CP et al. (2000): NIMH Diagnostic Interview Schedule for Children Version IV (NIMH DISC-IV): Description, differences from previous versions, and reliability of some common diagnoses. J Am Acad Child Adolesc Psychiatry 39:28–38.

Sherrill JT, Kovacs M (2000): Interview Schedule for Children and Adolescents (ISCA). J Am Acad Child Adolesc Psychiatry 39:67–75.

Smith GN, Honer WG, Kopala L, MacEwan GW, Altman S, Smith A (1995): Obstetric complications and severity of illness in schizophrenia. Schizophrenia Res 14:113–120.

State MW, Lombroso PJ, Pauls DL, Leckman JF (2000): The genetics of childhood psychiatric disorders: A decade of progress. J Am Acad Child Adolesc Psychiatry 39:946–962.

Steffenburg S, Gillberg C, Hellgren L, et al. (1989): A twin study of autism in Denmark, Finland, Iceland, Norway and Sweden. J Child Psycholo Psychiatry 30:405–416.

Steinhausen HC, Willms J, Spohr HL (1993): Long-term psychopathological and cognitive outcome of children with fetal alcohol syndrome. J Am Acad Child Adolesc Psychiatry 32:990–994.

Streissguth AP (1994): A long-term perspective of FAS. Alcohol Health Research World 18:74–81.

Sturm R, Ringel J, Bao C, Stein B, Kapur K, Zhang W, Zeng F (2001): National Estimates of Mental Health Utilization and Expenditures for Children in 1998. Journal of Behavioral Health Services and Research 28(3):319–333.

Turner SM, Beidel DC, Costello A (1987): Psychopathology in the offspring of anxiety disorders patients. J Consult Clini Psychology 55:229–35.

U.S. Department of Health and Human Services (1999): "Mental Health: A Report of the Surgeon General: Executive Summary." Rockville, MD: U.S. Department of Health and Human Services, Substance Abuse and Mental Health Services Administration, Center for Mental Health Services, National Institutes of Health, National Institute of Mental Health, 1999.

U.S. Department of Health and Human Services (2001): "Report of the Surgeon Generals Conference on Childrens Mental Health: A National Action Agenda." Rockville, MD: U.S. Department of Health and Human Services, Substance Abuse and Mental Health Services Administration, Center for Mental Health Services, National Institute of Health, National Institute of Mental Health, 2001.

U.S. Government (1993): "Federal Register" 58, 29425.

Verhulst FC, van der Ende J (1992a): Six-year developmental course of internalizing and externalizing problem behaviors. J Am Acad Child Adolesc Psychiatry 31:924–931.

Verhulst FC, van der Ende J (1992b): Six-year stability of parent-reported problem behavior in an epidemiological sample. J Abn Child Psychiatry 20:595–610.

Wamboldt MZ, Wamboldt FS (2000): Role of the family in the onset and outcome of childhood disorders: Selected research findings. J Am Acad Child Adolesc Psychiatry 39:1212–1219.

Wandersman A., Nation M (1998): Urban neighborhoods and mental health: Psychological contributions to understanding toxicity, resilience, and interventions. Am Psychologist 53:647–656.

Wechsler H, Pugh TF (1967): Fit of individual and community characteristics and rates of psychiatric hospitalization. Am J Sociology 73:331–338.

Weller EB, Weller RA, Fristad MA et al. (2000): Childrens Interview for Psychiatric Syndromes (ChIPS). J Am Acad Child Adolesc Psychiatry 39:76–84.

West MO, Prinz RJ (1987): Parental alcoholism and childhood psychopathology. Psycholo Bull 102:204–218.

Zahner GEP (1991): The feasibility of conducting structured diagnostic interviews with preadolescents: A community field trial of the DISC. J Am Acad Child Adolesc Psychiatry 30:659–668.

CHAPTER 24

Epidemiology of Mood and Anxiety Disorders in Children and Adolescents

KATHLEEN RIES MERIKANGAS[1,2] and SHELLI AVENEVOLI[1]

[1]Mood and Anxiety Program, Intramural Research Program, National Institute of Mental Health, Bethesda, MD; [2]Yale University School of Medicine, New Haven, CT

MOOD DISORDERS

Although researchers in the early and mid-1900s either denied the existence of depression during childhood (Rie, 1966) or believed that depression in children was masked by behaviors related to other childhood conditions (e.g., conduct disorder; Glaser, 1967), the existence of depression and other affective disorders in both children and adolescents has now been widely demonstrated in research and clinical settings (Rutter et al., 1970; Poznanski et al., 1976; Carlson, 1990). Since the early 1980s, hundreds of papers have been published on the phenomenology, assessment, magnitude, risk factors, and consequences of affective disorders first experienced in childhood and adolescence. Moreover, knowledge of the widely recognized biases of clinical samples of children has led to a substantial body of research in children selected from nonclinical samples. This chapter focuses on this body of work.

Definition and Assessment

In the research literature, the term "depression" describes a variety of related phenomena (Angold, 1988), including depression as a mood or affective state, a syndrome of symptoms, or a clinical disorder. These conceptualizations represent varying levels of impairment, different thresholds, and different approaches to measurement.

As an *affective state*, depression is characterized by the expression of sadness, unhappiness, or dysphoric mood. Depressed mood is often normative and has no conditions on the length of time it may last. Depressed affect is most often assessed with single-item or multi-item self-report checklists of emotions and

Textbook in Psychiatric Epidemiology, Second Edition, Edited by Ming T. Tsuang and Mauricio Tohen.
ISBN 0-471-40974-X

symptoms, employing Likert-type rating scales. Depression as a *syndrome* is defined as a constellation or pattern of behaviors and emotions that represent depression (Compas et al., 1993). Syndromes of depression may refer to subthreshold manifestations of clinical depression that fall below diagnostic criteria (i.e., shorter duration, fewer symptoms, or minimal impairment, e.g., Angst and Merikangas 1997); scores above clinical cut-points on scales and inventories (e.g., Child Depression Inventory, Center for Epidemiologic Studies of Depression Scale, Mood and Feelings Questionnaire) that assess diagnostic criteria; or an empirically derived cluster of anxiety and depressive symptoms (Achenbach 1991a, b, c). As a *disorder*, depression is conceptualized as a diagnostic category based on an already-identified grouping of symptoms (e.g., those established by the American Psychiatric Association or the World Health Organization) and the disability or impairment caused by these symptoms. Presently, affective disorders in children and adolescents are defined with the same criteria as those for adults, with minor exceptions as noted below.

Likewise, other affective states fall along a similar continuum. Subthreshold or hypomania, reflects an unusual pattern of behavior characterized by racing thoughts, grandiosity, and high activity levels that typically last for a short time, but that causes no notable impairment. Mania at the diagnostic level is characterized by changes in mood to euphoria or irritability, symptoms with impairment, and is often interspersed between episodes of depression.

Diagnostic criteria according to the *Diagnostic and Statistical Manual of Mental Disorders* (1994) defines two main groups of mood disorders–depressive disorders and bipolar disorders, each of which includes specific subtypes. The 10th edition of the International Classification of Diseases (World Health Organization 1993) has outlined similar categories and subtypes. Diagnostic criteria for all mood disorders are virtually identical for children and adults and are described in detail in this volume. The few exceptions include the following: in children and adolescents, irritable mood may be a proxy for depressed mood in the diagnoses of depressive disorders; failure to make expected weight gains may be a proxy for weight loss in major depression; and criteria for diagnosis of dysthymic disorder for children and adolescents requires a duration of one or more years, as opposed to two or more in adults.

Although it is generally agreed that the onset of bipolar disorder may occur during adolescence, the clinical manifestations and specific diagnostic criteria for bipolar disorder in children are controversial. A recent roundtable sponsored by the National Institute of Mental Health (NIMH, 2001) addressed the major issues regarding bipolar disorder in children and defined a research agenda for gathering evidence on the early signs, symptoms and course of bipolar disorder in youth. Most of the research presented in this chapter focuses on affective disorders, with reference to syndrome and mood only when relevant to discussion or when clinical data are lacking. Because of the dearth of information on bipolar disorder from community studies, this chapter will focus primarily on major depression and dysthymia in youth.

Magnitude of Mood Disorders

Although prevalence rates for depression were based previously on studies with small, unrepresentative, or primarily clinical samples of children and adolescents

(Gotlib and Hammen, 1992), larger, more representative, community samples and prospective cohorts have become increasingly available (see Table 1). Prevalence rates of major depression, dysthymic disorder, and bipolar disorder from 25 national and international studies (Anderson et al., 1987; Bird et al., 1988; Canals et al., 1995; Canals et al., 1997; Cohen et al., 1993; Costello et al 1988; Costello et al 1996; Deykin et al 1987; Feehan et al 1994; Fergusson et al., 1993a; Fleming et al., 1989; Frost et al., 1989; Giaconia et al., 1994; Goodyer and Cooper 1993; Johnson et al., 2000; Kashani and Simonds 1979; Kashani et al., 1983; 1987b; 1987a; 1989; Kessler and Walters 1998; Lewinsohn et al., 1991; 1993; 1995; 1998b; 2000a; 2000b; McGee and Williams 1988; McGee et al 1990; Newman et al 1996; Olsson and von Knorring 1999; Pine et al., 1998; Polaino-Lorente and Domenech 1993; Reinherz et al., 1993a; 1999; Rutter et al., 1970; Shaffer et al., 1996; Simonoff et al., 1997; Velez et al., 1989; Verhulst et al., 1985; 1997; Whitaker et al., 1990; Wittchen et al., 1998b) are listed in Table 2. Only studies that defined disorder according to standardized diagnostic criteria and that employed epidemiologic samples are included in these tables. Notably, there is wide variation in estimates of prevalence across studies. This is primarily attributable to methodological inconsistencies, such as use of different assessment instruments and sampling frames across studies (see Buka et al., in this volume).

Rates of Disorder

The most substantial amount of data on depression has been collected on the point prevalence of major depression. As evidenced in Table 2, point prevalence rates for major depression among school-age children (approximately 7–12 years) ranged from less than 1% (Costello et al., 1996) to 2% (Cohen et al., 1993; Kashani and Simonds, 1979; Polaino-Lorente and Domenech, 1993), with an average of approximately 1.5%. Point prevalence rates among adolescents (13–25) ranged from 1% (Fergusson et al., 1993a) to 7% (Garrison et al., 1997), with an average of 3.4%. Thirty-day prevalence in the National Comorbidity Study (NCS), the only nationally representative sample, was 5.8% (Kessler and Walters, 1998).

Rates for adolescents were somewhat higher in national compared to international studies. Six- and twelve-month prevalence rates ranged from 0.4% (Anderson et al., 1987; Costello et al., 1988) to 2.5% (Velez et al., 1989) in the three studies that assessed school-aged children, and from 3.6% (Verhulst et al., 1997; Wittchen et al., 1998) to 12.4% (Kessler and Walters, 1998) in 6 studies assessing adolescents. Twelve-month prevalence was higher for 21-year olds in the Dunedin study (Newman et al., 1996).

Lifetime rates of major depression in children were reported in only one study (1.1% at age 9; Kashani et al., 1983). Eight studies reported lifetime prevalence in adolescents; estimates ranged from 4.0% (Whitaker et al., 1990) to 24.0% (Lewinsohn et al., 1998b), with 15.3% in the NCS (Kessler and Walters, 1998). One-year incidence of major depression has been reported at 3.3% (Garrison et al., 1997) in adolescents ages 11–16 and 7.1% (Lewinsohn et al., 1998b) in adolescents ages 14–18.

Estimates of prevalence for dysthymic disorder follow this same general developmental pattern (i.e., rates are higher among adolescents than younger children); however, rates of dysthymic disorder were widely divergent across studies. Point

TABLE 1. Community Studies of Child and Adolescent Mood and Anxiety Disorders

Authors	Location	Wave	N	Age (years)	DX Criteria	DX Intv [a]	Period [b]
United States							
Bird et al. (1988)	Puerto Rico		386[c]	4–16	DSM-III	DISC	
Cohen et al. (1993)	New York State	T1	776	9–18	DSM-III-R	DISC	PT, 12M
Velez et al. (1989)		T2	760	11–20			
Pine et al. (1998)		T3	716	17–26			12M
Johnson et al (2000)							
Costello et al. (1988)	Pittsburgh		300[c]	7–11	DSM-III	DISC	12M
Costello et al. (1996)	North Carolina		1015	9, 11, 13	DSM-III-R	CAPA	3M
Deykin et al. (1987)	Boston		424	16–19	DSM-III	DIS	LT
Garrison et al. (1997)	Southeastern U.S.		359	11–16	DSM-III	K-SADS	PT
Kashani et al. (1987a, b)	Missouri		150	14–16	DSM-III (+tx)	DICA	PT
Kashani et al. (1989)	Missouri		210	8, 12, 17	DSM-III	CAS	PT
Kessler and Walters (1998)	United States		1769	15–24	DSM-III-R	CIDI	30D, 12M, LT
Kessler et al. (1994)							
Eaton et al. (1994)							
Magee et al. (1996)							
Wittchen et al. (1994)							
Lewinsohn et al. (1991; 1994; 1998b; 2000a, b)	Oregon	T1	1709	14–18	DSM-III-R	K-SADS-E	PT, LT
		T2	1507	15–19		LIFE	PT, LT
		T3	893[c]	24	DSM-IV	LIFE	PT, LT
Reinherz et al. (1993a; 1999);	Northeastern U.S.	T1	386	18	DSM-III-R	DIS	1M, 6M
		T2	375	21	DSM-III-R	DIS	LT
Giaconia et al. (1994)							
Shaffer et al. (1996)	Atlanta, New Haven, New York, Puerto Rico		1285	9–17	DSM-III-R	DISC	6M
Simonoff et al. (1997)	Virginia		2762 twins	8–16	DSM-III-R	CAPA	3M
Whitaker et al. (1990)	New Jersey		356[c]	13–18	DSM-III	Clinical Intw	LT
International							
Kashani et al. (1983)	Dunedin, New Zealand	B	189[c]	9	DSM-III	K-SADS-E	PT
Anderson et al. (1987)		T1	792	11	DSM-III	DISC	12M
McGee and Williams (1988)		T2	762	13	DSM-III	DISC	PT
Frost et al. (1989)							
McGee et al. (1990)		T3	943	15	DSM-III	DISC short	PT
Feehan et al. (1994)		T4	930	18	DSM-III-R	DIS-III-R	PT, 12M
Newman et al. (1996)		T5	961	21	DSM-III-R	DIS	12M
Canals et al. (1995; 1997)	Spain	T1	500	10–11	DSM-III-R		
		T2	290	18 (FU)	DSM-III-R	SCAN	PT
Fergusson et al. (1993)	Christchurch, New Zealand		1265	15	DSM-III-R	DISC	PT, 12M
Fleming et al. (1989)	Ontario, Canada		2852	6–16	DSM-III	SDI	6M
Bowen et al. (1990)							
Goodyer and Cooper (1993)	Cambridgeshire, England		1068 girls	11–16	DSM-III-R	DISC	PT, 12M 12M

TABLE 1. (*Continued*)

Authors	Location	Wave	N	Age (years)	DX Criteria	DX Intv [a]	Period [b]
Olsson et al. (1999)	Sweden		575[c]	16–17	DSM-III-R	DICA-R-A	LT
Polaino-Lorente and Domenech (1993)	Spain		1093[c]	8–11	DSM-III	CDRS-R	PT
Rutter et al. (1970)	Isle of Wight		2303	14–15	—	Clinical intvw	PT
Verhulst et al. (1997)	Netherlands		780[c]	13–18	DSM-III-R	DISC	6M
Verhulst et al. (1985)	Netherlands		116[c]	8, 11	DSM-III	CAS	
Wittchen et al. (1998a, b)	Munich, Germany		3021	14–24	DSM-IV	CIDI	12M, LT

[a]CAS = Child Assessment Schedule; CAPA = Child and Adolescent Psychiatric Assessment; CDRS-R = Children's Depression Rating Scale-Revised; CIDI = Composite International Diagnostic Interview; DICA = Diagnostic Interview for Children and Adolescents; DIS = Diagnostic Interview Schedule; DISC = Diagnostic Interview Schedule for Children; K-SADS = Schedule for Affective Disorders and Schizophrenia for School-Aged Children; SCAN = Schedules for Clinical Assessment in Neuropsychiatry; SDI = Survey Diagnostic Instrument (Boyle, Offord, and Hoffman, 1987).
[b]Prevalence definitions: PT = point, 30D = 30 days, 1M = 1 month, 6M = 6 months, 12M = 12 months, LT = lifetime.
[c]screened from larger population.

estimates were 0.1% (Costello et al., 1996) and 6.4% (Polaino-Lorente and Domenech, 1993; however, duration criteria were not applied) for children and ranged between 0.4% (Fergusson et al., 1993a) and 8.0% (Kashani et al., 1987a, b) among adolescent samples (see Table 2). Fewer studies reported 6-month and 12-month estimates. For children, estimates were 1.3% (Costello et al., 1988) and 1.8% (Anderson et al., 1987). For adolescents, rates were 2.3% (Verhulst et al., 1997), 2.9% (Wittchen et al., 1998), and 3.2% (Feehan et al., 1994). Lifetime estimates of dysthymia among adolescent samples ranged from 2.0% (Olsson and von Knorring, 1999) to 4.9% (Whitaker et al., 1990) with an average of 3.3%. One-year incidence rates have been reported at 3.4% (Garrison et al., 1997) in adolescents ages 11–16.

Manic episodes, bipolar disorder and hypomania are generally rare in children and adolescents. In the few studies reporting rates of these disorders, point, 12-month, and lifetime estimates ranged from 0% to 2.0% (Costello et al., 1996; Kashani et al., 1987a, b; Lewinsohn et al., 1998b; Pine et al., 1998).

Rates of Symptoms and Syndromes

Prevalence rates of depressed mood and symptoms derived from symptom checklists in community samples of children and adolescents suggest that depressed affect is more prevalent than depressive disorder. In the few studies of community samples of preadolescent children, prevalence rates ranged from approximately 10% to 18% (e.g., Kashani and Simonds, 1979; Rutter et al., 1986). Prevalence rates of depressed affect and symptoms among adolescents from the community ranged from about 21% to 50% (Petersen et al., 1992).

The prevalence of the anxious/depressed syndrome identified by Achenbach and colleagues and the depressive syndrome derived from the CES-D is estimated

TABLE 2. Rates of Depressive and Bipolar Disorders in Community Samples of Children and Adolescents

Authors	Age (years)	MDD[b, c]	Dysthymia[b, c]	Mania	Hypomania	Bipolar[c]
United States						
Bird et al. (1988)	4–16	5.9%[a] (I)				
Velez et al. (1989)	9–18	M: 2.3%, F: 4.7%				2.0% (T1 or T2)
Cohen et al. (1993)	11–20 (FU)	M: 1.6%, F: 4.2%				
Pine et al. (1998)	17–26 (FU)	M: 5.0%, F: 11.5%				1.4%
Johnson et al. (2000)						
Costello et al. (1988)	7–11	0.4%	1.3%	0%		0.2%
Costello et al. (1996)	9, 11, 13	0.03%	0.1%		0.1%	
Deykin et al. (1987)	16–19	6.8%				
Garrison et al. (1997)	11–16	T1: 7.0%	T1: 2.6%			
		T2: 5.4%	T2: 4.3%			
Kashani and Simonds (1979)	7–12	1.9%				
Kashani et al. (1987a, b)	14–16	4.7%	8.0%	0.7%		
Kashani et al. (1989)	8, 12, 17	1.5, 1.5, 5.7%				
Kessler and Walters (1998)	15–24	5.8% (30D)				
		12.4% (12M)				
		15.3% (LT)				
Lewinsohn et al. (1991;	14–18	2.9% (PT), 20.4% (LT)	3.2% (LT)			0.6% (PT), 0.9% (LT)
1994; 1998b; 2000a, b)	15–19 FU	3.1% (PT), 24.0% (LT)				0.5% (PT), 1.0% (LT)
	24 FU					0.6% (PT), 2.1% (LT)
Reinherz et al. (1993a; 1999)	18	2.9% (1M), 6.0% (6M)				
Giaconia et al. (1994)		9.4% (LT)				
	21 (FU)	10%				
Shaffer et al. (1996)	9–17	5.6% (I), 7.1% (noI)	7.2%[a] (I), 8.8%[a] (noI)			
Simonoff et al. (1997)	8–16	1.2% (I), 1.3% (noI)				
Whitaker et al. (1990)	13–18	4.0%	4.9%			

International						
Kashani et al. (1983)	9	1.8%, 1.1% (past)				
Anderson et al. (1987)	11	0.5%	1.8%[a]			
McGee and Williams (1988)	13	0.4%	1.6%			
Frost et al. (1989)						
McGee et al. (1990)	15	1.2%, 1.9% (past)	1.1%			
Feehan et al. (1994)	18	3.4%, 13.3% (past)	3.2%			
Newman et al. (1996)	21	16.8%	3.0%	2.0%		
Canals et al. (1997)						
	18	2.4%	5.8%		0%	
Fergusson et al. (1993a)	15	0.7% (PT) 4.2% (12M)	0.4% (PT)			
Fleming et al. (1989)	6–16	5.9%				
Goodyer and Cooper (1993)	11–16	3.6% (PT) 6.0% (12M)				
Olsson et al. (1999)	16–17	11.4%	2%			
Polaino-Lorente and Domenech (1993)	8–11	1.8%	6.4%			
Rutter et al. (1970)	14–15	1.5%				
Verhulst et al. (1997)	13–18	3.6%	2.3% (6M)			
Verhulst et al. (1985)	8, 11	8: M: 6.9%, F: 0% 11: M: 3.6%, F: 0%	8: M: 0%, F: 3.3% 11: M: 3.6%, F: 3.6%			
Wittchen et al. (1998b)	14–24	3.6% (12M) 9.3% (LT)	2.9% (12M) 3.0% (LT)		0.4% (12M) 0.4% (LT)	1.3% (12M) 1.4% (LT)

[a]Rate for any depression.
[b]I = with impairment; noI = without impairment.
[c]Prevalence definitions: PT = point, 30D = 30 days, 1M = 1 month, 6M = 6 months, 12M = 12 months, LT = lifetime, past = past episode.

at 5% in the normal population of both children and adolescents (Achenbach 1991c, d, e; Compas et al., 1993; Garrison et al., 1989). Rates of individual depressive symptoms in the Oregon Adolescent Depression Project (OADP) are given by Lewinsohn, Rohde, and Seeley (1998b).

Findings from cross-sectional studies of epidemiologic and clinical samples suggest a number of differences between children and adolescents in the prevalence of individual depressive symptoms. For example, preadolescent children are more likely to report somatic complaints than are adolescents (Kashani et al., 1989; Ryan 1987; Weiss et al., 1992). Other studies show that depressed children exhibit greater depressed appearance (Carlson and Kashani, 1988), less dysphoria, and less hopelessness (Ryan, 1987) than depressed adolescents. Depressed adolescents have been shown to exhibit a higher rate of hypersomnia than depressed children (Kovacs et al., 1989; Mitchell et al., 1988; Ryan, 1987) and more anhedonia, hopelessness, weight loss, and use of alcohol and illicit drugs, as well as greater lethality of suicide attempts (Garber, 1984; Ryan, 1987). Although Lewinsohn et al., (1998b) found no differences in rates of individual symptoms between those with onset before age 14 and those with onset after age 14, they did find that depressed adolescents are less likely to report weight or appetite changes and thoughts of death or suicide, and more likely to report feelings of worthlessness and guilt than adults in the ECA study (Lewinsohn et al., 1998b). Suicidal behavior is generally rare in the general population before the ages of 12–14 years (Rutter et al., 1986).

Comorbidity

Comorbidity between affective disorders and other disorders in children and adolescents has been documented extensively in clinical and community samples (see Angold et al., 1999; Brady and Kendall, 1992; Caron and Rutter, 1991; Merikangas and Angst, 1995a for reviews), suggesting that "comorbidity is the rule rather than the exception" in children and adolescents (Gotlib and Hammen, 1992) and that pure depression may be rare (Avenevoli et al., 2001; Lewinsohn et al., 1998b). Evidence from community samples of children and adolescents reveal that depression is associated with all major classes of disorders, including anxiety, behavior, eating, and substance use disorders (e.g., Gotlib and Hammen, 1992; Lewinsohn et al., 1993; Simonoff et al., 1997). Although most studies focus on either major depression or depression broadly defined (Rohde et al., 1991), those that examine dysthymia separately indicate that dysthymia is also comorbid with other emotional and behavioral disorders (Kovacs et al., 1994). Rates of comorbid conditions are generally lower in children and adolescents with bipolar symptomatology (Geller and Luby, 1997).

Anxiety disorders are the most common concomitant conditions with depression, ranging from approximately 20% to 75% in youth with depression drawn from community samples (median rate = 38.9%; median odds ratio = 20.3, range = 3.2–100.5, in Angold et al., 1999). Rates of depression in children and adolescents with anxiety disorders are generally lower, ranging from approximately 5% to 55% (median rate = 17.0%, in Angold et al., 1999). Lewinsohn et al., (1997b) reported that major depression was significantly associated with most of the major subtypes of anxiety disorder, including panic, separation anxiety, and overanxious disorders and social and simple phobias, but not obsessive–compulsive disorder. Rates of anxiety in youth with bipolar disorder are approximately 12% to 33% (Geller et al., 1995).

Conduct disorder is also frequently associated with affective disorders in community samples, with rates ranging from 0% to 83% (median = 27.3%; median odds ratio = 15.9, range = 1.4–52.5, in Angold et al., 1999) in youth with depression and approximately 20% in youth with bipolarity (Geller et al., 1995). ADHD and hyperactivity, broadly defined, are heavily comorbid with prepubertal-onset mania (Biederman et al., 1995; West et al., 1995; Geller et al., 1995). Associations between affective disorders and substance use disorders among children and adolescents are generally lower than associations between depression and anxiety and behavioral disorders, with rates ranging from 13% to 29% (Feehan et al., 1994; Newman et al., 1996; Lewinsohn et al., 1998b). An association between depression and somatic illnesses, particularly those involving the central nervous system (Rutter et al., 1976), such as migraine (Merikangas et al., 1990) have also been reported.

With respect to the temporal sequence of disorders, most evidence is based on retrospective reports of age of onset (Kessler and Walters, 1998), lifetime assessment in community-based studies (Lewinsohn et al., 1997b), family studies (e.g., Beidel and Turner, 1997), and clinical studies (Kovacs et al., 1989). Collectively, research suggests that conditions comorbid with depression typically onset prior to depression. Several longitudinal studies demonstrated that anxiety preceded the onset of depression in more than 60% of the persons with concomitant expression of the two syndromes (Orvaschel et al., 1995; Pine et al., 1998; Reinherz et al., 1989; Rohde et al., 1991). Simple phobia, separation anxiety, overanxious disorder, and social phobia all appear to precede diagnoses of major depression, whereas OCD and panic disorder may be more likely to follow the onset of depression (Lewinsohn et al., 1997b; Wittchen et al., 1999). There is also some indication that dysthymia is more likely to precede than follow anxiety (Lewinsohn et al., 1997b).

Studies assessing the average age of onset of anxiety and depressive disorders suggest not only a temporal relation between anxiety and depression, but a relation dependent upon developmental level. According to a review by Kovacs and Devlin (1998), anxiety disorders typically appear sometime during early to middle childhood (average age of onset across studies ranges from 6.7 to 11.3). Depressive disorders, in contrast, typically surface during early to middle adolescence (range = 10.8 to 14.9). In the vast majority of cases, the onset of conduct disorder precedes that of depression according to both retrospective and prospective studies (Kovacs et al., 1988; Harrington et al., 1991).

Substantial evidence reveals that comorbidity of affective and nonaffective disorders is associated with greater severity of depression. Adolescents with both syndromes have a greater number and severity of depressive symptoms (Mitchell et al., 1989; Kashani and Orvaschel, 1990), more severe anxiety symptoms (Strauss et al., 1988), a greater number of episodes of depression, more suicide attempts (Rohde et al., 1991); increased risk of recurrence (see Lewinsohn et al., 1991), longer duration of episodes, impaired role functioning (Lewinsohn et al., 1998b), and higher treatment and service utilization.

Risk Factors and Correlates of Mood Disorders

Gender. It has been well documented in national epidemiological studies that rates of depression are nearly 2:1 among adult females compared to adult males in developing countries (Culbertson, 1997; Merikangas, 2000). This finding holds for clinical diagnoses of major depression and dysthymia as well as subclinical levels of depressive symptoms (Nolen-Hoeksema and Girgus, 1994). Although this gender difference is not typically found in preadolescent children, rates of depression during adolescence are generally higher for girls than for boys.

Among preadolescents, researchers report either no gender differences in rates of depression (Angold and Rutter, 1992; Fleming et al., 1989; Kashani et al., 1983; Velez et al., 1989), or higher rates in preadolescent boys (e.g., Anderson et al., 1987; Nolen-Hoeksema and Girgus, 1994, Nolen-Hoeksema et al., 1991; Costello et al., 1988). During adolescence, however, rates of depression are greater among females than among males (Kessler and Walters, 1998; Cohen et al., 1993; Lewinsohn et al., 1993; McGee et al., 1990; Olsson and von Knorring, 1999; Reinherz et al., 1993a; Whitaker et al., 1990; Wittchen et al., 1998) with differences persisting into middle adulthood (Kessler et al., 1993).

Prospective studies of depression reveal that gender differences in the rates of depression emerge sometime during middle adolescence, around the age of 13 (Angold and Rutter, 1992; Ge et al., 1994; Hankin et al., 1998; Petersen et al., 1993; McGee et al., 1992; Nolen-Hoeksema and Girgus, 1994). In one study of 6th to 12th grade children, Petersen et al. (1991) reported that gender differences began to emerge in 8th grade, when children were 13–14 years of age. Similarly, in a longitudinal follow-up of a large community sample, McGee et al. (1992) reported a male to female sex ratio of 4.3:1 at age 11 and 0.4:1 at age 15. The change in the sex ratio is attributable to the increase in the incidence of depression among females after age 12. In the same birth cohort, Hankin et al. (1998) reported an even greater gender difference emerging between the ages of 15 and 18. Although rates of depression increase among both males and females during the middle adolescent years, the increase among females is far greater than that among males (Hankin et al., 1998). This is primarily explained by higher incidence rates among females across all ages between mid-to-late adolescence and not to a widening of the gender gap over time (Lewinsohn et al., 1993).

Most reviews of gender differences in rates of depression conclude that the sex effects are, at least to some extent, real and not fully accounted for by sampling or reporting bias (Merikangas, 2000a,; Merikangas and Pollock, 2000). Likewise, retrospective data from the National Comorbidity Study (Kessler et al., 1993) and prospective data from the Dunedin study (Hankin et al., 1998) showed no evidence that gender differences could be attributable to rates of recurrence among females. However, Lewinsohn et al. (1993) reported that females had greater relapse rates than males when evaluated prospectively. Additionally, two prospective longitudinal follow-up studies of children and adolescents have shown a greater stability of internalizing disorders in girls compared to boys (McGee et al., 1992; Feehan et al., 1993; Ferdinand and Verhulst, 1996), and a recent large-scale twin survey revealed that the sex difference in depression was minimal when the criteria for depression included impairment (Simonoff et al., 1997). Regardless of the conflicting findings, Piccinelli and Wilkinson (2000) argue that the inconsistencies across studies are nullified since lifetime prevalence rates are consistently higher in females after puberty.

A vast literature exists attempting to explain these gender differences. Among the leading contenders of factors explaining gender differences include adverse experiences in childhood, pre-existing anxiety disorders, sociocultural roles, vulnerability to life events, and coping skills (Nolen-Hoeksema and Girgus, 1994; Piccinelli and Wilkinson, 2000; Merikangas, 2000).

Much less evidence exists for gender differences in rates of mania, bipolar I and bipolar II. In the few epidemiological studies that reported rates of bipolar, rates were similar in males and females. Only Wittchen et al. (1998a, b) reported a female predominance of Bipolar II.

Age. There is great variability in estimates of age of initial onset of depression. Prior to the recent generation of studies of children and adolescents, estimates of the age of onset of depression were derived from retrospective studies of adults with depression (Angst, 1988) and suggested mid to late adolescence as the most common age of onset of first episode of major depression (Burke et al., 1990; Hammen and Rudolph, 1996; Lewinsohn et al., 1988), although the NCS suggests an average age of onset during early adulthood (i.e., 24 for men and 23.5 for women) (Kessler et al., 1993).

Longitudinal studies of treatment and epidemiologic samples of children and adolescents suggest an average age of onset between 11 and 14 years (Kovacs et al., 1984; Lewinsohn et al., 1993) for major depression and dysthymia. Evidence from prospective epidemiologic studies reveals a dramatic change in the prevalence of major depressive episodes after age 11 (McGee et al., 1992). According to incidence function of survival analyses in OADP, rates of depression onset increase from 1% to 2% at age 13 and from 3% to 7% at age 15 (Lewinsohn et al., 2000b). The incidence of depression continues to increase throughout early adulthood (Lewinsohn et al., 1986). There do not appear to be gender differences in the *average* age of onset of major depression in the NCS (Kessler et al., 1993).

Much less work has documented average age of onset of manic episodes and Bipolar disorders. According to retrospective studies, 20% to 40% of adults with bipolar disorder report that onset occurred during childhood (see Geller and Luby, 1997). A study of first admissions for bipolar depression in the United Kingdom revealed a dramatic increase in onset of bipolar among males and females after age 15 (Sibisi, 1990).

Social Class and Race or Ethnicity. Although studies of adult samples implicate social class effects on rates of depressive disorder and symptoms, findings from samples of children and adolescents are less consistent. Some studies assessing depressive disorders report a lack of association between depression and social class (Costello, 1988; Whitaker et al., 1990), while others report a significant association (Bird et al., 1988; Costello et al., 1996; Reinherz et al., 1993b). On the other hand, studies assessing depressive symptoms yield more consistent associations between elevated depressive symptoms and lower SES (see Fleming and Offord, 1990).

Most epidemiologic samples of children and adolescents are fairly homogenous and do not have the statistical power to test ethnic differences in rates of depression. The few studies that have compared rates across racial or ethnic groups yielded no differences in rates of disorder between Caucasian and African American children (Costello et al., 1988; Kandel and Davies, 1982; Kashani and Orvaschel, 1988) and between Caucasian and American Indian children (Costello et al., 1997). However, two studies reported higher rates of depressive symptoms in black adolescents (Schoenbach et al., 1982; Garrison et al., 1989, females only).

Familial and Genetic Risk. Despite the abundance of well-controlled family and genetic studies that have employed sophisticated methodology to investigate the transmission of affective disorders among adults, there are only a limited number of controlled family studies that have focused on the manifestation of affective disorders among adolescents. The results of family, twin, and adoption studies of mood disorders of adults have demonstrated conclusively that genetic factors are involved in the susceptibility to mood disorders, particularly bipolar disorder (Merikangas and Swendsen, 1996). The weighted average risk ratio (comparing the prevalence of mood disorders among relatives of cases compared to those of controls) for bipolar disorder among relatives of bipolar probands is 9.2, whereas the average risk ratio of major depression among relatives of bipolar probands compared to those of controls is 1.9. This indicates a very high magnitude of familial aggregation of bipolar disorder, similar to that found for many of the major diseases for which the genetic basis has been identified. In contrast, the average risk ratio for major depression among relatives of probands with major depression compared to those of controls was 2.0, indicating only a moderate influence of familial aggregation on nonbipolar mood disorders. Although sex, age, birth cohort, and socioeconomic status are differentially associated with major depression (greater risk among females, later birth cohorts, lower socioeconomic status), there is no evidence that they are differentially associated with the familial recurrence risk of mood disorders (Tsuang and Faraone, 1990; Merikangas et al., 1985).

Controlled family studies of adult relatives of children with depression as well as offspring of adults with depression provide consistent evidence that major depression has a strong familial component (Kovacs and Devlin, 1998; Beardslee et al., 1998; Neuman et al., 1997; Weissman, 1987). Children of depressed parents are three times more likely to have an episode of major depression than children whose parents are not depressed (Birmaher et al., 1996) and are four times more likely to develop an affective disorder (Lavoie and Hodgins, 1994). By the age of 25, children of affectively ill parents have a 60% chance of developing major depression (Beardslee et al., 1993). Risk to children is even greater when both parents exhibit a mood disorder (Merikangas et al., 1988). Studies of parents of children with major depression reveal a strong association between child and parent major depression (e.g., Puig-Antich et al., 1989; Williamson et al., 1995). Family studies assessing dysthymia suggest that dysthymia and major depression aggregate separately within families (Klein et al., 2001). Although several studies suggest that early age of onset is associated with increased familial aggregation of depression, the results of recent family and twin studies of youth conclude that prepubertal depression is less heritable than post-pubertal depression (Harrington et al., 1997; Silberg et al., 1999).

Controlled studies of offspring of parents with bipolar disorder exhibit wide variation in the frequency of affective disorders among offspring of affected parents (a range of 23% to 92%; Radke-Yarrow et al., 1992; Hammen et al., 1990), but collectively suggest a familial component. Rates of mania and bipolar disorder are generally low due to the young age of adolescent offspring in these studies; however, children of bipolar parents show greater specificity of transmission of affective disorders than do children of parents with unipolar depression (Merikangas and Angst, 1995a).

Although these studies provide evidence of familial influence in the etiology of affective disorders, they shed little light on possible mechanisms through which such factors may operate to produce affective psychopathology in children. Familial aggregation of depression may result from shared genes, common environmental factors, or a combination thereof.

The role of genetic factors underlying the familial aggregation of depression has been investigated by several twin studies of depressive symptoms and disorders among youth. Reports by Thapar and McGuffin (1994; 1995; 1997), Eley and Plomin (1997), Murray and Sines (1996), and O'Connor et al. (1998) conclude that there is a modest degree of genetic influence for childhood depressive symptoms, with greater heritability with age. However, some of these studies suggest that the age-related increase in heritability is limited to males, whereas the influence of the shared environment tends to increase with age in females (Eley and Stevenson, 1999). Finally, adoption studies of depression symptoms in children and adolescent found only negligible genetic influence (Eley and Stevenson, 1999; Van Den Oord et al., 1994).

Genetic factors may also play a role in the recurrence and stability of depression. The twin study of O'Connor et al. (1998) found that the stability of depressive symptoms over a three-year period was explained primarily by genetic influence; Silberg et al. (1999) found similar results among girls but not boys. Although a strong genetic component is implicated, O'Connor et al. (1998) warn that it is premature to accept the conclusion that the identified influence of heritability is, in fact, purely genetic, given that recent reports suggest strong and pervasive gene-environment correlations (e.g., evocation of stressful events based upon a genetic predisposition). Consistent with this, Silberg et al. (1999) found that individuals who inherited a genetic predisposition for depression also inherited a tendency to experience negative life events.

Although evidence suggests that the vulnerability for depression may be inherited, environmental stressors are likely necessary for the expression of affective disorders in offspring (Goldsmith et al., 1997; Warner et al., 1995). Indeed, the family environment of depressed adults is consistently characterized by family and parental discord, divorce, inattention, rejection, and abuse (Angold, 1988; Downey and Coyne, 1990; Rutter, 1989). Parker, Tupling, and Brown (1979) found that a parental discipline pattern of affectionless control was strongly associated with depressive disorders in adolescents; studies of bipolar depressives reveal normal parental levels on these dimensions (Parker, 1979). Community studies have documented associations between family dysfunction and depression in children and adolescents (Bird et al., 1988; Garrison et al., 1985; Kandel and Davies, 1982). These associations appear to be a reciprocal relationship between parental depression and child maladjustment (Downey and Coyne, 1990).

Hormonal Changes. Many of the biological changes associated with adolescence —including rises in levels of adrenal and gonadal hormones during the pubertal years—are related to increases in depressed affect and depression during this period. Negative affective tone has been linked to adrenal androgen levels among boys, and to follicle-stimulating hormone levels (FSH) among girls (Nottelmann et al., 1990; Susman et al., 1985). In addition, levels of testosterone and estradiol are both predictive of concurrent depressive disorder (Angold et al., 1999). Although the biological changes of puberty have been linked to concurrent depressed affect and, in some cases, the onset of depression, there is only indirect evidence regarding their relation to the stability or continuity of depression over the course of adolescence.

Although all adolescents experience hormonal changes during puberty, not all become depressed. This may be explained, at least in part, by examining whether and how hormonal change at puberty provokes changes in the adolescent's interpersonal world. For instance, studies of the relation between pubertal timing and depression indicate that early maturing girls experience more negative affect and internalizing problems (Graber et al., 1997; Petersen et al., 1991) and elevated rates of lifetime major depression (Graber et al., 1997) than do their average-maturing peers. Research also shows that pubertal maturation may interact with negative life events and psychosocial difficulties to explain increases in depression in adolescence, particularly among girls. Brooks-Gunn and Warren (1989), for example, found that negative life events, and the interaction between negative events and estrogen levels, accounted for much more of the variance in depressed affect than did variation in estrogen levels alone. Most of these studies are limited, however, by their focus on depressive symptoms and not disorder.

Neurobiologic Risk. Other biological factors in adolescence have been linked to depression as well. Although findings are less consistent in studies of children and adolescents than in studies of adults, research suggests that depression is related to dysregulation of neurotransmitters, sleep problems, and other neuroendocrine processes (e.g., Dahl et al., 1992). Additionally, there is preliminary evidence that the association between these factors and depression becomes more evident across the adolescent period (Dahl and Ryan in press). Although several other biologic parameters have been investigated among depressed adolescents, the studies have generally been small and inadequately controlled and have yielded inconsistent results. Studies of cortisol secretion, growth hormone, sleep electroencephalogram (EEG), and response to thyroid stimulating hormone provide mixed evidence regarding the biological underpinnings of adolescent depression. As in adult affective disorder, none has been confirmed as trait markers for depression (Kutcher and Marton, 1989).

Temperament. Specific temperaments or personality traits may also be associated with an increased risk of depression. Alternatively, such traits may constitute an early form of expression of depression or may be residual to depressive episodes.

In a prospective longitudinal study of 1,144 women, Rodgers (1990) showed that childhood neurosis was associated with adulthood psychopathology only in the presence of provocative events in adulthood. Kovacs and Devlin (1998) highlight that impairment in the ability to regulate negative affect, a trait that has at least some of its roots in aspects of temperament that are stable and observable long before adolescence, may be important for understanding the development of internalizing disorders and may explain the predictive validity of anxiety to depression. Individuals who manifest an internalizing disorder early in life may be at risk for depression during adolescence due to an underlying temperamental predisposition toward negative affectivity.

Cognitive Factors. Numerous studies have indicated an association between depression among children and adolescents (both in the normal population and in clinical settings) and a variety of cognitive factors including negative explanatory style and depressive attributional style (e.g., Seligman et al., 1984), tendency toward negativistic interpretations (e.g., Moyal, 1977), cognitive distortions (e.g., Haley et al., 1985), hopelessness (e.g., McCauley et al., 1988), and maladaptive attitudes (e.g., Nolen-Hoeksema et al., 1986). Moreover, research has consistently shown that depressed children display more cognitive errors, endorse more negative attributions, have greater external locus of control, and have lower self-esteem than do nondepressed children (Kandel and Davies, 1982; Kashani et al., 1983; Tems et al., 1993; Williams et al., 1989). Like biological factors, it appears that cognitive influences may act as predispositional factors that interact with exposure to stressful events to predict depression (Garber and Hilsman, 1992).

Despite the consistent finding that the presence of negative cognitions distinguish depressed individuals from those who are not, negative cognitions have not been shown conclusively to contribute to the onset or stability of depression. However, a recent study did find that adolescents with elevated levels of *both* dysphoric mood and dysfunctional thinking were at increased risk for recurrence of major depression (Lewinsohn et al., 1999a).

Life Events and Stressors. Exposure to stressful life events is one of the most widely studied risk factors for depressive symptoms and disorder. Numerous studies of clinical and community samples of children and adolescents have reported a significant relation between stressful life events and depression (e.g., Bird et al., 1988; Costello, 1988; Garrison et al., 1985; Williamson et al., 1995). The major events associated with depression in both retrospective and prospective studies are early separation from a parent by death or divorce, serious illnesses, and sexual and physical abuse (Reinherz et al., 1989; Roy, 1985). Many events and hassles associated with adolescence—including changes in family dynamics (Larson and Richards, 1991; Smetana 1995; Steinberg, 1988), friendships (Bukowski et al., 1993), romantic relationships (Monroe et al., 1999), and the transition from junior high school to high school (Isakson and Jarvis, 1999)—may also be stressful for some adolescents.

It appears, however, that adverse life events comprise nonspecific risk factors for depression. For example, Kendler et al. (1992) have shown that parental loss prior to age 17 years was significantly related to five of the six major psychiatric disorders investigated in their study of female twins. Similarly, Lewinsohn, Seeley,

Gotlib (1997a) found that daily hassles, major life events, and low social support did not distinguish those with depression from those with other disorders.

Studies assessing psychosocial stress as a predictor of the stability of depression have yielded mixed results. Many studies suggest that accumulation of negative life events is associated with subsequent depressed mood, syndromes, and disorder (e.g., Compas et al., 1989). In contrast, Lewinsohn et al. (1999a) argued that stressors are more important in predicting the onset of major depression than subsequent episodes of depression. Hammen (1991) has proposed a model of stress generation that suggests that stressful events generated by the depressed individual may trigger subsequent experiences of depression. Studies have shown that depressed children generate conflicts with parents and peers (Adrian and Hammen, 1993).

Persistence of Mood Disorders. According to a recent review of community and clinic studies, the average length of an episode of depression in children and adolescents is 7–9 months (Birmaher et al., 1996). However, comparison between community and clinical studies suggest shorter duration in nonclinical samples [e.g., 26 weeks (Lewinsohn et al., 1993, 1994)] than clinical samples [e.g., 36 weeks, (McCauley et al., 1993) and 44 weeks, (Kovacs, 1996)]. Longer episodes are typically associated with earlier onset (before age 15; Lewinsohn et al., 1998b). Mean length of dysthymic episodes is four years.

The stability of depressive disorders is typically assessed according to rate of recurrence, because clinical depression is episodic rather than unremitting over long periods of time. It is widely accepted that individuals who have experienced major depressive episodes are at increased risk for recurrence (Kovacs, 1996; Lewinsohn et al., 1994). The results of longitudinal studies of epidemiological samples suggest that children diagnosed with depression are likely to experience recurrences within a few years (e.g., Lewinsohn et al., 1993). In a review of longitudinal studies of clinical and epidemiological samples of children and adolescents, Birmaher et al. (1996) reported a cumulative probability of recurrence of 40% by two years and 70% by five years. Stability of depression appears greatest among those with early onset of depression, double depression a history of both (i.e., major depression and dysthymia) and other comorbid conditions (Kovacs et al., 1984) and when subthreshold levels are incorporated (Garrison et al., 1997). Follow-up of afflicted children and adolescents reveals that depressive disorder is characterized by considerable diagnostic specificity. In a review of internalizing disorders, Kovacs and Devlin (1998) concluded that youth who have a depressive disorder at one point are more likely to develop depression than another disorder at a subsequent point in time.

Although considerably less information is available on the stability of dysthymia, childhood onset dysthymia is associated with a more protracted course and increased risk for the development of major depression. Kovacs et al. (1984) estimated that 81% of children with dysthymia would develop major depression over time. Moreover, it is estimated that 20–40% of adolescents with major depression develop bipolar I within five years after onset of depression.

Emerging evidence on the stability of depressive disorders from childhood and adolescence to adulthood suggests some continuity of depression into adulthood. In a follow-up of clinically depressed children, Harrington et al. (1990) found that approximately 60% had experienced at least one recurrence of depression during adulthood. The five-year follow-up of the Oregon Adolescent Depression Project yielded evidence of considerable continuity from mid-adolescence to young adulthood (Lewinsohn et al., 1999b). In contrast, the prospective follow-up study of a New York cohort revealed that depression was more likely to switch to another disorder in adulthood than to remain stable over time (Pine et al., 1998). However, adult diagnoses in this study were based on the past year, thereby missing critical information on recurrence of depression during the interval period.

Depressed children and adolescents are at increased risk for more frequent and severe episodes of depression (Kovacs, 1996) and a more protracted course (Kovacs et al., 1984), and their social relationships and overall functioning remain markedly impaired even after recovery (Puig-Antich et al., 1985; Rao et al., 1995). Additionally, there is evidence suggesting that pre-pubertal depression is etiologically distinct from adolescent depression (Thapar and McGuffin, 1997; Silberg et al., 1999; Weissman et al., 1999). For example, there appear to be differences in both the specificity and risk factors for pre-adolescent and adolescent onset depression. Silberg (2000) suggests that genetic factors are associated solely with post-pubertal onset depression.

Consequences. The most severe consequence of depression in adolescents is suicide. Epidemiologic studies report rates of suicide attempts among adolescents between 3% and 15% (Lewinsohn et al., 1994). Forty-one percent of adolescents with depression in the OADP reported suicidal ideation and 21% of depressed youth in the NCS reported a suicide attempt (Kessler and Walters, 1998). Although depression is significantly associated with suicide attempts in adolescents, depression is rarely the sole disorder in suicidal adolescents (Hoberman and Bergmann, 1992). Comorbid substance abuse, anxiety disorders, and even personality disorders, when coupled with major depression, may be more predictive of suicide and repeated suicide attempts (Hoberman and Bergmann, 1992).

The other major consequence of depression in youth is the interruption of developmental tasks in the educational, social, and psychological spheres. Although not specific to depression, the most common sequelae of depression include impairment in school and work performance, relationships with family and friends (Reinherz et al., 1993b), and cognitive functioning (i.e., low self-esteem and dysfunctional attitudes). Thirty-six percent of depressed youth interviewed in the NCS reported that their depression interfered "much" in their lives and activities (Kessler and Walters 1998).

The long-term effects of interruption in social and psychological development and educational achievement have not been well established. It has been shown that depression during adolescence is associated with the following consequences in young adulthood: elevated level of stressful events; loss of social support from family and friends; low self-esteem; less satisfaction in life roles; lower income; lower educational aspirations, early marriage; early parenting, and decreased marital satisfaction (Gotlib et al., 1998; Rao et al., 1995). Recurrent depression is also associated with poorer long term outcome (Wittchen et al., 1998).

Treatment. Data from youth assessed in the NCS suggest that approximately 55% of those with lifetime depression seek treatment from a professional (Kessler and Walters, 1998). In the OADP, Lewinsohn, Rohde, Seeley (1998c) reported that 61% of those with major depression sought some kind of treatment. Wittchen

(1998b) reported that 24% of those with a single episode of depression, 40% of those with recurrent depression, 46% of those with dysthymia, and 35% of those with bipolar I or II sought treatment. Factors associated with service utilization include increased severity, comorbidity, prior history of depression, suicide attempt, academic problems, and female gender (Lewinsohn et al., 1998c; Kovacs, 1996).

ANXIETY DISORDERS

Anxiety is an ubiquitous human emotion. Its expression can range from a normal reaction to an acutely threatening stimulus to an anxiety attack with multiple physical sensations and fear of impending doom in response to an unknown stimulus. There are two properties that underlie the definitions of anxiety. It is generally unpleasant and future-oriented. It is distinguished from fear in that it either has no discernible source of danger or the emotion is disproportionate to the fear stimulus. Lader (1972) defines pathologic anxiety by subjective assessment of the individual patient that the symptoms are more frequent, more severe, or more persistent than those to which he or she is accustomed to or is able to tolerate.

Definitions and Assessment of the Anxiety Disorders

In this chapter, we consider the anxiety disorders as defined by the DSM-IV criteria including panic, phobias, and general anxiety. The major subtypes of anxiety include panic disorder (with or without agoraphobia), specific phobia, social phobia, and generalized anxiety disorder (GAD). Although obsessive–compulsive disorder and post-traumatic stress disorder are also included as anxiety disorders in the DSM-IV, they will not be included here due to differences in their prevalence rates and correlates. There are two additional subtypes of anxiety that are specific to youth: separation anxiety disorder and overanxious disorder. The DSM-IV did not include the category of overanxious disorder because of the purportedly substantial degree of overlap with GAD. However, as described below, there is emerging evidence that overanxious disorder does indeed provide coverage of anxiety disorder in youth who do not meet criteria for GAD.

Despite the biologic underpinnings of anxiety, there are no pathognomonic markers with which a presumptive diagnosis of an anxiety disorder may be made. Therefore, information for assessing the diagnostic criteria for anxiety disorders are strictly based on either a direct clinical interview or observation of objective manifestations of anxiety. Because of the broad meaning of the term "anxiety," numerous measures of anxiety have been employed. The most commonly used assessments include self-report checklists of both state and trait anxiety (e.g., State-Trait Anxiety Inventory, Spielberger et al., 1983); fears (Revised Fear Survey Schedule for Children, Ollendick et al., 1985); anxiety factors (Multidimensional Anxiety Scale for Children, March et al., 1997), as well as clinician-administered symptom checklists (e.g. Anxiety Rating for Children—Revised, Bernstein et al., 1996). In addition, the major structured and semistructured diagnostic interviews assess the diagnostic criteria for anxiety disorders. These include the lay interviewer administered Diagnostic Interview Schedule for Children (DISC) (Shaffer et al., 1996) and the clinician administered semistructured Schedule for Affective Disorders and Schizophrenia for School-Age Children Kiddie-(SADS) (Chambers et al., 1985); and the Diagnostic Interview for Children and Adolescents—Revised (DICA-R) (Welner and Rice, 1988, Welner et al., 1987). The Anxiety Disorders Interview Schedule for Children (Silverman et al., 1988) is the most comprehensive diagnostic interview of anxiety disorders for youth.

Several psychophysiologic indicators of anxiety have also been used in both adults and children. Experimental models which induce stress and measure autonomic output to test the human "fight or flight" response to threat have been used to study the range of triggers, correlates, and responses to fear-provoking situations. Behavioral tasks such as giving a speech or response to novelty, have been used to experimentally induce anxiety states in normals as well as those with anxiety disorders. Measures of changes in pulse, galvanic skin response, heart rate, and temperature regulation, as well as self-reported changes and observations of facial expressions, blushing, and other overt signs of anxiety are presumed to provide a more accurate depiction of anxiety than self-reports or interviews about typical response patterns to stress.

Magnitude of Anxiety Disorders

Table 3 presents the rates of anxiety disorders in children and adolescents in community surveys which applied either DSM-III-R or DSM-IV criteria (Anderson et al., 1987; Bird et al., 1988; Bowen et al., 1990; Canals et al., 1995, 1997; Cohen et al., 1993; Costello et al., 1996, 1988a, b; Feehan et al., 1993; Fergusson et al., 1993a; Kashani et al., 1987a; Kessler et al., 1994; Lewinsohn et al., 1993; Magee et al., 1996; McGee et al., 1990; Newman et al., 1996; Pine et al., 1998; Reinherz et al., 1993a; Simonoff et al., 1997; Velez et al., 1989; Verhulst et al., 1985; Whitaker et al., 1990; Wittchen et al 1994; 1998). Similar to community studies of adults, anxiety disorders are the most common disorder in the general population. However, there is a wide range in prevalence rates according to the specific anxiety subtypes as well as according to the study methodology. In general, approximately 20% of youth suffer from one of the anxiety disorders, and half as many have impairment in functioning resulting from anxiety or phobias (Shaffer et al 1996). The most common anxiety disorder is specific phobia (8%); followed by social phobia (5%), GAD (4%), and about 1–2% for all of the other anxiety disorders. Panic disorders were extremely rare; most of the community studies identified no cases of panic disorders among youth.

The findings vary dramatically by the source of information and age of the index child. However, no consistent trends emerge in terms of the direction of the differences between informants. For example, Fergusson et al (1993b) found that parents generally reported slightly higher rates of GAD and phobic states than did their 15 year old offspring, whereas Kashani et al. (1987a) found that across all ages from 8–17, the child report yielded substantially greater rates of disorder than the parental report. In the Methods for the Epidemiology of Child and Adolescent Mental Disorders study (Schaffer et al., 1996), informant differences for symptoms alone or those with impairment did not exhibit large differences. There was a weak trend for youth to report higher rates of anxiety than parents. With respect to prevalence period, there were no large differences between lifetime and 12- or

TABLE 3. Rates of Anxiety Disorders in Community Samples of Children and Adolescents

Study	Age (yeatrs)	Anxiety				Phobias			Total
		SAD	OAD	GAD	Panic Dx	Specific	Social	Agoraphobia	
United States									
Bird et al. (1988)	4–16	4.7%				2.6%			
Cohen et al. (1993)	9–18	M: 7.7%		M: 0%	M: 7.7%	M: 6.7%			
Velez et al. (1989)		F: 9.5%	F: 18.0%		F: 0%	F: 17.8%	F: 10.1%		
Pine et al. (1998)	11–20	M: 3.7%	M: 5.8%		M: 0%	M: 3.7%	M; 6.8%		
		F: 3.7	F: 10.3%		F: 0%	F: 8.2%	F: 12.6%		
	17–26			M: 2.2%	M: 0.3%	M: 12.0%	M: 1.7%		
				F: 7.8%	F: 1.7%	F: 32.1%	F: 9.5%		
Costello et al. (1988)	7–11	4.1%	4.6%		0%	9.2%	1.0%	1.2%	15.4%
Costello et al. (1996)	9, 11, 13	3.5%	1.4%	1.7%	0%	0.3%	0.6%	0%	5.7%
Kashani et al. (1987a)	14–16	4.1%				9.1%			8.7%
Kashani et al. (1989)	8, 12, 17								25.7, 15.7, 21.4%
Kessler (1994)	15–24			0.8% (30D)	1.9% (30D)	6.2% (30D)	7.3% (30D)	3.0% (30D)	
Eaton et al. (1994)				1.4% (12M)		10.8% (LT)	14.9% (LT)	7.7% (LT)	
Magee et al. (1996)				2.0% (LT)					
Wittchen et al. (1994)									
Lewinsohn et al. (1993)	14–18	0.2% (PT)	0.5% (PT)		0.4% (PT)	1.4% (PT)	0.9%	0.4% (PT)	3.2%
	15–19	0.1% (PT)	0.1% (PT)		0.3% (PT)	0.5% (PT)	0.2% (PT)	0.1% (PT)	1.3% (PT)
		4.3% (LT)	1.2% (LT)		1.2% (LT)	2.1% (LT)	1.5% (LT)	0.6% (LT)	9.2% (LT)
Shaffer et al. (1996)		6.5% (I)	11.4% (I)		21.6% (I)	15.1% (I)	6.5% (I)	6.5% (I)	39.5% (I)
		5.8% (noI)	7.7% (noI)		3.3% (noI)	7.6% (noI)	4.8% (noI)	4.8% (noI)	39.5% (I)
Simonoff et al. (1997)	8–16	1.5% (I)	4.4% (I)			4.4% (I)	2.5% (I)	1.1% (I)	
		7.2% (noI)	10.8% (noI)			21.2% (noI)	8.4% (noI)	2.7% (noI)	
Whitaker et al. (1990)	13–18			3.7%	0.6%				

International									
Anderson et al. (1987)	11	3.5%	2.9%			2.4%	0.9%		7.4%
McGee et al. (1990)	15	2.0%	5.9%			3.6%	1.1%		10.7%
Feehan et al. (1994)	18			1.8%	0.8%	6.1%	11.1%	4.0%	
Newman et al. (1996)	21			1.9%	0.6%	8.4%	9.7%	3.8%	
Bowen et al. (1990)	12–16	3.6%	2.4%						
Offord et al. (1989)	14–17			3.7%	0.6%				
Canals et al. (1995);	10–11								
(1997)	18			0%	0.3%	1.7%		0.7%	2.7%
Fergusson et al. (1993a)	15	0.5%	2.1%	1.7%		1.3%	0.7%		12.8%
Verhulst et al. (1997)	13–18	1.8%	3.1%	1.3%	0.4%	12.7%	9.2%	2.6%	23.5%
Wittchen et al. (1998)	14–24	—	—	4.3% (12M)	1.2% (12M)	1.8% (12M)	2.6% (12M)	1.6% (12M)	9.3% (12M)
				0.8% (LT)	1.6% (LT)	2.3% (LT)	3.5% (LT)	2.6% (LT)	14.4% (LT)

[a]I = with impairment; noI = without impairment.
[b]Prevalence definitions: PT = point, 30D = 30 days, 1M = 1 month, 6M = 6 months, 12M = 12 months, LT = lifetime.

6-month prevalence rates for most of the anxiety disorders (Lewinsohn et al., 1993; Reinherz et al., 1993a; Wittchen et al., 1998).

Patterns of Psychiatric Comorbidity

Comorbidity between anxiety disorders and other DSM-III-R or DSM-IV disorders are even more common in adolescents than in adults (Lewinsohn et al., 1993; Rohde et al., 1996). Anxiety disorders are associated with all of the other major classes of disorders including depression, disruptive behaviors, eating disorders, and substance use. In the Virginia Twin Study of Adolescent Behavioral Development (VTSABD), there was a significant degree of overlap within the subtypes of anxiety disorders as well as with depression. However, there was little overlap between anxiety disorders and behavior disorders (Simonoff et al., 1997). In older adolescents, anxiety disorders are more strongly associated with regular substance use including cigarettes, alcohol, and illicit substances in girls than in boys (Kandel et al., 1997). A review of comorbidity of anxiety and depression by Brady and Kendall (1992) suggests that anxiety and depression may be part of developmental sequence in which anxiety is expressed earlier in life than depression. Thus, although comorbidity between anxiety and both depression and substance problems is quite common in children and adolescents, further research on the mechanisms for links between specific disorders is necessary.

The magnitude of comorbidity in adults and adolescents with anxiety suggests that investigation of the role of other disorders in enhancing the risk for the development of anxiety disorders may be fruitful. The difficulty in dating onset of specific disorders, particularly from retrospective data, diminishes our ability to determine temporal relations between disorders. Nevertheless, some prospective studies have examined the links between anxiety disorders and earlier expression of other forms of psychopathology. For example, whereas some studies suggest that childhood depression may presage the onset of panic attacks, the results of a fairly large prospective study suggest a bilateral temporal association between panic attacks and depression (Hayward et al., 2000).

Other disorders that may enhance the risk for development of anxiety disorders include eating disorders (Bulik et al., 1997), depression, and substance use and abuse. With respect to substance use disorders, Rao et al. (1999) found that anxiety disorders may comprise a mediator of the link between depression and the subsequent development of substance use disorders in a clinical sample. The potential mechanisms through which anxiety may be associated with smoking in adolescents were examined by Patton et al. (1998) who found that both anxiety and depression were associated with smoking initiation through increased susceptibility to peer influences.

Conversely, some research suggests that substance use may trigger anxiety disorders in susceptible youth. For example, a prospective study of a community sample revealed that post-traumatic stress disorder may be triggered by substance abuse in about 50% of the cases (Giaconia et al., 2000). Similarly, Johnson et al (2000) found that adolescent smoking predicted adult onset of panic attacks, panic disorder, and agorophobia. Thus, although comorbidity between anxiety and both depression and substance problems is quite common in children and adolescents, further research on the mechanisms for links between specific disorders both across and within genders is necessary.

Both family and twin studies have been used to examine sources of overlap within the anxiety disorders, and between the anxiety disorders and other syndromes including depression, eating disorders, and substance abuse. Fyer et al. (1995; 1996) have demonstrated the independence of familial aggregation of panic and phobias. With respect to comorbidity, whereas panic disorder, generalized anxiety and depression have been shown to share common familial and genetic liability (Kendler, 1996; Maier et al., 1995; Merikangas et al., 1988), there is substantial evidence for the independent etiology of anxiety disorders and substance use disorders (Merikangas et al., 1988; Smoller and Tsuang, 1998; Kushner et al., 2000). Similar results have emerged from studies of symptoms of anxiety and depression in youth in which both anxiety and depression was found to result from common genetic diathesis (Thapar and McGuffin, 1997; Eley and Stevenson, 1999).

Risk Factors and Correlates

Gender. Although there is abundant literature on sex differences in depression, there is far less empirical research investigating the male–female differences in anxiety disorders. Similar to the sex ratio among adults, there is generally a lack of gender differences in treated samples of children and adolescents (Craske, 1997). By contrast, studies of community settings reveal that the sex difference in anxiety disorders is already apparent at ages 9–12. The average female-to-male gender ratio across studies in this review is 2.3.

A comprehensive review of community studies for all anxiety disorders by Orvaschel and Weissman (1986) revealed that fears tended to be more common in girls than in boys across all ages but that worries showed no particular sex difference. Several more recent community-based studies of children and adolescents have shown that the rates of anxiety are greater in girls across all ages (Whitaker et al., 1990; Feehan et al., 1993; Fergusson et al., 1993a; Verhulst et al., 1997.) Lewinsohn et al., (1998a) reported that despite the greater rates of anxiety in girls across all ages, there was no difference between boys and girls in the average age of onset of anxiety (mean for girls = 8.0 $\pm$ 3.9; mean for boys = 8.5 $\pm$ 3.8). With respect to prevalence period, Lewinsohn et al. (1998a) found that as compared to males, females had greater rates of current anxiety disorders (i.e., 12.2% vs. 8.5%), past anxiety disorders (5.2% vs. 2.7%), and anxiety symptom scores on a dimensional rating (M = 1.9 vs. 0.9).

Age. Retrospective reports of adults with anxiety disorders suggest that the onset of anxiety disorders generally occurs in childhood or adolescence. Although there is substantial variation across studies, the results of prospective community-based research reveal differential peak periods of onset of specific subtypes of anxiety: separation anxiety and specific phobias in middle childhood (i.e., ages 7 to 9); overanxious disorder in late childhood (i.e., 10–13); social phobia in middle adolescence (i.e., 15–16); and panic in late adolescence (i.e., 17–18) (Last et al., 1992; Cohen et al., 1993; Costello, 1989; Pine et al., 1998; Compton et al., 2000).

Examining the age at which the sex difference in anxiety becomes apparent and concomitant changes in the risk factors and correlates of anxiety across the period of risk for onset, may inform etiologic pathways to anxiety disorders. Inspection of incidence curves reveals a sharp increase in girls beginning as early as age five with a continuously increasing slope throughout adolescence. Although rates of anxiety among males also increase throughout childhood and adolescence, the rise is far more gradual than that of females, and they begin to level off in late adolescence. Thus, by age six, females have significantly greater rates of anxiety than males. Despite the far more rapid increase with age in girls than in boys, there was no sex difference in the mean age at onset of anxiety or in its duration (Lewinsohn et al., 1998a).

Social Class and Ethnicity. Rates of anxiety disorders in adults are greater among those at lower levels of socioeconomic status (Horwath and Weissman, 1995). Several community studies have yielded greater rates of anxiety disorders, particularly phobic disorders, among African-Americans (Eaton et al., 1991). With respect to children, Compton et al. (2000) found that white children were more likely to report symptoms of social phobia, whereas African-American children had more separation anxiety symptoms. Pine et al. (1998) reported that phobias were greater among those at lower levels of social class. The reasons for ethnic and social class differences have not yet been evaluated systematically; however, both methodologic factors as well as differences in exposure to stressors have been advanced as possible explanations.

Familial and Genetic Factors

Family and High Risk Studies. The familial aggregation of all of the major subtypes of anxiety disorders has been well established (Merikangas et al., 1998c). The results of more than a dozen controlled family studies of probands with specific subtypes of anxiety disorders converge in demonstrating a 3 to 5-fold increased risk of anxiety disorders among first-degree relatives of affected probands compared to controls. The importance of the role of genetic factors in the familial clustering of anxiety has been demonstrated by numerous twin studies of anxiety symptoms and disorders (Kendler et al., 1993; 1996). However, the relatively moderate magnitude of heritability also implicates environmental etiologic factors.

Studies of children of parents with anxiety have become an increasingly important source of information on the premorbid risk factors and early forms of expression of anxiety. Increased rates of anxiety symptoms and disorders among offspring of parents with anxiety disorders have been demonstrated by Turner et al. (1987), Biederman et al. (1991), Sylvester et al. (1988), Last et al. (1991), Beidel and Turner (1997), Capps et al. (1996), Warner et al., (1995), Merikangas et al., (1998a) and Unnewehr et al. (1998). Table 3 presents the risk of anxiety disorders among offspring of parents with anxiety disorders compared to those of controls averages 3.5 (range 1.3–13.3), suggesting specificity of parent-child concordance within broad subtypes of anxiety disorders.

The high rates of anxiety disorders among offspring of parents with anxiety suggest that there may be underlying psychological or biological vulnerability factors for anxiety disorders in general which may already manifest in children prior to puberty. Previous research has shown that children at risk for anxiety disorders are characterized by behavioral inhibition (Rosenbaum et al., 1988), autonomic reactivity (Beidel, 1988), somatic symptoms (Reichler et al., 1988; Turner et al., 1987), social fears (Sylvester et al., 1988; Turner et al., 1987), enhanced startle reflex (Merikangas and Swendsen, 1999) and respiratory sensitivity (Pine et al., 2000).

Twin Studies. There are also several studies of twins that have investigated the role of genetic factors in the etiology of anxiety symptoms. In general, the correlation among monozygotic twins for anxiety, worry, and social fears was approximately 0.34 for monozygotic and 0.18 for dizygotic twins, suggesting moderate heritability of anxiety symptoms. Tests of genetic and environmental influences revealed that both the shared environment and shared genes contribute to anxiety and fear symptoms (Stevensen et al., 1992; Thapar and McGuffin, 1995; Topolski et al., 1997). There was no sex difference in heritability in most of the studies; however, several studies reported stronger genetic influences for anxiety among girls at younger ages (Legrand et al., 1999); however, others showed only minimal effects on anxiety symptoms at very young ages (Warren et al., 2000). Lichtenstein and Annas (2000) concluded that the shared environment was associated with fearfulness in general, whereas genetic influences seem to contribute primarily to specific influences for the different fears.

Several methodologic features of the studies had strong influence on the findings. For example, Eaves et al. (1997) found that the heritability of both separation anxiety and overanxious disorder was far greater for parent-reported rather than child-reported disorder. In addition, because most of these studies employed self-reported or parental-reported symptom checklists, the generalizability to anxiety disorders is not known.

Temperament and Personality

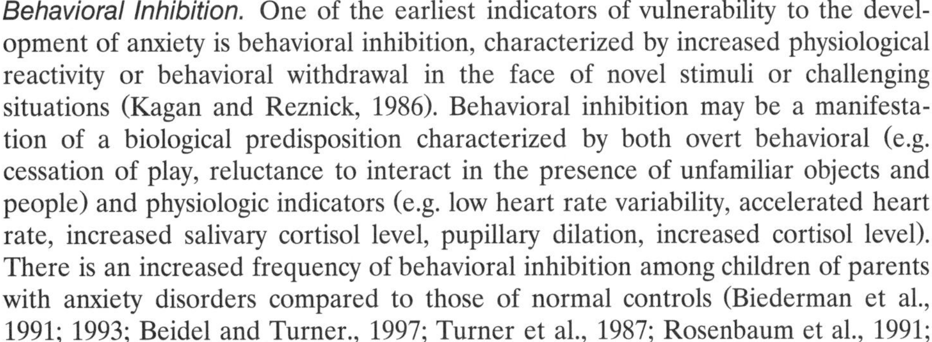

Behavioral Inhibition. One of the earliest indicators of vulnerability to the development of anxiety is behavioral inhibition, characterized by increased physiological reactivity or behavioral withdrawal in the face of novel stimuli or challenging situations (Kagan and Reznick, 1986). Behavioral inhibition may be a manifestation of a biological predisposition characterized by both overt behavioral (e.g. cessation of play, reluctance to interact in the presence of unfamiliar objects and people) and physiologic indicators (e.g. low heart rate variability, accelerated heart rate, increased salivary cortisol level, pupillary dilation, increased cortisol level). There is an increased frequency of behavioral inhibition among children of parents with anxiety disorders compared to those of normal controls (Biederman et al., 1991; 1993; Beidel and Turner., 1997; Turner et al., 1987; Rosenbaum et al., 1991; 1993; 1988; Sylvester et al., 1988).

Few studies have evaluated the differences in manifest inhibition and approach–avoidance in both clinical and nonclinical samples, leaving gaps in the conceptualization of the construct of inhibition. Some studies have shown that there is more stability of behavioral inhibition across early childhood among girls than among boys (Hirshfeld et al., 1992). The expression of behavioral inhibition studied prospectively may reveal patterns of anxiety symptomatology similar to those endorsed in adult populations. In a prospective study of a large community cohort of subjects from age 3 months to 13 years, Prior et al. (2000) found that maternal ratings of persistent shyness and shyness in late childhood were associated with the development of anxiety disorders in adolescence.

Anxiety Sensitivity. Anxiety sensitivity is another potential sensitive and specific trait marker for the development of anxiety disorders (Reiss et al., 1986; McNally, 1990; Schmidt et al., 1997). Anxiety sensitivity is characterized by beliefs that anxiety sensations are indicative of harmful physiological, psychological or social consequences (e.g. fainting or an impending heart attack). The misinterpretation of bodily cues that characterizes anxiety sensitivity may lead to a self-perpetuating "fear of fear" cycle. Of particular interest is the finding of the specificity of anxiety sensitivity with respect to development of anxiety disorders but not depression in a nonclinical sample (Schmidt et al., 1998). Likewise, Pollock et al. (in Press) reported that anxiety sensitivity appears to be specific to anxiety, as it did not contribute unique variance above self-rated anxiety symptoms in the prediction of depressive symptoms.

Anxiety sensitivity has been shown to be under genetic (Stein et al., 1999) and familial influence; anxiety sensitivity was found to constitute a potential premorbid marker for the development of anxiety disorders in high-risk but not low-risk youth (Pollock et al., in press). Prospective studies of youth have also demonstrated the prognostic significance of anxiety sensitivity in predicting the development of anxiety disorders. Based on the results of a five-year prospective study of adolescents, Hayward et al. (2000) concluded that anxiety sensitivity appeared to be a specific risk factor for the development of panic attacks in adolescents. These findings from prospective research, particularly the specificity with respect to anxiety, together with the importance of genetic and familial liability suggest that anxiety sensitivity is an important vulnerability factor that should be examined in future studies.

Perinatal Exposures. There is no evidence that either prenatal factors or delivery complications comprise risk factors for the development of anxiety disorders. The results of three studies that retrospectively assessed peri-natal events converged in linking such exposures to behavioral outcomes, but not to subsequent anxiety. For example, Allen et al. (1998) found that children who suffered from a variety of exposures ranging from prenatal substance use to postnatal injuries were more likely to develop behavior disorders, particularly attention deficit disorder and conduct problems, but not anxiety disorders. Likewise, the results of the Yale High Risk Study yielded no association between pre- and perinatal risk factors and the subsequent development of anxiety disorders (Merikangas et al., 1999).

Medical Symptoms and Disorders. Several studies have also suggested that there is an association between childhood medical conditions and the subsequent development of anxiety. Kagan et al. (1984) reported an association between allergic symptoms, particularly hay fever, and inhibited temperament in young children. In a retrospective review of pre- and perinatal and early childhood risk factors for different forms of psychiatric disorders in adolescence and early adulthood, Allen et al. (1998) found that anxiety disorders in adolescents were associated specifically with illness during the first year of life, particularly high fever. Taylor (1991) reported that immunologic diseases and infections were specifically associated with emotional disorders since children with developmental or behavioral disorders had no elevation in infections or allergic diseases. These findings suggest that it may be fruitful to examine links between immunologic function and the development of anxiety disorders.

The link between childhood allergies, eczema and behavioral inhibition was discussed by Kagan (1984), who proposed that the high levels of cortisol associated with anxiety may lead to immunologic sensitivity to environmental stimuli. Likewise, Allen et al. (1998) reported that adolescents and young adults with anxiety disorders were more likely to have suffered from infections during early childhood than others. The prevalence of high fevers in childhood along with diseases associated with the immune system were elevated among offspring of parents with anxiety disorders in the Yale High Risk Study (Merikangas et al., 1999). Taken together, these findings suggest future inquiry into the possible role of the immune system in anxiety states.

Prospective studies have revealed that the anxiety disorders may comprise risk factors for the development of some cardiovascular and neurologic diseases. Cohen et al. found that immunological illnesses in adolescents showed stronger associations with depressive as opposed to anxiety disorders. Haines et al. (1987), in contrast, reported that phobic anxiety was associated with ischemic heart disease, particularly with fatal ischemic events. Bovasso and Eaton (1999) employed cardiac and respiratory symptoms and illness to subtype panic attacks and their association with depression in a large community-based sample. They found that respiratory panic attacks were associated with the subsequent risk of myocardial infarction. Likewise, phobic disorder is strongly associated with migraine, with the onset of phobias predating that of migraine (Merikangas et al., 1998b; Swartz et al., 2000). The results of both family studies and prospective cohort studies suggest that there may be a subtype of migraine with shared liability for anxiety and depression (Merikangas et al., 1998b).

Autonomic and Psychophysiologic Reactivity. Autonomic physiologic profiles have been studied among children with behavior inhibiton (Kagan et al., 1995) and among individuals who face high risk for anxiety disorders due to parental anxiety disorders. In terms of family history, Bellodi et al. (1998) found similar temperamental and physiologic abnormalities among children of parents with panic disorder. Taken together, available data clearly delineate associations between acute anxiety and autonomic physiology profiles, but the implications of this work for the study of risk remain unclear. Moreover, the underlying assumption in this work posits an effect of perturbations in brain systems on both autonomic physiology and anxiety symptoms. As such, more work is also needed relating brain function to autonomic physiology.

Two studies have found startle abnormalities in children of adults with an array of anxiety disorders (Merikangas et al., 1999; Grillon et al., 1997); a third study found startle abnormalities in inhibited children, who face high risk for anxiety disorders (Kagan, 1994). In a high-risk study of offspring of parents with anxiety disorders compared to psychiatric and normal controls, the startle reflex and its potentiation by aversive states was used as a possible vulnerability marker to anxiety disorders in adolescent offspring of parents with anxiety disorders (Grillon et al., 1998). Startle was found to discriminate between children at high and low risk for anxiety disorders, as well as to discriminate between children at risk for anxiety compared to those at risk for alcoholism. However, different abnormalities in startle amplitude for high-risk males and females were observed. Startle levels were elevated among high-risk females, whereas high-risk males exhibited greater magnitude of startle potentiation during aversive anticipation. Two possible explanations for the gender differences in the high-risk groups were suggested by the authors: (1) differential sensitivity among males and females to explicit threat versus the broader contextual stimuli which are mediated by different neurobiologic pathways, (2) different developmental levels in males and females in which the vulnerability to anxiety may be physiologically expressed earlier in females.

Compared to the work on autonomic physiology, a larger body of research implicates abnormalities in respiration in risk or vulnerability for anxiety. Studies of asymptomatic adult relatives of patients with panic disorder (Coryell and Arndt, 1999; Perna et al., 1995; Griez et al., 1990; 1998) as well as patients with panic disorder with and without a family history of panic (Horwath et al., 1998; Perna et al., 1999) suggest that respiratory function serves as an index risk for anxiety, independent of any association between current state and respiratory function. Moreover, Pine et al. (2000) reported increased carbon dioxide sensitivity in children with anxiety disorders. Based on this work, abnormalities in respiration appear to provide some information on the vulnerability for anxiety states that are related to acute panic.

While these studies raise the possibility that indicate risk for anxiety may result at least partially from underlying neurochemical abnormalities, other studies are needed to confirm this possibility. For example, there are almost no studies of neurochemical function in high-risk youth, a key source of information regarding the underlying role of biologic parameters in the development of anxiety disorders. One exception is the study of Reichler et al, (1988) who assessed several biologic factors in their high-risk study of panic disorder including lactate metabolism, mitral valve prolapse, urinary catecholamines, and monoamine oxidase. Although none of these parameters discriminated high-risk from low-risk youth the lack of differences may have been attributable in part to low statistical power. Likewise, very few studies have compared neurochemical function in asymptomatic relatives of patients with and without anxiety disorders. Similarly, no studies have examined family loading for anxiety disorders in patients stratified in terms of their neurochemical functioning.

Life Events and Stressors. The role of life experiences in the etiology of anxiety states, particularly phobias and panic disorder, has been widely studied (Faravelli and Pallanti, 1989; Roy-Byrne et al., 1986; De Loof et al., 1989; Last et al., 1984). Life events have often been assigned a causal role in the onset of phobias, which are linked inherently to particular events or objects. More broadly, life experiences that to some extent threaten ones notion of safety and security in the world are often, at least retrospectively, perceived to trigger or precipitate the onset of anxiety disorders. In evaluating the evidence on the causal role of life experiences, it is critical to consider separately the subtypes of anxiety disorders. While it is likely that life stress may exacerbate phobic and generalized anxiety states, Marks (1986) concludes that phobic states resulting from exposure are far more rare than those that emerge with no apparent exposure. In contrast, post-traumatic stress disorder is defined as a sequela of a catastrophic life event.

The major impediment to evaluation of the causal role of life events in anxiety (or depression), is the retrospective nature of most research addressing this issue. For example, Lteif and Mavissakalian (1996) found that patients with panic or agoraphobia exhibited an increased tendency to report life events in general; this suggests that studies that limit assessment of life events to those preceding onset of a disorder may be misleading because they fail to provide comparison for the time period of onset. Moreover, stressful life events may interact with other risk factors such as family history of depression in precipitating episodes of panic (Manfro et al., 1996).

In terms of specific environmental risk factors, there has been abundant literature on the role of parenting in enhancing vulnerability to anxiety disorders. Based on Bowlby's (1960) theory that anxiety is a response to disruption in the mother–child relation, it has been postulated that maternal overprotection is related to anxiety, particularly separation anxiety. Using the Parental Bonding Instrument of Parker et al. (1979), several studies of clinical samples have found that adult patients with anxiety disorders recall their parents as less caring and more overprotective than did controls (Silove et al., 1991). These findings have been supported in nonclinical samples as well (Bennet and Stirling, 1998; Lieb et al., 2000). However, all of these studies caution that a causal link cannot be established because of the lack of independence of assessment of parent behaviors and offspring anxiety.

Another parental behavior that may enhance risk of anxiety in offspring is parental sensitization of anxiety through enhancing cognitive awareness of the child to specific events and situations such as bodily functions, social disapproval, the importance of routines, and necessity for personal safety (Bennet and Stirling, 1998). Bennet and Stirling (1998) found that subjects with anxiety disorders and those with high trait anxiety reported greater maternal and paternal overprotection and increased maternal sensitization to anxiety stimuli than controls.

Persistence. Anxiety disorders, particularly the phobias, tend to persist across the life course. However, there are major differences among the anxiety subtypes in terms of specificity and chronicity. Whereas the phobic states tend to be fairly stable and nonprogressive, generalized anxiety and panic tend to be less specific and less stable over time (Last et al., 1996; Pine et al., 1998).

Several follow-up studies of children and adolescents have shown that there is a high level of stability of anxiety disorders in general with some switching between categories of anxiety disorders over time (Cantwell and Baker, 1989; Ialongo et al., 1995). Newman et al. (1996) found that the stability of anxiety disorders from adolescence to adulthood was greater for anxiety disorders than for any other major diagnostic subtypes. Despite the high level of stability of anxiety symptoms, there are a substantial number of young adults who develop an initial episode of anxiety disorders after age 21 (Newman et al., 1996).

The stability of internalizing disorders in girls has been reported to be greater than that of boys in prospective longitudinal follow-up studies (McGee et al., 1992;

Feehan et al., 1993; Costello et al., 1993; Ferdinand et al., 1995). However, the results of other studies suggest a sex difference in the continuity of emotional problems. Bolognini et al. (1989) found that girls without emotional problems in childhood who developed new onset emotional problems in adolescence tended to have persistent problems into adulthood, whereas boys with emotional disorders in childhood tended to remit in adulthood.

A recent eight year follow-up study of a community sample of youth ages 9–18 at study entry provides compelling evidence for the stability of the subtypes of anxiety disorders (Pine et al., 1998). The stability of both social phobia and simple phobia was highly specific over time, whereas overanxious disorder was associated with major depression, social phobia and generalized anxiety in early adulthood.

Consequences

The majority of those with anxiety disorders in adolescence and early adulthood report significant impairment. The severe social consequences of anxiety symptoms and disorders are already apparent in grade school. Ialongo et al. (1995) reported that those children with anxiety in grade 1 tended to have lower academic achievement in grade 5 than those without anxiety. Prospective follow-up of adolescents with anxiety disorders by Woodward and Fergusson (2001) revealed that the life course outcomes were seriously impaired by anxiety disorders; adolescents with anxiety had greater risk for depression, illicit drug dependence, and failure to attend the university. Furthermore, the number of anxiety disorders was associated with increased severity of the outcomes. Despite the high magnitude of anxiety in the general population, less than one-third have sought treatment for their anxiety. The proportion of subjects with suicide attempts was higher than any of the other syndromes including depression, with the exception of eating disorders.

SUMMARY

Overlap Between Mood And Anxiety Disorders

Although this review considered the magnitude and risk factors for anxiety and depression independently, there is compelling evidence from prospective longitudinal studies, family studies, twin studies, and treatment studies that anxiety and depression have a common diathesis. There are now several reviews of comorbidity of anxiety and depression in youth that provide a comprehensive summary of the evidence for comorbidity as well as of the possible sources of comorbidity (Caron and Rutter, 1991; Angold et al., 1999). Their evaluation of methodologic issues, criterial overlap, common criteria, shared versus independent genetic and familial influences, and stability of course concluded that there is a common underlying genetic diathesis between anxiety and depression in general, but that there are also specific genetic and environmental factors that mold susceptibility to fear and anxiety.

Table 4 presents the risk factors for anxiety and depression divided by their unique associations with anxiety or depression as well as common risk factors that

TABLE 4. Vulnerability Factors for Anxiety Disorders and Depression

Both	Depression	Anxiety
Gender	Exposure to stress	Temperature:
Age	Pre-existing psychiatric disorders	Behavioral inhibition
Genetic/family history		Anxiety sensitivity
Temperament	Premorbid medical disorders:	Autonomic reactivity
Pre-existing medical disorders	e.g., migraine, diabetes	Respiratory function
		Premorbid medical disorders
Stress reactivity		e.g., asthma, allergies
Neuroendocrine factors		
Life events		
Parenting behaviors		
Family environment		

may influence either syndrome. This table illustrates the importance of considering each disorder alone, but also the importance of integration of research across anxiety and depression. There are numerous common risk factors for anxiety and depression, as well as several unique risk factors that affect one of the two syndromes specifically.

This chapter has reviewed the findings of community-based studies regarding the magnitude, risk factors, and consequences of anxiety and depression. Their magnitude renders these two syndromes as the most common mental disorders in the population. The persistence and serious social, personal, and economic consequences of the mood and anxiety disorders is alarming and highlights the need for intervention with these disorders on a community-wide basis. Although they are not as severe as schizophrenia and other major mental disorders, their high prevalence and associated impairment suggests that they should be a major target for early identification, prevention, and treatment.

The emerging neuroscience of mood and anxiety disorders and progress in classification and risk factor research should lead to major advances in our understanding of the mechanisms through which vulnerability to depression and anxiety subsequently translates into prevention and/or treatment. From a public health perspective, the devotion of substantial effort to enhance our understanding of the etiology of mood and anxiety disorders and to identify the most effective interventions would have major public health impact because of their high frequency and individual and community cost.

REFERENCES

American Psychiatric Association (1994): "Diagnostic and Statistical Manual for Psychiatric Disorders," 4th ed. Washington, DC: American Psychiatric Association Press.

Achenbach TM (1991a): The derivation of taxonomic constructs: A necessary stage in the development of developmental psychopathology. In Cicchetti D (ed), "Rochester symposium on developmental psychopathology: Models and integrations," Vol 3. Hillsdale: Erlbaum, pp 43–74.

Achenbach TM (1991b): "Integrative Guide for the 1991 CBCL/4 – 18, YSR, and TRF Profile." Burlington, VT: University of Vermont, Department of Psychiatry.

Achenbach TM (1991c): "Manual for the Child Behavior Checklist and 1991 Profile." Burlington, VT: University of Vermont, Department of Psychiatry.

Achenbach TM (1991d): "Manual for the Teacher Report Form and 1991 Profile." Burlington, VT: University of Vermont, Department of Psychiatry.

Achenbach TM (1991e): "Manual for the Youth Self-Report and 1991 Profile." Burlington, VT: University of Vermont, Department of Psychiatry.

Adrian C, Hammen C (1993): Stress exposure and stress generation in children of depressed mothers. Journal of Consulting and Clinical Psychology 61:354–359.

Allen NB, Lewinsohn PM, Seeley JR (1998): Prenatal and perinatal influences on risk for psychopathology in childhood and adolescence. Development Psychopathology 10:513–529.

Anderson JC, Williams S, McGee R, Silva PA (1987): DSM-III disorders in preadolescent children: Prevalence in a large sample from the general population. Archives of General Psychiatry 44:69–76.

Angold A (1988): Childhood and adolescent depression: I. Epidemiological and aetiological aspects. British Journal of Psychiatry 152:601–617.

Angold A, Rutter M (1992): Effects of age and pubertal status on depression in a large clinical sample. Development and Psychopathology 4:5–28.

Angold AE, Costello J, Erkanli A (1999): Comorbidity. Journal of Child Psychology and Psychiatry and Allied Disciplines 40:57–87.

Angst J (1988): Clinical course of affective disorders. In Helgason T, Daly RJ (eds), "Depressive illness: Prediction of course and outcome." Berlin: Springer-Verlag, pp 1–48.

Angst J, Merikangas KR (1997): The depressive spectrum: Diagnostic classification and course. Journal of Affective Disorders 45:31–40.

Avenevoli S, Stolar M, Li J, Dierker L, Merikangas KR (2001): Comorbidity of depression in children and adolescents: Models and evidence from a prospective high-risk family study. Biological Psychiatry 49:1071–1081.

Beardslee WR, Keller MP, Lavori PW, Staley J, Sacks N (1993): The impact of parental affective disorder on depression in offspring. Journal of the American Academy of Child and Adolescent Psychiatry 32:723–730.

Beardslee WR, Versage EM, Gladstone TRG (1998): Children of affectively ill parents: A review of the past 10 years. Journal of the American Academy of Child and Adolescent Psychiatry 37:1134–1141.

Beidel DC (1988): Psychophysiological assessment of anxious emotional states in children. Journal of Abnormal Psychology 97:80–82.

Beidel DC, Turner SM (1997): At risk for anxiety: I. Psychopathology in the offspring of anxious parents. Journal of the American Academy of Child and Adolescent Psychiatry 36:918–924.

Bellodi L, Perna G, Caldirola D, Arancio C, Bertani A, Di Bella D (1998): CO-sub-2-induced panic attacks: A twin study. American Journal of Psychiatry 155:1184–1188.

Bennet A, Stirling J (1998): Vulnerability factors in the anxiety disorders. British Journal of Medical Psychology 71:31–321.

Bernstein GA, Borchardt CM, Perwien AR (1996): Anxiety disorders in children and adolescents: A review of the past 10 years. Journal of the American Academy of Child and Adolescent Psychiatry 35:1110–1119.

Biederman J, Rosenbaum J, Bolduc-Murphy E, et al (1993): A three-year follow-up of children with and without behavioral inhibition. Journal of the American Academy of Child and Adolescent Psychiatry 32:814–821.

Biederman J, Rosenbaum JF, Bolduc EA, Faraone SV, Hirshfeld DR (1991): A high risk study of young children of parents with panic disorders and agoraphobia with and without comorbid major depression. Psychiatry Research 37:333–348.

Biederman J, Rosenbaum JF, Chaloff J, Kagan J (1995): Behavioral inihbition as a risk factor for anxiety disorders. In March J (ed), Anxiety Disorders in Children and Adolescents. New York: Guilford Press, pp 61–81.

Bird HR, Canino G, Rubino-Stipec M, et al. (1988): Estimates of the prevalence of childhood maladjustment in a community survey in Puerto Rico: The use of combined measures. Archives of General Psychiatry 45:1120–1126.

Bird HR, Gould MS, Yager T, Staghezza B, Canino G (1989): Risk factors for maladjustment in Puerto Rican children. Journal of the American Academy of Child and Adolescent Psychiatry 28(6):847–50.

Birmaher B, Ryan ND, Williamson DE, et al (1996): Childhood and adolescent depression: A review of the past 10 years. Part I. Journal of the American Academy of Child and Adolescent Psychiatry 35:1427–1439.

Bolognini M, Bettschart W, Plancherel B, Rossier L (1989): From the child to the young adult: Sex differences in the antecedents of psychological problems. A retrospective study over ten years. Social Psychiatry Psychiatric Epidemiology 24:179–186.

Bovasso G, Eaton W (1999): Types of panic attacks and their association with psychiatric disorder and physical illness. Comprehensive Psychiatry‘ 40:469–477.

Bowen RC, Offord DR, Boyle MH (1990): The prevalence of overanxious disorder and separation anxiety disorder: Results from the Ontario Child Health Study. Journal of the American Academy of Child Adolescent Psychiatry 29:753–758.

Bowlby J (1960): The making and breaking of affectional bonds. British Journal of Psychiatry 130:201–210.

Brady EU, Kendall PC (1992): Comorbidity of anxiety and depression in children and adolescents. Psychological Bulletin 111:244–255.

Brooks-Gunn J, Warren MP (1989): Biological and social contributions to negative affect in young adolescent girls. Child Development 60:40–55.

Bukowski W, Gauze C, Hoza B, Newcomb A (1993): Differences and consistency between same-sex and other-sex peer relationships during early adolescence. Developmental Psychology 29:255–263.

Bulik CM, Sullivan PF, Fear JL, Joyce PR (1997): Eating disorders and antecedent anxiety disorders: A controlled study. Acta Psychiatr Scand 96:101–107.

Burke KC, Burke JD, Regier DA, Rae DS (1990): Age at onset of selected mental disorders in five community populations. Archives of General Psychiatry 47:511–518.

Canals J, Domenech E, Carbajo G, Blade J (1997): Prevalence of DSM-III-R and ICD-10 psychiatric disorders in a Spanish population of 18-year olds. Acta Psychiatrica Scandinavica 96:287–294.

Canals J, Marti-Henneberg C, Fernandez-Ballart J, Domenech E (1995): A longitudinal study of depression in an urban Spanish pubertal population. European Child Adolescent Psychiatry 4:102–111.

Cantwell D, Baker L (1989): Stability and natural history of DSM-III childhood diagnoses. Journal of the American Academy of Child Adolescent Psychiatry 28:691–700.

Capps L, Sigman M, Sena R, Henker B (1996): Fear, anxiety and perceived control in children of agoraphobic parents. Journal of Child Psychology and Psychiatry and Allied Disciplines 37:445–452.

Carlson GA (1990): Bipolar disorders in children and adolescents. In Garfinkel BD, Carlson GA, Weller EB (eds), Psychiatric Disorders in Children and Adolescents. Philadelphia: W.B. Saunders Company, pp 21–36.

Carlson GA, Kashani JH (1988): Phenomenology of major depression from childhood through adulthood: Analysis of three studies. American Journal of Psychiatry 145:1222–1225.

Caron C, Rutter M (1991): Comorbidity in child psychopathology: Concepts, issues, and research strategies. Journal of Child Psychology and Psychiatry and Allied Disciplines 32:1063–1080.

Chambers W, Puig-Antich J, Tabrizi M, Davies M (1985): The assessment of affective disorders in children and adolescents by semi-structured interview: Test-retest reliability of the Schedule for Affective Disorders and Schizophrenia for school age children, present episode version. Archives of General Psychiatry 42:696–697.

Cohen P, Cohen J, Kasen S, et al. (1993): An epidemiological study of disorders in late childhood and adolescence-I: Age and gender-specific prevalence. Journal of Child Psychology and Psychiatry and Allied Disciplines 34:851–867.

Compas BE, Ey S, Grant KE (1993): Taxonomy, assessment, and diagnosis of depression during adolescence. Psychological Bulletin 114:323–344.

Compas BE, Howell DC, Phares V (1989): Risk factors for emotional/behavioral problems in young adolescents: A prospective analysis of adolescent and parental stress and symptoms. Journal of Consulting and Clinical Psychology 57:732–740.

Compton SN, Nelson AH, March JS (2000): Social phobia and separation anxiety symptoms in community and clinical samples of children and adolescents. Journal of the American Academy of Child and Adolescent Psychiatry 39:1040–1046.

Coryell W, Arndt S (1999): The 35% CO2 inhalation procedure: Test-retest reliability. Biological Psychiatry 45:923–927.

Costello EJ (1989): Developments in child psychiatric epidemiology. Journal of the American Academy of Child and Adolescent Psychiatry 28:836–841.

Costello EJ, Burns BJ, Angold A, Leaf PJ (1993): How can epidemiology improve mental health services for children and adolescents? Journal of the American Academy of Child and Adolescent Psychiatry 32:1106–1113.

Costello EJ, Costello AJ, Edelbrock C, et al. (1988a): Psychiatric disorders in pediatric primary care: Prevalence and risk factors. Archives of General Psychiatry 45:1107–1116.

Costello EJ, Burns BJ, Costello AJ, Dulcan MK, Brent D (1988b): Service utilization and psychiatric diagnosis in pediatric primary care: The role of the gatekeeper. Pediatrics 82(3 Pt2):435–41.

Costello EJ, Farmer E, Angold A, Burns B, Erkanli A (1997): Psychiatric disorders among American Indian and white youth in Appalachia: The Great Smoky Mountains study. American Journal of Public Health 87:827–832.

Costello J, Angold A, Burns BJ, et al. (1996): The Great Smoky Mountains Study of Youths: Goals, design, methods, and the prevalence of DSM-III-R Disorders. Archives of General Psychiatry 53:1129–1136.

Craske M (1997): Fear and anxiety in children and adolescents. Bulletin of the Menninger Clinic 61:4–36.

Culbertson FM (1997): Depression and gender: An international review. American Psychologist 52:25–31.

Dahl RE, Ryan ND (1996): The psychobiology of adolescent depression. In Ciccheti D, Toth SL (eds), "Rochester Symposium on developmental psychopathology: Adolescence: Opportunities and challenges," Vol 7. Rochester, NY: University of Rochester Press.

Dahl RE, Ryan ND, Williamson DE, et al. (1992): Regulation of sleep and growth hormone in adolescent depression. Journal of the American Academy of Child and Adolescent Psychiatry 31:615–621.

De Loof C, Zandbergen J, Lousberg H, Pols H, Griez E (1989): The role of life events in the onset of panic disorder. Behaviour research and therapy 27:461–463.

Deykin EY, Levy JC, Wells V (1987): Adolescent depression, alcohol and drug abuse. American Journal of Public Health 77:178–182.

Downey G, Coyne JC (1990): Children of depressed parents: An integrative review. Psychological Bulletin 108:1:50–76.

Eaton WW, Dryman A, Weissman MM (1991): Panic and phobia. In Robins LN, Regier DA (eds), "Psychiatric disorders in America: The epidemiological catchment area study." New York: Free Press, pp 155–179.

Eaton WW, Kessler RC, Wittchen HU, Magee WJ (1994): Panic and panic disorder in the United States. American Journal of Psychiatry 151(3):413–20.

Eaves LJ, Silberg JL, Meyer JM, et al. (1997): Genetics and developmental psychopathology: 2. The main effects of genes and environment on behavioral problems in the Virginia Twin Study of Adolescent Behavioral Development. Journal of Child Psychology Psychiatry Allied Disciplines 38:965–80.

Eley TC, Plomin R (1997): Genetic analyses of emotionality. Current Opinion in Neurobiology 7:279–284.

Eley TC, Deater-Deckard K, Fombonne E, Fulker DW, Plomin R (1998): An adoption study of depressive symptoms in middle childhood. Journal of Child Psychology and Psychiatry and Allied Disciplines 39(3):337–45.

Eley TC, Stevenson J (1999): Exploring the covariation between anxiety and depression symptoms: A genetic analysis of the effects of age and sex. Journal of Child Psychology and Psychiatry 40:1273–1282.

Faravelli C, Pallanti S (1989): Recent life events and panic disorder. American Journal of Psychiatry 146:622–626.

Feehan M, McGee R, Raja SN, Williams SM (1994): DSM-III-R disorders in New Zealand 18-year-olds. Australian and New Zealand Journal of Psychiatry 28:87–99.

Feehan M, McGee R, Williams SM (1993): Mental health disorders from age 15 to 18 years. Journal of the American Academy of Child and Adolescent Psychiatry 32:1118–1126.

Ferdinand RF, Van Der Reijden M, Verhulst FC, Fokko, Nienhuis J, Giel R (1995): Assessment of the prevalence of psychiatric disorders in young adults. British Journal of Psychiatry 166:480–488.

Ferdinand RF, Verhulst FC (1996): Psychopathology from adolescence into young adulthood: An 8-year follow-up study. American Journal of Psychiatry 152:1586–94.

Fergusson DM, Horwood LJ, Lynskey MT (1993a): Prevalence and comorbidity of DSM-III-R diagnoses in a birth cohort of 15 year olds. Journal of the American Academy of Child Adolescent Psychiatry 32:1127–1134.

Fergusson DM, Lynskey MT, Horwood LJ (1993b): The effect of maternal depression on maternal ratings of child behavior. Journal of Abnormal Child Psychology 21:245–269.

Fleming JE, Offord DR (1990): Epidemiology of childhood depressive disorders: A critical review. Journal of the American Academy of Child and Adolescent Psychiatry 29:571–580.

Fleming JE, Offord DR, Boyle MH (1989): Prevalence of childhood and adolescent depression in the community-Ontario Child Health Study. British Journal of Psychiatry 155:647–654.

Frost LA, Moffitt TE, McGee R (1989): Neuropsychological correlates of psychopathology in an unselected cohort of young adolescents. Journal of Abnormal Psychology 98:307–313.

Fyer AJ, Mannuzza S, Chapman TF, Lipsitz J, Martin LY, Klein DF (1996): Panic disorder and social phobia: Effects of comorbidity on familial transmission. Anxiety 2:173–178.

Fyer AJ, Mannuzza S, Chapman TF, Martin LY, Klein DF (1995): Specificity in familial aggregation of phobic disorders. Archives of General Psychiatry 52:564–573.

Garber J (1984): The developmental progression of depression in female children. In Cicchetti D, Schneider-Rosen K (eds), New Direction in Child Development (26, Dec, 1984).

Garber J, Hilsman R (1992): Cognition, stress, and depression in children and adolescents. Child and Adolescent Psychiatric Clinics of North America 1:129–167.

Garrison CZ, Schluchter MD, Schoenbach VJ, Kaplan BK (1989): Epidemiology of depressive symptoms in young adolescents. Journal of the American Academy of Child and Adolescent Psychiatry 28:343–351.

Garrison CZ, Schoenbach VJ, Kaplan BH (1985): Depressive symptoms in early adolescence. In Dean A (ed), "Depression and multidisciplinary perspective." New York: Brunner-Mazel, pp 60–82.

Garrison CZ, Waller JL, Cuffe SP, McKeown RE, Addy CL, Jackson KL (1997): Incidence of major depressive disorder and dysthymia in young adolescents. Journal of the American Academy of Child and Adolescent Psychiatry 36:458–465.

Ge X, Lorenz FO, Conger RD, Elder GH, Simons RL (1994): Trajectories of stressful life events and depressive symptoms during adolescence. Developmental Psychology 30:467–483.

Geller B, Luby J (1997): Child and adolescent bipolar disorder: A review of the past 10 years. Journal of the American Academy of Child and Adolescent Psychiatry 36:1168–1176.

Geller B, Sun K, Zimerman B, Luby J, et a.l (1995): Complex and rapid-cycling in bipolar children and adolescents: A preliminiary study. Journal of Affective Disorders 34:259–268.

Giaconia RM, Reinherz HZ, Hauf A, Paradis AD, Wasserman M, Langhammer DM (2000): Comorbidity of substance use and post-traumatic stress disorders in a community sampler of adolescents. American Journal of Orthopsychiatry 70:253–262.

Giaconia RM, Reinherz HZ, Silverman AB, Pakiz B, Frost AK, Cohen E (1994): Ages of onset of psychiatric disorders in a community population of older adolescents. Journal of American Academy of Child and Adolescent Psychiatry 33:706–717.

Glaser K (1967): Masked depression in children and adolescents. Annual Progress in Child Psychiatry and Child Development 1:345–355.

Goldsmith HH, Gottesmon I, Lemery K (1997): Epigenetic approaches to developmental psychopathology. Development and Psychopathology 9:365–387.

Goodyer I, Cooper P (1993): A community study of depression in adolescent girls II: The clinical features of identified disorder. British Journal of Psychiatry 163:374–380.

Gotlib IH, Hammen CL (1992): "Psychological aspects of depression: Toward a cognitive-interpersonal integration." Chichester,England UK: John Wiley Sons, pp 330.

Gotlib IH, Lewinsohn PM, Seeley JR (1998): Consequences of depression during adolescence: Marital status and marital functioning in early childhood. Journal of Abnormal Psychology 107:686–690.

Graber J, Lewinsohn PM, Seeley J, R, Brooks-Gunn J (1997): Is psychopathology associated with the timing of pubertal development? Journal of the American Academy of Child and Adolescent Psychiatry 36:1768–1776.

Griez E, Zandbergen J, Pols H, de Loof C (1990): Response to 35% CO2 as a marker of panic in severe anxiety. American Journal of Psychiatry 147:796–797.

Griez E, Schruers K (1998): Experimental pathophysiology of panic. Journal of Psychosomatic Research 45(6):493–503.

Grillon C, Dierker L, Merikangas KR (1998): Fear-potentiated startle in adolescent offspring of parents with anxiety disorders. Biological Psychiatry 44:990–997.

Grillon C, Dierker L, Merikangas KR. (1997): Startle modulation in children at risk for anxiety disorders and/or alcoholism. Journal of American Academy of Child and Adolescent Psychiatry 36:925–932.

Haines AP, Imeson JD, Meade TW (1987): Phobic anxiety and ischaemic heart disease. British Medical Journal 295:297–299.

Haley GM, Fine S, Marriage K, Morettei MM, Freeman RJ (1985): Cognitive bias and depression in psychiatrically disturbed children and adolescents. Journal of Consulting and Clinical Psychology 53:535–537.

Hammen C (1991): "Depression runs in families: The social context of risk and resilience in children of depressed mothers." New York: Springer-Verlag.

Hammen C, Burge D, Burney E, Adrian C (1990): Longitudinal study of diagnoses in children of women with unipolar and bipolar affective disorder. Archives of General Psychiatry 47:1112–1120.

Hammen C, Rudolph KD (1996): Childhood depression. In Mash EJ, Barkley RA (eds), "Child psychopathology." New York: Guilford Press, pp 153–195.

Hankin B, Abramson LY, Moffit TE, Silva PA, McGee R, Angell KE (1998): Development of depression from preadolescence to young adulthood: Emerging gender differences in a 10-year longitudinal study. Journal of Abnormal Psychology 107:128–140.

Harrington R, Fudge H, Rutter M, Pickles A, Hill J (1990): Adult outcomes of childhood and adolescent depression: I. Psychiatric status. Archives of General Psychiatry 47:465–473.

Harrington R, Fudge H, Rutter M, Pickles A, Hill J (1991): Adult outcomes of childhood and adolescent depression: II. Links with antisocial disorders. Journal of the American Academy of Child and Adolescent Psychiatry 30:434–439.

Harrington R, Rutter M, Weissman M, et al. (1997): Psychiatric disorders in the relatives of depressed probands. I. Comparison of prepubertal, adolescent and early adult onset cases. Journal of Affective Disorders 42:9–22.

Hayward C, Killen JD, Kraemer HC, Taylor CB (2000): Predictors of panic attacks in adolescents. Journal of the American Academy of Child and Adolescent Psychiatry 39:207–214.

Hirshfeld DR, Rosenbaum JF, Biederman J, et al. (1992): Stable behavioral inhibition and its association with anxiety disorder. Journal of the American Academy of Child Adolescent Psychiatry 31:103–111.

Hoberman HM, Bergmann PE (1992): Suicidal behavior in adolescence. Current Opinion in Psychiatry 5:508–517.

Horwath E, Wagner V, Wickramaratne P, Pine DS, Weissman MM (1998): Panic disorder and smothering symptoms: Evidence for increased risk in first degree relatives. Depression and Anxiety 6:147–153.

Horwath E, Weissman MM (1995): Epidemiology of depression and anxiety disorder. In Tsuang MT, Tohen M, Zahner GEP (eds), "Textbook in Psychiatric Epidemiology." New York: Wiley-Liss, Inc.

Ialongo N, Edelsohn G, Werthamer-Larsson L, Crockett L, Kellam S (1995): The significance of self-reported anxious symptoms in first grade children: Prediction to anxious symptoms and adaptive functioning in fifth grade. Journal of Child Psychology and Psychiatry and Allied Disciplines 36:427–437.

Isakson K, Jarvis P (1999): The adjustment of adolescents during the transition into high school: A short term longitudinal study. Journal of Youth and Adolescence 28:1–26.

Johnson J, Cohen P, Pine DS, Kassen S, Klein DF, Brook JS (2000): Association between cigarette smoking and anxiety disorders during adolescence and early adulthood. Journal of the American Medical Association. 284(18):2348–51

Johnson JG, Cohen P, Brook JS (2000): Associations between bipolar disorder and other psychiatric disorders during adolescence and early adulthood: A community-based longitudinal investigation. American Journal of Psychiatry 157:1679–1681.

Kagan J (1994): "Galen's Prophecy: Temperament in Human Nature." New York: Basic Books.

Kagan J, Reznick SJ (1986): Shyness and temperament. In Jones WH, Cheek JM, Briggs SR (eds), "Shyness: Perspectives on Research and Treatment." New York: Plenum Press.

Kagan J, Reznick SJ, Clarke C, Snidman N, Garcia-Coll C (1984): Behavioral inhibition to the unfamiliar. Child Development 55:2212–2225.

Kagan J, Snidman N, Arcus D (1995): The role of temperament in social development. In Chrousos GP, McCarty R (eds), Stress: "Basic mechanisms and clinical implications. Annals of the New York Academy of Sciences." New York: New York Academy of Sciences, pp 485–490.

Kandel DB, Davies M (1982): Epidemiology of depressive mood in adolescents. Archives of General Psychiatry 39:1205–1212.

Kandel DB, Johnson JB, Bird HR, et al. (1997): Psychiatric disorders associated with substance use among children and adolescents: Findings from the methods for the Epidemiology of Child and Adolescent Mental Disorders (MECA) study. Journal of Abnormal Child Psychology 25:121–132.

Kashani J, Beck N, Hoeper E, et al. (1987a): Psychiatric disorders in a community sample of adolescents. American Journal of Psychiatry 144:584–589.

Kashani J, Orvaschel H (1988): Anxiety disorders in mid-adolescence: A community sample. American Journal of Psychiatry 145:960–964.

Kashani J, Orvaschel H (1990): A community study of anxiety in children and adolescents. American Journal of Psychiatry 147:313–318.

Kashani J, Orvaschel H, Rosenberg T, Reid J (1989): Psychopathology in a community sample of children and adolescents: A developmental perspective. Journal of the American Academy of Child and Adolescent Psychiatry 28:701–706.

Kashani JH, Carlson GA, Beck NC, et al. (1987b): Depression, depressive symptoms, and depressed mood among a community sample of adolescents. American Journal of Psychiatry 144:931–934.

Kashani JH, McGee RO, Clarkson SE, et al. (1983): Depression in a sample of 9-year old children. Archives of General Psychiatry 40:1217–1223.

Kashani JH, Simonds JF (1979): The incidence of depression in children. American Journal of Psychiatry 136:1203–1205.

Kendler KS (1996): Major depression and generalised anxiety disorder: Same genes, (partly) different environments–revisited. British Journal of Psychiatry 168:68–75.

Kendler KS, Neale MC, Kessler RC (1993): Panic disorder in women: A population-based twin study. Psychological Medicine 23:397–406.

Kendler KS, Neale MC, Kessler RC, Heath AC, Eaves LJ (1992): A population-based twin study of major depression in women: The impact of varying definitions of illness. Archives of General Psychiatry 49:257–266.

Kendler KS, Neale MC, Kessler RC, Heath AC, Eaves LJ (1994–5): Clinical characteristics of familial generalized anxiety disorder. Anxiety 1(4):186–91.

Kessler R, McGonagle K, Swartz M, Blazer D, Nelson C (1993): Sex and depression in the National Comorbidity Survey I: Lifetime Prevalence, chronicity and recurrence. Journal of Affective Disorders 29:85–96.

Kessler RC, McGonagle KA, Zhao S, et al. (1994): Lifetime and 12-month prevalence of DSM-III-R psychiatric disorders in the United States: Results from the National Comorbidity Survey. Archives of General Psychiatry 51:8–19.

Kessler RC, Walters EE (1998): Epidemiology of DSM-III-R major depression and minor depression among adolescents and young adults in the National Comorbidity Survey. Depression and Anxiety 7:3–14.

Klein DN, Lewinsohn PM, Seeley JR, Rohde P (2001): A family study of major depressive disorder in a community sample of adolescents. Archives of General Psychiatry 58:13–20.

Kovacs M (1996): The course of childhood-onset depressive disorders. Psychiatric Annals 26:326–330.

Kovacs M, Akiskal HS, Gatsonis C, Parrone PL (1994): Childhood-onset dysthymic disorder: Clinical features and prospective naturalistic outcome. Archives of General Psychiatry 51:365–374.

Kovacs M, Devlin B (1998): Internalizing disorders in childhood. Journal of Child Psychology and Psychiatry and Allied Disciplines 39:47–63.

Kovacs M, Feinberg TL, Crouse-Novak MA, Paulauskas SL, Finkelstein R (1984): Depressive disorders in childhood: I. A longitudinal prospective study of characteristics and recovery. Archives of General Psychiatry 41:229–237.

Kovacs M, Gatsonis C, Paulauskas SL, Richards C (1989): Depressive disorders in childhood: IV. A longitudinal study of comorbidity with and risk for anxiety disorders. Archives of General Psychiatry 46:776–782.

Kovacs M, Paulauskas S, Gatsonis C, Richards C (1988): Depressive disorders in childhood: III. A longitudinal study of comorbidity with and risk for conduct disorders. Journal of Affective Disorders 15:205–217.

Kushner MG, Abrams K, Borchardt C (2000): The relationship between anxiety disorders and alcohol use disorders: A review of major perspectives and findings. Clinical Psychology Review 20:149–71.

Kutcher SP, Marton P (1989): Parameters of adolescent depression: A review. Psychiatric Clinics of North America 12:895–918.

Lader M (1972): The nature of anxiety. British Journal of Psychiatry 121:481–491.

Larson R, Richards MH (1991): Daily companionship in late childhood and early adolescence: Changing developmental contexts. Child Development 62:284–300.

Last C, Barlow D, O'Brien G (1984): Precipitants of agoraphobia: Role of stressful life events. Psychological Reports 54:567–570.

Last C, Hersen M, Kazdin A, Orvaschel H, Perrin S (1991): Anxiety disorders in children and their families. Archives of General Psychiatry 48:928–934.

Last CG, Perrin S, Hersen M, Kazdin A (1996): A propsective study of childhood anxiety disorders. Journal of the American Academy of Child Adolescent Psychiatry 35:1502–1510.

Last CG, Perrin S, Hersen M, Kazdin AE (1992): DSM-III-R anxiety disorders in children: Sociodemographic and clinical characteristics. Journal of the American Academy of Child and Adolescent Psychiatry 31:1070–1076.

Lavoie F, Hodgins S (1994): Mental disorders among children with one parent with a lifetime diagnosis of major depression. In Hodgins S, Lane C, Lapalme M, et al (eds), "A critical review of the literature on children at risk for major affective disorders." Ottawa: The Strategic Fund for Children's Mental Health, pp 37–82.

Legrand LN, McGue, Iacono WG (1999): A twin study of state and trait anxiety in childhood and adolescence. Journal of Child Psychological Psychiatry 40(6):953–958.

Lewinsohn PM, Allen NB, Seeley JR (1999a): First onset versus recurrence of depression: Differential processes of psychosocial risk. Journal of Abnormal Psychology 108:483–489.

Lewinsohn PM, Duncan EM, Stanton AK, Hautzinger M (1986): Age at first onset for nonbipolar depression. Journal of Abnormal Psychology 95:378–383.

Lewinsohn PM, Hoberman HM, Rosenbaum M (1988): A prospective study of risk factors for unipolar depression. Journal of Abnormal Psychology 97:251–264.

Lewinsohn PM, Hops H, Roberts RE, Seeley JR, Andrews JA (1993): Adolescent Psychopathology: I. Prevalence and incidence of depression and other DSM-III-R disorders in high school students. Journal of Abnormal Psychology 102:133–144.

Lewinsohn PM, Klein DN, Seeley JR (1995): Bipolar disorders in a community sample of older adolescents: Prevalence, phenomenology, comorbidity, and course. Journal of the American Academy of Child and Adolescent Psychiatry 34:454–463.

Lewinsohn PM, Klein DN, Seeley JR (2000a): Bipolar disorder during adolescence and young adulthood in a community sample. Bipolar Disorders 2:281–293.

Lewinsohn PM, Lewinsohn M, Gotlib IH, Seeley JR, Allen NB (1998a): Gender differences in anxiety disorders and anxiety symptoms in adolescents. Journal of Abnormal Psychology 107:109- 117.

Lewinsohn PM, Moerk KC, Klein DN (2000b): Epidemiology of adolescent depression. The Economics of Neuroscience 2:52–68.

Lewinsohn PM, Rhode P, Klein DN, Seeley JR (1999b): Natural course of adolescent major depressive disorder: I. Continuity into young adulthood. Journal of the American Academy of Child and Adolescent Psychiatry 38:56–63.

Lewinsohn PM, Rhode P, Seeley JR, Klein DN, Gotlib IH (2000): Natural course of adolescent major depressive disorder in a community sample: predictors of recurrence in young adults. American Journal of Psychiatry 157(10):1584–91.

Lewinsohn PM, Roberts RE, Seeley JR, Rhode P, Gotlib IH, Hops H (1994): Adolescent psychopathology: II. Psychosocial risk factors for depression. Journal of Abnormal Psychology 103:302–315.

Lewinsohn PM, Rohde P, Seeley JR (1998b): Major depressive disorder in older adolescents: Prevalence, risk factors, and clinical implications. Clinical Psychology Review 18:765–794.

Lewinsohn PM, Rohde P, Seeley JR (1998c): Treatment of adolescent depression: Frequency of services and impact on functioning in young adulthood. Depression and Anxiety 7:47–52.

Lewinsohn PM, Rohde P, Seeley JR, Hops H (1991): Comorbidity of unipolar depression: I. Major depression with dysthymia. Journal of Abnormal Psychology 100:205–213.

Lewinsohn PM, Seeley JR, Gotlib IH (1997a): Depression-related psychosocial variables: Are they specific to depression in adolescents? Journal of Abnormal Psychology 106:365–375.

Lewinsohn PM, Zinbarg R, Seeley JR, Lewinsohn M, Sack WH (1997b): Lifetime comorbidity among anxiety disorders and between anxiety disorders and other mental disorders in adolescents. Journal of Anxiety Disorders 11:377–394.

Lichtenstein P, Annas P (2000): Heritability and prevalence of specific fears and phobias in childhood. Journal of Child Psychology and Psychiatry 7:927–937.

Lieb R, Hans-Ulrich W, HoflerM., Fuetsch M, Stein M, Merikangas KR (2000): Parental psychopathology, parenting styles and the risk of social phobia in offspring: A prospective-longitudinal community study. Archives of General Psychology 57:859–866.

Lteif GN, Mavissakalian MR (1996): Life events and panic disorder/agoraphobia: A comparison at two time periods. Comprehensive Psychiatry 37:241–244.

Magee WJ, Eaton WW, Wittchen H-U, McGonagle KA, Kessler RC (1996): Agoraphobia, simple phobia and social phobia in the National Comorbidity Survey. Archives of General Psychiatry 53:159–168.

Maier W, Minges J, Lichtermann D (1995): The familial relationship between panic disorder and unipolar depression. Journal of Psychiatric Research 29:375–88.

Manfro GG, Otto MW, McArdle ET, et al. (1996): Relationship of antecedent stressful life events to childhood and family history of anxiety and the course of panic disorder. Journal of Affective Disorders 41:135–139.

March JS, Parker JD, Sullivan K, Stallings P, Conners CK (1997): The multidimensional anxiety scale for children (MASC): Factor sturcture, reliability, and validity. Journal of the American Academy of Child and Adolescence Psychiatry 36(4):554–565.

Marks IM (1986): Genetics of fear and anxiety disorders. British Journal of Psychiatry 149:406–418.

McCauley E, Mitchell JR, Burke P, Moss S (1988): Cognitive attributes of depression in children and adolescents. Journal of Consulting and Clinical Psychology 56:903–908.

McCauley E, Myers K, Mitchell J, Calderon R, et al (1993): Depression in young people: Intial presentation and clinical course. Journal of the American Academy of Child and Adolescent Psychiatry 32:714–722.

McGee R, Feehan M, Williams S, Anderson J (1992): DSM-III disorders from age 11 to age 15 years. Journal of the American Academy of Child and Adolescent Psychiatry 31:50–59.

McGee R, Feehan M, Williams S, Partridge F, Silva PA, Kelly J (1990): DSM-III disorders in a large sample of adolescents. Journal of the American Academy of Child and Adolescent Psychiatry 29:611–619.

McGee R, Williams S (1988): A longitudinal study of depression in nine-year-old children. Journal of the American Academy of Child and Adolescent Psychiatry 27:342–348.

McNally RJ (1990): Psychological approaches to panic disorder: A review. Psychological Bulletin 108:403–419.

Merikangas K, Swendsen J (1999): Contributions of epidemiology to the neurobiology of mental illness. In Charney D, Nestler E, Bunney B (eds), "Neurobiology of Mental Illness." New York: Oxford University Press, pp 100–107.

Merikangas KR (2000): Epidemiology of mood disorders in women. In Steiner M, Yonkers KA, Eriksson E (eds), "Mood Disorders in Women." London, UK: Martin Dunitz Ltd., pp 1–14.

Merikangas KR, Angst J (1995a): The challenge of depressive disorders in adolescence. In Michael R (ed), "Psychosocial disturbances in young people: Challenges for prevention:" Cambridge University Press, New York, NY, US, pp 131–165.

Merikangas KR, Angst J (1995b): Comorbidity and social phobia: Evidence from clinical, epidemiologic and genetic studies. European Archives of Psychiatry and Clinical Neuroscience 244:297–303.

Merikangas KR, Angst J, Isler H (1990): Migraine and psychopathology: Results of the Zurich Cohort Study of young adults. Archives of General Psychiatry 47:849–853.

Merikangas KR, Avenevoli S, Dierker L, Grillon C (1999): Vulnerablity factors among children at risk for anxiety disorders. Biological Psychiatry 46:1523–1535.

Merikangas KR, Dierker LC, Szatmari P (1998a): Psychopathology among offspring of parents with substance abuse and/or anxiety: A high risk study. Journal of Child and Adolescent Psychiatry 39:711–720.

Merikangas KR, Leckman JF, Prusoff BA, Pauls DL, Weissman MM (1985): Familial transmission of depression and alcoholism. Archives of General Psychiatry 42:367–372.

Merikangas KR, Mehta RL, Molnar BE, et al. (1998b): Comorbidity of substance use disorders with mood and anxiety disorders: Results of the international consortium in psychiatric epidemiology. Addictive Behaviors 23:893–907.

Merikangas KR, Pollock RA (2000): Anxiety disorder in women. In Goldman M, Hatch M (eds), "Women and Health." San Diego: Academic Press, pp 1010–1023.

Merikangas KR, Risch NJ, Merikangas JR, Weissman MM, Kidd KK (1988): Migraine and depression: Association and familial transmission. Journal of Psychiatric Research 22:119–129.

Merikangas KR, Stevens DE, Fenton B, et al. (1998c): Comorbidity and familial aggregation of alcoholism and anxiety disorders. Psychological Medicine 28:773–788.

Merikangas KR, Swendsen JD (1996): Genetic epidemiology of psychiatric disorders. Epidemiologic Reviews 19:1–12.

Merikangas KR, Swendsen JD, Preisig MA, Chazan RZ (1998): Psychopathology and temperament in parents and offspring: results of a family study. Journal of Affective Disorders 51(1):63–74.

Mitchell J, McCauley E, Burke P, Calderon R, Schloredt K (1989): Psychopathology in parents of depressed children and adolescents. Journal of the American Academy of Child and Adolescent Psychiatry 28:352–357.

Mitchell J, McCauley E, Burke PM, Moss SJ (1988): Phenomenology of depression in children and adolescents. Journal of the American Academy of Child and Adolescent Psychiatry 27:12–20.

Monroe SM, Rohde P, Seeley JR, Lewinsohn PM (1999): Life events and depression in adolescence: Relationship loss as a prospective risk factor for first onset of major depressive disorder. Journal of Abnormal Psychology 108:606–614.

Moyal BR (1977): Locus of control, self-esteem, stimulus appraisal, and depressive symptoms in children. Journal of Consulting and Clinical Psychology 45:951–952.

Murray KT, Sines JO (1996): Parsing the genetic and nongenetic variance in children's depressive behavior. Journal of Affective Disorders 38:23–34.

Neuman RJ, Geller B, Rice JP, Todd RD (1997): Increased prevalence and earlier onset of mood disorders among relatives of prepubertal versus adult probands. Journal of the American Academy of Child and Adolescent Psychiatry 36:466–473.

Newman DL, Moffitt TE, Caspi A, Magdol L (1996): Psychiatric disorder in a birth cohort of young adults: Prevalence, comorbidity, clinical significance, and new case incidence from ages 11–21. Journal of Consulting and Clinical Psychology 64:552–562.

NIMH (2001): National Institute of Mental Health Research Roundtable on prepubertal bipolar disorder. Bethesda. Journal of the American Academy of Child and Adolescent Psychiatry 40:871–878.

Nolen-Hoeksema S, Girgus JS (1994): The emergence of gender differences in depression during adolescence. Psychological Bulletin 115:424–443.

Nolen-Hoeksema S, Girgus JS, Seligman ME (1991): Sex differences in depression and explanatory style in children. Journal of Youth and Adolescence 20:233–245.

Nolen-Hoeksema S, Girgus JS, Seligman MEP (1986): Learned helplessness in children: A longitudinal study of depression, achievement, and explanatory style. Journal of Personality and Social Psychology 51:435–442.

Nottelmann ED, Inoff-Germain G, Susman EJ, Chrousos GP (1990): Hormones and behavior at puberty. In Bancroft J, Reinisch JM (eds), "Adolescence and puberty." New York: Oxford University Press, pp 88–123.

O'Connor TG, Neiderhiser JM, Neiderhiser DR, Hetherington EM, Plomin R (1998): Genetic contributions to continuity, change, and co-occurrence of antisocial and depressive symptoms in adolescence. Journal of Child Psychology and Psychiatry 39:323–336.

Offord DR, Boyle MH, Fleming JE, Blum HM, Grant NI (1989): Ontario Child Health Study: Summary of selected results. Canadian Journal of Psychiatry—Revue Canadienne de Psychiatric 34(6):483–91.

Ollendick TH (1983): Reliability and validity of the Revised Fear Surgery Schedule for Children (FSSC-R). Behaviour Research and Therapy 21(6):685–92.

Ollendick TH, Matson JL, Helsel WJ (1985): Fears in children and adolescents: Normative data. Behaviour Research Therapy 23:465–467.

Olsson GI, von Knorring A-L (1999): Adolescent depression: Prevalence in Swedish high-school students. Acta Psychiatrica Scandinavica 99:324–331.

Orvaschel H, Lewinsohn PM, Seeley JR (1995): Continuity of psychopathology in a community sample of adolescents. Journal of the American Academy of Child and Adolescent Psychiatry 34:1525–1535.

Orvaschel H, Weissman MM (1986): Epidemiology of anxiety disorders in children: A review. In Gittelman R (ed), Anxiety disorders of childhood. New York: The Guilford Press, pp 58–72.

Parker G (1979): Parental characteristics in relation to depressive disorders. British Journal of Psychiatry 134:138–147.

Parker G, Tupling H, Brown L (1979): A parental bonding instrument. British Journal of Medical Psychology 52:1–10.

Patton GC, Carlin JB, Coffey C, Wolfe GR, Hibbert M, Bowes G (1998): Depression, anxiety, and smoking initiation: A prospective study over 3 years. American Journal of Public Health 88:1518–1522.

Perna G, Cocchi S, Allevi L, Bussi R, Bellodi L (1999): A long-term prospective evaluation of first-degree relatives of panic patients who underwent the 35% CO-sub-2 challenge. Biological Psychiatry 45:365–367.

Perna G, Cocchi S, Bertani A, Arancio C, Bellodi L (1995): Sensitivity to 35% CO2 in healthy first-degree relatives of patients with panic disorder. American Journal of Psychiatry 152:623–625.

Petersen AC, Compas BE, Brooks-Gunn J (1992): "Depression in adolescence: Current knowledge, research directions, and implications for programs and policy." Washington, DC: Carnegie Council on Adolescent Development.

Petersen AC, Compas BE, Brooks-Gunn J, Stemmler M, Eye S, Grant KE (1993): Depression in adolescence. American Psychologist 48:155–168.

Petersen AC, Sarigiani PA, Kennedy RE (1991): Adolescent depression: Why more girls? Journal of Youth and Adolescence 20:247–271.

Piccinelli M, Wilkinson G (2000): Gender differences in depression. British Journal of Psychiatry 177:486–492.

Pine DS (1997): Cjildhood anxiety disorders. Current Opinion in Periatrics 9(4):329–38.

Pine DS, Cohen E, Cohen P, Brook JS (2000): Social phobia and the persistence of conduct problems. Journal of Child Psychology and Psychiatry, and Allied Disciplines 41:657–665.

Pine DS, Cohen P, Gurley D, Brook J, Ma Y (1998): The risk for early adulthood anxiety and depressive disorders in adolescents with anxiety and depressive disorders. Archives of General Psychiatry 55:56–64.

Polaino-Lorente A, Domenech E (1993): Prevalence of childhood depression: Results of the first study in Spain. Journal of Child Psychology Psychiatry 34:1007–1017.

Pollock RA, Carter AS, Avenevoli S, Dierker L, Chazan-Cohen R, Merikangas KR (In press): Anxiety sensitivity in children at risk for psychopathology. .

Poznanski EO, Krahenguhl V, Zrull JP (1976): Childhood depression: A longitudinal perspective. Journal of the American Academy of Child Psychiatry 15:491–501.

Prior M, Smart D, Sanson A, Oberklaid F (2000): Does shy-inhibited temperament in childhood lead to anxiety problems in adolescence? Journal of the American Academy of Child and Adolescent Psychiatry 39:461–468.

Puig-Antich J, Goetz D, Davies M, Kaplan T, et al. (1989): A controlled family history study of prepubertal major depressive disorder. Archives of General Psychiatry 46:406–418.

Puig-Antich J, Lukens E, Davies M, Goetz D, Brennan-Quattrock J, Todak G (1985): Psychosocial functioning in prepubertal major depressive disorders. Archives of General Psychiatry 42:500–507.

Radke-Yarrow M, Nottelmann E, Martinez P, Fox MB, et al. (1992): Young children of affectively ill parents: A longitudinal study of psychosocial development. Journal of the American Academy of Child and Adolescent Psychiatry 31:68–77.

Rao U, Ryan ND, Birmaher B, et al. (1995): Unipolar depression in adolescents: clinical outcome in adulthood. Journal of the American Academy of Child and Adolescent Psychiatry 34:566–578.

Rao U, Ryan ND, Dahl RE, et al. (1999): Factors associated with the development of substance use disorder in depressed adolescents. Journal of the American Academy of Child and Adolescent Psychiatry 38:1109–1117.

Reichler RJ, Sylvester CE, Hyde TS (1988): Biological studies on offspring of panic disorder probands. In Dunner DL, Gershon ES, Barrett JE (eds), "Relatives at risk for mental disorders." New York: Raven Press, Ltd.

Reinherz HZ, Giaconia RM, Carmola Hauf AM, Wasserman MS, Silverman AB (1999): Major depression in the transition to adulthood: Risks and impairments. Journal of Abnormal Psychology 108:500–510.

Reinherz HZ, Giaconia RM, Lefkowitz ES, Pakiz B, Frost A (1993a): Prevalence of psychiatric disorders in a community population of older adolescents. Journal of the American Academy of Child and Adolescent Psychiatry 32:369–377.

Reinherz HZ, Giaconia RM, Pakiz B, Silverman AB, Frost AK, Lefkowitz ES (1993b): Psychosocial risks for major depression in late adolescence: A longitudinal community study. Journal of the American Academy of Child and Adolescent Psychiatry 32:1155–1163.

Reinherz HZ, Stewart-Berghauer G, Pakiz B, Frost AK, Moeykens BA, Holmes WM (1989): The relationship of early risk and current mediators to depressive symptomatology in adolescence. Journal of the American Academy of Child and Adolescent Psychiatry 28:942–947.

Reiss S, Peterson RA, Gursky DM, McNally RJ (1986): Anxiety sensitivity, anxiety frequency and the prediction of fearfulness. Behaviour Research Therapy 24:1–8.

Rie HE (1966): Depression in childhood: A survey of some pertinent contributions. Journal of the American Academy of Child Psychiatry 5:653–685.

Rodgers B (1990): Behaviour and personality in childhood as predictors of adult psychiatric disorder. Journal of Child Psychology and Psychiatry 31:393–414.

Rohde P, Lewinsohn PM, Seeley JR (1991): Comorbidity of unipolar depression: II. Comorbidity with other mental disorders in adolescents and adults. Journal of Abnormal Psychology 100:214–222.

Rohde P, Lewinsohn PM, Seeley JR (1996): Psychiatric comorbidity with problematic alcohol use in high school students. Journal of the American Academy of Child and Adolescent Psychiatry 35:101–109.

Rosenbaum JF, Biederman J, Bolduc-Murphy EA, et al. (1993): Behavioral inhibition in childhood: A risk factor for anxiety disorders. Harvard Review of Psychiatry 1:2–16.

Rosenbaum JF, Biederman J, Gersten M (1988): Behavioral inhibition in children of parents with panic disorder and agoraphobia: A controlled study. Archives of General Psychiatry 45:463–470.

Rosenbaum JF, Biederman J, Hirshfeld DR, et al. (1991): Further evidence of an association between behavioral inhibition and anxiety disorders: Results from a family study of children from a non-clinical sample. Journal of Psychiatric Research 25:49–65.

Roy A (1985): Early parental separation and adult depression. Archives of General Psychiatry 42:987–991.

Roy-Byrne P, Uhde TW, Sack DA (1986): Plasma HVA and anxiety in patients with panic disorder. Biological Psychiatry 21:847–849.

Rutter M (1989): Isle of Wight revisited: Twenty-five years of child psychiatric epidemiology. Journal of the American Academy of Child and Adolescent Psychiatry 28:633–653.

Rutter M, Izard CE, Read PB (1986): "Depression in young people." New York: Guilford Press.

Rutter M, Tizard J, Whitmore K (1970): "Education, health, and behaviour." New York: Longman,Inc.

Rutter M, Tizard J, Yule W, Graham P, Whitmore K (1976): Isle of Wight Studies, 1964–1974. Psychological Medicine 6:313–332.

Ryan ND (1987): The clinical picture of major depression in children and adolescents. Archives of General Psychiatry 44:854–861.

Schmidt N, Lerew D, Jackson R (1997): The role of anxiety sensitivity in the pathogenesis of panic: Prospective evaluation of spontaneous panic attacks during acute stress. Journal of Abnormal Psychology 106:355–364.

Schmidt NB, Lerew DR, Joiner TE, Jr. (1998): Anxiety sensitivity and the pathogenesis of anxiety and depression: Evidence for symptom specificity. Behavior Research and Therapy 36:165–177.

Schoenbach VJ, Kaplan BH, Grimson RC, Wagner EH (1982): Use of a symptom scale to study the prevalance of a depressive syndrome in young adolescents. American Journal of Epidemiology 116:791–800.

Seligman MEP, Peterson C, Kaslow NJ, Tanenbaum RL, Alloy LB, Abramson LY (1984): Attributional style and depressive symptoms among children. Journal of Abnormal Psychology 93:235–238.

Shaffer D, Fisher P, Dulcan MK, Davies M (1996): The NIMH Diagnostic Interview Schedule for Children Version 2.3 (DISC-2.3): Description, acceptability, prevalence rates, and performance in the MECA study. Journal of the American Academy of Child Adolescent Psychiatry 35:865–877.

Sibisi CDT (1990): Sex difference in the age of onset of bipolar affective illness. British Journal of Psychiatry 156:842–845.

Silberg J, Pickles A, Rutter M, et al. (1999): The influence of genetic factors and life stress on depression among adolescent girls. Archives of General Psychiatry 56:225–232.

Silberg JL (2000): Genetic (and environmental) risk factors in chil"The Unmet Needs in Diagnosis and Treatment of Mood Disorders in Children and Adolescents." Washington DC: National Depressive and Manic-Depressive Association.

Silove D, Parker G, Hadzipavlovic D, Manicavasagar V, Blaszczynski A (1991): Parental representations of patients with panic disorder and generalised anxiety disorder. British Journal of Psychiatry 159:835–841.

Silverman WK, Cerny JA, Nelles WB, Burke AE (1988): Behavior problems in children of parents with anxiety disorders. Journal of the American Academy of Child Adolescent Psychiatry 27:779–784.

Simonoff E, Pickles A, Meyer J, et al. (1997): The Virginia twin study of adolescent behavioral development: Influences of age, sex, and inpairment on rates of disorders. Archives of General Psychiatry 47:487–496.

Smetana JG (1995): Parenting styles and conceptions of parental authority during adolescence. Child Development 66:299–316.

Smoller JW, Tsuang MT (1998): Panic and phobic anxiety: Defining phenotypes for genetic studies. American Journal of Psychiatry 155:1152–1162.

Spielberger C, Gorsuch R, Lushene R, Vagg P, Jacobs G (1983): "Manual for the State-Trait Anxiety Inventory." Palo Alto, CA: Consulting Psychologists Press.

Stein MB, Jang KL, Livesley WJ (1999): Heritability of Anxiety Sensitivity: A twin study. American Journal of Psychiatry 156:246–251.

Steinberg L (1988): Reciprocal relation between parent-child distance and pubertal maturation. Developmental Psychology 24:122–128.

Stevensen J, Batten N, Cherner M (1992): Stevenson, Jim; Batten, Nicki; Cherner, Mariana. Fears and fearfulness in children and adolescents: A genetic analysis of twin data. Journal of Child Psychology and Psychiatry and Allied Disciplines 33:977–985.

Strauss CC, Last CG, Hersen M, Kazdin AE (1988): Association between anxiety and depression in children and adolescents with anxiety disorders. Journal of Abnormal Child Psychology 16,1:57–68.

Susman EJ, Nottelmann ED, Inoff-Germain GE, et al. (1985): The relation of relative hormonal levels and physical development and socio-emotional behavior in young adolescents. Journal of Youth and Adolescence 14:245–264.

Susman EJ, Nottlemann ED, Inoff-Germain G, Dorn LD, Chrousos GP (1987): Hormonal influences on aspects of psychological development during adolescence. Journal of Adolescent Health Care 8(6):492–504.

Swartz KL, Pratt LA, Armenian HK, Lee LC, Eaton WW (2000): Mental disorders and the incidence of migraine headaches in a community sample. Archives of General Psychiatry 57:945–950.

Sylvester CE, Hyde TS, Reichler RJ (1988): Clinical psychopathology among children of adults with panic disorder. In Dunner DL, Gershon ES, Barrett JE (eds), "Relatives at Risk for Mental Disorder," Vol 26. New York: Raven Press, Ltd., pp 87–102.

Taylor EA, Sandberg SJ, Thorley G, Giles S (1991): "The epidemiology of childhood hyperactivity:"Oxford University Press/Maudsley Monographs.

Tems CL, Stewart SM, Skinner JR, Hughes CW, Emslie G (1993): Cognitive distortions in depressed children and adolescents: Are they state dependent or traitlike? Journal of Consulting and Clinical Psychology 22:316–326.

Thapar A, McGuffin P (1994): A twin study of depressive symptoms in childhood. British Journal of Psychiatry 165:259–265.

Thapar A, McGuffin P (1995): Are anxiety symptoms in childhood heritable? Journal of Child Psychology and Psychiatry and Allied Disciplines 36:439–447.

Thapar A, McGuffin P (1997): Anxiety and depressive symptoms in childhood–A genetic study of comorbidity. Journal of Child Psychology and Psychiatry and Allied Disciplines 38:651–656.

Topolski TD, Hewitt JK, Eaves LJ, et al. (1997): Genetic and environmental influences on child reports of manifest anxiety and symptoms of separation anxiety and overanxious disoders: A community-based twin study. Behevior Genetics 27:15–28.

Tsuang MT, Faraone SV (1990): "The genetics of mood disorders." Baltimore: Johns Hopkins University Press.

Turner SM; Beidel DC, Costello A (1987): Psychopathology in the offspring of anxiety disorders patients. Journal of Consulting and Clinical Psychology 55:229–235.

Unnewehr S, Schneider S, Florin I, Margraf J (1998): Psychopathology in children of patients with panic disorder or animal phobia. Psychopathology 31:69–84.

Van den Oord EJ, Boomsma I, Verhulst FC (1994): A study of problem behavior in 10- to 15-year-old biologically related and unrelated international adoptees. Behavior Genetics 24:193–205.

Velez C, Johnson J, Cohen P (1989): A longitudinal analysis of selected risk factors for childhood psychopathology. Journal of the American Academy of Child and Adolescent Psychiatry 28:861–864.

Verhulst FC, Berden GFMG, Sanders-Woudstra JAR (1985): Mental health in Dutch children: (II) The prevalence of psychiatric disorder and relationship between measures. Acta Psychiatrica Scandinavica (Supplement) 72,324:1–45.

Verhulst FC, van der Ende J, Ferdinand RF, Kasius MC (1997): The prevalence of DSM-III-R diagnoses in a national sample of Dutch adolescents. Archives of General Psychiatry 54:329–336.

Warner V, Mufson L, Weissman M (1995): Offspring at high risk for depression and anxiety: Mechanisms of psychiatric disorder. Journal of the American Academy of Child and Adolescent Psychiatry 34:786–797.

Warren SL, Schmitz S, Emde RN (2000): Behavioral genetic analyses of self-reported anxiety at 7 years of age. Journal of the American Academy of Child and Adolescent Psychiatry 38:1403–1408.

Weiss B, Weisz JR, Politano M, Carey M, Nelson WM, Finch AJ (1992): Relations among self-reported depressive symptoms in clinic-referred children versus adolescents. Journal of Abnormal Psychology 101:391–397.

Weissman MM (1987): Children of depressed parents: Increased psychopathology and early onset of major depression. Archives of General Psychiatry 44:847–853.

Weissman MM, Warner V, Wickramaratne PJ, Kandel DB (1999): Maternal smoking during pregnancy and psychopathology in offspring followed to adulthood. Journal of the American Academy of Child Adolescent Psychiatry 38:892–899.

Welner Z, Reich W, Herjanic B, Jung KG, et al. (1987): Reliability, validity, and parent-child agreement studies of the Diagnostic Interview for Children and Adolescents (DICA). Journal of the American Academy of Child and Adolescent Psychiatry 26:649–653.

Welner Z, Rice J (1988): School-aged children of depressed parents: a blind and controlled study. Journal of Affective Disorders 15:291–302.

West SA, McElroy SL, Strakowski SM, Keck PEJ, McConville BJ (1995): Attention deficit hyperactivity disorder in adolescent mania. American Journal of Psychiatry 152:271–273.

Whitaker A, Johnson J, Shaffer D, et al. (1990): Uncommon troubles in young people: Prevalence estimates of selected psychiatric disorders in a nonreferred population. Archives of General Psychiatry 47:487–496.

Williams S, McGee R, Anderson J, Silva PA (1989): The structure and correlates of self-reported symptoms in 11-year-old children. Journal of Abnormal Child Psychology 17:55–71.

Williamson DE, Ryan ND, Birmaher B, Dahl RE, Nelson B (1995): A case-control family history study of depression in adolescents. Journal of the American Academy of Child and Adolescent Psychiatry 34:1596–1607.

Wittchen HU, Perkonigg A, Lachner G, Nelson CB (1998a): Early developmental stages of psychopathology study (EDSP): Objectives and design. European Addiction Research 4(1-2):18–27.

Wittchen HU, Stein MB, Kessler RC (1999): Social fears and social phobia in a community sample of adolescents and young adults: Prevalence, risk factors and co-morbidity. Psychological Medicine 29:309–323.

Wittchen H-U, Nelson CB, Lachner G (1998): Prevalence of mental disorders and psychosocial impairments in adolescents and young adults. Psychological Medicine 28:109–126.

Wittchen H-U, Zhao S, Kessler RC, Eaton WW (1994): DSM-III-R generalized anxiety disorder in the National Comorbidity Survey. Archives of General Psychiatry 51:355–364.

Woodward LJ, Fergusson DM (2001): Life course outcomes of young people with anxiety disorders in adolescence. Journal of the American Academy of Child and Adolescent Psychiatry 40:1086–1093.

World Health Organization (1993): ICD-10 "Classification of mental and behavioural disorders." Geneva: World Health Organization.

INDEX